Magnetic Resonance Imaging

Allen D. Elster, M.D.

Department of Radiology
Bowman Gray School of Medicine
Wake Forest University
Winston-Salem, North Carolina

IN COLLABORATION WITH

Stanley F. Handel, M.D.

NMR Associates;
Clinical Professor of Radiology
University of Texas System Cancer Center
M.D. Anderson Hospital and Tumor Institute
Houston, Texas

Arnold M. Goldman, M.D.

NMR Associates;
Clinical Associate Professor of Radiology
University of Texas System Cancer Center
M.D. Anderson Hospital and Tumor Institute
Houston, Texas

Magnetic Resonance Imaging

A REFERENCE GUIDE AND ATLAS

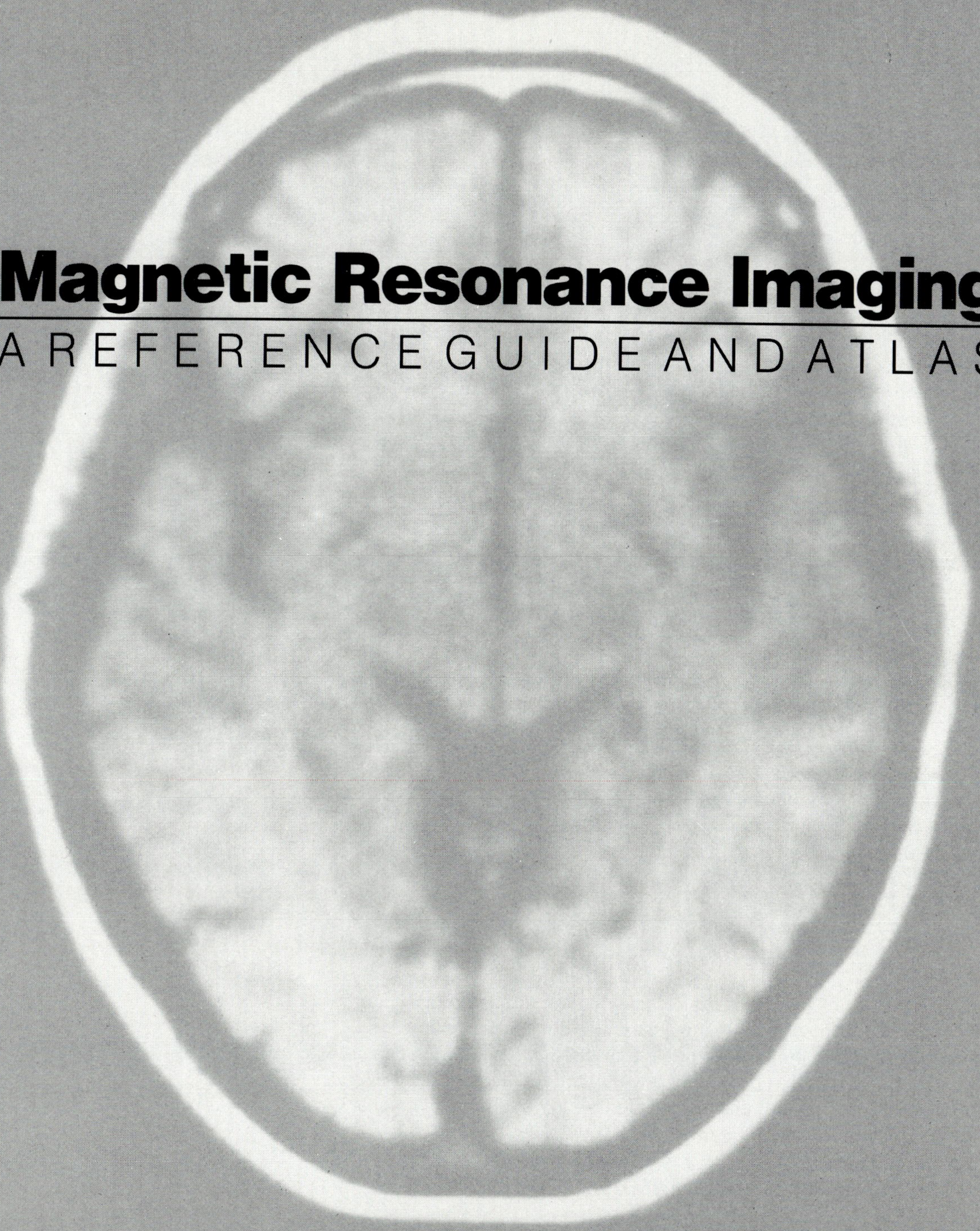

J. B. LIPPINCOTT COMPANY □ PHILADELPHIA

LONDON MEXICO CITY NEW YORK ST. LOUIS SÃO PAULO SYDNEY

Acquisitions Editor: Robert W. Reinhardt
Sponsoring Editor: Sanford J. Robinson
Manuscript Editor: Helen Ewan
Indexer: Alexandra Weir
Art Director/Designer: Tracy Baldwin
Production Supervisor: Kathleen P. Dunn
Production Coordinator: George V. Gordon
Compositor: Ruttle, Shaw & Wetherill, Inc.
Printer/Binder: Halliday Lithograph

 Printed in the United States of America. For information write J. B. Lippincott Company, East Washington Square, Philadelphia, Pennsylvania 19105.

6 5 4 3

Library of Congress Cataloging-in-Publication Data

Elster, Allen D.
Magnetic resonance imaging.

Bibliography: p.
Includes index.
1. Magnetic resonance imaging—Atlases. 2. Anatomy, Human—Atlases. I. Goldman, Arnold M., 1934– II. Handel, Stanley F. III. Title. [DNLM: 1. Anatomy. 2. Nuclear Magnetic Resonance. QS 4 E49m]
RC78.7.N83E57 1986 616.07′54 86-2898
ISBN 0-397-50766-6

The authors and publisher have exerted every effort to ensure that drug selection and dosage set forth in this text are in accord with current recommendations and practice at the time of publication. However, in view of ongoing research, changes in goverment regulations, and the constant flow of information relating to drug therapy and drug reactions, the reader is urged to check the package insert for each drug for any change in indications and dosage and for added warnings and precautions. This is particularly important when the recommended agent is a new or infrequently employed drug.

To Allen William Elster, II and his families:
You are the heirs and scions to a legacy of the heart, where greatness lies not in intellectual advancement, but in emotional commitment.

PREFACE

Welcome to the exciting world of magnetic resonance imaging!

By opening this book you have entered a new dimension in medicine, which will have profound impact on the diagnosis and treatment of disease for years to come. Before you can fully utilize this powerful new technology, however, you must first develop some new skills and acquire new perspectives on the human body.

In the 1970s the advent of computed tomography (CT) forced radiologists and other physicians to rethink and rediscover the importance of certain anatomic relationships within the human body. Viewing the human body in axial cross section led to a new appreciation for the anatomic basis of disease and the pathways by which disease spreads.

In the 1980s magnetic resonance imaging (MRI) will carry this process of anatomic rediscovery one step further. MR scanners are capable of easily and routinely imaging the human body in multiple planes, including the axial, sagittal, and coronal. The use of MR will call upon the diagnostician to understand complex anatomic relationships in multiple directions. No matter how familiar one is with the human body, at least a few of the anatomic relationships revealed by MR in *Magnetic Resonance Imaging* should be surprising.

Magnetic resonance technology will also expand our ability to recognize anatomic structures and pathology never before imaged by any other modality. For example, the substantia nigra of the brain stem is now routinely visualized on coronal MR scans. Magnetic resonance, therefore, has the potential to show us anatomic structures and relationships never before seen, except at the dissection table.

The impact of MRI is at more than an anatomic level. While on one hand drawing us more deeply towards a realization of the importance of anatomic relationships, MRI will also draw us away from the realm of simple anatomy into the physiology and biochemistry of disease. The imaging characteristics of a particular organ will depend as much on its microscopic composition and physiology as on its gross morphology. The interaction of electromagnetic radiation at the molecular level must be appreciated. The physician who masters MRI, therefore, is the one who has a grasp of anatomy, physiology, and physics. This book will attempt to lead you along this path.

Here are a few of the goals you will attain from completion of this book. First, you will gain a good appreciation for the current state of MR technology. You will know what parts of the body can and cannot be imaged well. You will have some concept of the potential of MR in imaging pathology in each body region. Second, you will learn the imaging characteristics of most tissues in the body and how various pulse sequence techniques generate signals from these tissues. You will learn how to predict with reasonable accuracy the relative signal intensity of each tissue, given a certain pulse sequence technique. You will also come to appreciate how common pathologic processes such as hemorrhage, edema, infection, and infarction affect the imaging characteristics of each tissue. Finally, you will gain knowledge of the complex anatomic relationship of the entire human body in axial, coronal, sagittal, and oblique planes.

This book can also serve as a reference guide for those involved in the performance or interpretation of MR scans. Up-to-date specifications are available for each of the major MR scanners in clinical use in the United States. A complete bibliography of MRI from 1980 to 1985 is also included. For each body part discussed, specifically recommended pulse sequences and imaging techniques are suggested. The multiple full-page images may serve as a ready reference atlas for the detailed anatomy of each region of the body.

Before you embark upon your study of MRI, a final word of encouragement and advice. Do not be frightened away from this field by so-called experts who make it appear complicated or imply that a Ph.D. in physics is required to understand it. Actually, MRI is relatively simple. After a few pages of simplified physics instruction, this book will quickly lead you into familiarity with the appearance of the normal human body and its common variations shown by MR. You will then be ready to select image sequences, perform scans, and begin learning the fine art of their interpretation.

For the very reason that many novices to the field become lost or bogged down in the physics of MRI, the presentation of physical principles is very abbreviated. Only those most basic concepts and conclusions that directly affect the performance of MR scans are included. Just as the physician performing CT scans does not really need to know much about scan geometry or reconstruction algorithms, so the physician performing MR scans does not have to know quantum mechanics or Fourier waveform analysis.

This very cursory approach to physics, however, does require some compromises. Many facts and equations will have to be accepted on blind faith. Occasionally, you will be told some "facts" that are really only partial truths or oversimplifications, which may not hold up under rigorous mathematical analysis. You will have time at a later date to learn the finer points of physics and the many exceptions to the rules. While the others are plodding through a mire of physics, you will be learning the business of interpreting MR scans.

Congratulations again on your interest in and courage to enter this exciting new field. You will not be disappointed with what it holds.

Allen D. Elster, M.D.

ACKNOWLEDGMENTS

> . . .I will keep this Oath and this stipulation—to reckon him who taught me this Art equally dear to me as my parents. . . . to look upon his offspring in the same footing as my own brothers, and to teach them this Art, if they shall wish to learn it, without fee or stipulation; and that by precept, lecture, and every other mode of instruction, I will impart a knowledge of the Art to my own sons, and those of my teachers, and to disciples bound by a stipulation and oath according to the law of medicine. . . .
>
> —Hippocrates

Arnold Goldman and Stanley Handel instructed me in the "Art" of magnetic resonance imaging when no scanner was available at our academic institutions. They did so without fee or stipulation. They inspired me and allowed me to experience with them the development of an exciting new field. Without their encouragement and teaching this book would not have been possible. As they have honored Hippocrates by embodiment of his Oath, so I wish to honor these two thoughtful and principled physicians here.

Several manufacturers involved in MR technology were very helpful in supplying a number of high-resolution images that appear in this book. In particular, I would like to express my appreciation to Sheldon I. Schaffer of Technicare Corporation, John Cassese of Fonar Corporation, Barbara K. Baker of Picker International, Inc., Peggy Driefke and Dr. John F. Schenck of General Electric, Dr. J. D. Coil and Dr. W. Steinbrich of Philips Medical Systems, Inc., Anne Deery of Siemens Medical Systems, Inc., and Joe Och of Thomson-CGR Medical Corporation.

Finally, and most importantly, I would like to thank two special members of my family for their many hours of loving labor and support. My father, Allen William Elster, spent countless tiring days and nights in his photographic laboratory working and reworking nearly a thousand illustrations for potential use in this book. This is only one small example of the innumerable important yet unrecorded acts of devotion to his family that he has performed throughout his life. I can only hope that his grandson and namesake will be half as great a man.

My wife, Jeanine, has also spent uncounted tiring hours typing and editing, in addition to her most important role as baby Allen's wonderful mother. I thank her for these things specifically, but even more for the devotion and encouragment she has given me in our difficult decisions to change careers (and addresses) to enter radiology. Such total love and support represent a rare combination of human qualities, which is only a part of what makes her such an extraordinary wife, companion, and Mommy.

CONTENTS

SECTION I **Physical Foundations**

CHAPTER 1 Instrumentation *3*

CHAPTER 2 Physical Principles of Magnetic Resonance *15*

CHAPTER 3 Imaging Sequences and Parameters *29*

CHAPTER 4 Effects of Pathology on the MR Image *51*

CHAPTER 5 Artifacts in MR Scanning *57*

SECTION II **Imaging Guide and Atlas of the Human Body**

CHAPTER 6 The Brain *71*

CHAPTER 7 The Head and Neck (Excluding Brain) *127*

CHAPTER 8 The Chest *173*

CHAPTER 9 The Abdomen *199*

CHAPTER 10 Pelvis and Hips *215*

CHAPTER 11 Surface Coil Applications: Spine, Breast, and Knee *233*

APPENDIX A Specifications of Nine Major Commercial MR Scanners, 1985 *253*

APPENDIX B Glossary of MR Terminology *259*

APPENDIX C Abbreviations Commonly Used in MR Imaging *263*

Bibliography *265*

Index *287*

SECTION I

Physical Foundations

CHAPTER 1

Instrumentation

At the end of 1985, more than 220 magnetic resonance (MR) scanners were in operation in the United States. In the next 2 years, that number is easily expected to double. The rapid deployment and acceptance of this new technology is a tribute both to its proven capabilities and to the promise MR holds for the future of diagnostic imaging.

The rapid proliferation of MR technology is similar to that experienced by computed tomography (CT) in the 1970s. In several respects, however, the development and deployment of MR have been more dramatic than that of CT. Many of the companies involved in the development of CT scanners also took the lead in MR technology. Some basic features of CT systems (such as display consoles and array processor computers) could be directly transferred with modification to the new MR systems. Moreover, the intellectual climate in the medical community was ready to accept the multiplanar format offered by magnetic resonance imaging (MRI). A decade of CT experience had laid the basic foundations for interpretation of cross-sectional images.

TABLE 1-1

Some Advantages and Disadvantages of MR Compared With CT

Advantages

No ionizing radiation

Fewer artifacts from dense bone and metal clips

Imaging in multiple planes without moving the patient

Signals from tissues are dependent on several chemical and physical properties, which may be studied independently

Future potential for flow measurements, spectroscopy, biochemical characterization, and physiologic monitoring

Disadvantages

Slower scanning times than CT

High initial cost of the scanner ($1.1 to $2.1 million)

Special site planning and shielding ($100,000 to $500,000)

Danger to patients with cerebral aneurysm clips, pacemakers

Unknown effects of high magnetic fields

Claustrophobia in magnet

MR also offers a promise, yet to be fulfilled, for greater specificity in the diagnosis of disease. Similar hopes were held for CT at its inception, but it is now well recognized that many varied disease processes may have identical CT appearances. MRI seems once again to have renewed hope that an infallible method of diagnosis has been devised. We wait expectantly to see to what degree MR spectroscopy, physiological monitoring, and tissue characterization will fulfill this prophesy.

It seems only natural to compare briefly the capabilities of CT and MR, since they have arisen from a common source and have similar goals and applications. Keep in mind, however, that such a comparison is a little unfair, because CT represents a mature technology whereas MR is still new. Nevertheless, a few valid generalizations can safely be made (Table 1-1).

As an initial comparison, MR requires no ionizing radiation to produce an image, whereas CT scanning exposes the patient to relatively high doses of x-irradiation. There is yet no definite proof that the strong magnetic fields used in MRI are harmful. No detectable or lasting adverse effects of MRI have been reported in the more than 80,000 clinical MR scans that have been performed to date. More subtle effects, such as those on cell membrane glycoproteins or on embryogenesis, might still occur. At present, therefore, pregnant women are not routinely scanned by MR unless clinically indicated. Future research will clarify the risks, if any, that MR holds for this class of patients.

At the current time, there are only two absolute contraindications to MR scanning. Patients with ferromagnetic cerebral aneurysm clips should not be placed in the scanner (although the author is aware of at least one such patient who was inadvertently but safely scanned). The rapidly changing magnetic fields might induce motion in such an aneurysm clip, shearing the vessel or causing other problems. Metallic clips elsewhere in the body should present no danger, nor should other metallic prostheses.

The second absolute contraindication to MRI involves patients with cardiac pacemakers. Once again, the rapidly changing magnetic fields might induce dysfunction or reset an implanted pacemaker. Induced currents in pacer lead wires might also precipitate an arrhythmia.

A few relative contraindications to MR scanning

TABLE 1-2
Contraindications to MR Scanning

Absolute	
Patients with cerebral aneurysm clips	
Patients with cardiac pacemakers	
Relative	
Claustrophobic or uncooperative patients	
Pregnant patients	
Metallic prosthetic heart valves	
Ferromagnetic foreign bodies in critical locations (*e.g.*, eye)	
Implanted stimulator wires for pain control	
No Contraindications	
Surgical clips outside the brain	
Metallic prostheses	

may also be considered, in addition to pregnant patients, discussed above. Claustrophobic patients may acutely decompensate in the narrow bore of the scanner; this may occur to some degree in 1% to 3% of patients scanned, requiring premature termination of the examination. Uncooperative patients are also difficult to scan. Patient motion may degrade an entire study rather than merely specific slices, as in CT; this depends on the MRI sequence used and the degree of patient motion. Table 1-2 lists these relative and absolute contraindications to MR scanning.

MRI has another great advantage compared with CT in that MR is relatively little affected by artifacts from dense materials such as bone, dental fillings, or metallic prostheses. A major limitation of CT in the spine and posterior fossa has been the presence of beam-hardening bone streak artifacts, which degrade image quality. Because dense cortical bone has few mobile hydrogen atoms to produce an MR signal, such artifacts are not seen with MRI. This advantage has already made MR the imaging modality of choice in preference to CT for the posterior fossa and brain stem.

Metallic prostheses, dental fillings, and clips often severely degrade CT images. MR images will demonstrate either little or no artifact from these devices, depending on their composition. When an artifact is present on MRI, it is usually localized near the metallic device and does not send streaks across the whole image. Examples of metallic artifacts on MR images are shown in Chapter 5.

Perhaps the greatest advantage of MR relative to CT is the potential that MR holds for tissue characterization. The information obtainable by CT is at the gross anatomic level. CT can detect differences only in tissue x-ray attenuation. MRI, on the other hand, holds the potential for characterization of tissue at the molecular level. A variety of electromagnetic interactions within tissue can be distinguished by MR. By varying pulse sequences, magnetic fields, and detection modes, it may be possible to image a variety of separate molecules and atoms. Spectroscopy, as performed with laboratory MR units, may one day be possible with clinical MR scanners in human patients. There is also the potential to perform physiological monitoring and flow measurements by MR as well. No one really knows to what degree these developments will prove useful, although the promises are tremendous.

All of the fascinating advantages of MR must be weighed against two realities of everyday life—money and time. MR scanners remain rather expensive (more than $2 million for the machine and siting), although prices should come down in the future with competition and increased supply. A second practical disadvantage is the time required to obtain and process images. In most instances, the scanning time compared with CT is about 150% to 200% longer. Nevertheless, improvements are constantly being made, and scanning times for MR are already becoming shorter.

The Magnet

The strength of the magnetic field and how that field is produced lie at the heart of MR technology. It is necessary to know a little about the various magnet types and sizes in order to be conversant in the field. All magnets used in MRI can be placed in one of three categories—permanent, resistive, or superconductive (Table 1-3).

Permanent magnets are giant versions of the hand-held horseshoe magnet used as children's toys. Permanent MR magnets are very stable and produce

TABLE 1-3

Types of Magnets Used for MRI

Permanent Magnet

Field strength: 0.05 T to 0.35 T

Field homogeneity: Good

Advantages: Very stable. No electric power or coolant consumption. Low fringe field requiring minimal shielding.

Disadvantages: Weight (up to 100 tons for a 0.35 T magnet). Requires strict room temperature ($\pm 1^\circ$C) and humidity ($\pm 5\%$) control to maintain field stability.

Example: Fonar Beta 3000

Resistive Magnet

Field strength: <0.2 T

Field homogeneity: Fair

Advantages: Low price. Low fringe field.

Disadvantages: Sensitivity to temperature fluctuations. High cooling costs. High electricity power consumption.

Example: Technicare 0.15-T Resistive scanner

Superconductive Magnet

Field strength: 0.3 T to 2.0 T

Field homogeneity: Excellent

Advantages: High field strength. Very stable. Little electricity expense.

Disadvantages: Most expensive to build. Requires cryogens which are expensive. Danger of quenching (sudden loss of superconductivity with explosive boiling off of liquid helium).

Examples: Siemens Magnetom, Diasonics MT/S, Technicare Teslacon

a uniform magnetic field. They are cheap to operate, since they require no power source or cooling system. The major disadvantage is their weight, which may be as great as 100 tons for a large magnet. The Fonar Beta 3000 scanner is the most popular example of a permanent magnet imager (Fig. 1-1).

Resistive magnets were the earliest type used in MRI. Relatively cheap to build, these magnets are giant ferromagnetic cores with electric wire windings that produce their fields as solenoids (electromagnets). The fields obtained are relatively low and nonuniform. Resistive magnets also require a large amount of electric power to operate. Several companies continue to make resistive MR scanners, but their popularity is decreasing.

Superconductive magnets are the type used in most clinical MR centers in the United States today. Their principle of operation is based on the phenomenon of superconductivity that occurs in certain metals when they are cooled to low temperatures (4°K) by liquid helium. At these temperatures near absolute zero, electric resistance in solenoid winding disappears, and a strong, uniform magnetic field is produced with no significant loss of energy. Superconductive magnets produce the strongest fields of any magnet, and the fields are very uniform. Disadvantages include expense of construction and expense of cryogens (liquid helium and nitrogen), which must be replenished every few weeks at a cost of several thousand dollars. Examples of MR scanners that use superconducting magnets include the Technicare Teslacon, the Diasonics MT/S, and the Siemens Magnetom (Fig. 1-2).

The strength of a magnetic field by which magnets are rated is measured in units called *gauss* (G) or *tesla* (T). The term tesla is now preferred over the older term gauss. For purposes of conversion, 1 T equals 10,000 G. The magnetic field strength of magnets in most of today's MR scanners lies in the range of 0.15 to 2.0 T.

It is difficult to appreciate the size of the magnetic fields used in MR scanners, since the units gauss and tesla have little meaning except to physicists. As a point of reference, the strength of the earth's magnetic field on its surface is about ½ G, or 0.00005 T. The strength of a 1.5-T MR scanner magnet can be appreciated by the force it would exert on nearby metallic objects.

If proper precautions were not taken, magnetic credit cards would be erased and the tiny gears in a wristwatch would become magnetized when a person entered the scanning suite door 15 feet away from such a magnet. At 10 feet away, a metal wheelchair would roll forward toward the magnet. At 7 feet, hairpins would be pulled from hair and metal fountain pens would be pulled from pockets. At a distance of 4 feet away, a metal object such as a wrench or screwdriver would be lifted from the floor. A metal oxygen tank, if pulled toward and stuck to the magnet, would be impossible to remove by hand.

Nine major companies produce most of the MR scanners in clinical use in the United States today—Diasonics, Fonar, Elscint, General Electric, Philips, Picker, Technicare, and Thompson-CGR. Appendix A lists the current specifications and options available on each of these scanners.

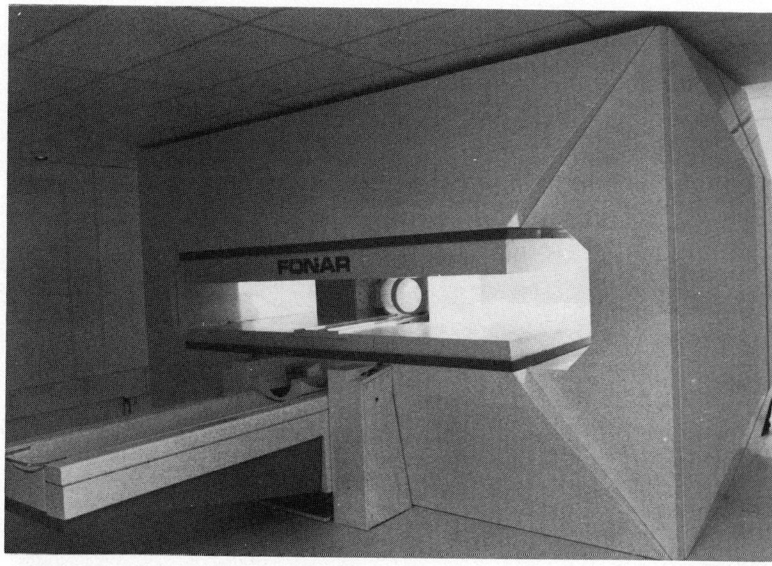

FIGURE 1-1

Fonar Beta 3000 permanent magnet MR scanner has a field strength of 0.3 T. (Courtesy of Fonar Corp., 110 Marcus Drive, Melville, NY 11747)

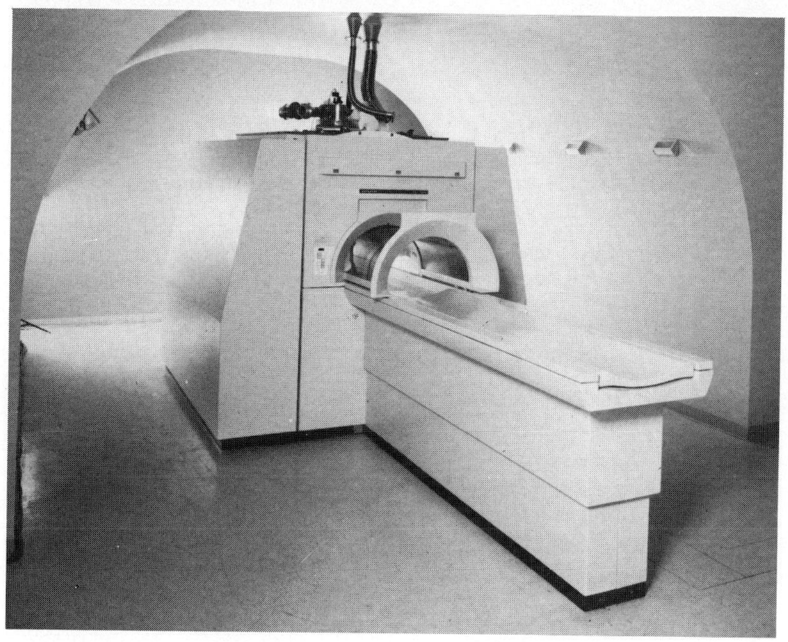

FIGURE 1-2

Philips Gyroscan S15 superconducting magnet offers a field strength of 1.5 T. (Courtesy of Philips Medical Systems, Inc.)

The MR Scanner and System Components

For those readers unfamiliar with MR scanning, it may be instructive to look at the various components of an MR system, including the scanner, coils, peripheral devices, and siting construction. Some of the illustrations used have been supplied by various manufacturers and represent part of the spectrum of MR equipment now on the market. Other illustrations have been obtained from an imaging center in Houston, NMR Associates-Kirby, which may be considered a typical community MRI facility.

The main MR magnet is housed within a large rectangular or cylindrical frame, measuring as much as 15 or 20 feet in its greatest dimension (Fig. 1-3).

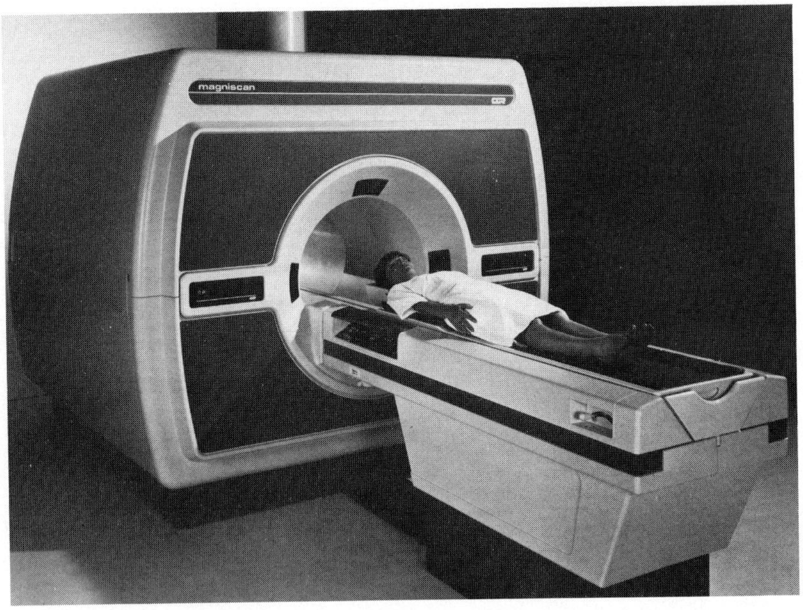

FIGURE 1-3

Patient is shown on the gantry of a Thomson-CGR Magniscan 5000 superconductive magnet. (Courtesy of Thomson-CGR Corporation)

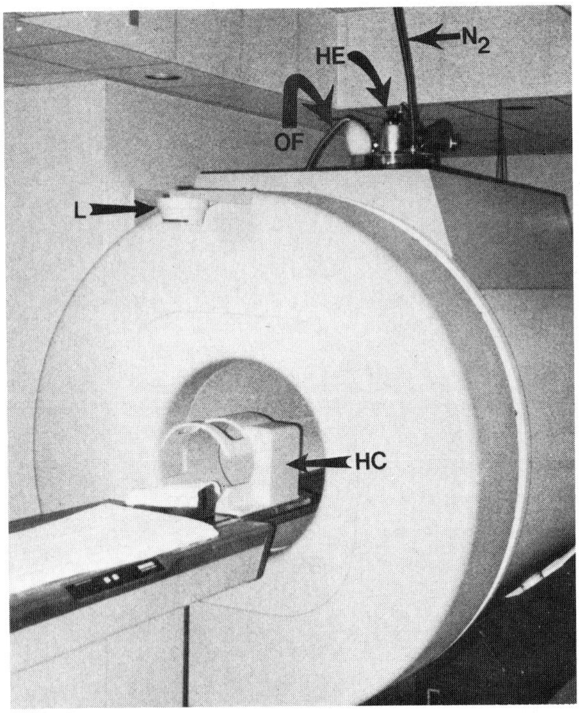

FIGURE 1-4

Components of the Diasonics MT/S superconductive MR scanner. HC = head coil; L = laser alignment light; OF = overflow valve; HE and N_2 = portals for instilling liquid helium and nitrogen, respectively.

As with a CT scanner, the patient lies on a gantry that can be moved into the center of the magnet. At the top of most superconductive magnets, several valves and pipes may be seen (Fig. 1-4). Through these, liquid helium and nitrogen are added every few weeks to maintain the low temperatures necessary for superconduction.

Hidden within the magnet housing are several sets of wire coils (Fig. 1-5). The main magnet windings are usually made of a niobium-titanium alloy covered by copper. The niobium-titanium functions as the superconductor, when cooled to 4°K by the liquid helium. The copper layer retains some resistance and acts as an insulator. The copper coating also protects the magnet from overheating (quenching) if a leak occurs and superconductivity is lost.

Two sets of smaller magnet coils are also present within the main housing. **Shim coils** are small electromagnets that are adjusted after siting to correct irregularities in the field of the main magnet. **Gradient coils** consist of three to six sets of small electromagnets that are mutually perpendicular (orthogonal). The purpose of these gradient coils is to superimpose additional small magnetic fields that vary predictably within the patient during the scan. The function of these magnetic gradients is to allow for spatial encoding of MR signals and hence slice selection.

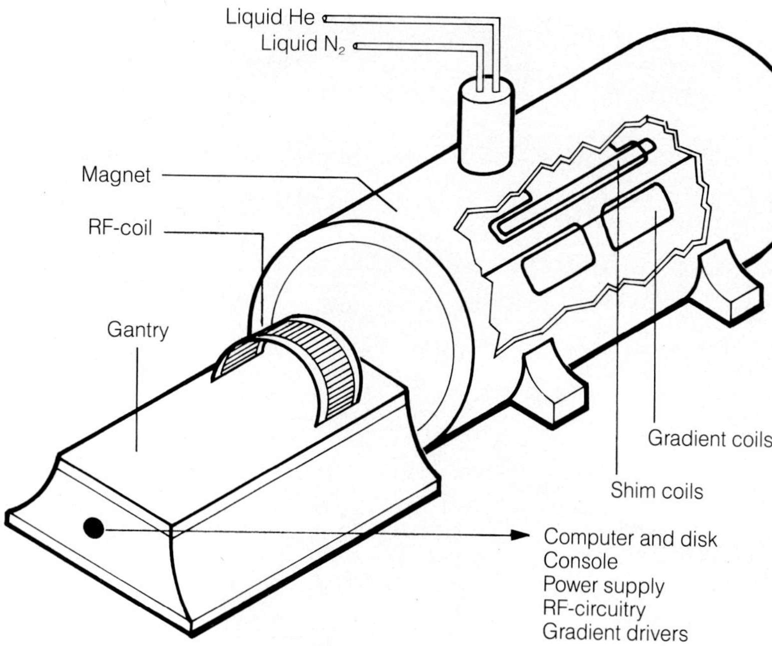

FIGURE 1-5
Components of a typical superconductive MR scanner.

The main magnet and acessory magnets establish and finely regulate the powerful magnetic fields required for magnetic resonance to take place. However, a much smaller device known as a **radio-frequency coil (RF coil)** must be placed close to the patient in order to stimulate and record an MR signal. An example of such an RF coil is shown in Figure 1-6.

The RF coil has two functions: as a transmitter and as a receiver of electromagnetic radiation (radio waves). During scanning, the RF coil first sends a burst of electromagnetic radiation through the patient's body. As will be described in the next chapter, the burst of radiation stimulates hydrogen nuclei in the patient's tissues into resonance. As these stimulated nuclei relax from resonance, they release absorbed energy as electromagnetic radiation. This emitted radiation can be detected as the MR signal. The same RF coil that was originally used as a transmitter is then used as an antenna to record the emitted MR signal. Alternatively in some systems, separate transmitter and receiver RF coils may be employed.

Different sizes and shapes of RF coils are used, depending on what part of the body is being scanned. The RF coil shown in Figure 1-6 has a diameter of approximately 30 cm. This is suitable for head and neck imaging and is sometimes called the

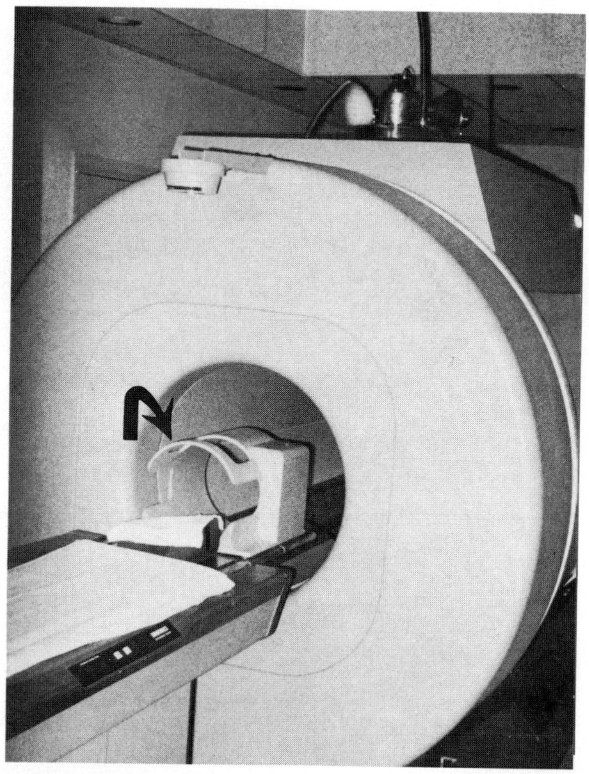

FIGURE 1-6
RF coil used in head and neck imaging (*head coil*).

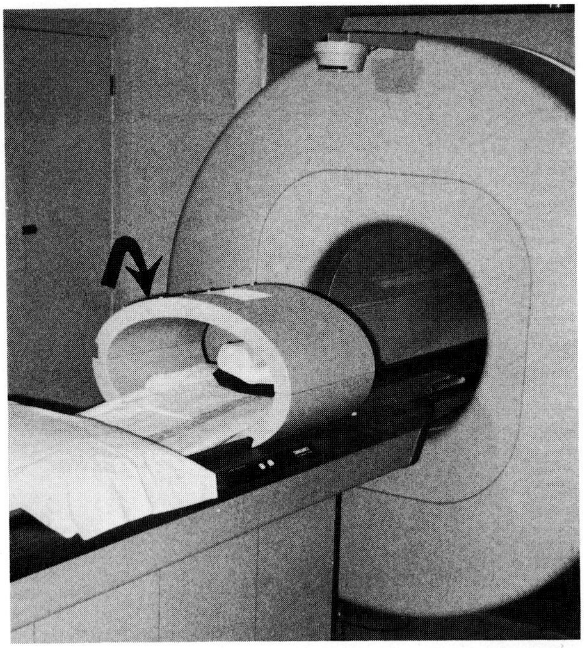

head coil. A larger coil measuring about 55 cm in diameter is used to image the chest and abdomen; this is sometimes called the **body coil** (Fig. 1-7). The patient is first positioned on the gantry with the RF coil around him or her. Then the patient and RF coil are moved together into the scanner for imaging.

In order to improve image quality and signal strength for anatomic structures that are superficial, a variety of much smaller **surface coils** have been developed. Surface coils have found applications for the orbit, temporal bone, neck, spine, breast, heart,

FIGURE 1-7

RF coil for chest and abdomen imaging (*body coil*).

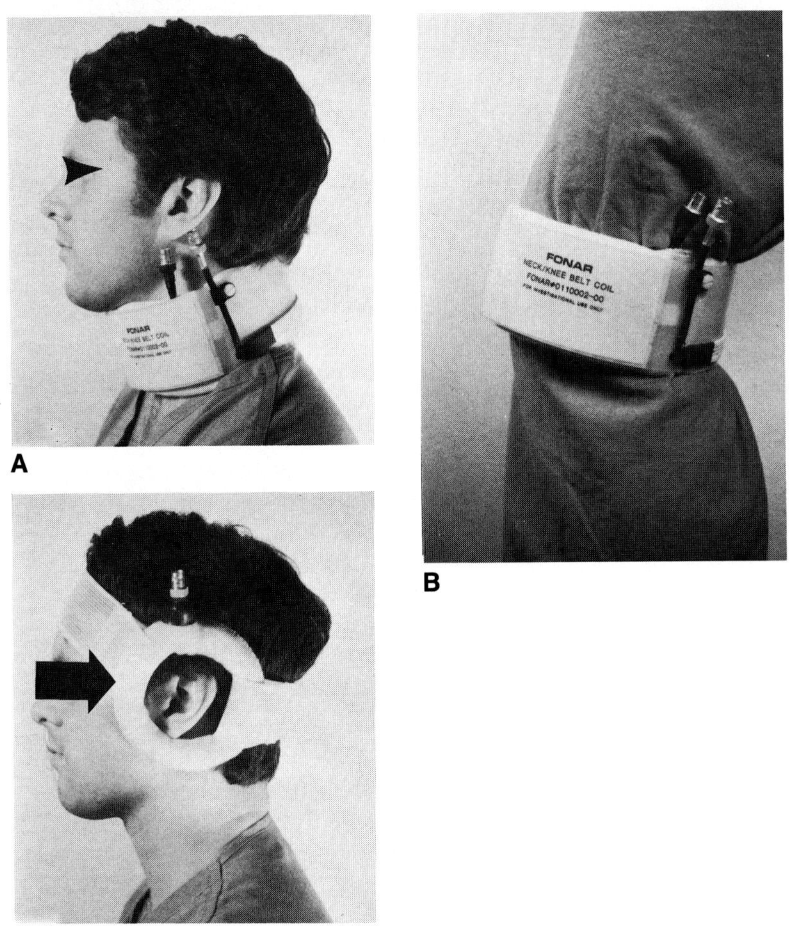

FIGURE 1-8

Examples of surface coils. (A) neck coil; (B) knee coil; (C) temporal bone coil. (Courtesy of Fonar Corp., 110 Marcus Drive, Melville, NY 11747)

and knee. These surface coils are placed directly on or very near the body part being examined. For imaging they function as receivers in conjunction with a larger transmitter RF coil. For spectroscopy separate transmitter and receiver surface coils may be employed. Examples of surface coils are shown in Figure 1-8, and examples of images obtained by surface coils appear in the chapters on the head and neck, chest, spine, and extremities.

As would be expected, a substantial number of peripheral devices are needed in addition to the magnet and gantry. The scan is directed and controlled from an operator's console similar in design to that of a CT scanner (Fig. 1-9). A second physician's console may be purchased for remote reviewing of images. A large number of available software options allow magnification of images, measurements, and selection of regions of interest for chemical analysis.

Computers, disk drives, and power supplies may usually be found in a separate air-conditioned room (Fig. 1-10). These machines control the magnetic

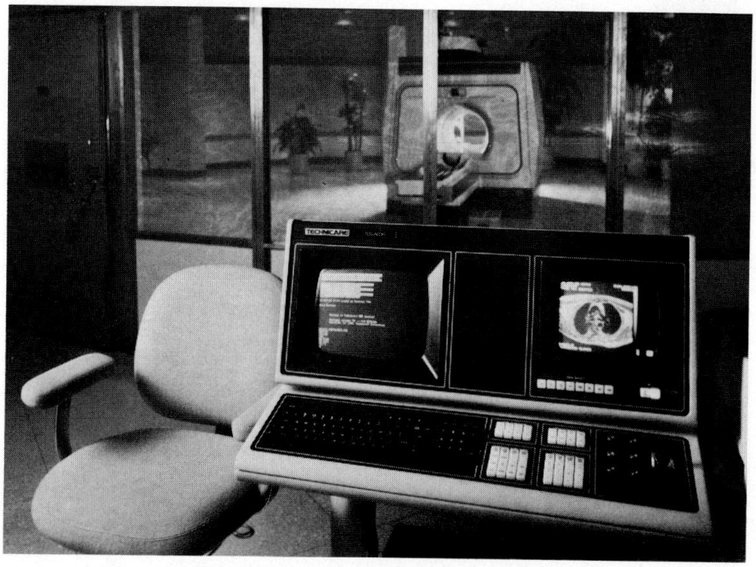

FIGURE 1-9

Operator's console and MR scanner at the Cleveland Clinic. The wavy effect on the wall behind the console is due to copper wire mesh screen, which acts as a shield for radio-frequency magnetic fields. (Courtesy of Technicare Corporation and Cleveland Clinic, Technicare Corp. © 1985)

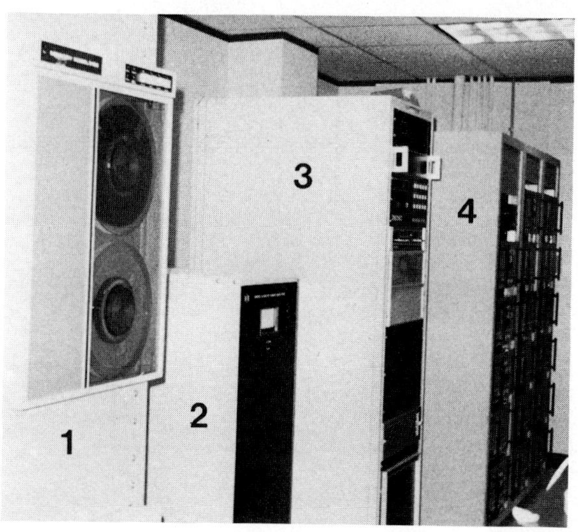

FIGURE 1-10

Some peripheral electronic equipment needed to operate an MR scanner from NMR Associates-Kirby in Houston, Texas. 1 = operator's computer, disk drives, and tape drive; 2 = RF power amplifier; 3 = transmitter/receiver, frequency synthesizer, and computer for pulse sequence control; 4 = gradient power supplies.

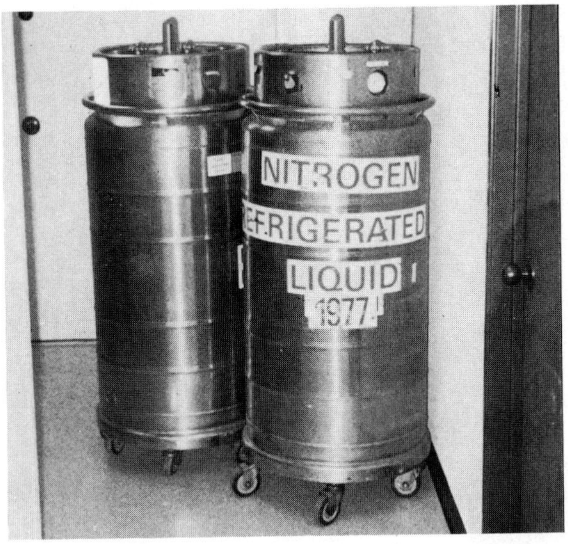

FIGURE 1-11

Storage tanks for cryogens must be aluminum, since they are taken into the scanning room when replenishment is needed.

fields and monitor and process the MR signal. Large aluminum tanks for storing liquid helium and nitrogen are found in an adjoining room or closet. In most superconductive scanners, liquid helium must be replenished every three to six weeks, whereas liquid nitrogen must be added more frequently (Fig. 1-11).

The room containing the magnet must be specially designed and shielded for two reasons. First, the fringe magnetic fields produced by the large magnet might interfere with nearby electronic equipment (like a computer or an employee's pacemaker). Second, extraneous electromagnetic radiation from televisions, passing automobiles, or elevators might interfere with the production and detection of small MR signals from within the body.

It is not easy or cheap to design and build such a shielded room. No structural iron may be present in the building within 15 or 20 feet of the magnet. A special copper wire mesh grounded cage must surround the entire room. No magnetizable (ferromagnetic) materials are allowed within the magnet room. This means that every nail, screw, light fixture, pipe, and wire within the room must be made of a nonferrous metal-like aluminum. Figure 1-9 shows the copper screen and door as well as the predominantly wood construction of the magnet room at the Cleveland Clinic. The floor plan for an entire MRI suite is illustrated in Figure 1-12.

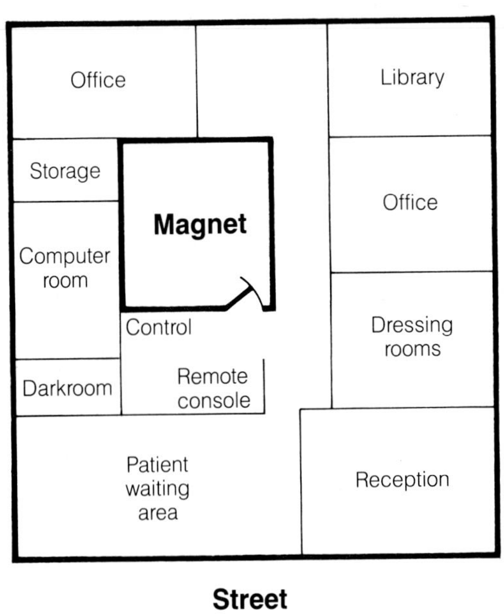

FIGURE 1-12

Layout of a typical MR scanning site, modeled after NMR Associates-Kirby in Houston, Texas.

Performance of a Typical MR Scan

The reader may find it instructive to follow the performance of a typical MR scan from start to finish, in order to understand the steps necessary to scan a patient. Let us assume our patient is a young man with leg weakness. His physician has requested an MR scan of the brain to rule out a diagnosis of multiple sclerosis.

First, the patient is taken to a dressing area, where he removes his watch, metallic jewelry, and clothes. After donning a hospital gown, he is led into the magnet room and lies supine on the gantry. The plastic and wire head coil (Fig. 1-6) is now positioned over his head. Together the patient and RF coil are pushed along the gantry into the center of the magnet.

With the patient and RF coil in the center of the magnet, the MR technologist must now perform a maneuver known as *tuning the coil.* On some scanners, this is done automatically, but on others it must be done by hand. This tuning process involves at most turning a few knobs on the control panel or RF coil. The purpose of tuning is to optimize the electronic circuitry to provide maximal resonance signal for the particular body part being imaged. When tuning is finished, the technologist will leave the magnet room, close the door, and return to the operator's console. From the operator's console, the technologist will type in commands to perform the scan.

Several parameters must be selected in order to perform an MR scan. These parameters will be discussed in detail in Chapter 3, and at that time the reader will gain considerable facility in understanding how each parameter changes the MR image. There are about six parameters that must be specified by the operator in order to perform an MR scan: the plane of imaging, slice thickness, matrix (pixel) size, number of signal averages, pulse sequence, and pulse time intervals. A typical set of values for this patient that might be useful in detecting multiple sclerosis would be obtained by selecting the coronal plane, slice thickness of 7 mm, 128 × 256 matrix, two signal averages, and a spin-echo pulse sequence with time intervals of TR = 2.0 seconds and TE = 28 msec. The criteria for selecting these parameters are discussed in Chapter 3.

With the imaging parameters selected, the scan is ready to begin. The technologist pushes a few buttons, and image acquisition is under way. In about 15 minutes, the computer presents us with a set of 12 coronal images of the patient's brain, which demonstrate several high-intensity white matter lesions compatible with multiple sclerosis (Fig. 1-13).

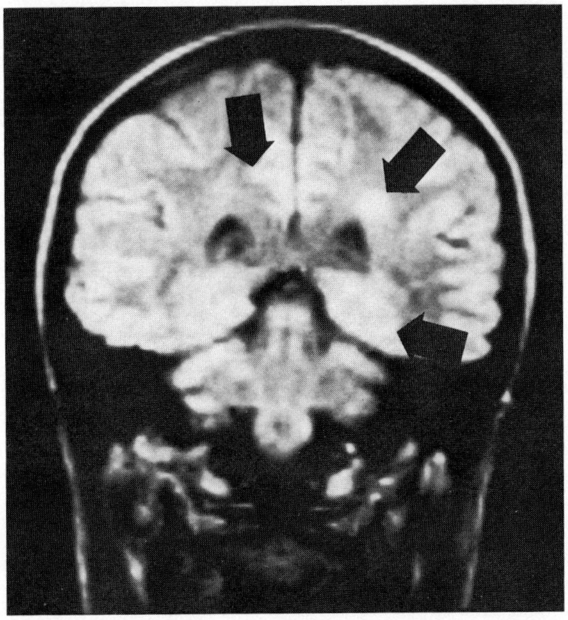

FIGURE 1-13

Coronal spin-echo image of a patient with several high-intensity white matter lesions (*arrows*) compatible with multiple sclerosis.

At this point, the radiologist or diagnostician may desire to repeat the scan, this time using different pulse sequence, plane of imaging, or sequence timing parameters. It is not necessary for the patient to be moved or repositioned. All of this is done electronically. At the display console, the physician may modify the image and perform special measurements, such as proton density or T1 time constant calculations in selected regions of interest. Note that the physician should not use the CT-derived terms *density* or *attenuation* in describing the MR image. He should report that he sees several "high-intensity" lesions on the MR image.

When the scan is completed, the patient is led out of the room and back to the dressing area. Before he leaves, he may be asked to pay for the scan or give his insurance number. A typical charge for such a brain MRI scan in 1985, including the interpretation fee, was about $800. At this rate, most imaging centers and hospitals believe they can pay for their scanner and staff over a five-year period, if they do eight scans per day, based on a five-day week.

CHAPTER 2

Physical Principles of Magnetic Resonance

This chapter presents those basic principles required for performing and interpreting MR scans and aids the reader in gaining a simple, working knowledge of MR for clinical use.

The physical concepts of MR are no more difficult to understand than those of ordinary x-radiation; they are only different. It is not necessary for physicians to fully understand Compton scattering or filtered back-projection mathematics to interpret intelligently the images from a CT scanner. Likewise, it is not necessary to know quantum physics or Fourier analysis to work with MRI.

In the discussion that follows, it will be necessary to oversimplify some of the physical concepts presented, for the sake of greater understanding. Likewise, some principles must be accepted on blind faith. When at all possible, we will avoid analogies to compass needles, merry-go-rounds, and wobbling tops. These analogies are only large-scale approximations to phenomena that occur at the subatomic level. The problem with using such large-scale analogies is that they are based on classic principles of electromagnetism—angular momentum and magnetic moments—which are incorrect at the subatomic level. Strict adherence to these analogies may lead to paradoxes and incorrect conclusions. Accordingly, the physics of MR will be presented from the more abstract but more accurate quantum mechanical viewpoint, invoking large-scale physical analogies only incidentally.

Do not despair if such an approach does not allow you to feel comfortable with the physical processes of MR. The behvior of matter on such a small scale is very different from what we experience at an ordinary level. Even the great physicist Professor Richard Feynman of the California Institute of Technology has expressed that he still feels somewhat ill at ease about the subatomic world. No one, including famous physicists, ever comfortably perceives the rules of quantum mechanics that explain MR as being "natural." Of course, the rules are indeed natural, but not to our experience in the larger world.

With this approach and philosophy in mind, let us now conduct a brief overview of the process of magnetic resonance.

The Meaning of Nuclear Magnetic Resonance

Before delving into physics, it is important to have a simplified but clear idea of what MR involves. Let us first begin by analyzing the very name, Nuclear Magnetic Resonance.

The term **nuclear** reminds us that we are dealing with a process that involves the atomic nucleus, not the electron cloud surrounding it. In research centers using special scanners, it is possible to image by MR a number of different atoms, including hydrogen, sodium, potassium, and fluorine. In general

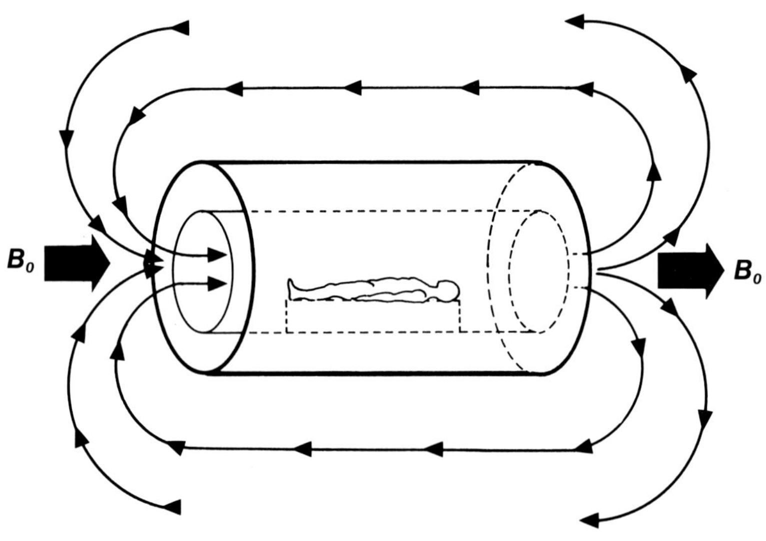

FIGURE 2-1
Diagram of a superconductive MR scanner showing the direction of the static (constant) magnetic field, B_0.

clinical use today, however, only hydrogen imaging is performed. Since the most abundant hydrogen isotope contains only a single proton in its nucleus, we may conclude that MRI in clinical practice today involves only hydrogen protons.

The term **magnetic** refers to two things. First of all, the process of MR takes place within the bore of a large magnet, as described in Chapter 1. This magnet produces a tremendously powerful **static field**, denoted B_0 in Figure 2-1. This static magnetic field has a strength many thousands of times that of the earth's own magnetic field. The B_0 field remains on at all times throughout the imaging process. Additional smaller gradient and radio-frequency magnetic fields are at times superimposed on the static field for purposes of spatial encoding and nuclear stimulation, but the B_0 field remains constant and is never shut off.

The second magnet that MR refers to is the hydrogen proton itself. Quantum theory imbues each proton with certain magnetic physical properties, allowing it to interact with energy in the electromagnetic spectrum. In the classic description, each proton may be thought of as a tiny spinning magnet (Fig. 2-2), which may interact with other nuclear magnets in neighboring atoms, as well as with externally applied magnetic fields. Quantum theory limits this proton magnet to certain fixed energy levels and orientations. By jumping between these fixed (quantized) energy levels and orientations, each proton may absorb, store, and emit electromagnetic energy in the form of radio waves. These emitted radio waves are detected as the MR signal. MR signals from each small volume element (voxel) of tissue are assembled to produce the final MR image.

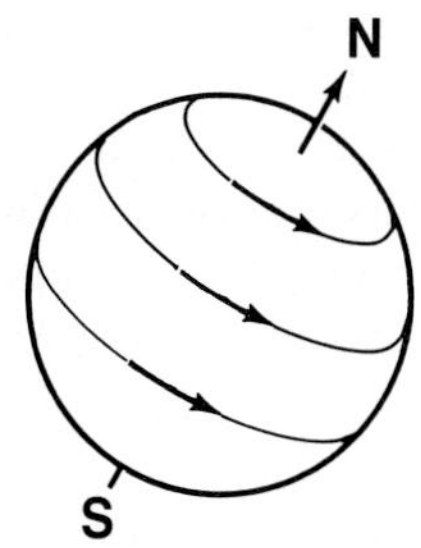

FIGURE 2-2

A hydrogen proton can be thought of as a tiny spinning magnet, with north and south poles as illustrated.

The term **resonance** is used to describe any physical system that oscillates between high- and low-energy states. In the world of MR, this involves hydrogen protons absorbing and releasing energy in the electromagnetic spectrum by transitions between quantized energy levels. As will be described, such transitions can occur only when energy is supplied or absorbed at a specific frequency in the range of radio waves, called the **Larmor resonance frequency**.

Although this oscillation of proton energy states is somewhat difficult to visualize, many examples of the resonance phenomenon surround us in the larger world. Well-recognized examples of resonance include a vibrating tuning fork, a swinging pendulum, a plucked guitar string, and a child on a pogo stick. A fundamental property of these larger mechanical systems as well as the nuclear proton electromagnet system is that such oscillations occur at very specific frequencies, unique for each system. The tuning fork, when struck, will vibrate only at a certain pitch, its **resonance frequency**. This frequency is determined by the shape and composition of the tuning fork, as well as by the fork's external environment. Changing either the composition or the environment will change the resonance frequency.

For example, a tuning fork made out of plastic or wood would vibrate with a different pitch from one made of steel. Similarly, the proton in a hydrogen nucleus would be expected to resonate a a different frequency from one in a sodium-23 nucleus or one in a phosphorus-31 nucleus.

Placing the runing fork under water would cause it to vibrate with a different frequency from the same tuning fork in air. Similarly, changing the strength of the static magnetic field might be expected to alter the resonance frequency of a hydrogen proton.

A tuning fork, when placed in front of a speaker, will not vibrate unless sound waves of its particular resonance frequency (pitch) strike it. Likewise, a hydrogen proton in a magnetic field B_0 cannot be stimulated to undergo resonance unless electromagnetic energy of its intrinsic resonance frequency

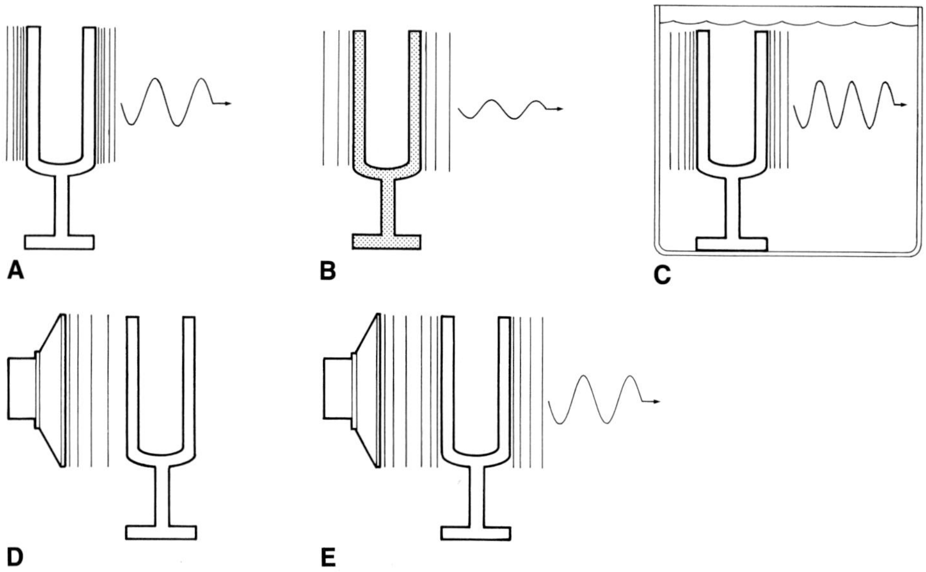

FIGURE 2-3

Resonance of a tuning fork. (A) A tuning fork, when struck, vibrates only at its characteristic resonance frequency. (B) If this tuning fork were made of a different material, it would have a different resonance frequency. (C) The same tuning fork in (A), placed under water, vibrates at a different frequency. Resonance frequency may be altered by changing the external environment. (D) A tuning fork placed in front of a speaker will not vibrate when an arbitrary sound wave strikes it. (E) The same tuning fork will vibrate (resonate) if sound waves of its specific resonance frequency strike it.

stimulates it. These phenomena are illustrated in Figure 2-3.

The process of MR signal generation can be thought of in two steps: (1) *stimulation* to resonance and (2) *relaxation* from resonance. We will now discuss these two stages in more detail.

Stimulation to Resonance

Quantum mechanics presents a complicated but accurate representation of the hydrogen proton. This model ascribes to the proton a set of fixed (quantized) energy levels and electromagnetic states. The proton can be thought of as having properties similar, but not identical, to the magnetism, angular momentum, and spinning we observe in the larger world.

Because such a description is so difficult to visualize except for physicists and mathematicians, a few large-scale physical analogies are sometimes helpful. As mentioned previously, we may think of each proton as a tiny spinning magnet (Fig. 2-2). The entire sample of tissue being imaged may be thought of as a collection of spinning magnets, represented as tiny balls with arrows to indicate the direction of the magnetic poles. In a sample of tissue far away from all external magnetic fields, each tiny proton magnet is randomly oriented, as shown in Figure 2-4.

When this sample of tissue is placed in a strong static magnetic field (B_0) as in the bore of an MR magnet, many of these small proton magnets will align with the external field. These many tiny magnetic poles will add together and produce a small magnetic field of their own within the tissue. This small magnetic field is called the macroscopic **magnetization** of the tissue, represented by the vector M in Figure 2-5. Note that this magnetization is parallel to the static field, B_0 although it is millions of times smaller. The baseline value for this magnetization is denoted M_0.

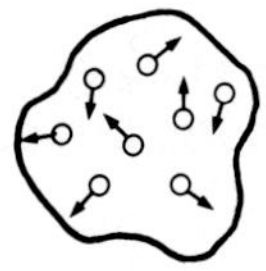

FIGURE 2-4

In a sample of tissue far away from external magnetic fields, the tiny proton magnets are randomly oriented.

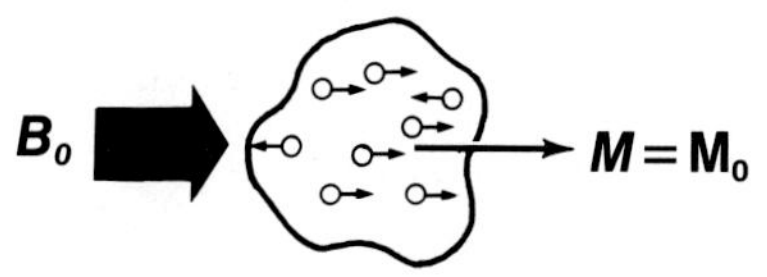

FIGURE 2-5

When this tissue is placed in a strong magnetic field, B_0, the tiny proton magnetic moments will tend to align with the field, producing a small field of their own, *M*. This small induced field within the tissue is called the magnetization vector, *M*, whose baseline value is M_0.

Now consider what happens when a second oscillating magnetic field is applied at right angles to the static field (Fig. 2-6). This second magnetic field, denoted B_1, is generated by electric currents in the RF coil, shown in Figure 1-6. There are several differences between the B_0 and B_1 fields. The B_0 field is about 10,000 times more powerful than the B_1 field. For example, the strength of the B_0 field might be about 1 T, whereas the B_1 field is on the order of 1 G (0.0001 T). Second, the B_0 field is constant and is always directed along the bore of the magnet. The B_1 field, however, is rapidly rotating but is always perpendicular to the direction of the static field, B_0.

The rotation frequency of the B_1 field is very carefully chosen. The B_1 field must rotate many millions of times per second. If an arbitrary frequency is selected for B_1, there will be little or no effect on the sample tissue or its magnetization vector, *M* (Fig. 2-6*A*). This is equivalent to the analogy with the tuning fork, which will not vibrate in front of a speaker unless stimulated at its specific resonance frequency.

If the frequency of B_1 is chosen to match precisely a frequency known as the **Larmor resonance frequency**, a remarkable phenomenon takes place. The tiny proton magnets within the tissue being imaged are able to absorb energy from the B_1 field. When these protons absorb energy, they jump to higher quantum levels and orientations. Because they have absorbed this extra energy, they are no longer so tightly aligned with the static B_0 field. This disruption and change in magnetic alignment can be thought of as a shift in the size and direction of the net magnetization vector *M* (Fig. 2-6*B*).

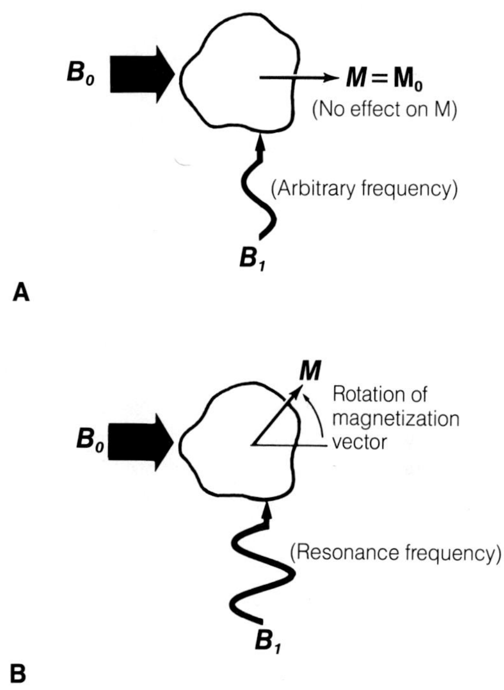

FIGURE 2-6

Stimulation by a radio-frequency field, B_0. (A) When an arbitrary frequency is chosen for B_1, there is little or no effect on the magnetization vector, *M* (equivalent to tuning fork analogy Figure 2-3D). (B) When B_1 is chosen to match the Larmor resonance frequency of the hydrogen proton-magnet system, MR occurs and the magnetization vector rotates away from its original alignment (equivalent to tuning fork analogy Figure 2-3E).

In addition to absorbing energy, the protons in the tissue can also release energy, when they fall from higher to lower quantum levels and orientations. Once again, the energy they release can be emitted only at the specific Larmor resonance frequency. This absorption and re-emission of electromagnetic energy is the process of **nuclear magnetic resonance.**

We can calculate the Larmor resonance frequency if the strength of the static field (B_0) is known. We use a formula known as the **Larmor equation**, which is written

$$\omega_0 = \gamma B_0 \qquad \text{(Eq. 2-1)}$$

where ω_0 = the resonance frequence in megahertz (MHz) and B_0 = the strength of the static magnetic field in tesla. The symbol γ is a constant called the **gyromagnetic ratio**, which for the hydrogen nucleus has a value 42.58 MHz/T.

As an example of the use of this equation, consider a Siemens Magnetom scanner, which operates at a static field strength of 0.5 T. The resonance frequency used in this scanner would be approximately ω_0 = (42.58 MHz/T) × (0.5 T) = 21.3 MHz. This frequency is very close to that used for certain mobile telephones and citizens' band (CB) radios. This is the reason we have called the B_1 field the radio-frequency field and the coil that produces it the RF coil.

The Larmor equation has several practical consequences for MRI. First of all, magnetic field strength will determine at which radio frequencies the scanner will operate. For example, a General Electric Signa scanner that operates at 1.5 T will have a resonance frequency of approximately ω_0 = (42.58 MHz/T) × (1.5 T) = 63.9 MHz. Thus the 1.5 T Signa scanner would operate at a base frequency about three times as high as the Magnetom scanner at 0.5 T. This linear relationship between field strength and resonance frequency is shown in Table 2-1.

A second consequence of the Larmor equation is that certain nuclei other than hydrogen nuclei may undergo nuclear magnetic resonance. The frequency at which this occurs is not the same as for hydrogen, because the gyromagnetic ratios of other nuclei are different (Table 2-2). Thus by stimulating the patient's tissues at different frequencies, it is possible for nuclei other than hydrogen to undergo resonance. MRI using sodium and phosphorus nuclei is already undergoing clinical trials in some centers.

TABLE 2-1

Resonance Frequency of Hydrogen in Different Magnetic Fields*

Field Strength of MR Scanners in Common Use	Resonance Frequency
0.15 T	6.4 MHz
0.3	12.8
0.5	21.3
0.6	25.5
1.0	42.6
1.5	63.9
2.0	85.2

*Based on the Larmor equation $\omega_0 = \gamma B_0$

Where ω_0 = resonance frequency

γ = gyromagnetic ratio, which for hydrogen is 42.58 MHz/T

B_0 = magnetic field strength

TABLE 2-2

Gyromagnetic Ratios for Certain Paramagnetic Nuclei

Nucleus	Gyromagnetic Ratio (γ)
^{1}H	42.58 MHz/T
^{19}F	40.05
^{31}P	17.23
^{23}Na	11.26
^{13}C	10.71

A third consequence of the Larmor equation is that small changes in the static field will result in small changes in the resonance frequency, ω_0. If the static field is altered in a small, predictable manner in space, the resonance frequency of protons in the tissue will also be changed in a small, predictable way. The *gradient coils* discussed in Chapter 1 produce small fields that superimpose on the static field. The small changes in frequency and phase produced by the gradient coil magnetic fields allow us to localize accurately from which point in the tissue an MR signal arises.

Relaxation from Resonance

The relaxation process begins at the time the stimulating field (B_1) is turned off. At this time, the macroscopic magnetization vector has been rotated and changed in size, so that it is no longer parallel to the static field (B_0). This situation is depicted in Figure 2-7A.

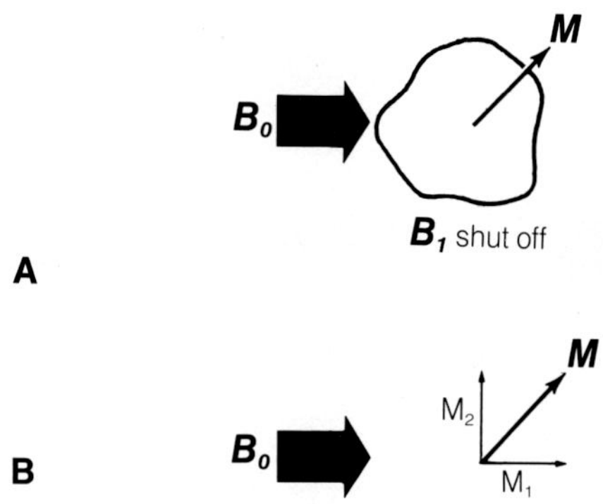

FIGURE 2-7

(A) Position of magnetization vector, *M,* immediately after B_1 field is shut off. (B) This vector, *M,* may be decomposed into two components, M_1 and M_2, parallel and perpendicular respectively to B_0.

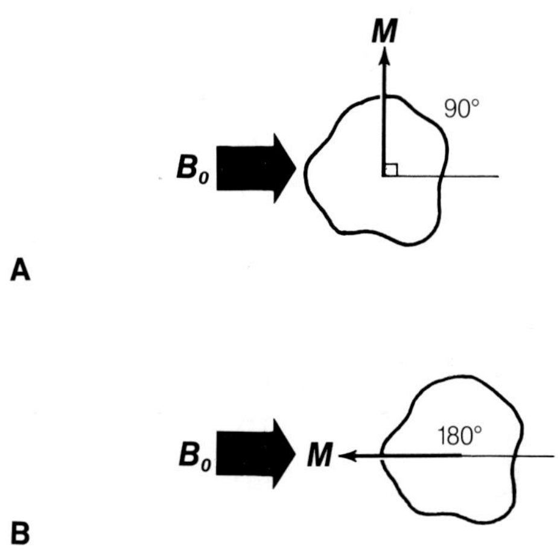

FIGURE 2-8

Position of magnetization vector, *M,* after a 90° pulse (A) or 180° pulse (B).

The obliquely oriented *M* vector may be decomposed into two components, represented as M_1 and M_2 in Figure 2-7*B*. M_1 represents the component of *M* parallel to the static field, and M_2 represents the transverse (perpendicular) component. In some books, these components are denoted M_z and M_{xy}, respectively. The significance of considering the M_1 and M_2 components is that it allows us to discriminate between two separate modes of relaxation. These two relaxation processes are known as T1 and T2 relaxation, respectively.

As the stimulated protons undergo relaxation, they release the energy they absorbed. As a basic principle of quantum physics, this energy must be re-emitted only at the same frequency at which it was absorbed (*i.e.,* the Larmor resonance frequency). Several things may happen to the energy that is released: (1) It may be released as radio waves and recorded as the MR signal, using the RF coil as an antenna receiver; (2) it may be lost irreversibly to the surrounding tissue "lattice," in the form of heat or induced molecular motion (T1 relaxation); or (3) it may be transferred reversibly to other protons undergoing resonance, although phase uniformity may be lost (T2 relaxation).

By varying the strength and duration of the B_1 field, it is possible to synchronize the quantum transitions of the resonating hydrogen nuclei. This synchronization can be thought of as rotation of the magnetization vector (*M*) relative to the static magnetic field (B_0). If the B_1 field is left on for about 50 μsec, the magnetization vector will rotate so that it is oriented at 90° relative to the B_0 field (Fig. 2-8*A*). If the B_1 field is made twice as strong or left on for twice as long (*e.g.,* 100 μsec), the vector *M* will continue to rotate so that it now points directly opposite to the B_0 field (Fig. 2-8*B*). Since these are relatively short bursts of energy supplied by the B_1 field at radio-wave frequencies, they are called **RF pulses.** The RF pulses that cause 90° and 180° rotations of the magnetization vector *M* are called a **90° pulse** and a **180° pulse**, respectively. It can be seen that by changing the strength and duration of the RF pulse it is possible to rotate the magnetization vector in any direction.

When the B_1 field is shut off, the process of *stimulation* to resonance is completed. During the next several seconds, the stimulated protons will re-emit their absorbed energy. As these protons give up their energy, they will return to their original stable alignment with the static field. This can be monitored as a return of the rotated magnetization

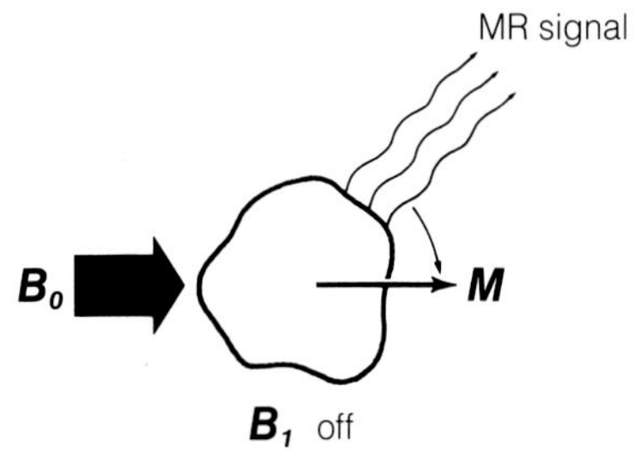

FIGURE 2-9

When the RF field is turned off, the magnetization vector, *M*, returns to its original alignment parallel to B_0. An MR signal is recorded as this magnetization vector changes alignment.

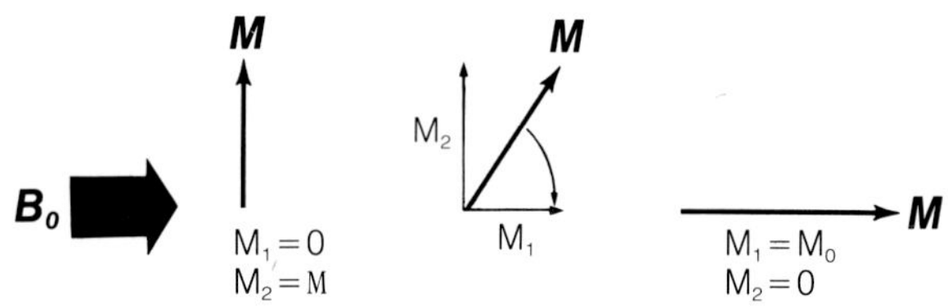

FIGURE 2-10

Relaxation after a 90° pulse. Immediately after the 90° pulse, the M_1 component is zero and M_2 component is at a maximum. As relaxation occurs, M_2 shortens and M_1 lengthens until final realignment takes place.

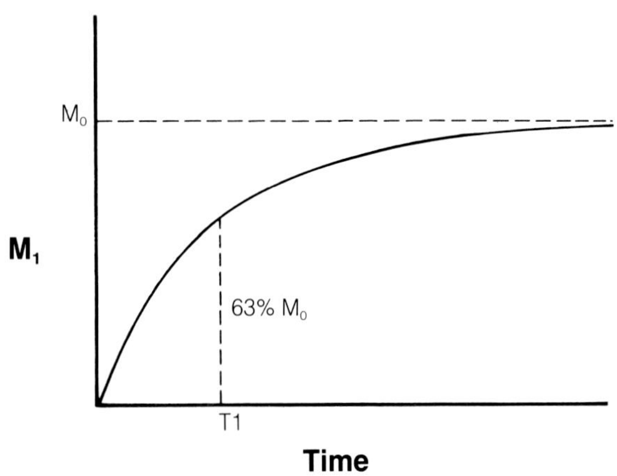

FIGURE 2-11

Measurement of T1 relaxation time. T1 is defined as time for M_1 to recover 63% of its original value (M_0) after a 90° pulse.

vector *M* back to its original orientation parallel to B_0 (Fig. 2-9). The process by which stimulated protons release their energy and return to their original alignment is known as **relaxation.**

The release of energy in the form of radio waves is the basis for MRI. Only energy components perpendicular to the static field may be recorded by the RF coil, since the components parallel to B_0 are changing too slowly to induce an appreciable signal in the coil. The MR signal from each small volume of tissue is a little different, because it has been coded to have a slightly different frequency and phase by the gradient magnetic fields. By a complex mathematical process known as **Fourier transformation,** the location of each signal from within the sample may be computed. This signal is then represented as a bright dot on the video display, with stronger signals producing brighter dots.

Loss of MR energy parallel to the external field (B_0) is known as **T1 relaxation.** Other names for this process include *longitudinal relaxation, thermal relaxation,* and *spin-lattice relaxation.* T1 relaxation may be determined by measuring the changes in the M_1 component of *M* following an RF pulse. This is illustrated in Figures 2-10 and 2-11.

After cessation of a 90° pulse, the *M* vector is at right angles to B_0. At this point, the M_1 component is zero. As longitudinal relaxation occurs, the *M* vector will rotate so that it returns to its equilibrium position with length M_0 maximal and parallel to B_0. The relaxation process in the M_1 direction can be graphically depicted as an exponential growth curve. The characteristic time constant of such an exponential curve can be defined as the time required for the curve to grow from zero to $(1 - 1/e)$, or 63% of its final value. For the M_1 curve shown in Figure 2-11, this time constant is labeled T1. As will be discussed later, tissues of varying composition may be uniquely characterized by the values of their T1 time constants.

The value of T1 in a tissue is a measure of how efficiently energy of resonating protons is dispersed into that tissue during relaxation. Neighboring atoms and molecules in the tissue ("the lattice") have their own local magnetic fields, which fluctuate because of thermal motion. These fluctuating magnetic fields may interact with and absorb energy from the resonating protons. This energy transfer can occur only at frequencies near the Larmor frequency. The primary mechanism for this energy transfer is by intermolecular dipole–dipole interaction, producing rotational motion and heat in the neighboring molecules.

Certain molecules are very efficient at absorbing and interacting with protons near the Larmor frequency. Fats and cholesterol have multiple hydrogen-laden side chains and are remarkably efficient at T1 relaxation. As such, fat and fatty tissues have among the shortest values of T1 time constants in the body. Small molecules like water tumble too quickly and are inefficient at spin-lattice interactions. Large molecules like proteins tumble too slowly. Thus the measured T1 values of water and proteins are quite long.

T2 relaxation is also known as *transverse* or *spin–spin relaxation.* T2 relaxation is a measure of how long transverse magnetization would last in a perfectly homogeneous external magnetic field. Equivalently, T2 relaxation represents how long it would take resonating protons to fall out of phase or lose coherence with each other in a uniform field following a 90° pulse.

Assuming a perfectly uniform external static field and an ideal 90° pulse, all resonating protons would oscillate in phase with one another. This would produce a net tissue magnetization vector *M* directed at right angles to the static field. Immediately after the 90° pulse, the M_2 component of *M* is at a maximum. As relaxation occurs, the M_2 component decays toward zero, since there is no transverse magnetization at equilibrium (Fig. 2-10). In other words, the phase coherence between resonating protons is lost. This M_2 decay process, like that for M_1, is an exponential curve, with a characteristic time constant, T2 (Fig. 2-12). This T2 time constant, (the *transverse* or *spin–spin relaxation time*) is the time it takes for the transverse magnetization to decay to 1/e, or 37% of its initial value. As with the T1 time constant, different tissues may be characterized by their T2 values.

In contrast to T1 relaxation processes, T2 relaxation does not involve energy transfer from resonating nuclei to the lattice. T2 interactions only result in a change of phase between resonating protons (*i.e.,* the protons lose coherence). The resonating nuclei exchange energy only with each other, so no energy is lost.

In general, the value of T2 is more closely related to tissue state (solid or liquid) than is T1. The tightly held and closely packed hydrogen nuclei in solids are more efficient at spin–spin interactions

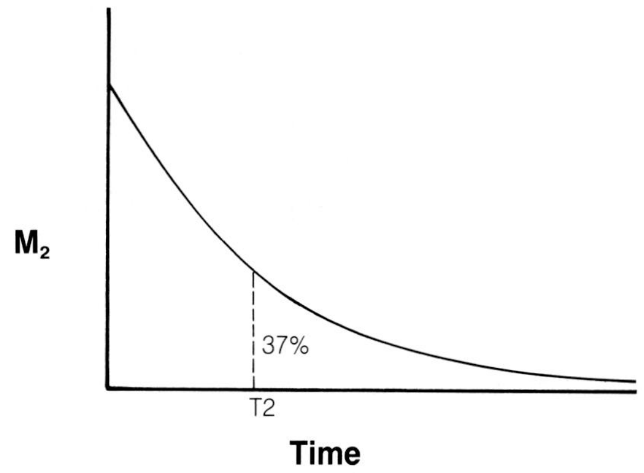

FIGURE 2-12

Measurement of T2 relaxation time. T2 is defined as the time for M_2 to fall to 37% of its highest value after a 90° pulse.

than are those in loosely structured liquids. Accordingly, dense, solid tissues with large proteins (like skeletal muscle) have the shortest values of T2. Watery tissues and fluids like cerebrospinal fluid have very long values of T2.

It should be noted that the T2 relaxation illustrated in Figures 2-10 and 2-12 was described for an ideal, perfectly uniform external magnetic field. In all magnets, however, inhomogeneities in the field exist. This results in a more rapid decay of transverse magnetization than would be expected from spin–spin interactions alone. The reason for more rapid decay in nonuniform fields is that certain nuclei will experience locally stronger fields than others in resonance. These nuclei in the stronger field areas will precess (resonate) faster than those in the lower field areas. As such, phase coherence established by the original 90° pulse will be more rapidly lost in such inhomogeneous fields. A clever technique called spin echo for correcting such inhomogeneities is described in the next chapter.

Four Properties Determine MR Signal Strength

How bright a dot appears on the final MR image is directly proportional to MR signal strength recorded from the volume element of tissue represented by that dot. In general, four physical characteristics of a tissue being imaged will determine how strong a signal that tissue emits when stimulated into magnetic resonance. These four properties are (1) the concentration of hydrogen protons in the tissue, (2) the velocity at which these protons are moving, (3) T1 relaxation effects, and (4) T2 relaxation effects.

Hydrogen Concentration. Since MR is a phenomenon involving hydrogen protons, it is not surprising that the recorded signal intensity from a tissue should be directly proportional to hydrogen concentration in that tissue. The relative hydrogen density in several body tissues has been measured, and the results are displayed in Table 2-3. An interesting pattern is seen. For most tissues of the body, the concentration of hydrogen is remarkably similar, varying at most by 10% to 15%. In the head, for example, only 3% difference in hydrogen concentration is noted between brain and cerebrospinal fluid. For many areas of the body, therefore, imaging by proton density alone would not allow much contrast resolution.

Hydrogen concentration difference alone, however, does adequately explain the imaging characteristics of two types of tissues. First, air and air-containing structures like the lungs and bowel have very low concentrations of hydrogen. Second, cortical bone, which is composed mostly of calcium and phosphate, also contains little hydrogen. Therefore, air-containing spaces and cortical bone will always have little signal and appear dark on MR images, no matter what pulse sequence is used. The lungs will have slightly higher signals than an empty air-containing space, because lung parenchyma has appreciable hydrogen density. Bone containing marrow or fat may have an intensely bright signal centrally in its medullary cavity, although its hydrogen-deficient cortex will remain dark.

TABLE 2-3

Relative Hydrogen Density of Body Tissues

Tissue	Relative H Concentration
White matter	100
Muscle	100
Fat	98
Cerebrospinal fluid	97
Kidney	95
Gray matter	94
Spleen	93
Liver	91
Blood	91
Pancreas	87
Cortical bone	<10
Lungs	<10
Air	< 1

Approximations from several sources. Note that the relative hydrogen spin density is within 10% to 15% for most tissues in the body except bone, lung, and air.

Velocity Effects. Most organs and tissues in the body are relatively stationary, and velocity considerations play no role in their MRI characteristics. The appearance of flowing blood, however, is markedly dependent on its velocity, as well as other features including plane of imaging, imaging sequence, slice acquisition mode, turbulence of flow, and the angle at which the blood vessel intersects the plane of imaging.

Although the appearance of flowing blood depends on many factors and is difficult to predict, two basic generalizations usually hold true. Rapidly flowing blood or blood with turbulence often has little MR signal and appears dark on most imaging sequences. Slowly flowing blood, on the other hand, often has an intense signal. This may be particularly marked on even-numbered echoes when the spin-echo pulse technique is used.

Why does rapidly flowing blood appear dark? At least two factors may contribute to high velocity signal loss. The **fast transition phenomenon** is illustrated in the first part of Figure 2-13. In this diagram, nuclei in slice 1 are stimulated to resonance by an RF pulse. Before their relaxation signal can be recorded, however, these nuclei have flowed downstream out of the slice. Hence no signal is recorded from these nuclei in slice 1. A second factor contributing to signal loss in rapidly flowing blood is **turbulence.** The effects of turbulence remain to be investigated more thoroughly, but it is thought that the random motion of fluids in turbulence produces a more rapid loss in phase coherence and disappearance of the signal.

Why may slowly flowing blood appear bright?

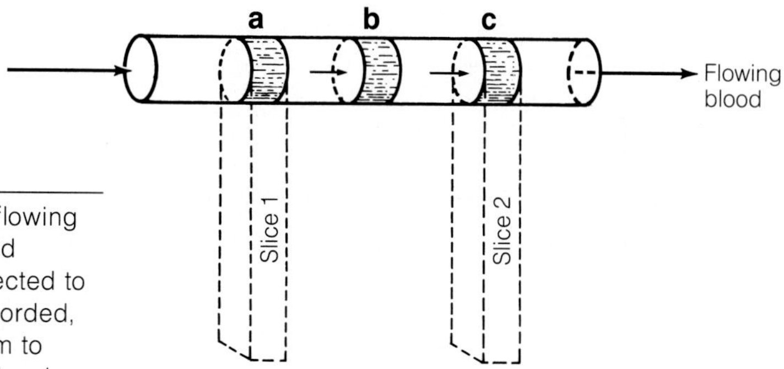

FIGURE 2-13

Simplified diagram showing some effects of flowing blood on the MR signal. At *a*, fully magnetized flowing blood enters slice 1, where it is subjected to an RF pulse. Before an MR signal can be recorded, some of these nuclei have moved downstream to point *b*. This can produce loss of signal in slice 1 (fast transition phenomenon). If the partially saturated blood at *b* has not fully recovered its magnetization by the time it reaches point *c*, repeated RF stimulation in slice 2 will yield a weaker signal than from the nuclei in slice 1. The signal in slice 1 is "paradoxically enhanced" with respect to slice 2 although the same blood is flowing at the same rate through both slices. The degree to which MR signal is diminished (fast transition) or augmented (paradoxical enhancement) depends on flow rate and other factors such as turbulence, direction of flow, and pulse sequence.

Originally called "paradoxical enhancement," this phenomenon can be considered to arise from two processes. An **entry phenomenon** can produce signal enhancement in slowly flowing blood that enters the first slice of multislice imaging volume. The entering blood contains fully magnetized, unsaturated protons. By contrast, blood and stationary tissue already within the imaging volume are partially saturated, having not yet fully recovered from previous RF excitations. As a result, the entering unsaturated blood can produce a higher signal than adjacent partially saturated blood or stationary tissue.

A second mechanism producing paradoxical enhancement is known as **even echo rephasing.** This phenomenon occurs only in slowly flowing blood subjected to successive 180° RF pulses in a pulse sequence known as multiple spin echo (described in Chap. 3). In this pulse sequence, multiple 180° pulses are applied at regular intervals to the tissue and signals recorded after each pulse. In this situation, every two consecutive 180° pulses add together to produce a 360° rotation of the magnetization vector *M*. If there were no motion and if the external magnetic field were perfectly uniform, the two 180° pulses would largely cancel each other except for the normal signal decay, which would occur in the time between them. However, additional gradient fields are superimposed on the static magnetic field for spatially encoding the MR signal. The presence of flow in the readout gradient magnetic field introduces nonlinearities that are not canceled by pairs of 180° pulses. As a result, the signal from slowly flowing blood is augmented and appears brighter on images recorded after even-numbered echoes than after odd-numbered ones.

In conclusion, therefore, the effects of blood flow on the MR signal are complex and difficult to predict. In general, rapidly flowing or turbulent blood will have little signal, whereas slowly flowing blood may be intense, particularly on even-echo images. Research is currently under way in a number of centers to quantitate blood flow based on MR signal.

T1 Effects. The signal strength from all imaging sequences currently in use depends in some way on the T1 relaxation time of the tissue being imaged. The T1 time is not specific for a particular tissue, because many tissues may have values of T1 that overlap. Furthermore, the calculated value of T1 is methodology dependent, and absolute values are not important. The measured value of T1 for a tissue depend on the strength of the static magnetic field as well. Values of tissue T1 measured at 1.5 T are approximately twice as long as measurements made at 0.2 T. Despite this variation with field strength and methodology, the relative values of T1 among different tissues are remarkably constant. A list of T1 and T2 values of various tissues obtained at 0.15 T is

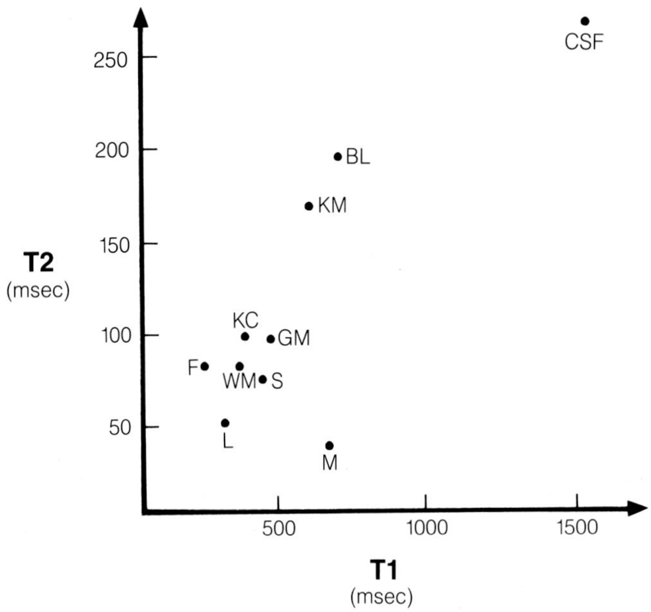

FIGURE 2-14

A T1-T2 graph demonstrating the location of various body tissues measured at 0.3 T. Note that values are only approximate and derived from numerous sources, since calculation of T1 and T2 parameters is methodology dependent. (CSF = cerebrospinal fluid, BL = blood, KM = medulla of kidney, KC = cortex of kidney, GM = gray matter, WM = white matter, F = fat, S = spleen, L = liver, M = skeletal muscle).

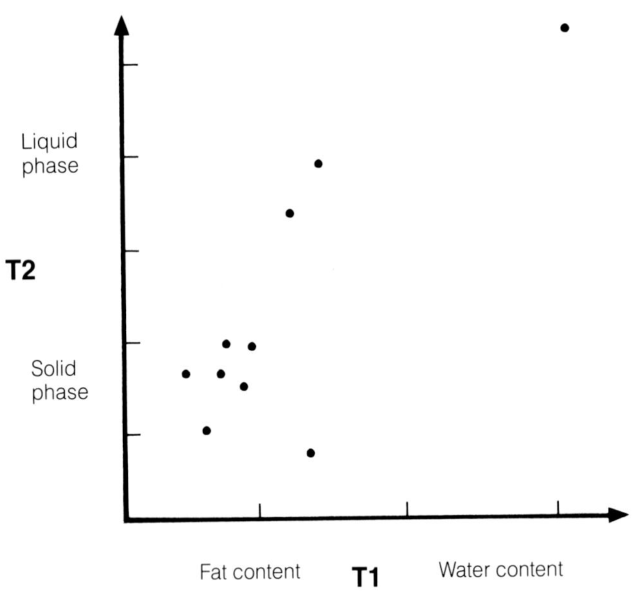

FIGURE 2-15

Schematic representation of Figure 2-14 demonstrating trends in T1 and T2 as they relate to phase and content of water or fat.

TABLE 2-4

T1 and T2 of Tissues at 0.15 T*

Tissue	T1 (msec)	T2 (msec)
Fat	170	80
Liver	250	50
Brain—white matter	350	80
—gray matter	500	100
Spleen	450	75
Kidney—cortex	340	70
—medulla	650	130
Muscle	580	40
Blood	720	175
Cerebrospinal fluid	1500	260
Water	2500	2500

* Values of T1 and T2 are only approximations from numerous sources, since measurements are methodology dependent.

presented in Table 2-4. A graphic presentation of the same data is shown in Figure 2-14.

As mentioned in the previous section, the values of tissue T1 depend strongly on relative content of fat and free water in that tissue. Fat and fatty tissues have short values of T1, because the structure of fat is remarkably efficient at spin-lattice interactions near the Larmor frequency. Tissues containing high water content (like body fluids and the renal medulla) have very long values of T1, since they are inefficient at these interactions.

T2 Effects. T2 relaxation is an important determinant of signal strength from the spin-echo pulse sequence and is less important in other pulse techniques. Changes in tissue T2 may be among the most discriminating features of tissue contrast and in the detection of pathologic conditions. As was previously noted, the value of T2 is more closely related to tissue state than is any other single feature. Solids are efficient at spin–spin interactions and have short values of T2. Liquids are inefficient and have long values.

The general trends for predicting tissue values of T1 and T2 are shown in Figure 2-15. It is very important to have a good understanding of this figure as well as the approximate positions of various body tissues as shown in Figure 2-14. Note the general trends and also the relative values of T1 and T2. In general, values for tissue T2 are roughly 1/10 of the values for tissue T1. It is not possible to predict a value of T2 if the value of T1 is known, nor vice versa.

Several hints may be helpful for remembering the relation and trends on this T1–T2 graph. For example, it is easy to think of cerebral white matter as having more fat (myelin) and less water than gray matter, as well as being more dense. Thus you can remember that the T1 and T2 values of white matter are slightly lower than those of gray matter. In a similar manner, you can think of there being more water in the renal medulla than in the renal cortex, since the former contains more urine. Thus you can remember that the medulla will have longer T1 and T2 values than the renal cortex.

Although such reasoning is not infallible, it allows one for the most part to keep certain important relations between the T1 and T2 values of various tissues in perspective. This working knowledge of tissue characteristics and their effects on the MR signal will be directly applicable to the understanding of MR scans in health and disease. In the final analysis, the person who understands the relative values of T1 and T2 and how they effect the MR image will be a more effective diagnostician than one who studies quantum physics.

CHAPTER 3

Imaging Sequences and Parameters

The first two chapters of this book provided the physical science background necessary for understanding MR. Although important as a foundation, this knowledge alone does not allow one to predict how a given tissue will appear on an MR scan. The purpose of this chapter is to bridge the gap between MR physics and clinical imaging by describing those parameters that must be specified in order to perform an MR scan and the effect that changing those parameters has on the final image. The spin-echo pulse technique and several other pulse sequences, including partial saturation and inversion recovery, will be discussed in detail.

Parameters That Must Be Specified to Perform an MR Scan

Table 3-1 lists seven basic parameters and options that must be specified by the machine operator in order to perform an MR scan.

Plane of the Image

On all MR scanners in use today, an option exists for specifying the plane of imaging: axial, coronal, or sagittal. At least two manufacturers (Technicare and Fonar) have developed programs to allow image acquisition and display in oblique planes as well. In the usual imaging situation today, acquisition of MR images is performed in a two-dimensional mode, similar to planar slices obtained with a CT scanner. The advantage of MR over CT is that these slices may be directly obtained in any of the three major imaging planes without moving the patient or incurring the noisy inaccuracy of reformatting. When this two-dimensional image acquisition mode is used in MRI, as it nearly always is, the desired plane of imaging must be specified in advance. It takes some clinical experience to know the optimum plane for viewing certain anatomic structures and for interpreting certain pathological conditions. The second half of this book will be devoted to such considerations.

TABLE 3-1

Parameters That Must Be Specified to Perform an MR Scan

Parameter	Typical Options	Comments
Plane of image	Axial Coronal Sagittal	Oblique plane option available on some scanners.
Slice thickness	3 mm 7 mm 5 mm 10 mm	Thinner slices give better anatomic detail but require longer imaging times for same signal-to-noise ratio.
Matrix size	128 × 128 128 × 256 256 × 256	Better resolution with 256 × 256, but markedly longer imaging time (see Fig. 3-2).
Number of signal averages	1, 2, 4, 8, or 16	More averages improve image but require more time (see Fig. 3-2).
Pulse sequence	Partial saturation Inversion recovery Spin-echo	See Chapter 3. Spin-echo is most popular and versatile.
Pulse time intervals	TI = 200–800 msec TR = 250–4000 msec TE = 20–120 msec	Selection of TI and TR specify an IR sequence uniquely. TR and TE specify a spin-echo sequence.
Special options	Respiratory gating Cardiac gating Combined gating	Respiratory rate and heart rate gating prolong imaging time but are virtually required when detailed imaging of chest or upper abdomen is needed.

It should be noted that some commercial scanners have an option that permits three-dimensional image acquisition of data. In this situation, data are collected over the entire imaging volume simultaneously. This is made possible by stimulating the body part being imaged with a broad-band (nonselective) radio-frequency pulse. (In the two-dimensional image acquisition mode, a narrow-band [slice-selective] RF pulse is used, which stimulates nuclei only in the narrow plane of imaging.) The advantages of the three-dimensional mode of imaging are an improved signal-to-noise ratio and the ability to produce images in any plane retrospectively. The disadvantages of the three-dimensional mode are increased scan time and sensitivity to patient motion. At the present two-dimensional imaging seems to be the preferred method and the only mode commercially available on several scanners.

Slice Thickness

Several slice thicknesses are available on commercial MR scanners, varying from about 2 mm to 10 mm. Slices in the 1-mm range may be obtained with specialty surface coils. A trade-off exists between slice thickness, signal intensity, and scanning time. Thinner slices improve visualization of anatomic detail but require longer scanning times to maintain equivalent signal-to-noise ratios.

Matrix (Pixel) Size

Most commercial MR scanners built in 1985 do not offer as large an image matrix as the best CT scanners. For example, a General Electric 9800 CT scanner offers a 512 × 512 matrix. Most MR scanners, on the other hand, offer matrices from 128 × 128 to 256 × 256. Trade-offs similar to those noted with slice thickness exist with the selection of finer matrices. Figure 3-1 shows the effect of varying matrix size on the final image. Clearly, 256 × 256 matrices show finer anatomic detail than the 128 × 128 matrix. However, scanning time is longer for the 256 × 256 matrix and more signal averages must be taken in order to maintain the same signal-to-noise ratio. Using standard fields of view for the head, a 128 × 128 matrix produces pixels that measure 1.7 mm, whereas a 256 × 256 matrix produces pixels of 0.8 mm.

Number of Signal Averages

Signal averaging is the single best technique to improve MR image quality. Although quite acceptable images may be obtained without signal averaging, most MR diagnosticians find that at least two and sometimes four signal averages provide superior images. Advanced spin-echo processing techniques and further improvements in coil design will reduce the need for signal averaging in the future. Figure 3-2 shows the improvement in image quality that is possible with signal averaging. It is clear from this figure that signal averaging improves the image significantly. However, as is the case with other techniques to improve image quality, the benefits of signal averaging must be weighed against the increased scanning time required. Also, it is surprising to note that the incremental gain in image clarity is marginal for large numbers of signal averages. When many signal averages are taken, scan time is prolonged and patient motion may erase the gain of more signal averages.

Pulse Sequence

Virtually unlimited combinations of radio-frequency pulses may be applied to a tissue to generate an MR signal. The selection of such pulse sequences lies at the heart of MRI and research, and the rest of this chapter is devoted to a consideration of those in common use. All pulse sequences in current use involve tissue stimulation by combinations of 90° and 180° radio-frequency pulses, which rotate the tissue magnetization vector M by 90° or 180°, respectively, as described in Chapter 2. What makes the various pulse sequences unique is the order of these pulses and the time intervals between them.

Table 3-2 lists the three pulse sequences most frequently used today: partial saturation (PS), inversion recovery (IR), and spin-echo (SE). Two other techniques, free induction decay (FID) and steady-state free precession (SSFP) are seldom used and will not be discussed here. Even the partial saturation and inversion recovery techniques have lost popularity since their inception. It is safe to say that, across the country, most clinical imaging is performed today using the spin-echo technique or one of its variants. For this reason, most of the images in this book are from spin-echo sequences.

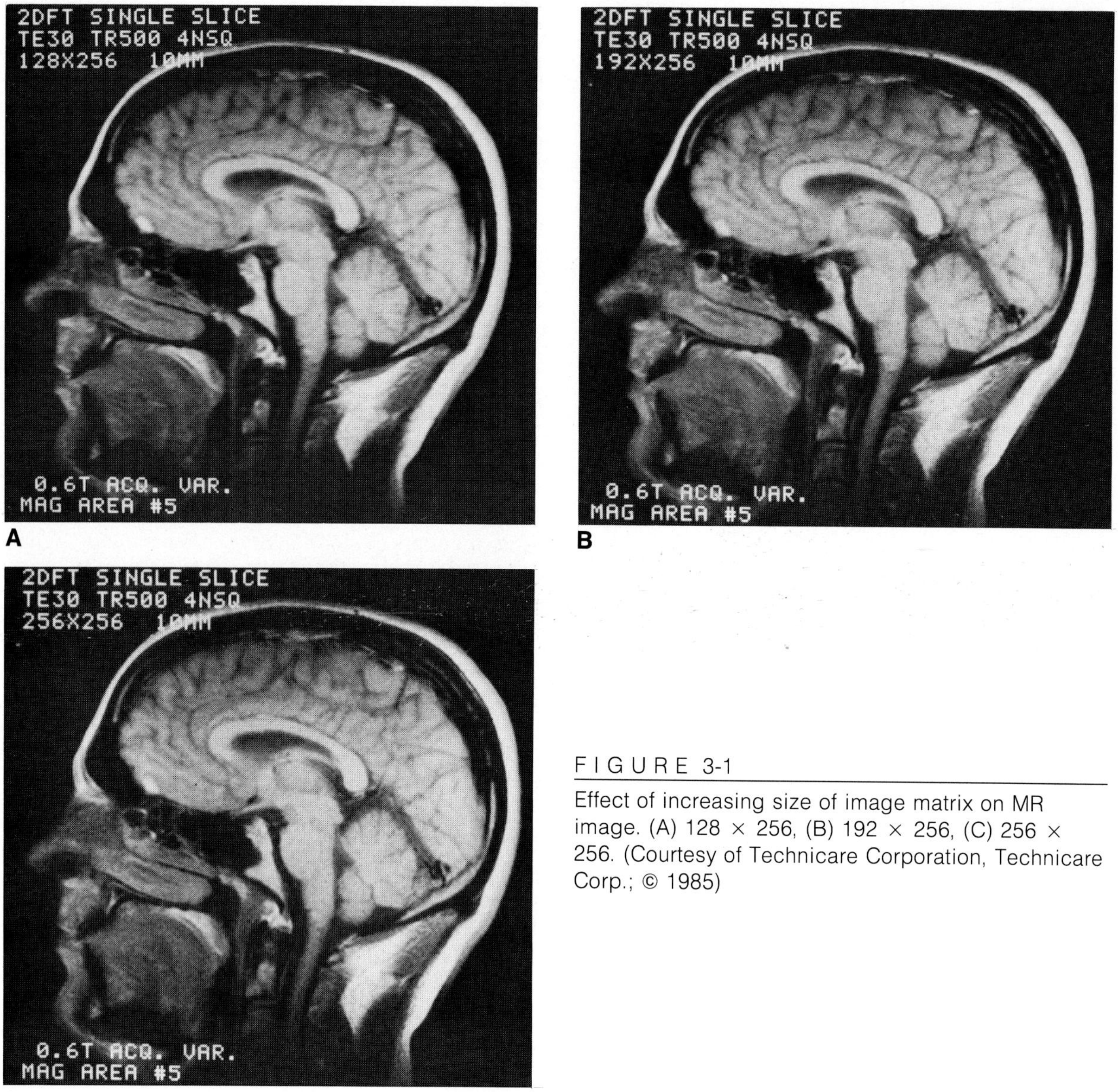

C

FIGURE 3-1

Effect of increasing size of image matrix on MR image. (A) 128 × 256, (B) 192 × 256, (C) 256 × 256. (Courtesy of Technicare Corporation, Technicare Corp.; © 1985)

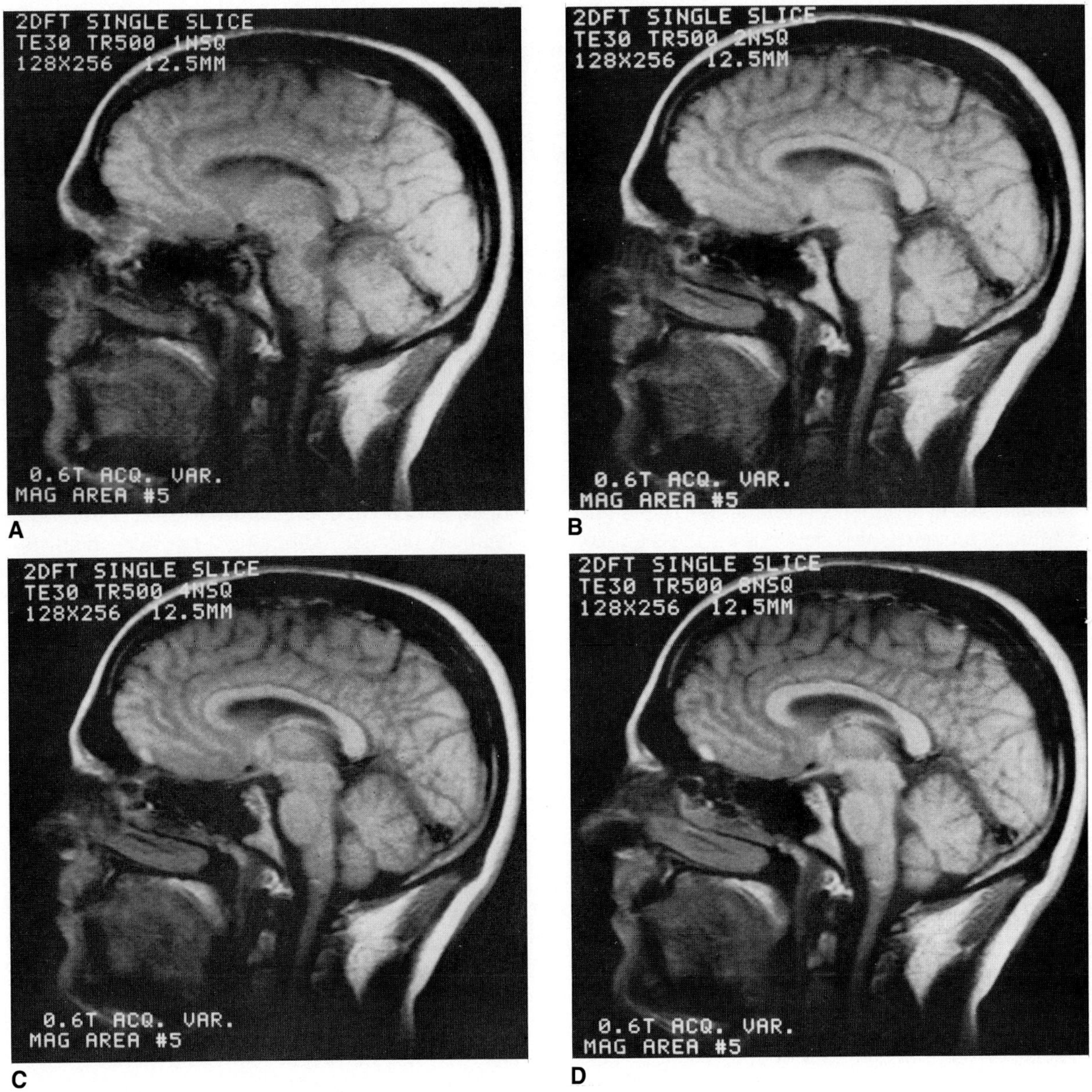

FIGURE 3-2

Effect of number of signal average on MR image. (A) one average, (B) two averages, (C) four averages, (D) eight averages. Note that incremental gain between four and eight averages is less than between one and two averages. (Courtesy of Technicare Corporation, Technicare Corp.; © 1985)

TABLE 3-2

How Tissue Parameters Affect MR Signal Intensity

Pulse Sequence	[Hydrogen]	T1	T2
Partial saturation	Directly proportional	Inversely proportional	Little effect
Inversion recovery	Directly proportional	Inversely proportional, except in contrast reversal zone	Little effect
Spin-echo	Directly proportional	Inversely proportional	Directly proportional

Table 3-2 shows that each of the pulse sequences listed generates MR signals whose intensity is proportional to hydrogen concentration. The signal from each sequence also depends on the T1 relaxation time of the tissue being imaged. This dependence on T1 is an inverse relation. That is, tissues with longer T1 values generally produce less signal (appear darker) in the MR image than tissues with shorter T1 values, assuming all other factors (hydrogen concentration, T2, velocity effects) are equal. In their classic description, neither the partial saturation nor the inversion recovery techniques produce signals that depend on tissue T2 values.* Only the spin-echo sequence produces a signal that depends on the tissue T2 relaxation time. This is a significant advantage the spin-echo technique holds over the other pulse sequences listed. It has been found that changes in tissue T2 values may be among the earliest and most sensitive indicators of tissue pathology. Since only spin-echo provides T2 information about a tissue being imaged, it has come to occupy the premier position in clinical MRI in the United States today.

The Spin-Echo Sequence

Although it may appear somewhat complicated at first, the spin-echo sequence is merely a train of alternating 90° and 180° RF pulses, as shown in Figure 3-3. The effect of this series of pulses is to rotate intermittently the tissue magnetization vector, *M*, and monitor its rate of return to equilibrium. As described in Chapter 2, this return toward equilibrium alignment parallel to the static magnetic field, B_0, depends on the inherent tissue relaxation times, T1 and T2.

The initial 90° pulse, when applied to the sample tissue, rotates the magnetization vector of that tissue perpendicular to the static magnetic field. This pulse also has the property of aligning and bringing the resonating hydrogen nuclei in phase with one another. The 90° pulse lasts less than a millisecond, then is shut off. A graphic representation of this situation immediately after the 90° pulse is shown in Figure 3-4.

As described in Chapter 2, the process of relaxation from resonance can now take place, as the magnetization vector attempts to realign itself with the static field. This occurs in two directions: perpendicular and parallel to the B_0 field. For the moment, let us consider relaxation in the transverse plane (*i.e.,* that perpendicular to the B_0 field).

The component of M in the transverse plane is directly related to the phase coherence between resonating nuclei. As an aid to visualization, think of the nuclei stimulated by the 90° pulse as all vibrating in an upward direction (Fig. 3-5 *A,B*).* Within a few

* Note: As they are implemented on many commercial scanners, partial saturation and inversion recovery employ an additional 180° pulse for readout purposes. This departs from the classic description of these techniques and causes them to possess some T2 dependence.

* Note: It should be remembered that no actual "tipping" of protons takes place. The diagrams presented here are only macroscopic analogies. What happens on the subatomic scale is that the distribution of nuclear spins in the upper and lower energy levels fluctuates in a harmonious, time-dependent fashion that is determined quantum mechanically. The small arrows (spin isochromats) are visual aids to represent the principal vector components of each proton's magnetic wave equation at the quantum level.

FIGURE 3-3

The spin-echo pulse sequence. (A) Single spin-echo sequence consists of a 90° pulse followed at time ½ TE by an 180° pulse, with an echo signal recorded. Sequence is repeated at time TR later. (B) Multiple spin-echo sequence. Successive 180° pulses may be applied with multiple echoes recorded. Note that each echo is weaker than its predecessor because of T2 decay.

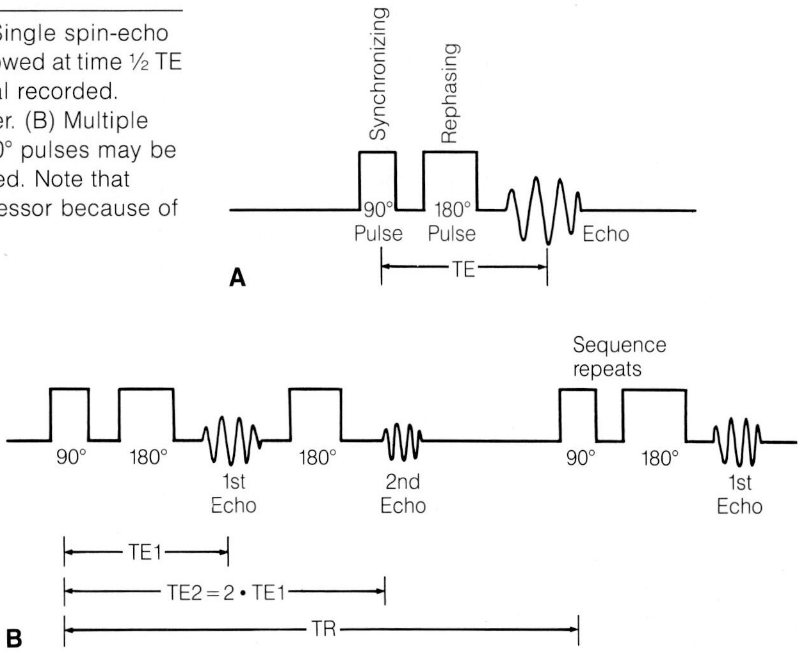

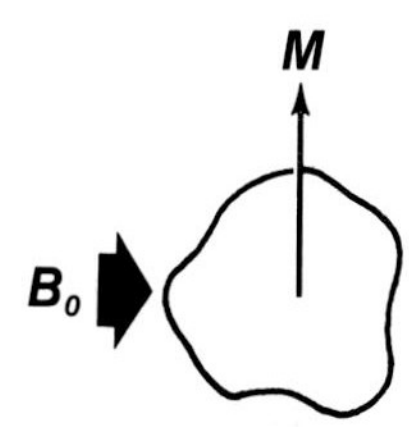

FIGURE 3-4

Immediately after the 90° pulse, the magnetization vector, *M,* is at right angles to the static field, B_o.

milliseconds after the 90° pulse is shut off, these harmoniously resonating nuclei begin to lose their phase coherence or uniformity (Fig. 3-5 *C,D*). Two factors are responsible for this loss of coherence: T2 interactions and irregularities in the static field.

T2 interactions, previously discussed, can be thought of as magnetic interactions between tiny proton magnets in neighboring atomic nuclei. These interactions are inescapable and cannot be corrected for or controlled. Indeed, this would not even be desirable, because the measurement of these T2 relaxation processes is part of what provides image contrast and diagnostic information in MRI.

Irregularities (inhomogeneities) in the static magnetic field, however, are undesirable and only confuse useful diagnostic MR signals. The reason static field irregularities cause problems can be explained in terms of the Larmor equation (Eq. 2-1). Since it is impossible to design a magnet with a perfectly uniform static magnetic field, certain areas within the imaging region will have a slightly higher than average magnetic field, whereas other areas will experience a slightly lower magnetic field. Nuclei in the areas of slightly lower field will resonate at slightly lower frequencies than those in the higher field areas. The more slowly resonating nuclei will fall out of phase with the more rapidly resonating nuclei. This produces loss of phase coherence established by the 90° pulse and loss of the transverse component of magnetization.

Fortunately, a clever technique known as spin-echo has been devised to correct for this loss of coherence because of static field irregularities. The principle of spin-echo is to apply a second *rephasing* pulse a few milliseconds after the initial 90° or *synchronizing* pulse. This rephasing pulse is also known as a 180° pulse because it flips the individual proton magnetic moments by 180° (as well as their summation, the tissue magnetization vector, *M*). A few

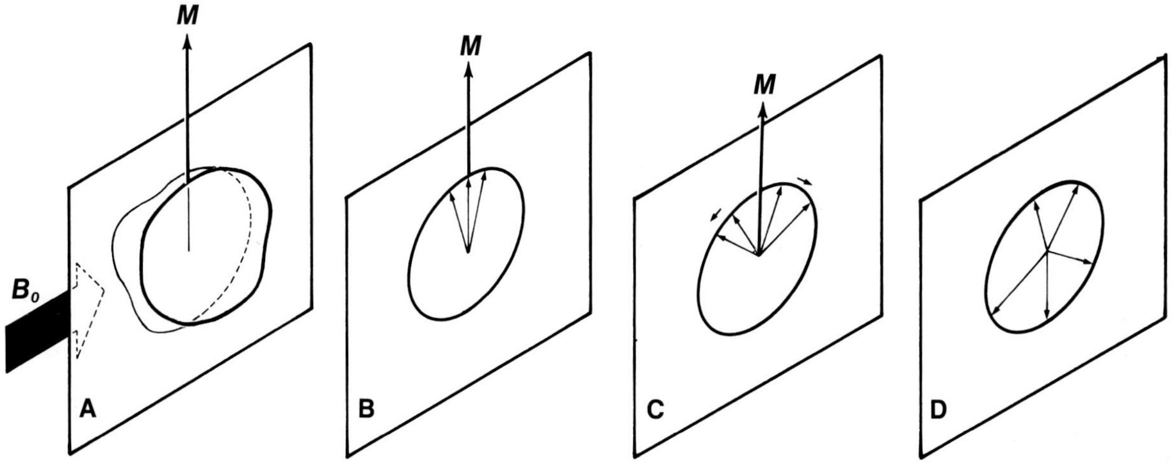

FIGURE 3-5

Transverse relaxation. (A) Three-dimensional representation of the plane transverse to B_0. (B) Immediately after 90° pulse, the individual proton magnetic moments are all in phase. Small arrows represent these individual magnetic moments, also called spin-isochromats. (C) With transverse relaxation, the individual magnetic moments fall out of phase with one another, because the synchronizing stimulus of the RF pulse is no longer present. This results in a decrease in magnitude of the magnetization vector, *M,* which is merely the vector sum of individual proton magnetic fields. (D) With further decay, the spin-isochromats are now randomly dispersed in phase. The transverse component of *M* is now 0.

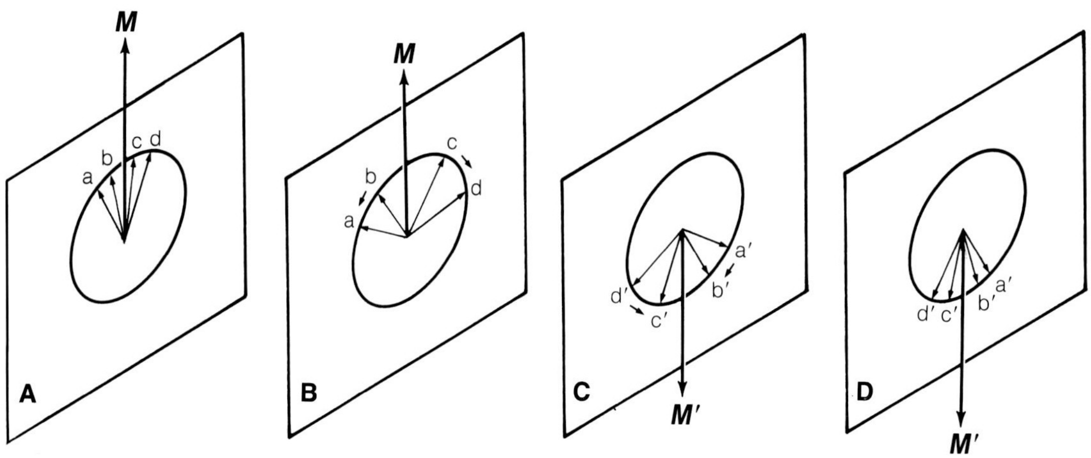

FIGURE 3-6

How the 180° pulse forms an echo. (A) and (B) Individual proton moments *a, b, c, d* fall out of phase with one another, resulting in a decreased magnitude for *M.* This falling out of phase results from two processes: T2 decay and irregularities in the static field. (C) After 180° pulse, each individual magnetic moment has been rotated 180°. (D) Continued precession of the individual spins causes them to come back into phase at time TE, with a maximal value *M′* in opposite direction to original *M.* This 180° pulse has corrected for irregularities in the static field that produce loss of transverse phase coherence. Pure T2 interactions between nuclei cannot be corrected for, and the ratio of *M′* to *M* is a measurement of T2 interactions.

milliseconds later, the nuclei that fell out of coherence with each other because of magnetic field irregularities have now come back into phase with one another. They have been "refocused," and it is now possible to record a MR signal from them, known as the *echo* (Fig. 3-6).

In order to understand better how this 180° pulse creates a spin-echo, the following analogy to a foot race is sometimes helpful. Consider a number of runners lined up at the starting blocks, ready to begin a race along a circular track. The runners represent individual proton magnetic moments, and their dispersion along the track represents loss of coherence during the MR transverse relaxation process. When the runners are close together (as at the start), they are in perfect and total coherence. This is the situation that exists immediately after the initial 90° pulse (the starting gunshot).

As the race progresses, certain slower runners will eventually fall behind the faster runners. This is equivalent to loss of MR phase coherence, as more slowly resonating nuclei fall behind the more rapidly resonating nuclei.

After a certain period of time, the runners are told that the gun will be fired again (the 180° pulse). When this shot is fired, the runners will reverse their direction and run back toward the starting line. The end result is that all runners will arrive back at the starting line at the same time, regardless of their speeds of progression. This simultaneous return of all the runners to the starting line corresponds to the refocused echo signal recorded from the proton ensemble. This spin-echo principle has corrected for local magnetic field irregularities, which have caused certain nuclei to resonate faster than others.

The time delay between the original 90° or synchronizing pulse and the echo signal is known as the *echo time* (TE). In general, the echo time is twice the interval between the 90° pulse and the 180° pulse. In usual practice, TE ranges from about 20 msec to 120 msec and is selected by the machine operator prior to scanning.

On most MR scanners, it is possible to apply a second 180° pulse at a variable time after the first echo and to record a second echo. This multiple echo technique is illustrated in Figure 3-3 *B*. Note that the second echo is weaker than the first because of T2 decay. As is illustrated, it is possible to define first and second echo times, denoted TE1 and TE2, respectively. Usually TE2 is twice as long as TE1.

The echo process may be repeated indefinitely, by continuing to apply 180° pulses and recording echoes. However, the signals from the third, fourth, and later echoes soon become too weak to detect. (Recall that the echo process corrects only for transverse decay due to magnetic field irregularities; T2 decay proceeds unabated.) In common practice, therefore, only two to four echoes are usually recorded.

The entire pulse sequence can be repeated at a certain interval later, called the *repetition time* (TR), which is defined as the time between 90° pulses, as shown in Figure 3-3 *B*. In common practice, TR is usually chosen in the range of 500 msec to 2000 msec (0.5 sec to 2.0 sec).

In summary, therefore, the spin-echo pulse sequence can be defined by two timing parameters, the TE and the TR. A shorthand notation is sometimes applied to describe a spin-echo technique with parameters TR and TE, written SE TR/TE. For example, a spin-echo technique with TR = 1500 msec and TE = 30 msec can be denoted SE 1500/30. When multiple echoes are recorded from a spin-echo sequence, these will be denoted SE TR/TE1, TE2. For example, with TR = 1000 msec and echoes at 30 msec and 60 msec, the sequence will be denoted SE 1000/30,60.

What makes the spin-echo technique so useful and appealing is the relative ease by which varying TR and TE parameters brings out physical properties of the tissue being imaged. For convenience, let us consider values of TE and TR "short" if they are below 25 msec and 500 msec, respectively. Let us consider values of TE and TR "long" if they are above 75 msec and 2500 msec, respectively. Table 3-3 illustrates how the final MR signal is weighted depending on choice of TR and TE.

If both TR and TE are short, sometimes called a *short spin-echo sequence*, the relative signal intensities recorded from two tissues depend primarily on their T1 relaxation time constants. Proton concentration differences and T2 differences do not have much effect when both TR and TE are short. Furthermore, T1 contributions are inversely proportional to signal strength in the spin-echo technique. That is, a tissue with a long T1 will have lower MR signal and appear darker than a tissue with a short T1, when the sequence is T1 weighted.

If TE is short and TR is long, the relative T1 and T2 effects are less important, and the sequence be-

TABLE 3-3

Parameter Weighting in Spin-Echo

TE	TR	Weighting
Short	Short	T1
Long	Long	T2
Short	Long	Hydrogen density
Other	Other	Mixed effects; use Bloch equation (Eq. 3-1)
Short TE means <25 msec		Short TR means <0.5 sec
Long TE means >75 msec		Long TR means >2.5 sec

comes more dependent purely on hydrogen proton density. This is particularly the case if TR is much greater than the longest tissue T1 value and if TE is much shorter than the shortest tissue T2 value.

For values of TR and TE in intermediate ranges, it is not possible to remember easily to what degree T1, T2, and proton density will contribute to MR signal strength and tissue contrast. A rather complicated equation has been derived for us in predicting the MR signal intensity obtained from a tissue subject to a spin-echo sequence. Known as the **Bloch equation,** this formula allows us to understand readily and to predict imaging characteristics of various tissues, although it is only an approximation to complex molecular interactions:

$$S_{SE} = f(H)\, g(V)\, [1 - e^{-TR/T1}]\, e^{-TE/T2} \quad \text{(Eq. 3-1)}$$

where

S_{SE} = MR signal strength for a spin-echo sequence
$f(H)$ = a function of hydrogen proton concentration in the tissue
$g(V)$ = a function of tissue velocity; for stationary tissues, $g(V) = 1$
TR, TE = repetition time and echo time, selected by the operator
T1, T2 = longitudinal and transverse relaxation times, tissue-specific

It is not necessary to memorize this equation. It is presented only for reference and as a semiquantitative approach to understanding the spin-echo process. Several features of this equation should be considered.

First, remember that MR signal strength, S_{SE}, determines directly how bright a dot appears in the final MR image. Weak signals are represented as black dots. Strong signals appear as white dots. Intermediate signals are represented as shades of gray.

The term f(H) represents a function of hydrogen proton concentration in the tissue being imaged and has already been discussed in Chapter 2. Recall again that for most tissues, f(H) has a value of 90% to 100%. Contrast between many tissues purely based on differences in proton density is not very good. The very low values of f(H) for cortical bone and air do represent the dominant imaging factor for these substances. Tissues like lung, cortical bone, tendon, and air-containing loops of bowel contain few hydrogen protons and appear dark on all imaging sequences.

The term g(V) is a velocity term, which has a value of unity for all stationary tissues. This term becomes important only to explain the imaging characteristics of flowing blood. To review from Chapter 2, flowing blood may either appear bright or dark, depending on velocity, plane of imaging, imaging technique, and other factors. Rapidly flowing blood usually appears dark for two reasons: (1) turbulence and (2) high-velocity signal loss. Slowly flowing blood may appear bright for two reasons: (1) even-echo rephasing and (2) flow-related enhancement. At imtermediate velocities, the appearance of flowing blood is difficult to predict.

The exponential terms $[1 - e^{-TR/T1}] \cdot e^{-TE/T2}$ describe a somewhat complicated interaction of two tissue characteristics (T1 and T2) and two operator-selected variables (TR and TE). It is important to have a good understanding of how changes in each of these four parameters affect signal strength. Figure 3-7 graphically illustrates signal intensity as a function of T1, T2, TR, and TE.

One may use the Bloch equation to deduce the conclusions already made in Table 3-3 concerning extreme values of TR and TE and spin-echo weighting. For example, picking TR >> T1 causes the term $e^{-TR/T1}$ to approach 0. This results in an equation (and signal) that depends only on TE and T2 and is independent of T1. Picking TE << T2 causes the term $e^{-TE/T2}$ to approach 1. Equation 3-1 then simplifies to a form dependent on T1 and TR but independent of T2. With an intermediate range of TR and TE values, say TR = 1000 msec and TE = 30 msec, we may use the Bloch equation together with values

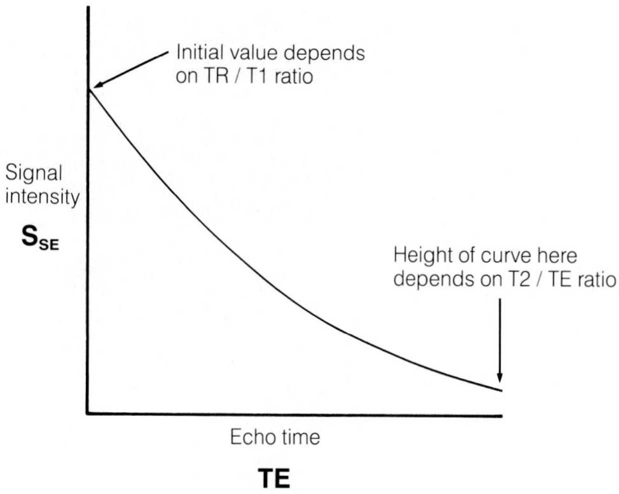

FIGURE 3-7

MR signal intensity of a spin-echo sequence. In general, signal intensity is directly proportional to TR and T2 but indirectly proportional to T1 and TE.

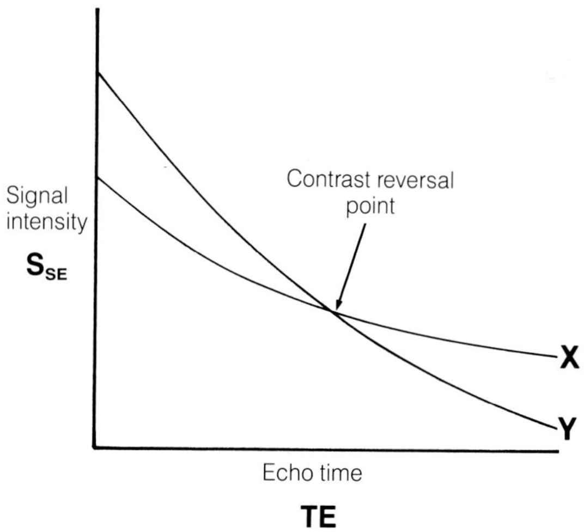

FIGURE 3-8

Contrast reversal may occur between two tissues, X and Y, as TE is increased.

of T1 and T2 from Table 2-3 to produce a typical relative brightness scale (Table 3-4).

Consideration of the Bloch equation also leads to a somewhat surprising relationship between the signal strengths of two tissues as either TR or TE is increased. For certain values of TE and TR, the relative signal strengths between two tissues may reverse. That is, a tissue that appears black may become white and one that appears white may become black. This is known as the *contrast reversal phenomenon*. This may be better understood by way of an example.

Consider two tissues, X and Y, which have different values of T1 and T2. For the sake of argument, let us assume that both the T1 and T2 relaxation times of tissue X are greater than the corresponding relaxation times of tissue Y. This might be the case if tissue X represented cerebrospinal fluid and tissue Y represented brain parenchyma. Figure 3-8 illustrates a graph of signal intensity for tissues X and Y as a function of TE, as predicted by the Bloch equation (Eq. 3-1).

Note that for short values of TE, the signal intensity of tissue Y is greater than that of tissue X. This is because for short values of TE the signal is T1 weighted. Thus, tissue X with a longer T1 value than tissue Y will have lower signal intensity in accordance with the inverse relationship between S_{SE} and T1 described above.

For long values of TE, however, T2 effects begin to predominate. Since signal strength is directly proportional to T2, tissue X with a longer T2 will now appear brighter than tissue Y. In other words, a contrast reversal has taken place. This is demonstrated

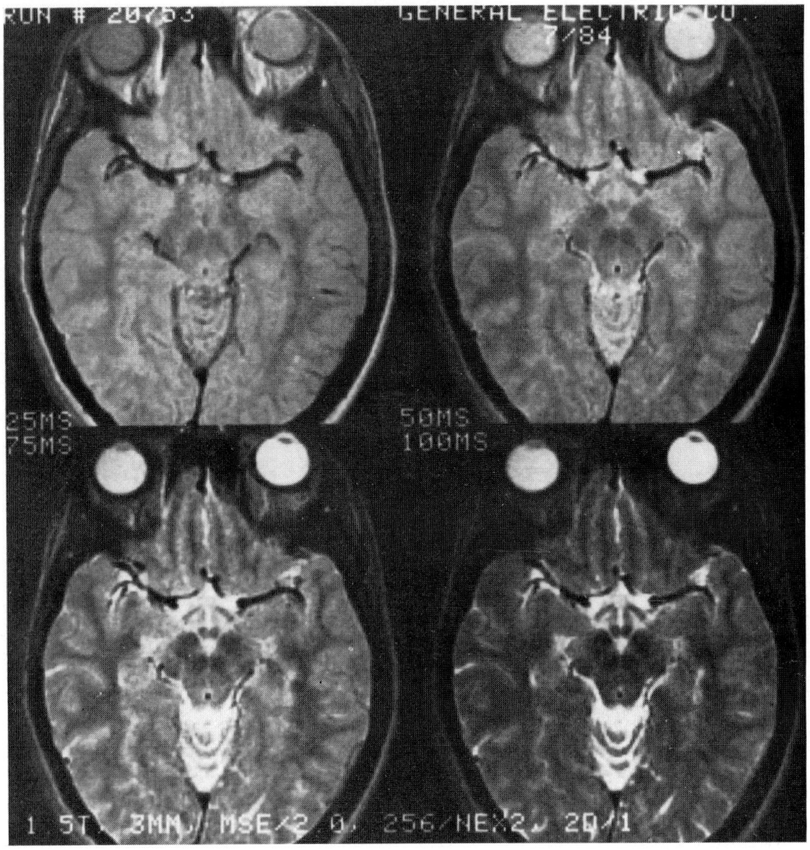

FIGURE 3-9

Example of contrast reversal phenomenon between brain and cerebrospinal fluid in a spin-echo sequence as TE is increased from 25 to 50 to 75 to 100 msec. Note that cerebrospinal fluid goes from black to gray to white relative to brain parenchyma. (Courtesy of General Electric)

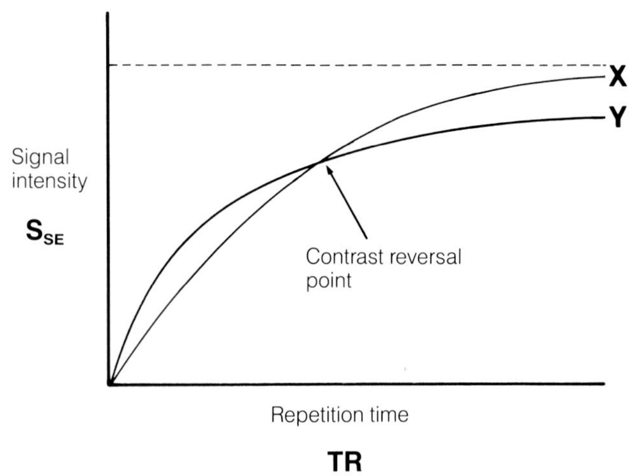

FIGURE 3-10

A contrast reversal phenomenon may also occur between two tissues, X and Y, as TR is increased.

TABLE 3-4

Relative Brightness of Body Tissues Seen on a T1-Weighted Spin-Echo Sequence*

Tissue	Brightness
Fat	White
Bone marrow	↑
Brain	
Abdominal viscera	Gray
Muscle	
Body fluids	
Cortical bone	↓
Air	Black

* For example: TE = 30 msec, TR = 500 msec

in the MR scan of a brain shown in Figure 3-9. With TR held constant, TE is increased from 25 msec to 100 msec. The cerebrospinal fluid is seen to go from black to gray to white relative to brain parenchyma, thus demonstrating the contrast reversal phenomenon.

A similar contrast reversal phenomenon can be observed by increasing TR while holding TE constant. This is illustrated in Figure 3-10. The Bloch equation (Eq. 3-1) predicts a different sort of exponential relationship between S_{SE} and TR. Nevertheless, the same basic principles apply as in the previous example.

For short values of TR, T1 effects predominate, and hence the signal from tissue X with a long T1 is smaller than that from Y with a short T1. As TR increases, T2 effects will begin to predominate. Tissue X, with a longer value of T2, now has a stronger signal than tissue Y, with a shorter T2. Figure 3-11 illustrates this contrast reversal phenomenon between brain and cerebrospinal fluid as TR is increased, holding TE constant.

The precise contrast reversal point can be determined for two tissues by using the Bloch equation (Eq. 3-1). It should be noted that not all tissue pairs will exhibit this behavior; it depends on specific relationships between the values of T1, T2, and the timing parameters. Second, once a contrast reversal occurs, further increase in the value of TR or TE will not return the tissues to their initial contrast relationship. Contrast reversal phenomena may also be seen with other pulse sequences, such as inversion recovery.

In summary, several features about the spin-echo sequence should be remembered:

1. The spin-echo pulse sequence is uniquely specified by two timing parameters, the echo time (TE) and the repetition time (TR). In the usual case, TE = 20 − 120 msec and TR = 300 − 3000 msec.
2. The spin-echo technique can provide T1-weighted, T2-weighted, or proton-weighted images, depending on the choice of timing parameters.
3. Picking TR and TE short produces a T1-weighted image, in which the relative signal strength of two tissues is inversely related to their values of T1.
4. Picking TR and TE long produces a T2-weighted image, in which the relative signal strength of two tissues is directly related to their values of T2.
5. Picking TR long and TE short produces a proton-weighted image, in which the relative signal strength of two tissues is directly proportional to their hydrogen proton concentrations.
6. The Bloch equation (Eq. 3-1) provides a quantitative relationship to explain the spin-echo imaging characteristics of various tissues.
7. A contrast reversal phenomenon may occur between two tissues as either TE or TR is increased.

Other Imaging Sequences

Because of its adaptability, wide range of sensitivity, and relative speed of image acquisition, the spin-echo technique has overwhelmingly become the most popular imaging sequence in general use today. A variety of other imaging sequences are also available and may be useful in certain clinical situations. These other sequences include partial saturation, free induction decay, and inversion recovery.

It should be noted that some confusion frequently arises in discussing these other pulse sequences because their classic description may vary from their mechanism of implementation on commercial scanners. For example, virtually all major manufacturers have added a final 180° *readout pulse* to each of these sequences, making them in reality spin-echo techniques. This additional 180° pulse has been added for a variety of technical reasons, including the need for a time delay for the phase-encoding gradient pulse for direct Fourier spatial encoding. The 180° pulse thus imparts some T2 de-

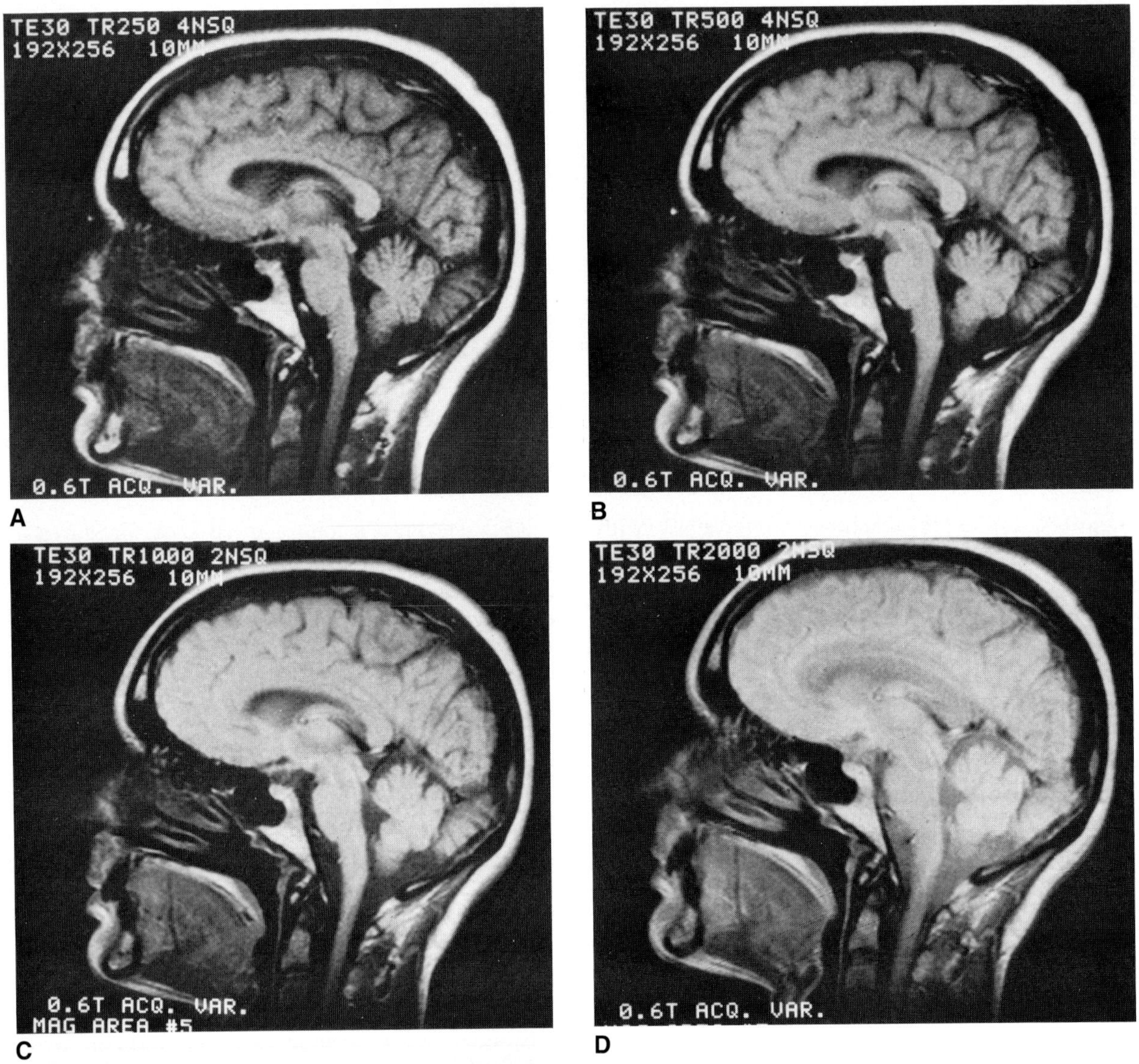

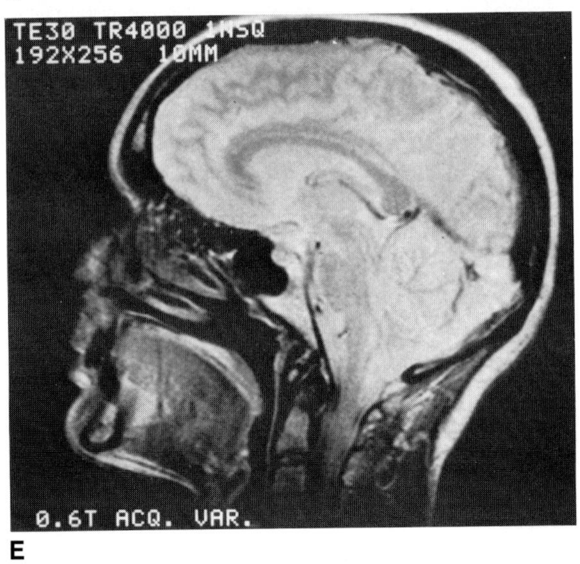

FIGURE 3-11

Example of contrast reversal phenomenon between brain and cerebrospinal fluid as TR is increased and TE held constant at 30 msec. (A) TR = 250 msec; (B) TR = 500 msec; (C) TR = 1000 msec; (D) TR = 2000 msec; (E) TR = 4000 msec. (Courtesy of Technicare Corporation, Technicare Corp., © 1985)

pendence on the final MR signal. This important fact has often been ignored in many articles and discussions that have appeared in the literature.

The **free induction decay sequence** (FID) is now rarely used and is presented more for historical reasons. Ideally, it can be thought of as a spin-echo sequence where TE = 0. However, it is technically impossible to turn off the radio-frequency coil and begin recording a signal instantaneously. In reality, therefore, FID imaging is performed with TE = 10 msec to 20 msec. Thus, the FID sequence is really spin-echo with TE very short.

The **partial saturation sequence** (PS) is known by a variety of names, including saturation recovery (SR), repeated FID, or progressive saturation. In the classic description, it consists of a single 90° pulse repeated at a constant interval (TR), as shown in Figure 3-12. The effect of these repeated 90° pulses is to convert the longitudinal components of tissue magnetization into transverse components for signal generation. In common practice, TR is usually chosen to be relatively short, say 200 msec to 400 msec, although occasionally longer sequences such as PS 1000 (*i.e.,* PS with TR = 1000 msec) may be used.

The PS sequence produces images whose tissue contrasts depends primarily on tissue T1 and proton density. When TR is short, image contrast is dominated by T1 effects in an inverse manner, as with spin-echo. Tissues with long T1 values will appear darker than tissues with short T1 values. When TR is long, image contrast is dominated by hydrogen proton concentration effects.

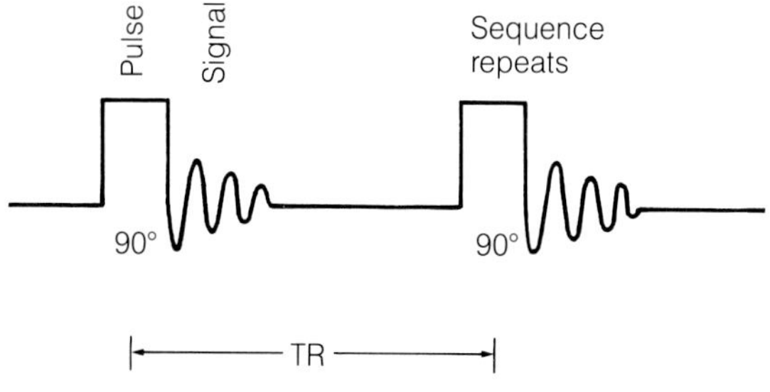

FIGURE 3-12

The PS pulse sequence. A free-induction decay signal is recorded after each 90° pulse. The sequence repeats at period TR.

A form of the Bloch equation has been derived for the PS pulse sequence:

$$S_{PS} = f(H) \cdot g(V) \cdot [1 - e^{-TR/T1}] \qquad \text{(Eq. 3-2)}$$

where

S_{PS} = MR signal strength for a partial saturation sequence
f(H) = a function of hydrogen proton concentration in the tissue
g(V) = a function of tissue velocity, significant only for blood
TR = pulse repetition time, selected by the operator
T1 = longitudinal relaxation time, tissue specific

An example of several slices through the brain performed with a PS 400 technique is presented in Figure 3-13.

When TR is chosen in a short range (less than 400 msec), the PS sequence has the advantage of acquisition of a large number of data points in a very short time. Unfortunately, using a very short TR also results in a weak signal and impairment of multisection imaging capabilities.

The **inversion recovery sequence** (IR) is perhaps the most widely used technique after spin-echo. In its classic description, IR is a two-pulse sequence as shown in Figure 3-14*A*. The tissue magnetization vector, *M*, is first inverted by a 180° pulse. This rotates *M* so that it now points opposite to the static field.

The receiver antenna coils can only detect magnetization perpendicular to the static field. Therefore, a second pulse of 90° is applied at a time (T1) called the *inversion time*, a few hundred milliseconds after the initial inverting pulse. The effect of this 90° pulse is to rotate the partially recovered magnetization vector into the transverse plane, so that a signal may be detected by the receiver coil. The entire process may be repeated at a variable time later, called the repetition time (TR).

The IR sequence produces images that can be made highly sensitive to differences in tissue T1 values. The effect of inverting the magnetization vector by the initial 180° pulse allows tissue to relax over twice the dynamic range possible with the 90° PS pulse. Because of this expanded range in the longitudinal direction, superb image contrast based on differences in tissue T1 values may be produced.

A form of the Bloch equation has been derived for the IR technique as well:

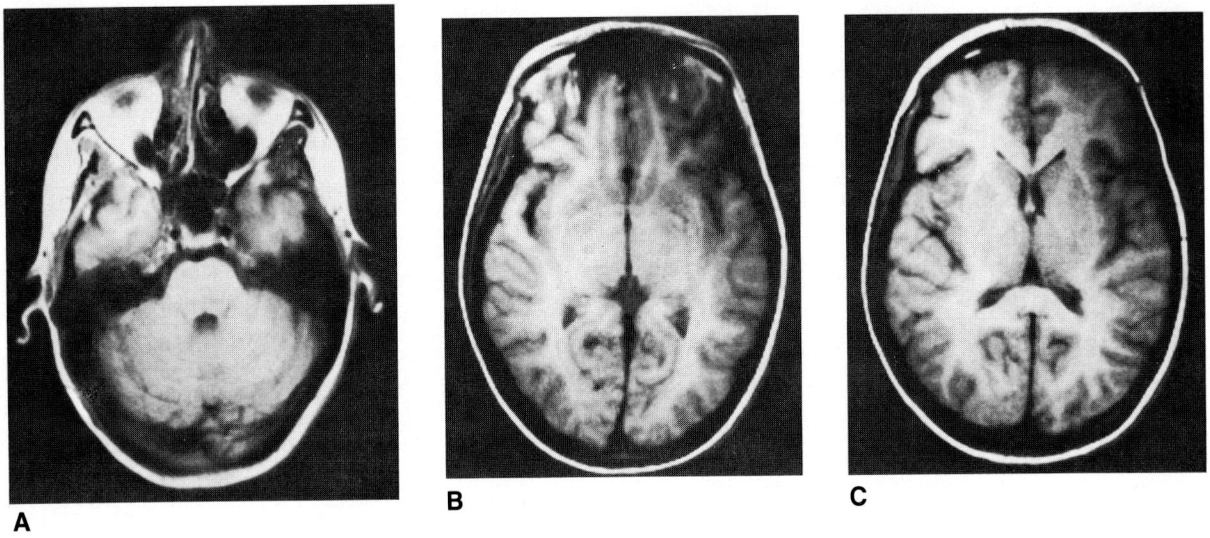

FIGURE 3-13

MR brain images obtained with PS technique. (PS 400). (Courtesy of General Electric)

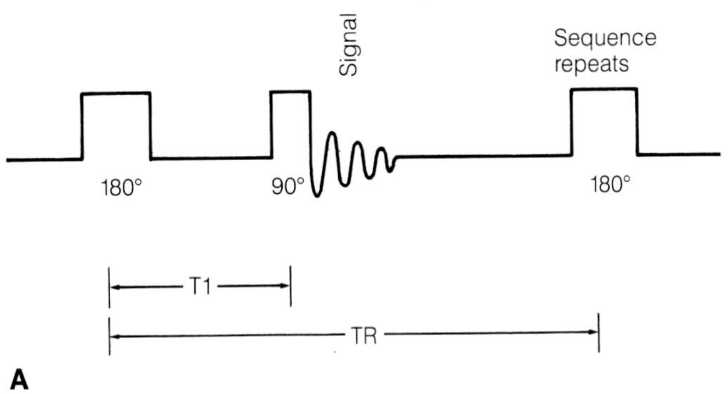

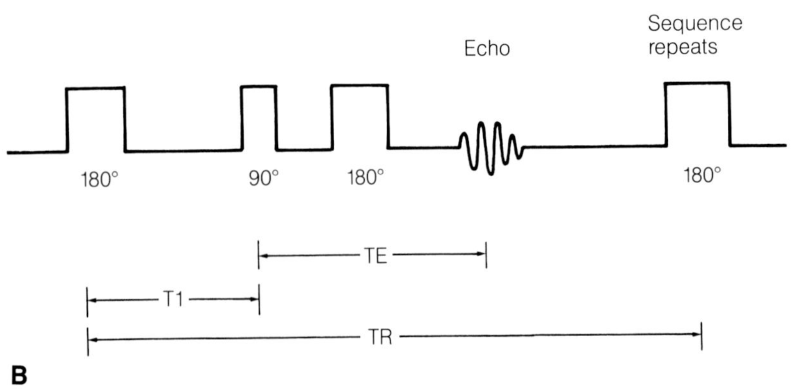

FIGURE 3-14

The IR pulse sequence. (A) In the classic description, a 90° pulse follows the 180° ("inversion") pulse at time TI. A FID signal is then recorded. (B) As implemented on most commercial scanners, a second 180° ("rephasing") pulse is applied shortly after the 90° pulse. The IR signal is then recorded as an echo. This hybrid technique is sometimes called inversion spin-echo.

$$S_{IR} = f(H)\,g(V)\,[1 - 2e^{-TI/T1} + e^{-TR/T1}] \quad \text{(Eq. 3-3)}$$

where

S_{IR} = MR signal strength from an inversion recovery sequence
f(H) = a function of hydrogen proton density, as before
g(V) = a function of tissue velocity, as before
TI, TR = inversion time and repetition time, selected by the operator
T1 = longitudinal relaxation time, tissue specific

The bracketed term $[1 - 2e^{-TI/T1} + e^{-TR/T1}]$ produces a somewhat complicated relationship between two operator selected variables, TI and TR, and a tissue-specific factor, T1. The fact that this term may be negative for certain values of TR, TI, and T1 leads to some interesting complexities. Depending on the type of scanner used, the receiver coils and circuits may or may not be able to distinguish negative from positive signals. Thus may be seen complex patterns of contrast reversal, which disappear and then reappear again.

A second major point of confusion is that most commercial MR scanners today employ an additional 180° *refocusing pulse* at a variable time after the 90° read-pulse. This pulse sequence is still called IR, but in reality it is also a spin-echo technique (Fig. 3-14*B*). The effect of this additional 180° pulse is to make the IR image somewhat dependent on tissue T2 as well as on T1. In this situation, the Bloch equation (Eq. 3-3) must be amended by inserting an additional term, $e^{-TE/T2}$, as a multiplicand on the right. Sometimes this modified IR technique is called *inversion spin-echo*.

A shorthand notation for the IR technique has been proposed, similar to that for spin-echo. For example, an IR sequence with TR = 1500 msec and TI = 400 msec can be denoted IR 1500/400. If the scanner also employs a refocusing pulse with an echo signal recorded at time TE = 30 msec, this IR sequence may be designated IR 1500/400/30. A typical range of parameter values for IR might be TI = 200 – 800 msec, TR = 500 – 2500 msec, and TE = 25 – 50 msec. Note that by definition, TR must be longer than TI.

It is possible to choose IR parameters to produce a very high degree of image contrast between two tissues, if one knows their approximate T1 relaxation times. Choosing the inversion time parameter (TI) equal to the average T1 time of the two tissues produces optimum contrast distinction between these tissues. The TR value is usually chosen to be about 3 × TI for optimum signal-to-noise ratio. An example of serial axial sections through the brain is presented in Figure 3-15, with an IR technique designed to produce high contrast between gray and white matter.

The IR technique can thus be used to produce superb image contrast between tissues. Unfortunately, outside of the narrow range for which it is designed, the IR sequence provides relatively poor tissue differentiation. As an example of the limited dynamic range of IR, consider the sagittal head image in Figure 3-16. Designed for imaging the brain parenchyma, this IR does an excellent job. Notice, however, that the reminder of the head is inadequately visualized, with poor image contrast and low signal-to-noise ratio.

An extension of this concept, let us reconsider the Bloch equation for IR (Eq. 3-3). As was mentioned previously, the bracketed term $[1 - 2e^{-TI/T1} + e^{-TR/T1}]$ may have any value—positive, negative, or 0. If it so happens that a particular combination of parameters and tissue T1 make this term 0, no MR signal will be recorded. Thus it is possible to miss large masses completely with the IR technique, if by chance the selected combination of parameters added to 0. Several examples have appeared in the MR literature of tumors that were invisible with an IR technique.

Imaging Time Considerations

A major remaining drawback of MR is the time required to acquire and process images. Patient tolerance in the magnet usually limits examination of each part of the body to about three or four pulse sequences or planes. Since the standard mode of image acquisition on most commercial MR scanners today is two-dimensional (planar), this discussion will center around this technique.

Total imaging time is the sum of image acquisition time (t_{ac}) and image reconstruction time (t_{re}). Image acquisition time accounts for the bulk of total imaging time and covers that period between the beginning of RF stimulation and the end of MR signal recording in a given plane. Image reconstruction

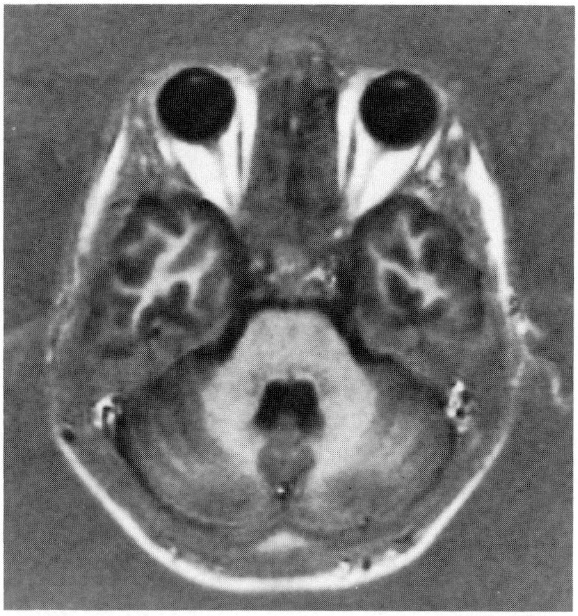

A

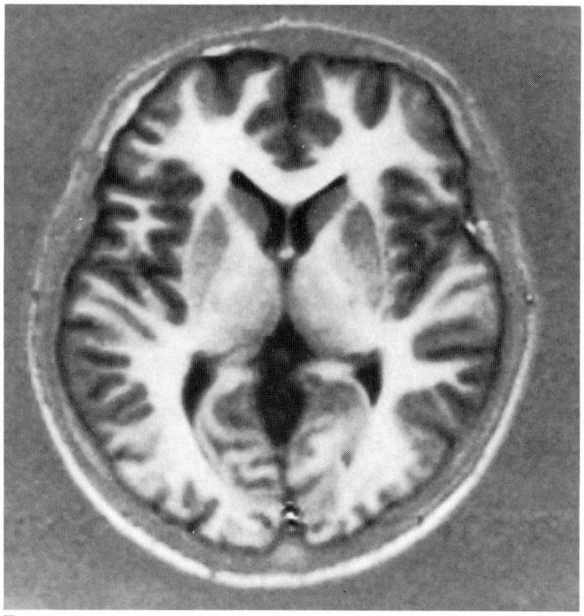

B

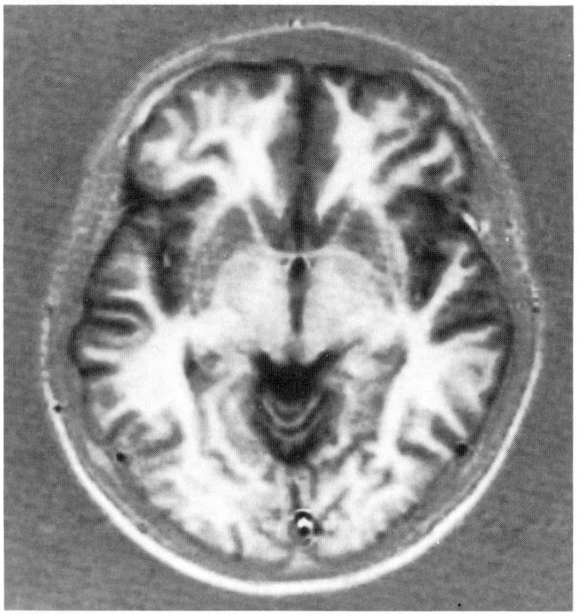

C

FIGURE 3-15

MR brain images obtained with IR technique. (IR 2500/400/43). (Courtesy of Siemens)

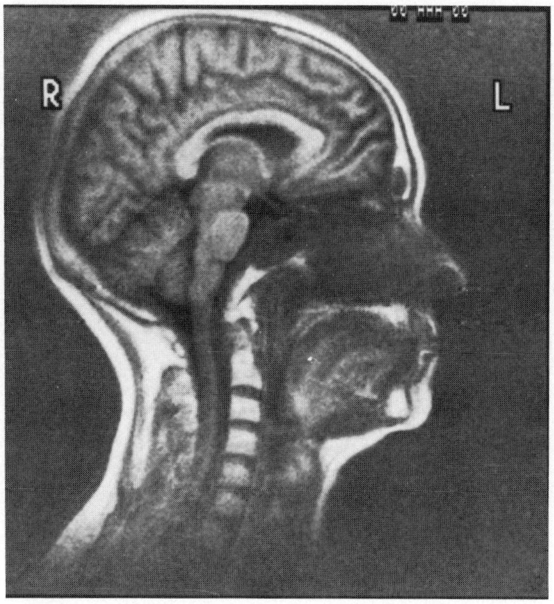

FIGURE 3-16

IR image (IR 2500/400/43) shows excellent brain contrast. The face and nasopharynx, however, are poorly imaged, with low contrast and low signal-to-noise ratio. Outside of the limited range for which it is designed, the IR sequence provides poor images. (Courtesy of Philips Medical Systems, Inc.)

time is the time it takes the computer and array processor to convert raw MR signal into a proper image.

Image acquisition time in planar imaging depends on three factors: (1) the number of signal averages, n; (2) the matrix size, m, which is the number of signal lines sampled; and (3) the pulse sequence repetition time, TR. The image acquisition time for a single slice can be written

$$t_{ac} = n \times m \times TR$$

For example, for a 256 × 256 matrix, two signal averages, and TR = 3.0 seconds, single-slice image acquisition time would be $t_{ac} = 2 \times 256 \times 3.0 =$ 1536 seconds, or about 26 minutes. If only single slices are acquired in this fashion, examining an entire brain would take several hours.

Fortunately, a clever technique known as *slice interleaving* has been developed to circumvent these long examination times. Only about 30 msec of time is actually required to stimulate and record the MR signal from a given slice. The remainder of the pulse period is silent, until a repeat train of pulses occurs at time TR later. By slice interleaving, the computer stimulates another slice while waiting in the silent period of the first slice. It is possible to stimulate 10 or 20 slices in this staggered but simultaneous fashion. Accordingly, image acquisition time is reduced by a factor of 10 or 20.

With short TR times, as in PS sequences, there is little or no time for slice interleaving. With IR sequences, slice interleaving is impaired by the presence of the inversion interval (between the 180° and 90° pulses). Therefore, imaging times for IR, and to a lesser degree for PS, are prolonged relative to spin-echo. Table 3-5 illustrates average image acquisition times for a typical commercial MR scanner using planar, multislice interleaving.

TABLE 3-5

Average Image Acquisition Times for a Typical MR Scanner*

Pulse Sequence	No. of Slices	Image Acquisition Time
IR 1000/300/30	1	8.6 min
PS 300/25	1	2.6 min
SE 1000/30, 60	10	8.6 min
SE 1600/30, 60	16	13.0 min

*Typical scan times obtained on Magniscan 5000 using 256 × 256 matrix and two signal averages. (Modified from manufacturer's literature, Thomson-CGR Corp.)

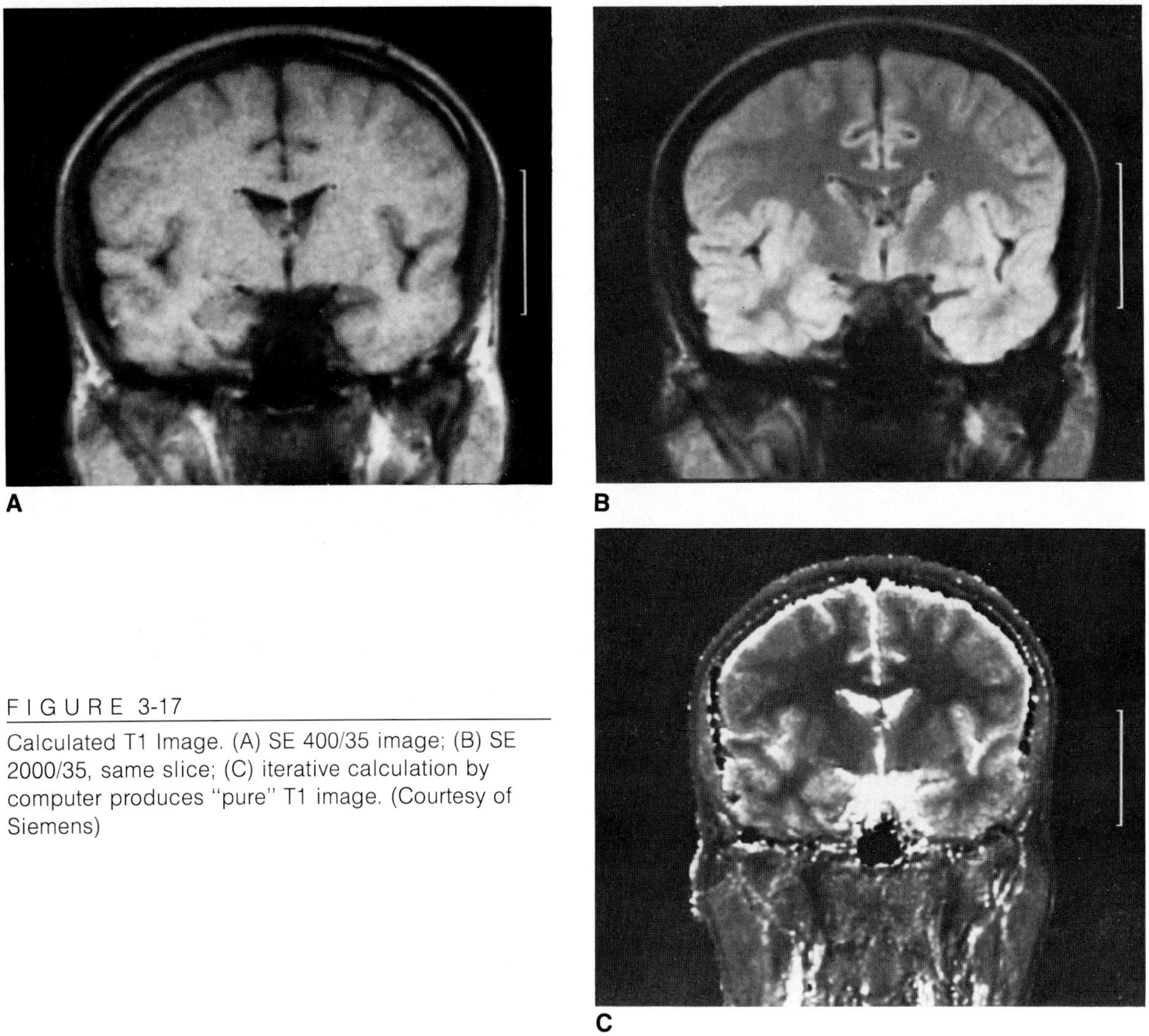

FIGURE 3-17

Calculated T1 Image. (A) SE 400/35 image; (B) SE 2000/35, same slice; (C) iterative calculation by computer produces "pure" T1 image. (Courtesy of Siemens)

Image reconstruction time is relatively short compared with image acquisition time. Image reconstruction time depends primarily on the matrix size. For most commercial scanners, image reconstruction time for a 256 × 256 matrix is on the order of 5 seconds per image. For larger matrices, such as a 512 × 512, reconstruction time is significantly prolonged and is on the order of 30 seconds per image.

Postprocessing: T1 and T2 Images

Using the spin-echo technique and software available on most clinical MR scanners, it is possible to calculate "pure" T1 and "pure" T2 images. Although it is not clear whether these techniques will provide meaningful diagnostic information, the reader should have some familiarity with these techniques.

Figure 3-17 illustrates a calculated pure T1 image. To generate this image, the same slice is imaged by spin-echo two times. TE is kept constant while TR

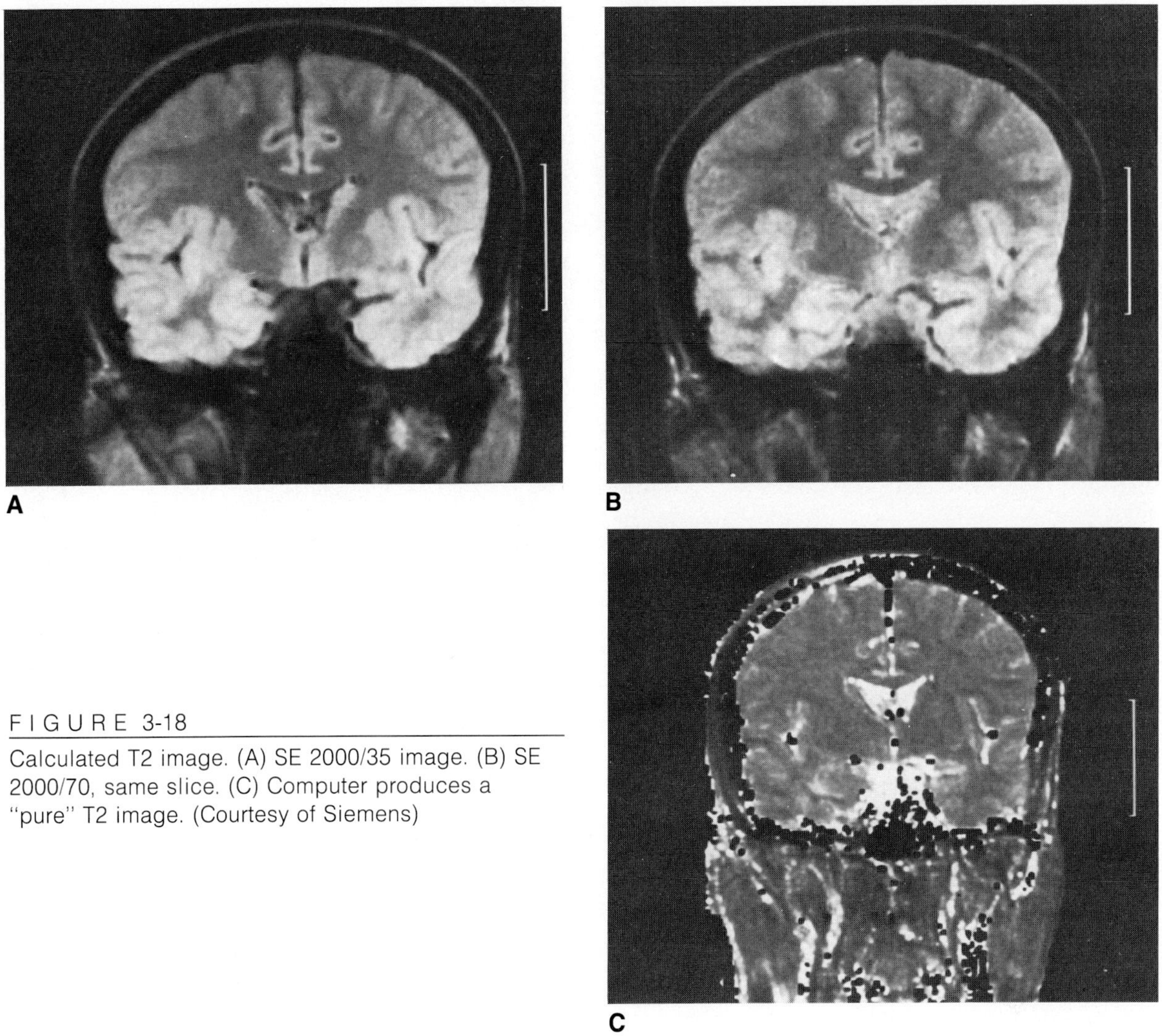

FIGURE 3-18

Calculated T2 image. (A) SE 2000/35 image. (B) SE 2000/70, same slice. (C) Computer produces a "pure" T2 image. (Courtesy of Siemens)

is varied. An iterative calculation by the computer then solves Eq. 3-2 for T1.

Figure 3-18 illustrates the calculation of a pure T2 image. To generate a pure T2 image, the same slice is again imaged twice by a spin-echo sequence. This time TR is kept constant while TE is varied. Once again the computer solves Eq. 3-2 for T2.

It should be noted once more that the actual values of T1 and T2 computed are methodology dependent and should not be taken as absolute values. For example, calculated T1 strongly depends on the strength of the B_0 (static) magnetic field. T1 will also vary within the tissue because of nonuniformity in the magnetic field. Calculated T2 values are even more inaccurate. Predicted values of T2 vary with RF nonuniformity as well as with interactions with gradient pulses. Therefore, keep in mind that although it is possible to produce calculated T1 and T2 images, they should be considered qualitatively and not quantitatively accurate.

CHAPTER 4

Effects of Pathology on the MR Image

The primary purpose of this book is to present normal anatomy and its variations on MR images. No single book could comprehensively and adequately discuss the myriad of pathological conditions that might be imaged by MR. It also seems a little premature to attempt to describe at this time the classic MR appearance of different diseases, since experience in all centers is still limited. References are available at the end of the text for interested readers who want to know about MR of pathological conditions.

Instead of discussing specific diseases, this chapter will approach MRI of pathological processes from a more general standpoint. The discussion that follows will center on the T1 and T2 changes one might expect in a variety of generalized disease processes: edema, tumor, ischemia, hemorrhage, fatty infiltration, calcification, and accumulation of paramagnetic substances. If these basic principles and patterns are understood, it will be relatively easy to remember and predict the imaging characteristics of tissues affected by each type of pathology.

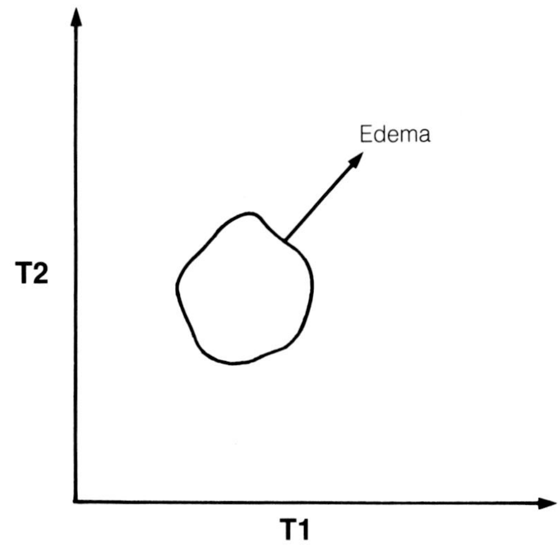

FIGURE 4-2

Effect of edema. Lengthening of both T1 and T2 characteristics of an edematous tissue is seen as edema (water) acculculates.

Edema

As is well known to every physician, a large number of varied diseases may manifest themselves by the production of edema. These diseases include infection, tumor, trauma, infarction, and demyelinization. Although the diseases vary, the end result, edema, has a remarkably similar appearance on MR images.

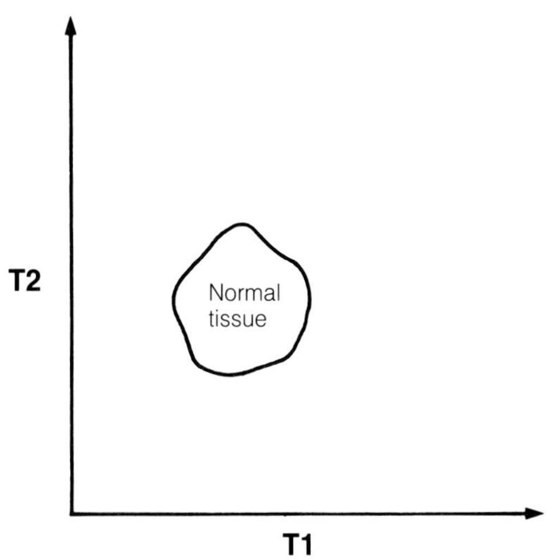

FIGURE 4-1

Representation of normal tissue in terms of T1 and T2 characteristics.

As a memory aid, it is helpful to represent disease processes by changes in position on the T1–T2 graph, as originally presented in Chapter 2 (Fig. 2-14), and in Figure 4-1, this chapter. Recall that water, and hence edema fluid, has exceedingly long values for T1 and T2. This is because the small free-water molecules tumble rapidly and are inefficient at spin–spin and spin-lattice interactions.

For any tissue, therefore, the presence of edema shifts its T1–T2 point upward and to the right, toward larger values of T1 and T2 (Fig. 4-2). This produces expected imaging characteristics as discussed in the previous chapter.

On T1-weighted images, tissues with edema will have lower signal than the surrounding normal area. On T2-weighted images, edematous tissues will have an intense signal. This can be remembered by observing how tissues known to have high water content and body fluids (cerebrospinal fluid, urine) change between images. Edema can be expected to change in a similar fashion.

Tumor

When MRI was first developed, it was originally hoped that changes in tissue T1 and T2 would specifically lead to the diagnosis of tumors. As more information is gained, however, it has become increasingly clear that tumors present a variety of largely unpredictable changes in their imaging characteristics. Although we cannot at present diagnose tumors by tissue type through MRI, certain general principles apply.

First of all, most tumors in some way differ from surrounding normal tissue in molecular structure or in the ratio of free/bound water. Thus it is conceivable that some imaging sequences will produce optimal contrast between normal and abnormal tissues. What these sequences are, however, is still being researched.

Although not without exception, many investigators have observed that tumors in laboratory animals and humans are best imaged with techniques that emphasize both T1 and T2 characteristics of tissue. Thus, spin-echo sequences have been recommended for the detection of tumor. Tumor contrast may be more marked with spin-echo sequences receiving intermediate contributions from T1 and T2 (for example with TE = 30 msec and TR = 1000 msec). However, certain tumors are best seen on heavily T2-weighted images (for example, TE = 80 msec and TR = 2000 msec).

In general practice, therefore, when tumor is suspected, a variety of spin-echo sequences that weight T1 and T2 characteristics in varying degrees are currently used. As more information is accumulated by research, it may one day be possible to know in advance the optimal imaging strategies to apply when a particular differential diagnosis is considered.

Fluid-filled cystic tumors behave in such a fashion as would be expected by their contents. Most fluid-filled cysts contain water and varying degrees of protein and fat. Thus, most cysts behave like water, with long values of T1 and T2 that change in intensity in the appropriate direction with variation in imaging parameters. Cystic and solid lesions may thus be distinguished by MR.

Calcification in tumors, an important characteristic of CT, is difficult or impossible to detect by MR. This is because areas of calcification, like cortical bone, produce no appreciable MR signal because of their low hydrogen content. Large areas of calcification may be recognized, however, by the region of signal dropout, which does not change significantly, even by changing the pulse sequence or sequence parameters.

It is still not clear how well MR can differentiate tumor from its surrounding edema. Indeed, much of what we identify as tumor intensity on MR scans may merely represent tumor edema in uninvolved tissues. It is therefore possible to overestimate the size of a given tumor by MR, just as with angiography or CT, because of its associated edema mass effect.

As a final note, it is not currently possible to differentiate reliably benign from malignant tumors on the basis of their T1 and T2 imaging characteristics. Associated anatomic alterations and invasion or destruction of neighboring tissues remain the major clues to the appropriate diagnosis. These somewhat varied tumor-imaging characteristics are represented graphically in Figure 4-3.

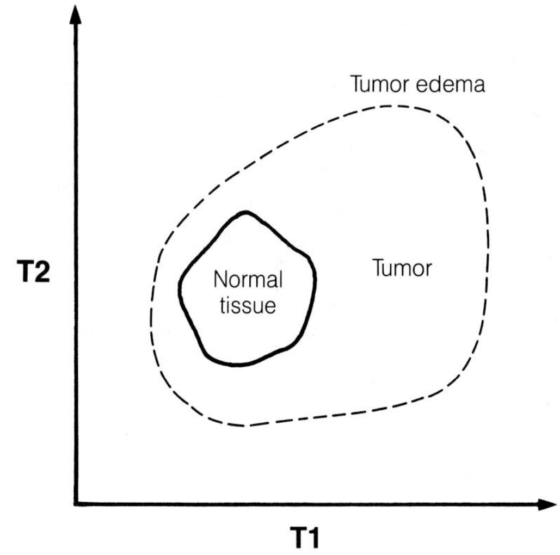

FIGURE 4-3

Effect of tumor. Tumor effects are variable. Edema surrounding tumor produces long T1 and T2.

Ischemia and Infarction

The MR tissue changes in ischemia and infarction have been studied in a large number of animal models, as well as in clinical studies of humans. The

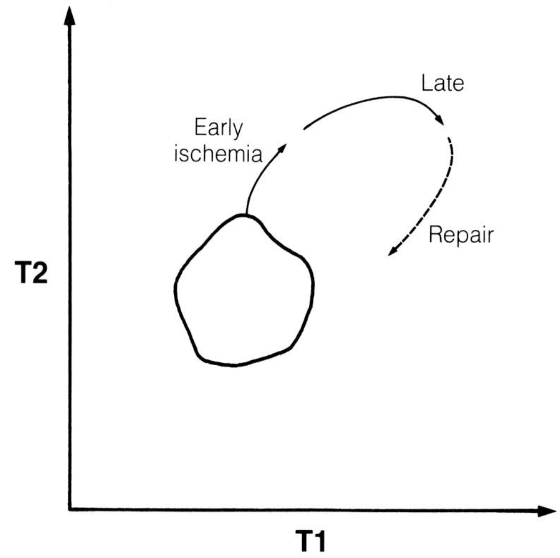

FIGURE 4-4

Effect of ischemia varies with organ studied. In general, in the first 24 hours of ischemia, T2 is prolonged with little effect on T1. Later, both T1 and T2 are prolonged.

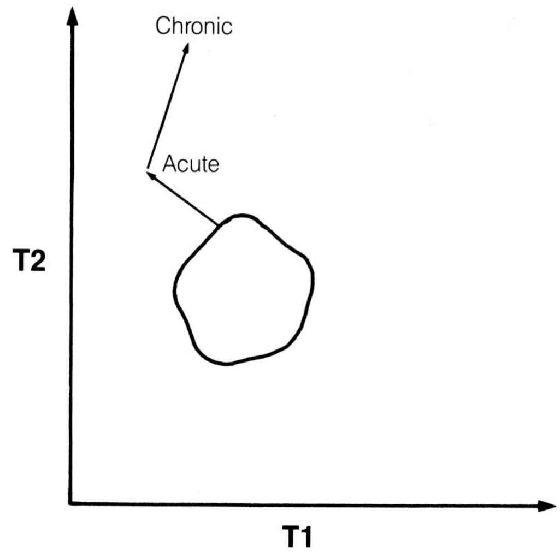

FIGURE 4-5

Effect of hemorrhage. Acute hemorrhage may shorten T1 with little effect on T2. More chronic hemorrhage shows prolonged T2.

precise imaging characteristics depend on the time after ischemia or infarction, as well as the particular tissue studied. It has now been demonstrated that MR can detect, often earlier than CT, ischemia and infarction in the brain, muscle, heart, and kidneys.

As a general principle, areas of ischemia or infarction in tissues may be detected as early as 3 to 6 hours following onset. The earliest changes seen are in the values of T2, which presumably become prolonged because of tissue edema. In certain tissues like the heart, T1 values may never change significantly at any stage of the infarction. In most other tissues, however, including brain and skeletal muscle, both T1 and T2 become prolonged, although T1 changes may not be seen until after 24 hours. Depending on the completeness of infarction and degree of revascularization, T1 and T2 values may remain elevated for months or years after injury. These changes in ischemia and infarction are represented graphically in Figure 4-4.

Hemorrhage

As with the other pathological processes mentioned, the imaging characteristics of hemorrhage in the body will depend on their location, age, resorption rate, and presence or absence of rebleeding. Furthermore, some controversy exists concerning the T1 and T2 changes that an aging hematoma may undergo.

Figure 4-5 illustrates a fairly typical pattern of changes in an aging intracerebral hematoma. During the acute phase, the T2 value is moderately prolonged but the T1 is often moderately shortened. After a few days, the T2 value becomes further prolonged. The T1 value will either remain the same or become longer.

At this stage (very late after the initial hemorrhage, say greater than one week), what happens to the T1 and T2 values depends on what happens to the hematoma. With complete resorption of the hematoma, T1 and T2 values may return to normal. In the event that the hematoma remains as a chronic fluid collection, it becomes more like water, with resorption of its hemoglobin and protein components. In this situation, both the T1 and T2 values may lengthen.

Fatty Infiltration

Fatty infiltration is a well-known tissue response to injury and is commonly noted in the liver and skeletal muscle. Because of its molecular configuration with multiple hydrogen-laden side chains, fat is very efficient at T1 interactions. Accordingly, fat has very short values of T1. The T2 values of fat are intermediate and nonspecific.

Figure 4-6 illustrates the effect of fatty infiltration of normal tissue. This curve represents a shortening of the T1 value of the infiltrated tissue with little change in the T2 value. Knowing this pattern of change allows one to predict the imaging characteristics of such tissue. Because T1 values are shortened, such infiltrated tissues will have an intense signal on T1-weighted sequences, such as short spin-echo or partial saturation.

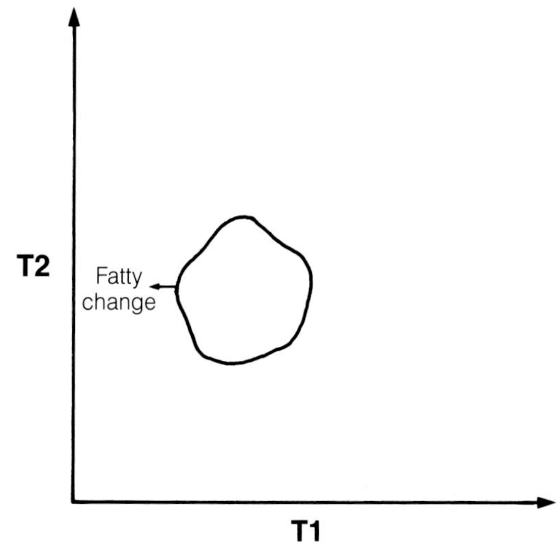

FIGURE 4-6

Effect of fatty change. Fatty infiltration shortens T1 with little effect on T2.

Calcification

Calcification in tissue is among the easiest conditions to detect by CT. The differential diagnoses of many diseases by CT and plain radiography are based on the presence or absence of calcification. Unfortunately, MRI is able to detect only very large foci of calcification. This is because calcified tissue has a paucity of free hydrogen protons to participate in resonance and produce an MR signal.

Figure 4-7 illustrates graphically what happens to the signal characteristics of tissue with large amounts of calcification. Instead of shifting the tissue T1–T2 graph, calcification results in areas of signal dropout. These areas of calcification will be of low intensity regardless of the pulse sequence parameters used. Similar signal dropout may also be seen in areas of dense scarring or fibrosis, without gross calcification.

Paramagnetic Substances: Endogenous and Exogenous

A paramagnetic substance is defined as a material that has a small positive magnetizability. This means that when placed in a strong magnetic field, such a material will have a tendency to align its net magnetization vector in the direction of that field. By definition, the hydrogen proton has these properties. The ^{1}H atom can therefore be considered a paramagnetic substance. Other atoms with unpaired protons or neutrons may also be considered paramagnetic substances; these include ^{13}C, ^{14}N, ^{17}O, ^{19}F, and ^{31}P. Such paramagnetic substances with *unbalanced nuclear spins* may undergo resonance and be used for imaging.

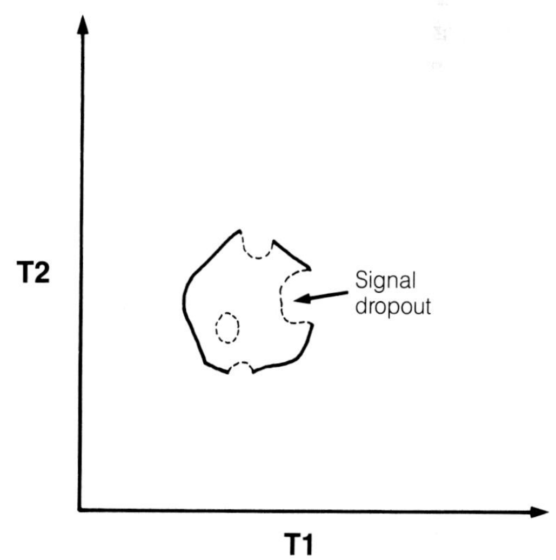

FIGURE 4-7

Effect of calcification. Areas of signal dropout due to low hydrogen density in calcified (or scarred) areas.

Other classes of paramagnetic substances have *unbalanced electron spins.* These electron-unbalanced paramagnetic substances include ions of certain transition elements as well as larger molecules. Like paramagnetic substances with unbalanced nuclear spins, these electron-unbalanced substances may interact with external magnetic fields. When a resonating hydrogen proton is brought close to one of these paramagnetic substances, the proton may interact and release its energy more efficiently. Therefore, if paramagnetic substances with unbalanced electron spins accumulate in a tissue in MR, the relaxation times of that tissue are noticeably shortened. This is represented in Figure 4-8, where the arrow illustrates that T1 and T2 are decreased in tissues that accumulate paramagnetic substances.

How does a tissue accumulate paramagnetic substances? The answer is that paramagnetic substances may accumulate in certain disease processes (endogenous source), or they may be administered to the patient orally or intravenously as an MR contrast agent (exogenous source). Each of these sources will now be discussed.

Both ferrous (Fe^{2+}) and ferric (Fe^{3+}) ions contain unbalanced electron spins and are strongly paramagnetic. Certain disease states (such as hemochromatosis and iron overload) result in the accumulation of ferritin, hemosiderin, and low-molecular-weight iron fractions in organs like the liver and pancreas. The accumulation of these iron-containing molecules results in marked shortening of tissue T1 and T2 values of organs affected by these diseases.

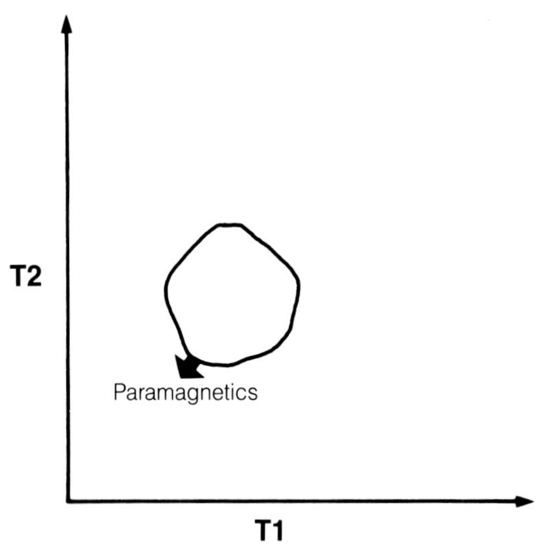

FIGURE 4-8

Effect of paramagnetics. Paramagnetic accumulation (exogenous or endogenous) results in shortening of both T1 and T2.

TABLE 4-1

Paramagnetic Substances Potentially Useful for MRI

Transition Metal Ions	
	Manganese (Mn^{2+})
	Iron (Fe^{2+}, Fe^{3+})
	Copper (Cu^{2+})
	Nickel (Ni^{2+})
	Chromium (Cr^{3+})
Lanthanide Series Ions	
	Gadolinium (Gd^{3+})
Stable Free Radicals	
	Nitroxides (R_2NO)

Hemoglobin and its degradation products may also be paramagnetic. It is possible that MRI changes in a maturing hematoma are partially a function of the paramagnetic properties of ferrous compounds released from hemoglobin. Similarly, melanin and its derivatives may have paramagnetic properties. It has been said that melanoma metastases may have short relaxation times based in part on paramagnetic effects of melanin.

A number of paramagnetic substances are being investigated as exogenous agents to be used as contrast materials for MRI. A few of the more promising agents are listed in Table 4-1. Most of these substances are derivatives of certain rare earth and transition elements, such as manganese and gadolinium. When administered orally or intravenously, these paramagnetic agents may accumulate in certain target organs such as the liver, kidney, or brain. Where they accumulate, these agents will reduce the T1 and T2 relaxation times of the tissue, as shown in Figure 4-8. A great deal of research into these agents and others is being conducted at a number of medical centers.

CHAPTER 5

Artifacts in MR Scanning

It is important for the interpreter of MR scans to have some knowledge about the common artifacts encourtered. These artifacts are different from those seen in other branches of diagnostic imaging. Some artifacts are easily explainable and correctable; others are difficult to understand and remove. The artifacts discussed in this chapter will be considered to be of several origins: motion, ferromagnetic objects, the imaging system itself, and those intrinsic to the tissues being scanned.

Motion Artifacts

Motion artifacts remain some of the most common, easily identifiable, and easily correctable phenomena that degrade the MR image. Gross patient motion (Figs. 5-1 and 5-2) results in multiple ghosted images. More subtle patient motion may produce degraded image quality without obvious ghosting (Fig. 5-3). Motion artifacts are more prominent on sequences requiring long image acquisition time (*i.e.,* long TR intervals). If interleaved slice acquisition mode is used, certain images in a sequence may be normal and others degraded. Commonsense methods to reduce patient motion and anxiety (*e.g.,* explaining the importance of remaining motionless, comfortable gantry and patient positioning, soft lights, music via headphone, sedation) may all be used to reduce the incidence of gross patient motion artifacts.

When surface coils are used, motion of either the surface coil or the patient will produce ghost artifacts. Motion of the surface coil and the patient in unison will also produce artifacts that are as degrading as either motion separately. It has been suggested that rigidly mounting the surface coil off the patient eliminates coil motion and improves image quality, even if patient motion continues. It remains to be seen how practical a technique this will be in clinical practice (Fig. 5-4).

Respiratory and cardiac motion artifacts will be discussed more completely in Chapter 8, The Chest. An example of degraded image quality on a nongated scan is shown in Figure 5-5. Note that most artifact is seen in a vertical direction from the moving

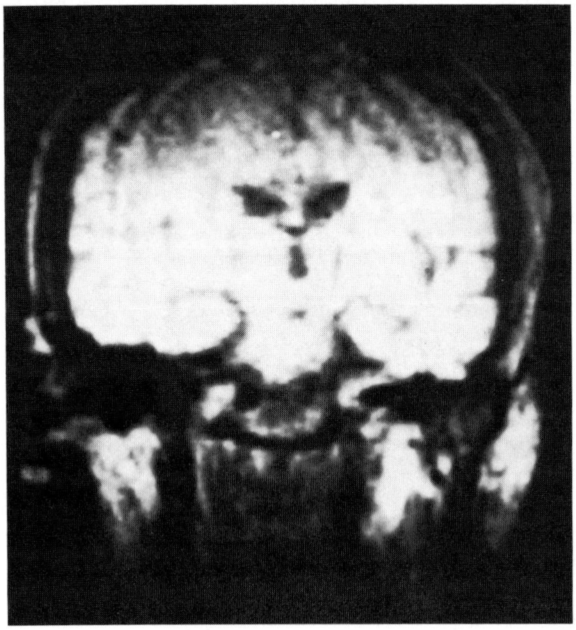

FIGURE 5-1

Gross patient motion produces multiple ghosted images.

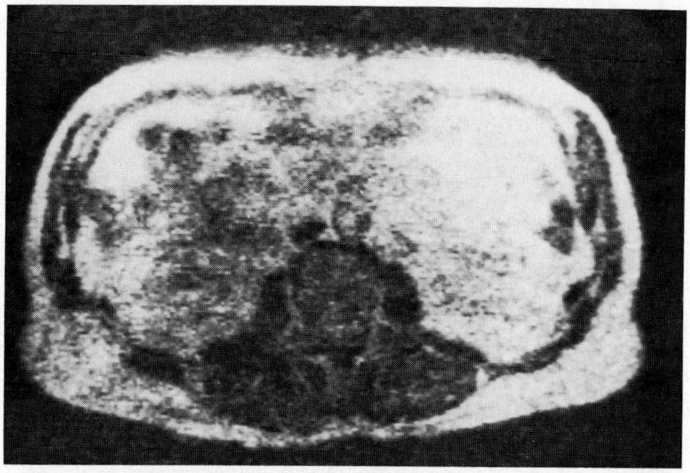

FIGURE 5-2

Periodic patient motion such as respiratory motion produces ghosting and snow along the phase-encoded axis.

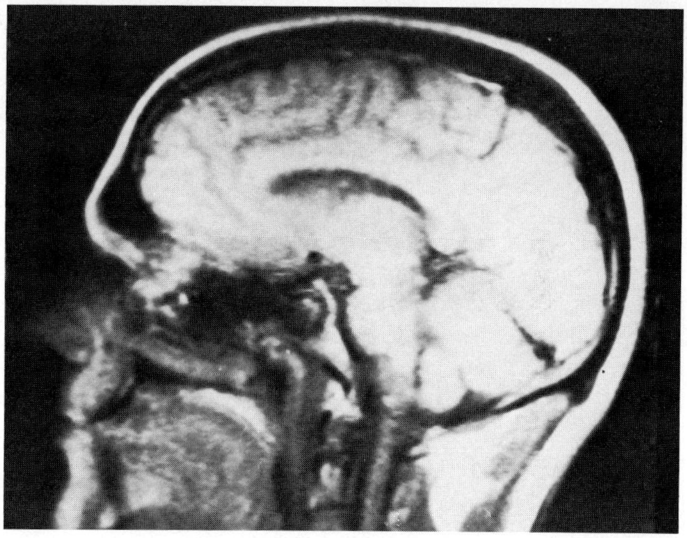

FIGURE 5-3

Smaller degrees of patient motion may degrade image quality without obvious ghosting.

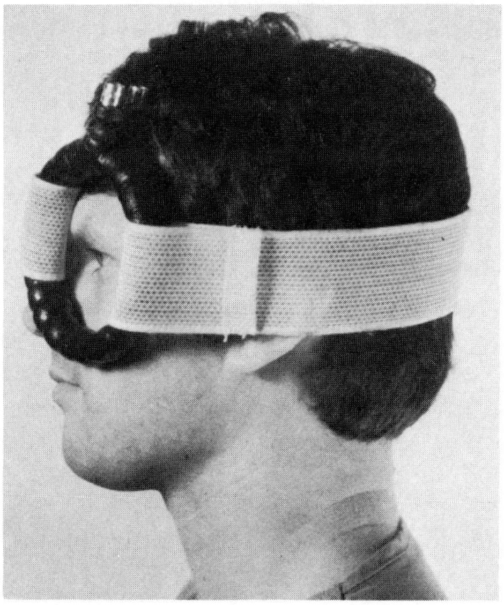

A

FIGURE 5-4

Two possible methods of surface coil mounting. In (A), the surface coil is connected to patient. (Courtesy of Fonar Corp., 110 Marcus Drive, Melville, NY 11747). In (B) the orbital surface coil is mounted independently from the patient. (Courtesy of Siemens)

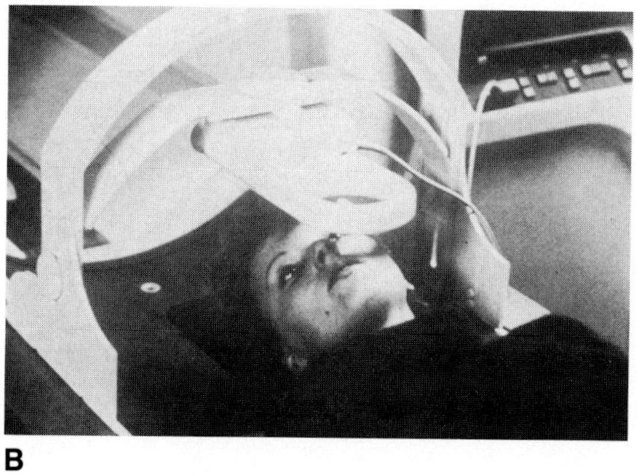

B

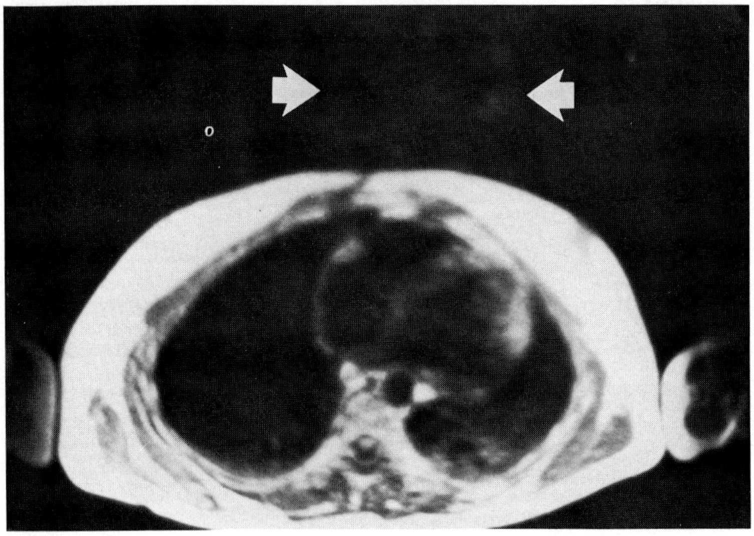

FIGURE 5-5
Cardiac motion causes artifacts along the phase-encoded axis (arrows).

heart. This is a result of signal distortion along the phase-encoding axis, which is in the vertical direction on this axial scan.

Ferromagnetic Objects

A number of ferromagnetic objects, both within and outside the patient, may degrade image quality. Examples of such objects include hairpins, dental bridgework, surgical clips and sutures, and prostheses. In contrast to high-density scatter artifacts produced by these objects in CT, often in MRI the effect is only a local distortion of the image. Examples of wire suture in a craniotomy and dental bridgework inducing image distortion are shown in Figure 5-6. When the object is external to the patient, the obvious solution is to remove it. When the object is internal to the patient, one must merely accept and recognize the distortion it produces.

System Artifacts

Several characteristic image artifacts relate primarily to design flaws, field inhomogeneities, and improper patient-machine tuning. These will be discussed in turn.

External electromagnetic radiation may induce interference in the recording or processing of the image. Radio-frequency interference produces a characteristic set of short parallel lines across the image (Fig. 5-7). Low-frequency electric interference may occur as the image is displayed on the television monitor for filming. Repeating the slice acquisition or refilming the image, respectively, will correct these problems.

Characteristic herringbone or crisscross patterns (Fig. 5-8) may occur as an error in array processing the signal information. This results from a computer malfunction during reconstruction of signal data. It is usually not necessary to repeat slice acquisition. Often, only reprocessing the data will correct the problem.

Improper tuning of the RF coil with respect to the body part being scanned may result in a noisy image (Fig. 5-9). A similar effect may be seen at the extremes of the part being scanned (*e.g.,* the first and last slice), where the edges of the body part may lie at the edge of the coil (Fig. 5-10). A noisy, distorted image may be formed when a part of the body touches the RF coil. This results in an impedance mismatch and mistuning of the coil with respect to the body part scanned.

Error may occur during filming of the image. Improper level and window settings produce suboptimal display of detail (Fig. 5-11). The camera may be out of focus as well (Fig. 5-12).

(Text continues on p. 64.)

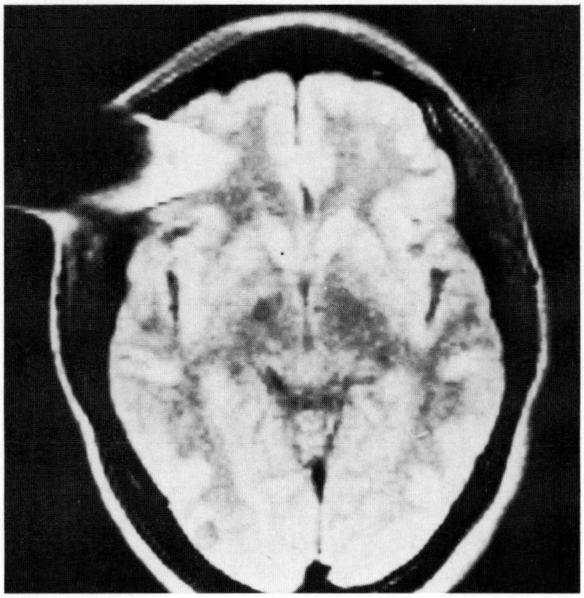

A

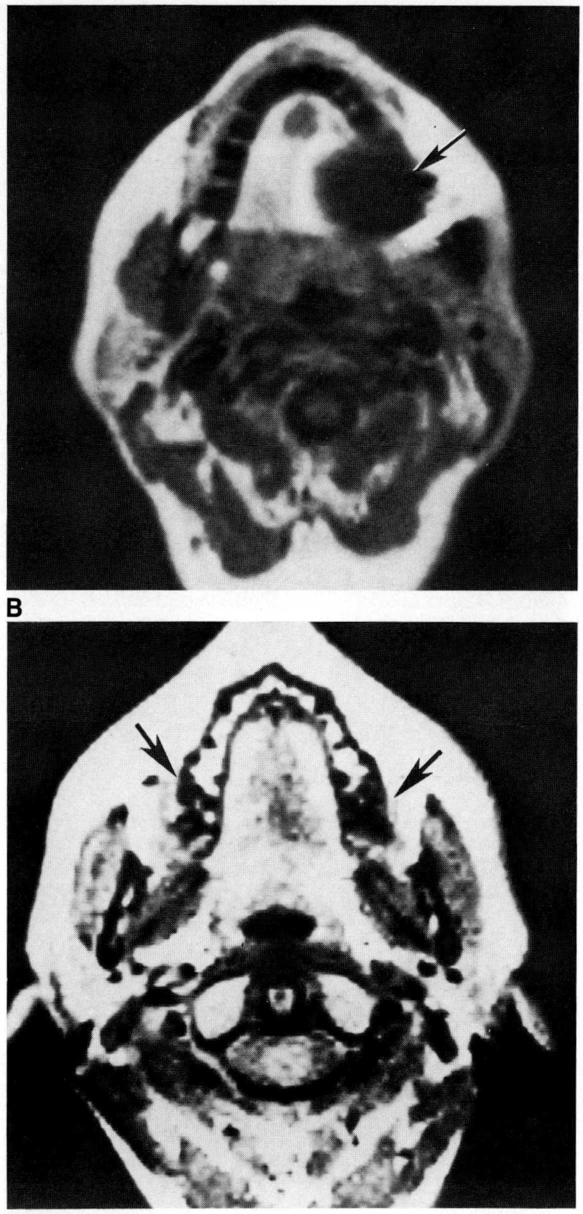

B

C

FIGURE 5-6

(A) Regional image distortion from wire sutures in a craniotomy bone flap. (B) Marked distortion due to ferromagnetic dental bridgework. (C) Routine fillings in teeth usually produce little artifact.

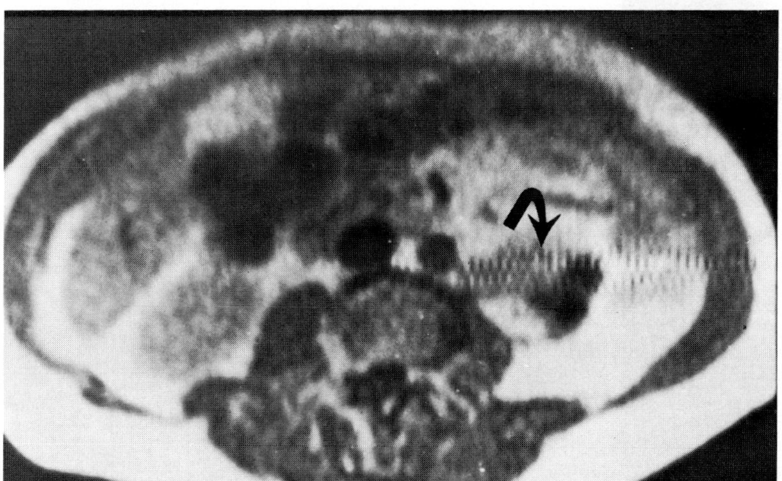

FIGURE 5-7

Radio-frequency interference produces a set of short parallel lines through the image (arrow).

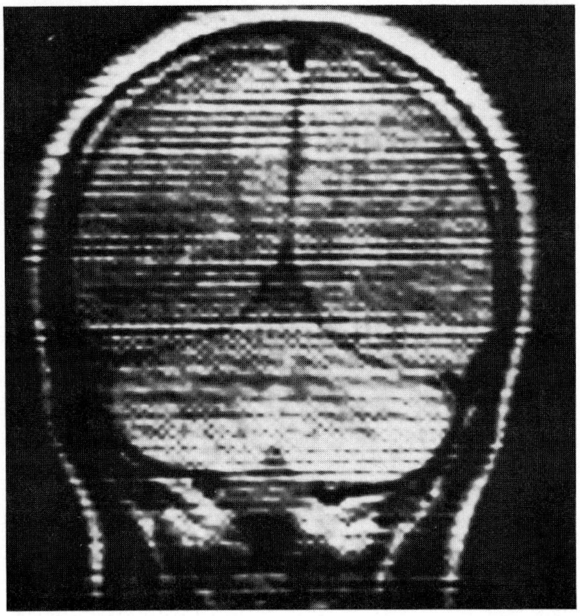

A

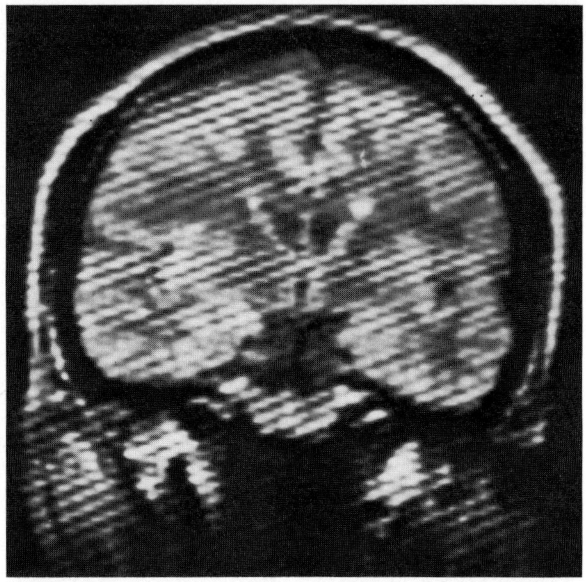

B

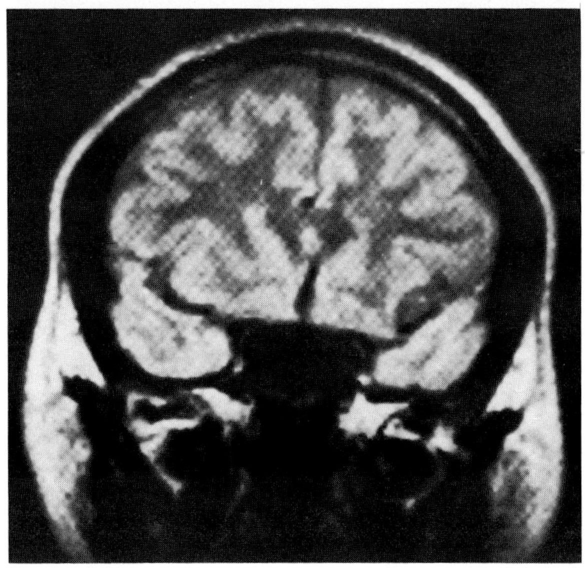

C

FIGURE 5-8

Array processor artifacts are crisscross or herringbone.

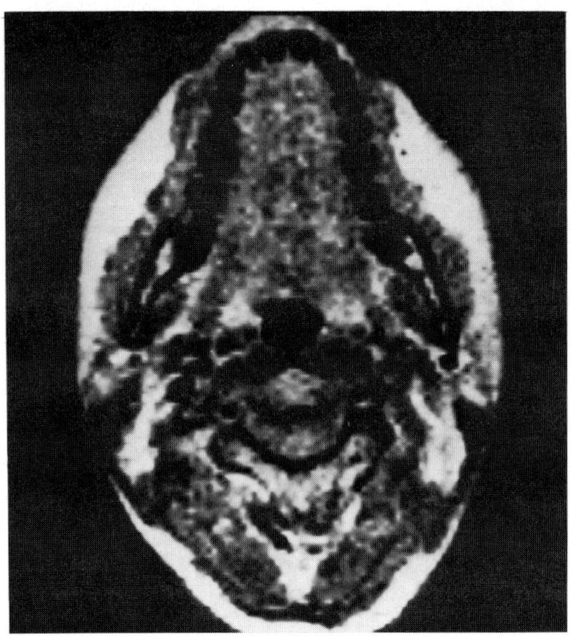

FIGURE 5-9

Improper tuning of RF coil produces a dark, noisy image.

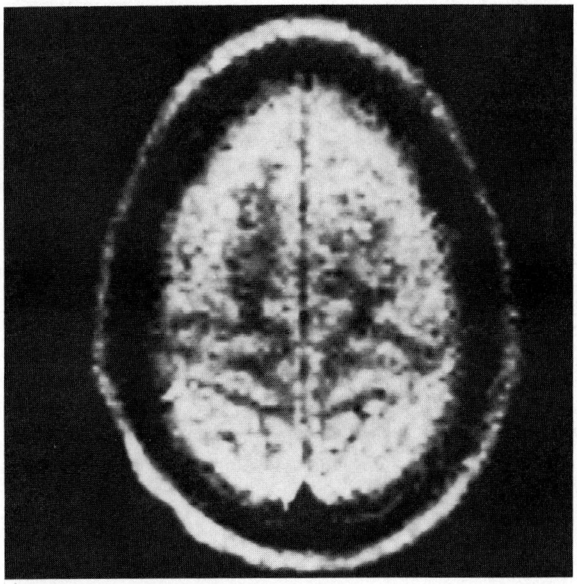

FIGURE 5-10

The body part at the edge of the RF coil is less well tuned than parts centrally.

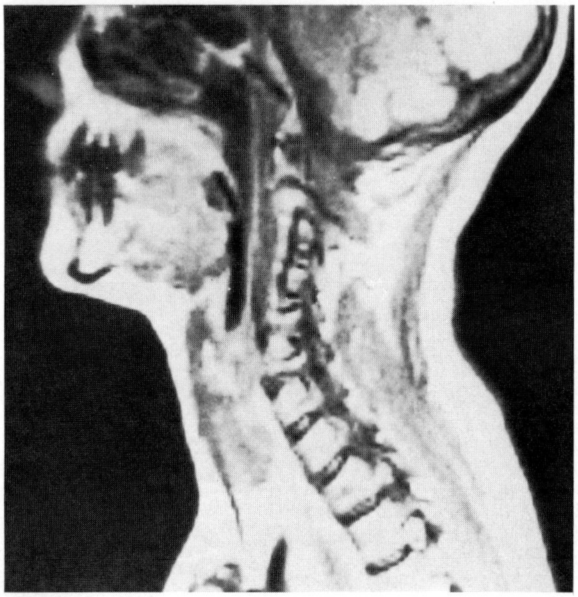

FIGURE 5-11

Improper level and window settings for display.

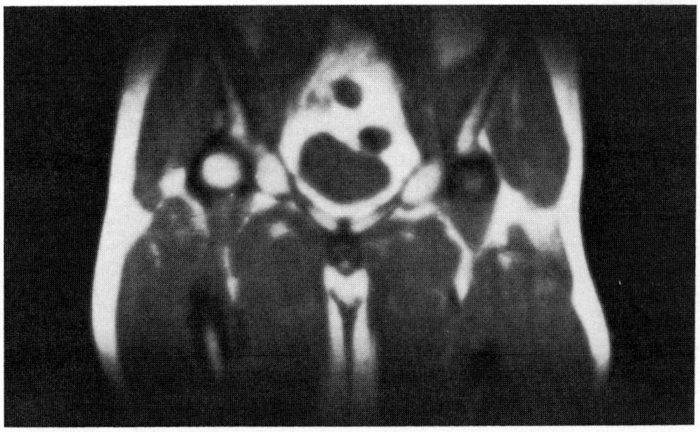

FIGURE 5-12

Camera out of focus during filming.

Multiecho nonuniformities may occasionally be encountered on certain MR scanners (Fig. 5-13). These represent a variation of area intensity seen on long TE images from a multiecho acquisition. Believed to be due to gradient coil–shim coil interactions, these may be corrected by improved coil design and shielding.

Nonuniformity of image signal intensities may result from a variety of patient- and machine-related factors. Asymmetric patient positioning within the RF coil may result in an abnormally low signal from the side of the patient farthest from center (Fig. 5-14). Improper gradient or RF coil fields may result in a linearly decreasing signal strength across an image (Fig. 5-15). Imhomogeneities in the RF field may cause protons to be "flipped" different amounts for the same pulse. This may result in focal changes in signal intensity (Fig. 5-16). Nonlinearities in the RF coil may produce a so-called *pincushion distortion* at the extremes of an image. This is often noted with large patients in body RF coils (Fig. 5-17).

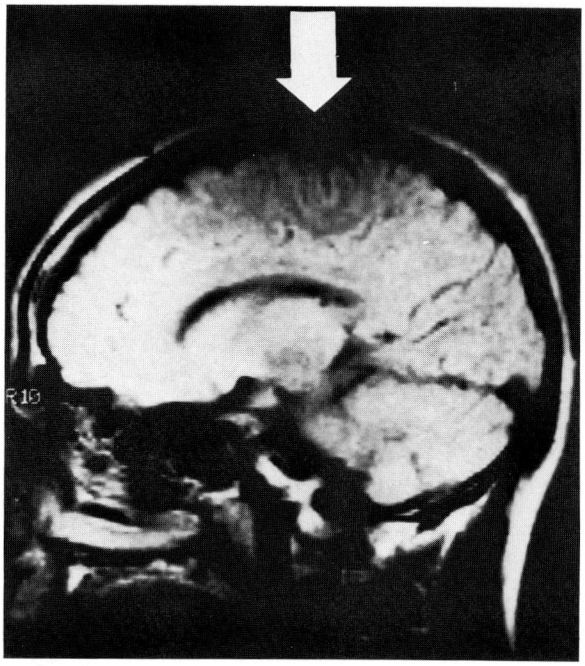

FIGURE 5-13

Multiecho nonuniformities (arrow) due to shim coil–gradient coil interactions on late echoes.

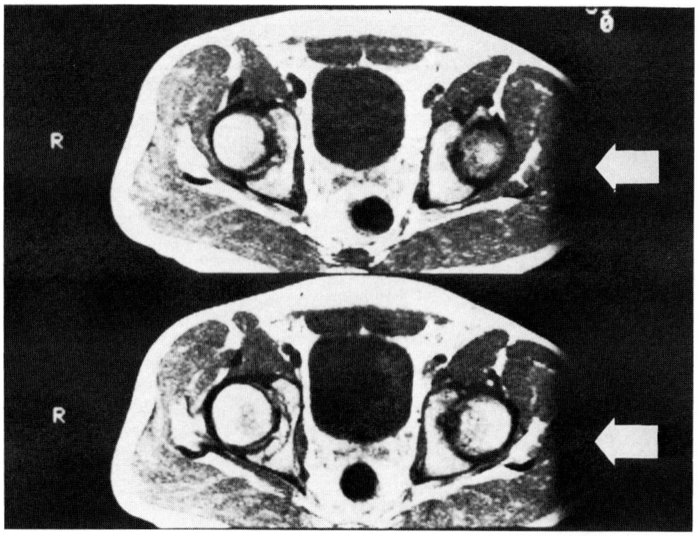

FIGURE 5-14

Asymmetric patient positioning causes low signal from one side of image (arrows).

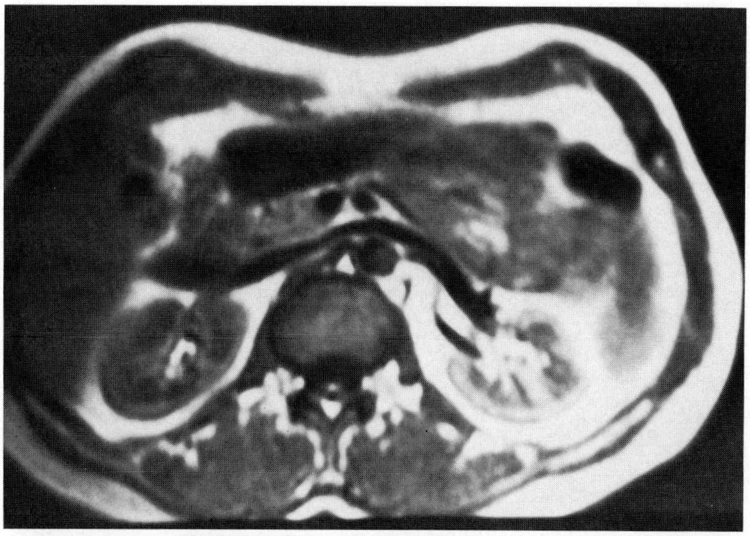

FIGURE 5-15

Field asymmetries produce linear gradient of intensity change across an image. Improper setting of resonance "flip angles" may have similar appearance.

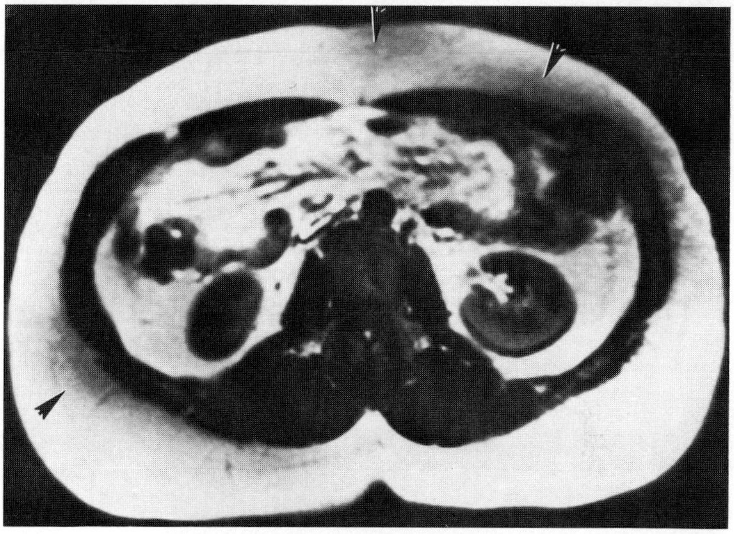

FIGURE 5-16

Focal changes in signal intensity in fat (arrows) due to inhomogeneities in the RF field.

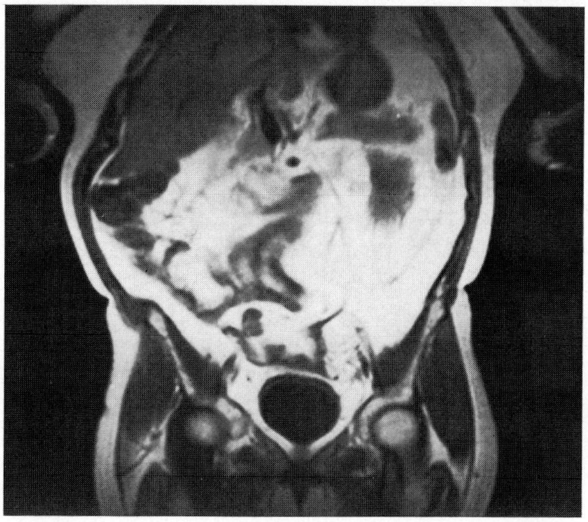

FIGURE 5-17

Pincushion distortion is seen at the extremes of large patients in the body coil. Note the distortion of the chest and upper abdomen.

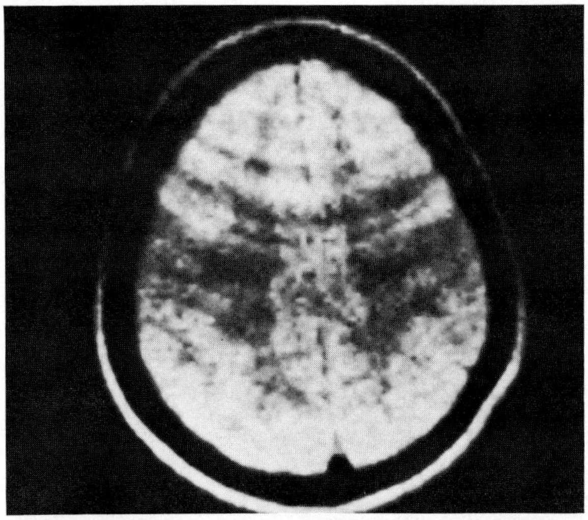

FIGURE 5-18

X-axis control maladjustment superficially looks similar to patient motion artifact.

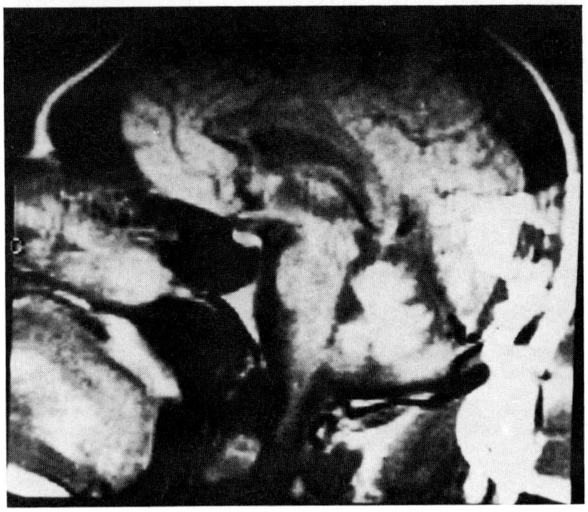

FIGURE 5-19

Wraparound artifact due to improper aspect ratio setup.

At least two artifacts may arise from improper adjustment of internal machine circuitry by the MR service technician. In Figure 5-18, the x-axis setup controls have been maladjusted, resulting in a ghosting in the vertical direction similar to patient motion artifact. Figure 5-19 illustrates an artifact known as *wraparound,* which results from the technician's incorrectly adjusting circuitry controlling the *aspect ratio* of the image. The nature of this artifact is somewhat complex but can be thought of in the following simplistic fashion.

In general, all points in an image are phase encoded over a range of 0° to 360°, which corresponds to the extremes of the image. If incorrect adjustments are made in setting up this process, the ensemble of phases may extend over a range greater than 360°. Typically, this occurs only in larger patients. For example, the location of the patient's nose in Figure 5-19 might be encoded to 370°. When this is displayed on the console, 370° is not distinguishable from 10°, so a wraparound of the image occurs. This artifact typically occurs only with larger patients who occupy the extremes of the scanning volume; it may thus be seen intermittently and requires servicing by the machine technician.

Frequency Shift Artifacts

The frequency shift (chemical shift) artifact is unique to MR scanning. In planar imaging techniques that use a two-dimensional Fourier transform method, spatial information is encoded in terms of phase in one axis and in terms of frequency in the other. Chemical shifts in frequency of the MR signal between tissues of varying compositions may be expressed as distortions or displacements of the MR image. This is particularly noted at interfaces of tissues of widely varying fat content, such as in the retroperitoneum.

Figure 5-20 shows an example of such a frequency shift artifact commonly seen around the kidney. In the scanner used for this image, frequency encoding is performed along the vertical axis. Note that a black band is seen posterior to the kidney, whereas anterior to the kidney there is a white band. These bands represent frequency shift artifacts.

As a semiquantitative approach to understanding this artifact, let us consider that the retroperitoneal fat is homogeneous and that its chemical composition is such that the resonating hydrogen protons within it are more shielded by protein side chains than those protons in the adjacent kidney. As a result of this shielding, the protons in the fat experience a slightly lower local magnetic field than would be expected. As such, according to the Larmor equation, these protons will resonate at a lower frequency than would be expected. This frequency shift is small and is on the order of 3 parts per million (ppm). If the resonance center of the scanner is 64 MHz (typical for a 1.5-T machine), the frequency shift would be 64 MHz $\times$ 3 ppm = 192 Hz. Assuming a readout gradient of 400 Hz/cm, this 192-Hz frequency shift would result in a spurious displacement of the kidney of 192/400, or 0.5 cm.

Spurious overlap of kidney on retroperitoneal fat at the upper margin of the kidney in Figure 5-20 accounts for the white band of increased signal. Spurious separation of kidney from fat at the lower margin produces a crescent of decreased signal intensity (the dark band). Similar artifacts may be seen at other interfaces, particularly where fat abuts an organ. Other places frequency shift artifacts may be seen include the optic nerve, at the junction between the intervertebral disk and end-plate, at the wall of the bladder, and near the capsule of the spleen (see Fig. 9-3*F*).

The physical nature of this artifact may be verified by placing the patient on his side and repeating the scan. In this situation, the black and white crescents would be seen to lie along the medial and lateral margins of the kidney, always in the direction of the frequency encoding gradient. Because the frequency shift is proportional to base frequency, increasing the strength of the magnetic field would be

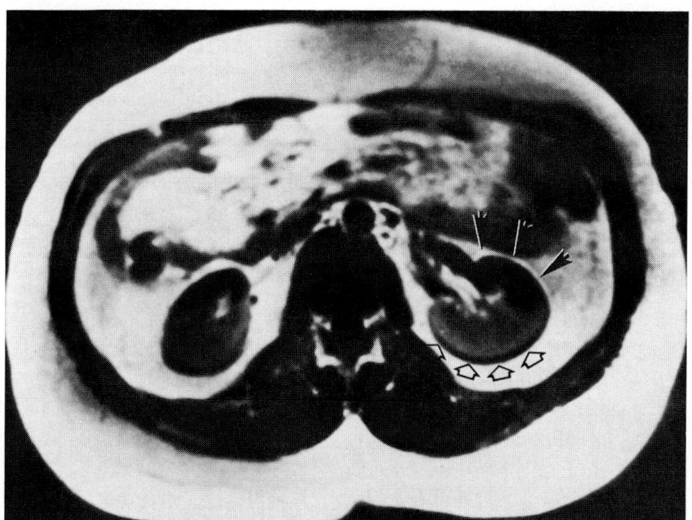

FIGURE 5-20

Frequency (chemical) shift artifact around the kidney (arrows) appears as a black band posteriorly and as a white band anteriorly. (Courtesy of Picker International, Clinical Sciences Center)

expected to increase the size of these artifacts. Appropriate changes must be made in the data acquisition window or field gradients to limit these artifacts in the high-strength scanners (*i.e.,* 1.5 to 2.0 T).

Finally, it should be noted that only frequency shift artifacts within the plane of imaging have been discussed. A similar problem may exist in three dimensions, however, since frequency gradients are used to define planes of imaging. Therefore, certain structures that lie outside the plane of imaging may be included in that plane because of chemical shift effects. In this manner, frequency shift artifacts between planes of imaging may be an occult cause of degraded image quality.

SECTION II

Imaging Guide and Atlas of the Human Body

CHAPTER 6

The Brain

The early success and current wide acceptance of MRI can be largely attributed to its spectacular ability to image the central nervous system (CNS). In only a few years, MR has equaled or surpassed CT as an imaging modality for a number of disease processes in the brain. MRI has proved particularly valuable in evaluating the posterior fossa and brain stem because it is not plagued by streak artifacts from the bony skull base so commonly seen with CT.

MRI has also demonstrated an exquisite sensitivity for detection of brain pathology. As discussed in Chapter 4, MRI is very sensitive to changes in tissue free-water content. In the brain, such changes in the ratio of free and bound water may represent the earliest manifestation of a variety of disease processes, such as edema, ischemia, demyelination, tumor, and infection. Intensely bright signals can be recorded from these areas of increased free water on T2-weighted pulse sequences. The use of paramagnetic contrast agents that cross the blood–brain barrier may further increase MR sensitivity.

Imaging Strategies

There is at present no agreement among world authorities about optimal imaging strategies and MR techniques for use in scanning the brain. Imaging strategies by necessity will vary depending on preexisting diagnostic probabilities, as well as knowledge of CT scan and angiographic and clinical findings. Selection of imaging plane depends largely on the anatomic structures under consideration. Selection of pulse sequences depends on the T1 and T2 relaxation values in the region of interest, as well as the pathological conditions encountered. We will now consider separately the advantages and disadvantages of various planes and pulse sequences for MRI of the brain.

An important first question one might ask is, What is the optimal imaging plane in which to view the brain—axial, coronal, or sagittal? Because of the familiar anatomic relationships seen on axial sections, a routine MR brain scan should probably include at least one set of axially oriented images. This will also allow relative ease of comparison with past or future CT scans in the same patient. In addition to axial images, an additional set of images in a second plane, either coronally or sagittally, may be of benefit. The use of this second plane will often confirm or clarify equivocal frindings seen on axial images. This second plane can also provide an improved appreciation of the anatomic relations of the disease process discovered.

As will be shown in forthcoming illustrations, coronal sections of the brain are particularly useful in demonstrating a number of anatomic structures and relationships. These include the pituitary, the optic tract, the cavernous sinus, the basal ganglia, the substantia nigra, the ventricular system, and the deep white matter tracts of the cerebrum. Coronal images may occasionally detect lesions not well visualized on axial sections.

Sagittally oriented images are also helpful in a number of situations, although in general we have not found them as helpful as axial and coronal projections. Sagittal images are preferred, however, when pathology in the brain stem, base of skull, or at the cervicocranium is encountered. When pathological conditions involve higher regions of the brain, however, we have found sagittal images often add little if any information to that already obtained from the axial and coronal sections. It is reasonable, therefore, to limit routine acquisition of sagittal images to those cases in which lesions of the brain stem or base of skull are suspected.

A second important question one might pose is, Which imaging sequences and parameters are optimal for demonstrating pathological conditions of the brain? Unfortunately, world experts in MRI still disagree about the anwer to this question. At least a part of the answer depends on what type of lesion one expects to find. Since there is no final answer to this question, we will settle with a few reasonable generalizations and suggested approaches.

First, it is important to have a general knowledge of normal T1 and T2 values in the CNS (Table 6-1). As would be expected, cerebrospinal fluid (CSF) has very long T1 and T2 values, because it is primarily water. Brain parenchyma has significantly shorter T1 and T2 values than CSF. Gray matter may be conveniently thought of as having more water and less fat than white matter. Accordingly, gray matter has slightly longer T1 and T2 values than white matter. (This explanation is not entirely accurate but can serve as a mnemonic device.) Note in Table 6-1 that there is also some difference in T1 and T2 values between various gray and white matter nuclei and tracts within the brain.

As discussed in Chapters 3 and 4, pathological

TABLE 6-1

T1 and T2 Values of the Brain*

Region	T_1 (msec)	T_2 (msec)
Cortical gray matter	700	60
Cerebellar gray matter	650	60
Caudate head	660	59
Lenticular nucleus	600	56
Thalamus	610	56
Subcortical white matter	420	53
Posterior internal capsule	440	54
Cerebellar white matter	460	57
Orbital fat	290	57
Ocular vitreous	2800	160
CSF	2700	170

*Modified from Kjos BO et al: Reproducibility of relaxation times and spin density calculated from routine MR Imaging sequences: Clinical study of the CNS. AJR 144:1165–1170, 1985.

processes may affect T1 and T2 independently. It seems reasonable, and indeed necessary, to use both T1-weighted and T2-weighted sequences to detect and screen for brain lesions. The T1-weighted sequence may be either partial saturation (PS), inversion recovery (IR), or short spin-echo (SE). T1 weighting allows good differentiation of anatomic interfaces of brain and CSF. Additionally, excellent gray matter–white matter distinction may be obtained, particularly with inversion recovery sequences designed for this purpose (*e.g.,* IR 1500/500/25, Fig. 6-1).

Although T1-weighted pulse sequences provide superior anatomic delineation, T2-weighted sequences usually are more sensitive in detecting brain lesions. The long spin-echo technique has been found best for this purpose (*e.g.,* SE 3000/60 or SE 1000/100). With short spin-echo sequences, brain and CSF are easily distinguished (Fig. 6-2*A*). With T2 weighting, the CSF becomes isointense or slightly more intense than brain parenchyma (Fig. 6-2*B*). It may be difficult to distinguish accurately the brain–CSF interface. With very heavily T2-weighted sequences, the brain–CSF interface is easily seen, with the contrast reversal now complete (Fig. 6-2C).

Suggested Protocols for CNS Imaging

In this and the following chapter, a set of imaging protocols will be presented for MRI of the anatomic regions of interest. It should be realized that in no case is there universal agreement about "optimal" or "best" imaging strategies for each organ. Optimal imaging strategies depend on a number of factors, including time constraints, the implementation of pulse sequences on a particular scanner, as well as clinical suspicion of a particular disease process.

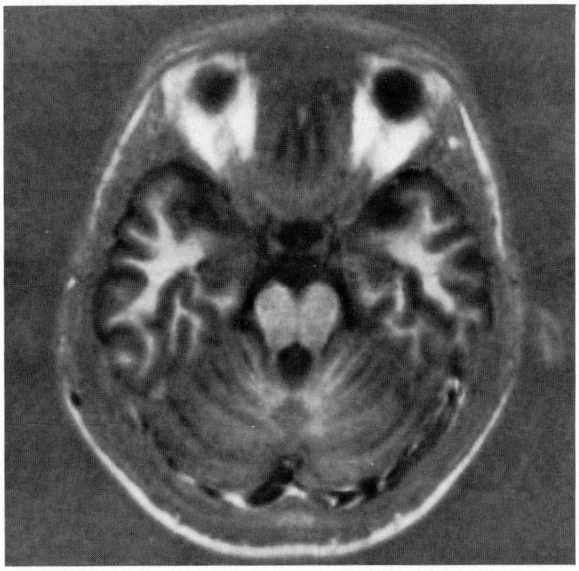

FIGURE 6-1

Inversion recovery image of the brain. Specially designed sequences such as this IR 1500/500/25 technique provide superb gray matter–white matter differentiation. (Courtesy of Siemens)

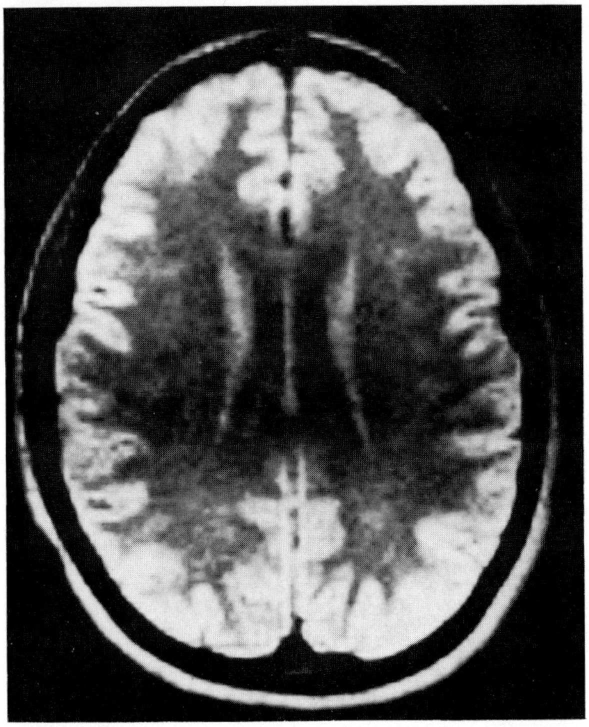

A

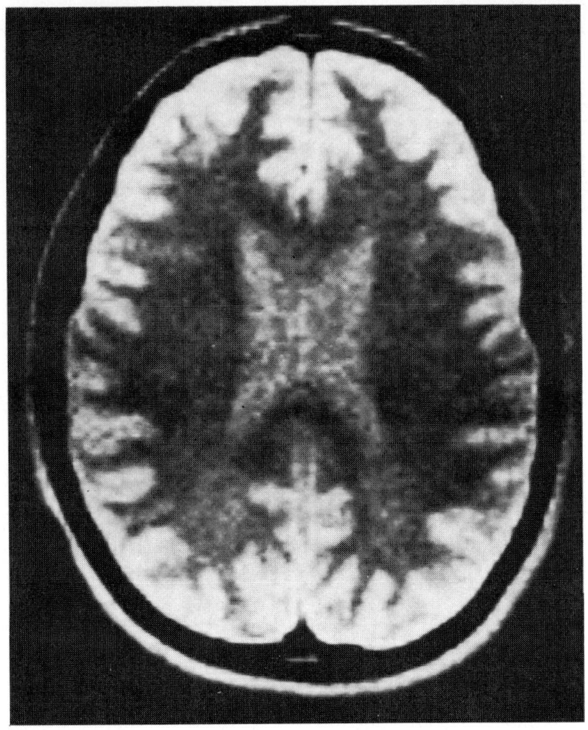

B

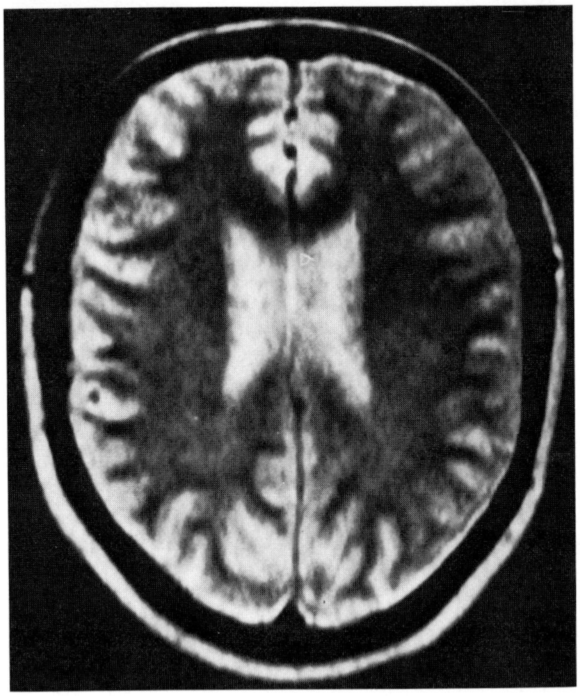

C

FIGURE 6-2

Effect of T2-weighting on spin-echo images. (*A*) SE 2000/28; (*B*) SE 2000/56; (*C*) SE 2000/100. Progressive T2-weighting with increase in TE parameter causes contrast reversal between brain and CSF.

What we have found to be efficient and accurate on our Diasonics MT/S scanner may be relatively inefficient on another brand of scanner. The imaging protocols presented, therefore, should not be considered dogmatic. Rather they should be used as a guide around which a particular MR center may base its own imaging strategies, modified by time constraints, cost factors, brand of scanner, and patient poulation. Suggested protocols for brain MRI are presented in Table 6-2.

TABLE 6-2

Possible Protocols for Brain MRI

Routine Screen for Brain Lesions

Indications: Nonspecific complaints and no focal neurologic findings

Dizziness (without vestibulocochlear dysfunction)

Headaches

Confusion

Normal CT scan

Protocol: Axial plane, SE 2500/40, 80

Axial plane, SE 300/25 or IR 1500/400

Trauma or Extraparenchymal Hemorrhage

Indications: Note that CT scanning instead of MRI is the modality of choice for acute trauma or suspected bleeding

Evaluate possible isodense subdural

Evaluate degree of brain parenchymal injury from shearing, contusion, anoxia, edema

Protocol: Axial plane, SE 2500/40,80

Coronal plane, SE 1000/30

Seizures

Indications: Focal or generalized

Protocol: Axial plane, SE 1500/30,60

Coronal plane, SE 2500/40,80

Note that coronal plane is particularly valuable for suspected temporal lobe pathology

Focal Parenchymal Lesions

Indications: Neurologic deficit explainable in terms of a single specific lesion

Tumor

Arteriovenous malformation

Hemorrhage

Stroke

Protocol 1 (supratentorial lesion suspected):

Axial plane, SE 300/25 or PS 400 or IR 1500/400

Axial plane, SE 2000/100

Coronal plane, SE 2500/40,80

Protocol 2 (brain stem or vermian lesion suspected):

Axial plane, SE 300/25 or PS 400

Axial plane, SE 2500/40,80

Sagittal plane, SE 1000/30,60

Protocol 3 (cerebellar hemisphere lesion suspected):

Axial plane, SE 2500/40,80

Coronal plane, SE 500/30

Suspected Multifocal Disease

Indications: Multiple sclerosis

Other demyelinating disease

Multiple focal neurologic lesions separated in space or time, not explainable by a single focus

Multiple white matter infarcts

Metastases

Emboli

Infections

Protocol: Axial plane, SE 3000/40,80

Coronal plane, SE 1000/30,60

For suspected multiple sclerosis or demyelinating disease, be sure to cover upper cervical spinal cord on axial slices

Juxtasellar Lesions

Indications: Pituitary tumor

Lesion of optic nerves or chiasma

Parasellar masses, tumors, aneurysms, granuloma

Protocol: Requires thin slice capabilities (1 to 3 mm) for optimal delineation, although larger lesions may be reliably imaged with 5-mm to 7-mm-thick slices

Sagittal SE 750/30,60 or PS 500

Coronal SE 2000/30,60,90

Cerebellopontine Angle Lesions

Indications: Acoustic neuroma

Meningioma

Other mass lesion

Protocol: Thin slice (2.5 to 5.0 mm) preferred

Axial SE 500/30 or PS 400

Axial SE 2500/40,80

Coronal SE 1500/30,60

See temporal bone protocol in Chapter 7

Cervicocranial Junction Lesions

Indications: Chiari malformation

Basilar invagination

Syrinx

Mass lesion/arteriovenous malformation/ stroke at the foramen magnum level

Protocol: Sagittal SE 500/30 or PS 400

Axial SE 1500/30,60,90

Bones and Soft Tissues of the Skull

Although the parts of the brain are easily recognized even by persons unfamiliar with MRI, a number of MR signals from the rest of the head may be confusing. From the outside inward, scalp fat is the first bright substance encountered (Fig. 6-3). Occasionally, superficial scalp vessels may also be recognized as areas of signal dropout due to flowing blood. Musculature attached to the skull has characteristically low intensity, but the individual muscle groups are easily distinguished because they are separated by high-intensity fat.

The inner and outer tables of the skull are poorly visualized because they are composed of cortical bone with little MR signal. A bright signal is commonly detected from the diploic space, which contains fatty marrow and slowly flowing blood (Fig. 6-3). Occasionally, the diploic space may be quite thick as a normal variant (Fig. 6-4*A*). Hyperostosis frontalis interna should also be recognized and distinguished from other pathological conditions such as bilateral subdural hematomas (Fig. 6-4*B*).

The skull base includes the petrous portions of the temporal bones, the sphenoid bone, and the basiocciput. The petrous temporal bones contain a number of important structures, including the internal carotid arteries, jugular veins, seventh and eighth cranial nerves, and the vestibulocochlear apparatus. MR images of the complicated anatomy of this region are presented in Chapter 7. MRI of the orbit will also be considered at that time.

A few aspects of the skull base must be considered here, because certain structures produce signals that may be confused with brain lesions. In axial section, signal from slowly flowing blood in a jugular vein is commonly noted (Fig. 6-5). Fat in the petrous pyramid tips often produces bright signals that are usually symmetrical (Fig. 6-6). The basiocciput forms a characteristic C shape of high intensity on axial images (Fig 6-7).

Centrally, the basiocciput and sphenoid bone join to form a base on which the brain stem rests. The superior surface of this bony complex is called the clivus. Sagittal images through the clivus produce a characteristic bright white triangle due to signal from fatty marrow (Fig. 6-8). Any disruption or irregularity of the sharp edges of this triangle should arouse suspicion of a lesion in the clivus, sphenoid

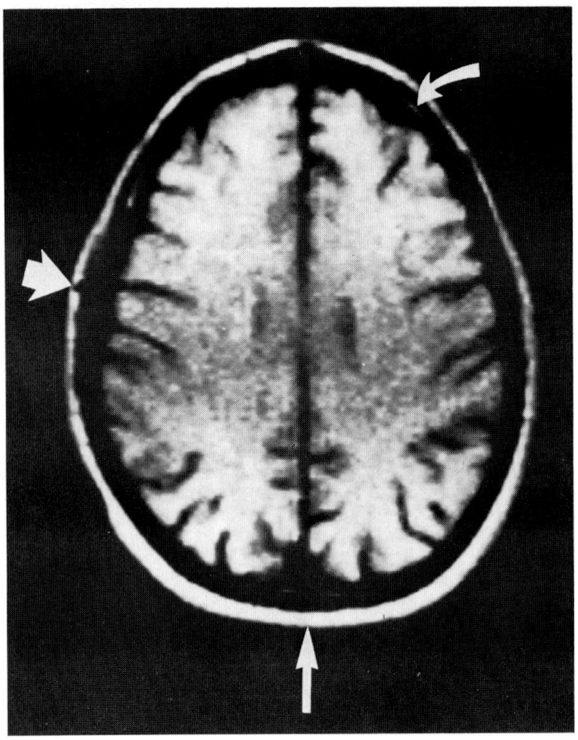

FIGURE 6-3

Normal skull on SE 500/28. Scalp fat (white arrow, inferiorly) is the first bright MR signal encountered. Superficial scalp vessels (short arrow on left) appear dark because of signal dropout. Fatty marrow and blood in the diploic space may produce a signal (curved arrow).

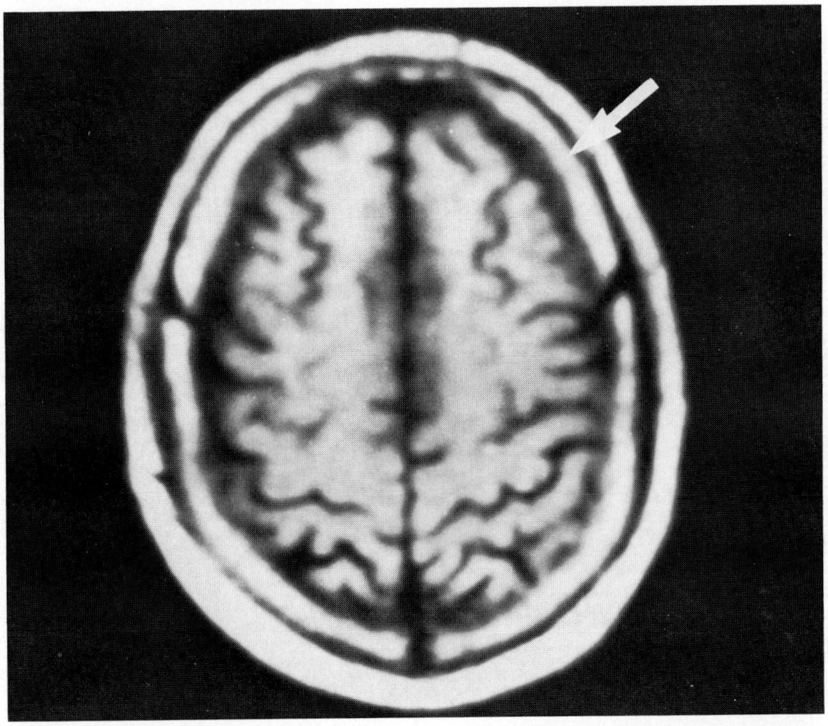

A

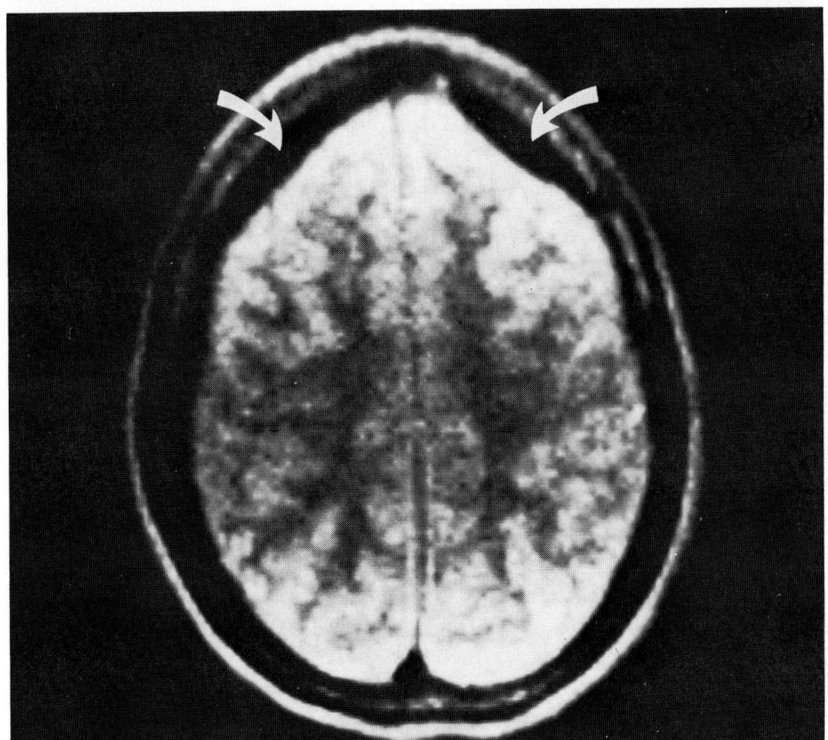

B

FIGURE 6-4

Normal skull variants. (*A*) Very thick diploic space (arrow); (*B*) hyperostosis frontalis interna (arrows).

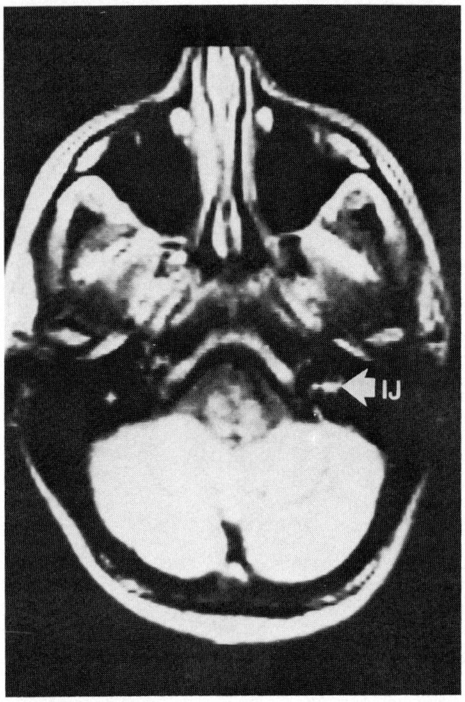

FIGURE 6-5

Blood in the internal jugular vein (IJ) often produces a bright signal in the skull base because of its slow flow.

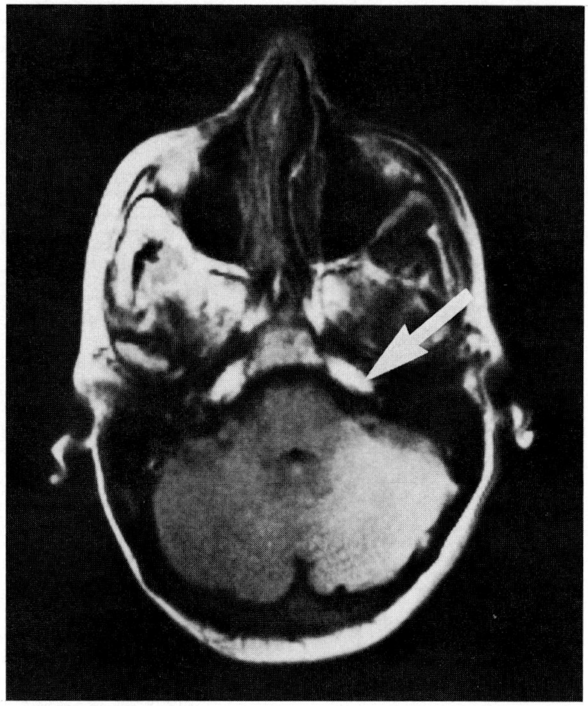

FIGURE 6-6

Fat in the petrous pyramid tips produces a bright signal (arrow).

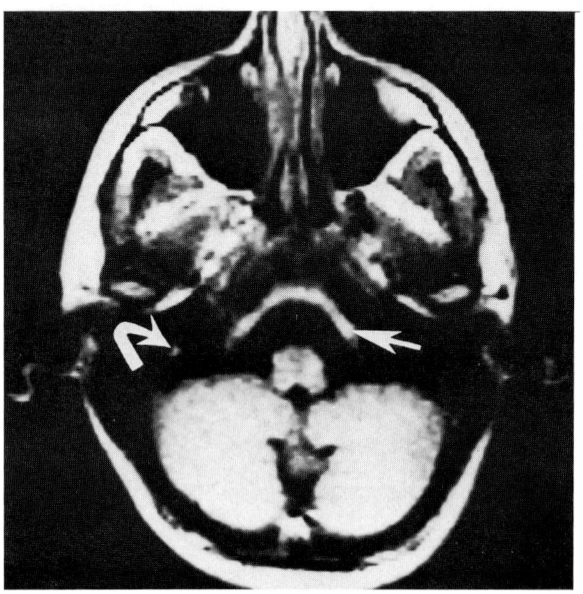

FIGURE 6-7

The basiocciput (straight arrow) forms a characteristic C shape on axial MR images of the skull base. Note also the signal from the right internal jugular vein (curved arrow).

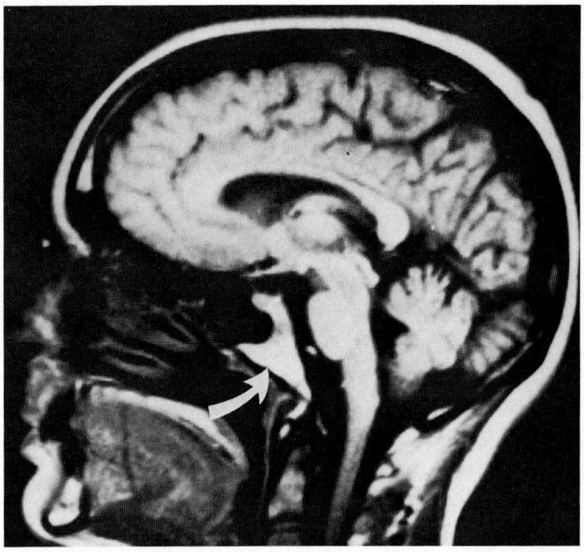

FIGURE 6-8
The clivus (arrow) forms a sharp white triangle at the skull base, composed of the sphenoid bone and basioccipital bone.

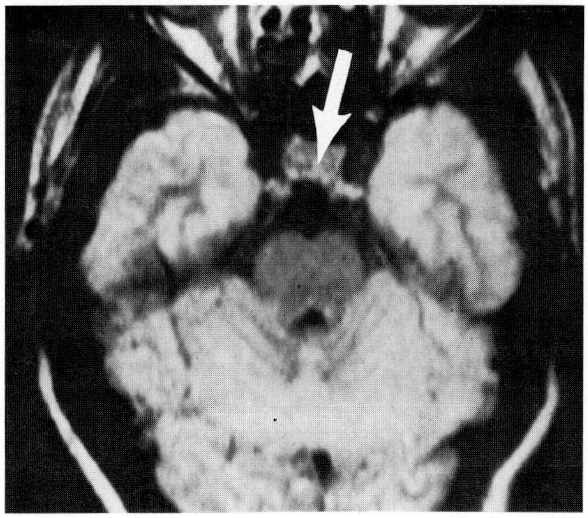

FIGURE 6-9
Partial volume effect with fat in the sphenoid body (arrow) may simulate a pituitary mass.

FIGURE 6-10
The spheno-occipital synchondrosis (arrows) is a normal finding in younger patients, not to be mistaken for fracture or other lesions. (Courtesy of Fonar Corp., 110 Marcus Drive, Melville, NY 11747)

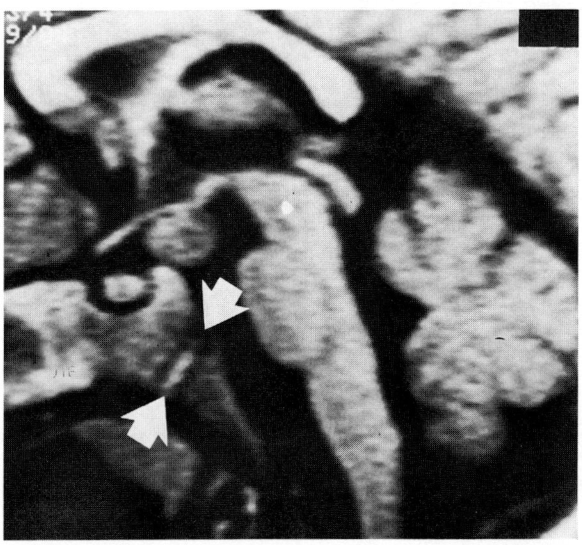

sinus, or adjacent brain stem and dura. Partial voluming of the marrow in the body of the sphenoid bone might simulate a pituitary mass (Fig. 6-9). In younger patients, the shpeno-occipital synchondrosis may be visualized as a dark band and may be mistaken as a fracture or other pathological condition (Fig. 6-10).

CSF-Containing Spaces in the Brain

CSF, by virtue of its long T1 value, appears black on most inversion recovery and spin-echo sequences with short timing parameters. With the use of appropriate inversion recovery parameters or with very long TR and TE values in spin-echo, the CSF may be made to appear isodense or even white compared with brain parenchyma. Although pure white CSF is aesthetically pleasing because of its resemblance to myelographic contrast, it is unclear whether the increased acquisition times required to produce such images are justified by the added diagnostic information obtained. For visualizing blood vessels such as the basilar artery (as well as disk herniation in the spine), sequences producing pure white CSF may be valuable. For routine imaging, however, many investigators believe that obtaining this bright white CSF produces no more diagnostic information than other sequences with shorter image acquisition times and a slightly muddy CSF. Figures 3-9, 3-11, and 6-2 have illustrated the effects of TR and TE on CSF signal intensity.

The ventricular system of the brain is well visualized on all imaging sequences, having the expected configurations in the axial, coronal, and sagittal planes. The lateral ventricles and third ventricle may be well evaluated in axial or coronal planes. The cerebral aqueduct and fourth ventricle are particularly well seen in sagittal section (Fig. 6-11).

The cisterns surrounding the brain can be well visualized on the T1-weighted images. Multiple named sulci, gyri, and fissures of the cerebral cortex are silhouetted against black CSF and can be easily identified. These structures may be identified on atlas plates A, C, and S at the end of this chapter.

Cerebral Vasculature

A number of cerebral blood vessels are routinely visualized in MRI of the brain. In general, rapidly flowing blood in the larger arteries will appear black, for reasons discussed in Chapter 2. Similarly, slowly flowing blood in the larger venous sinuses and in smaller vessels on the brain surface may exhibit enhancement, particularly on second echo images. These characteristics of flowing blood in the brain on occasion make the diagnosis of certain vascular lesions like arteriovenous malformations and aneurysms possible without arteriography.

The basilar artery, which is surrounded by CSF on three of four sides, is best identified with pulse sequences that render the CSF relatively white. Figure 6-12 illustrates the appearance and location of the basilar artery and its major division into the posterior cerebral and superior cerebellar arteries. Occasionally, the branches of the posterior and anterior inferior cerebellar arteries may also be identified.

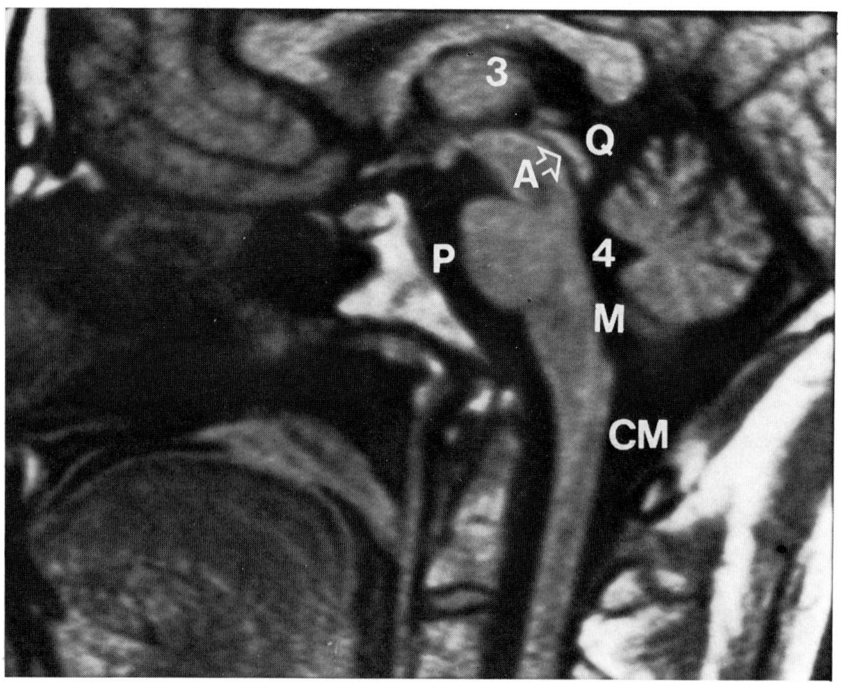

FIGURE 6-11

CSF-containing spaces around the brain stem. Short SE 500/30 produces good contrast. 3 = third ventricle; 4 = fourth ventricle; A = cerebral aqueduct; Q = quadrigeminal plate cistern; M = foramen of Magendie; CM = cisterna magna; P = prepontine cistern. (Courtesy of Fonar Corp., 110 Marcus Drive, Melville, NY 11747)

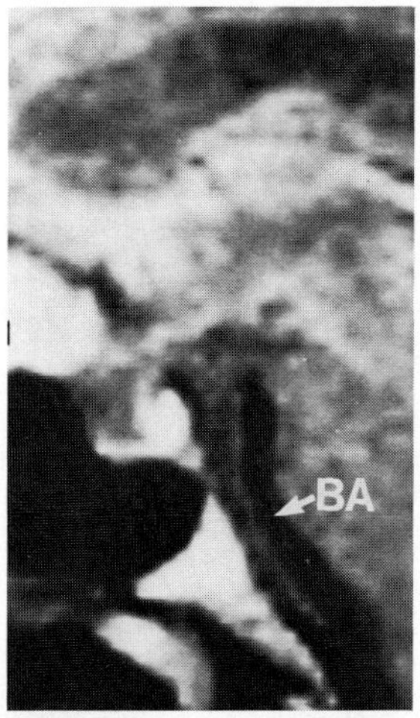

A

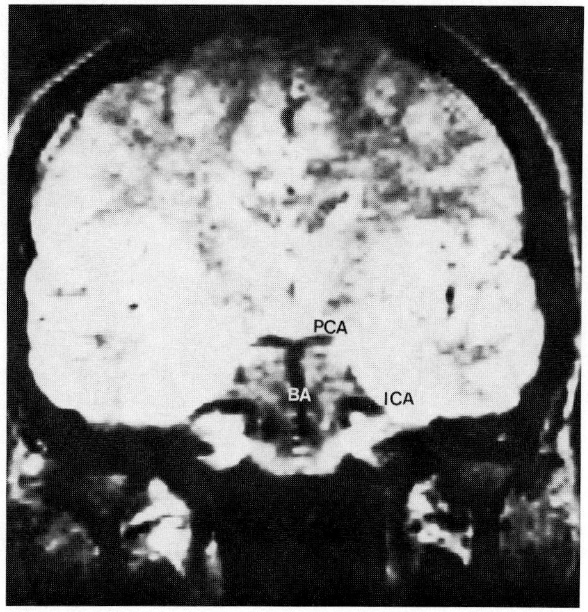

B

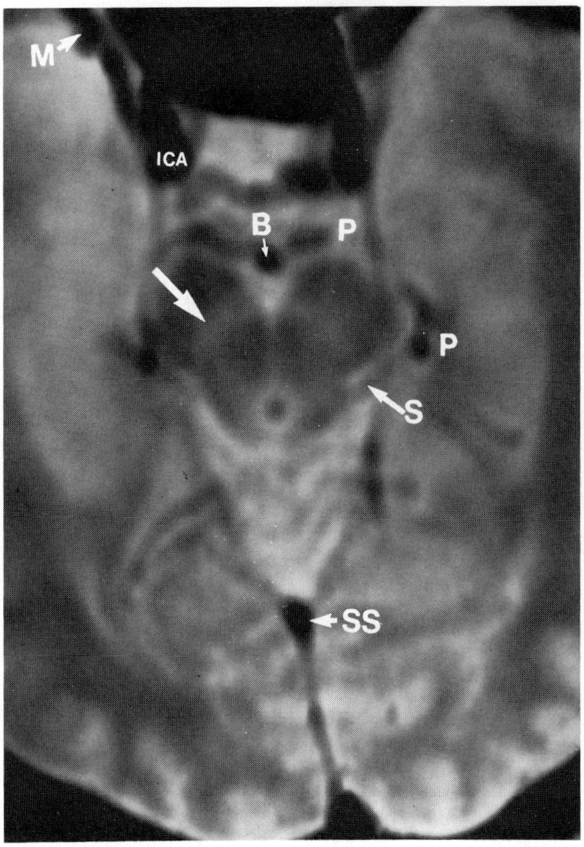

C

FIGURE 6-12

The basilar artery and its branches. (*A*) Sagittal SE 2000/56 shows the dark basilar artery (BA) against a whiter CSF. (*B*) Coronal SE 2000/56 image shows the basilar artery (BA) dividing into posterior cerebral arteries (PCA). Note also the internal carotid arteries (ICA). (*C*) M = middle cerebral artery; ICA = internal carotid artery; B = basilar artery; P = posterior cerebral artery; S = superior cerebellar artery; SS = straight sinus. Incidentally, note the arrow pointing to the substantia nigra.

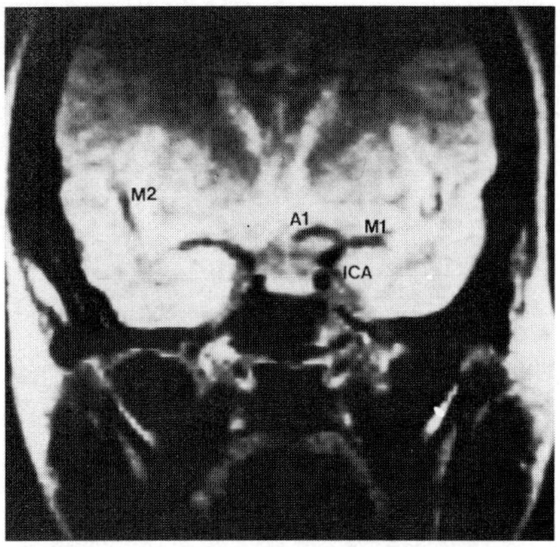

A

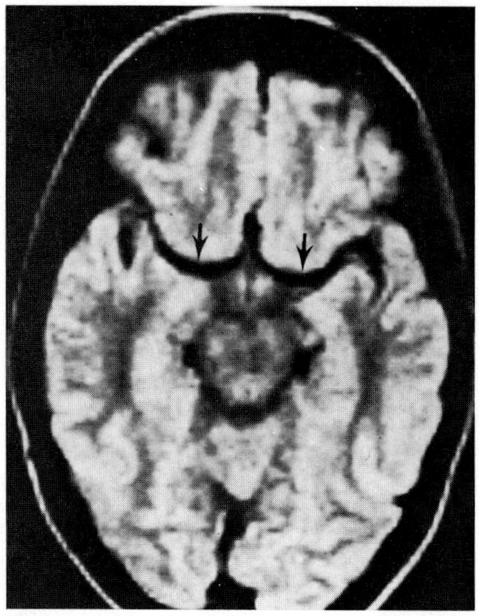

B

FIGURE 6-13

Branches of the internal carotid artery (ICA). (*A*) Coronal SE 2000/56 shows division of the ICA into M1 and A1 segments. M2 segment of the MCA also seen. (*B*) Axial SE 1500/28 image shows the middle cerebral arteries (arrows).

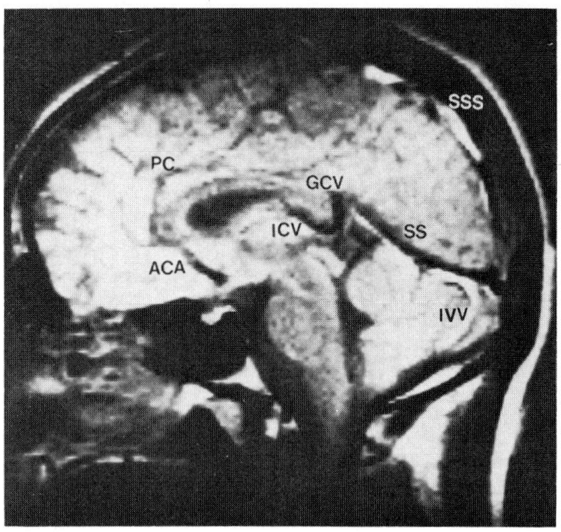

A

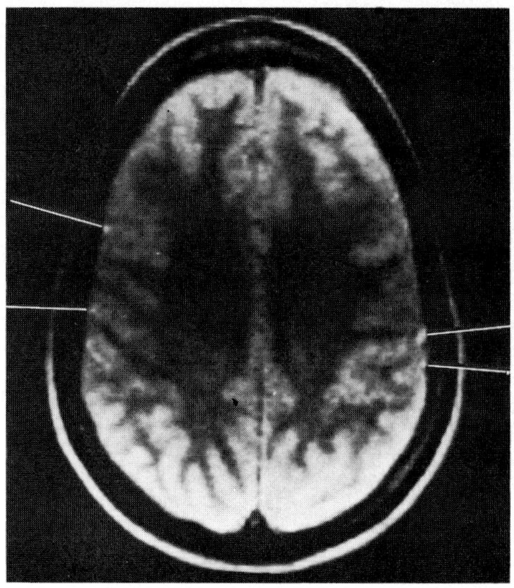

B

FIGURE 6-14

Veins and surface vessels. Second echo images produce increased intensity of blood flowing in large veins and in surface vessels. (*A*) SSS = superior sagittal sinus; SS = straight sinus; IVV = inferior vermian vein; ICV = internal cerebral vein; GCV = great cerebral vein; ACA = anterior cerebral artery; PC = pericallosal artery. (*B*) White lines point to high-intensity blood in surface vessels. These bright spots on the brain surface on second echo images should not be confused with intensifying lesions.

The major divisions of the internal carotid artery are also easily seen in appropriate projection as areas of signal void. Figure 6-13 shows its division into the anterior and middle cerebral arteries. Smaller branches may occasionally be identified and are shown in the atlas pages at the end of this chapter.

The major venous sinuses are especially well visualized on the sagittal brain second echo image (Fig. 6-14*A*). The great cerebral vein and internal cerebral vein are commonly imaged. Small vessels on the brain surface should not be confused with intensifying pathological lesions (Fig. 6-14*B*).

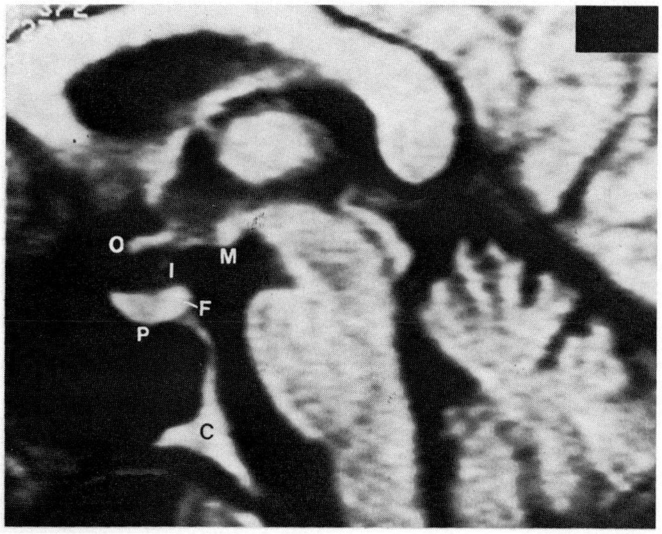

FIGURE 6-15

Pituitary fossa in sagittal SE 500/28· section. O = optic chiasm; I = infundibulum; M = mamillary body; P = pituitary gland; F = fat in sella posterior to pituitary; C = clivus. (Courtesy of Fonar Corp., 110 Marcus Drive, Melville, NY 11747)

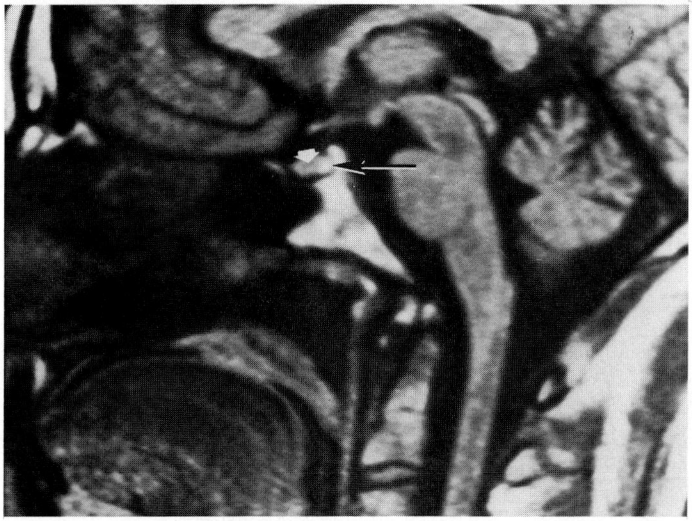

FIGURE 6-16

Fat pad (black arrow) in the posterior sella produces a high-intensity signal of T1-weighted sequences such as this SE 400/28 sagittal image. Also note the normal slightly lower intensity centrally in the pituitary (white arrow). (Courtesy of Fonar Corp., 110 Marcus Drive, Melville, NY 11747)

The Pituitary and Parasellar Regions

The sella and adjacent regions are adequately imaged by MR, although spatial resolution is still somewhat limited on most commercial scanners. Further refinements in MR technology with thinner slices will overcome these limitations.

The pituitary gland itself is best imaged in the coronal or sagittal planes using a short spin-echo or partial saturation technique (SE 500/25 or PS 300). In agreement with CT, the height of the pituitary gland should be less than 8 mm, and its upper surface should be flat or concave (Fig. 6-15). The pituitary is normally nonhomogeneous. The most posterior portion of the pituitary fossa has been shown to contain a fat pad, identifiable in about 95% of patients. This fat pad gives a high-intensity signal on sagittal images performed with partial saturation or spin-echo techniques (Fig. 6-16). The midportion of the gland on sagittal images is commonly observed to be of lower intensity (Fig. 6-16). It has been speculated that this low-intensity area represents partial volume averaging between the pituitary gland and

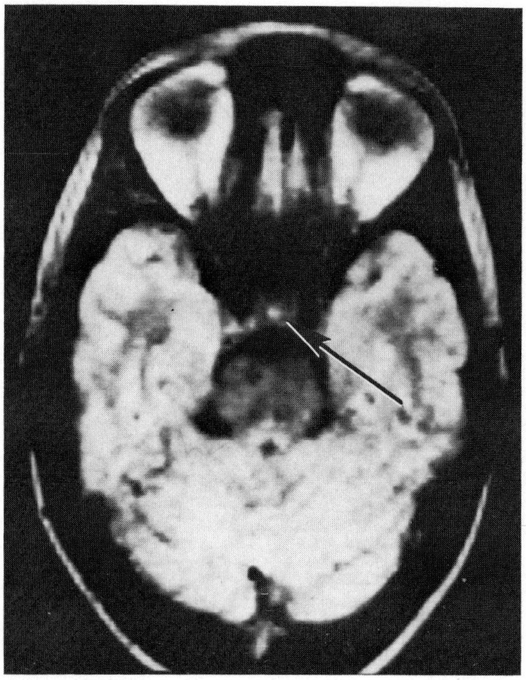

A

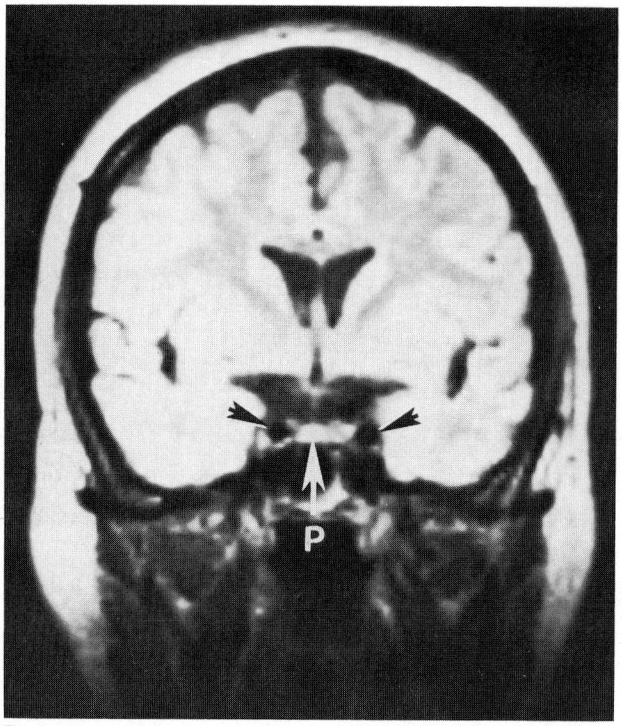

B

FIGURE 6-17

The infundibulum is seen as a dot on axial images (arrow in *A*) and as a line on sagittal or coronal images (*B*). Note also in *B* the pituitary gland (P) and cavernous carotid arteries (arrows).

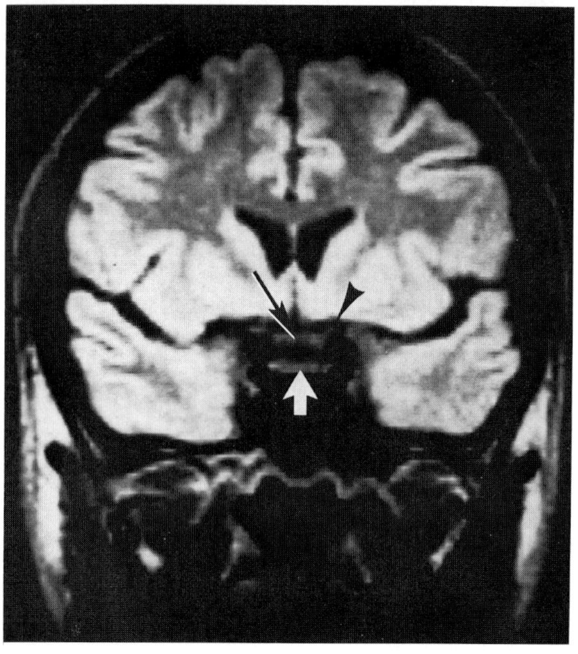

FIGURE 6-18

The optic chiasm (black arrow) and optic tract (arrowhead) are well seen on coronal images. Note also the pituitary gland (white arrow), which should be flat or concave on its upper surface.

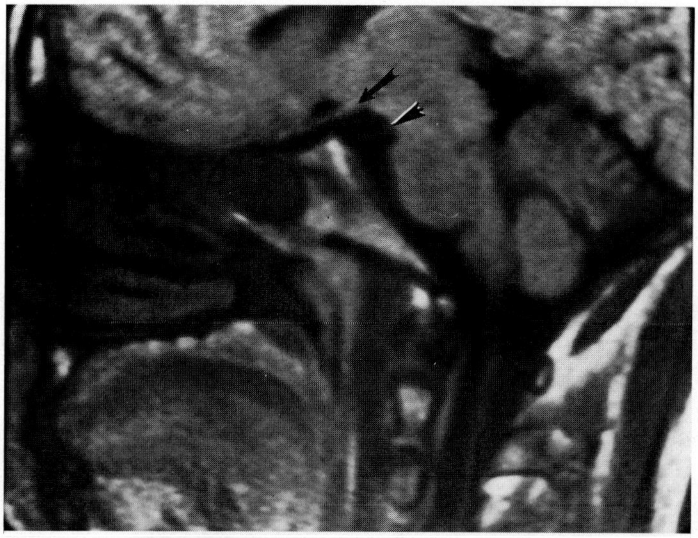

FIGURE 6-19

Sagittal SE 400/28 image demonstrates the optic tract (arrow) and oculomotor nerve (arrowhead). (Courtesy of Fonar Corp., 110 Marcus Drive, Melville, NY 11747)

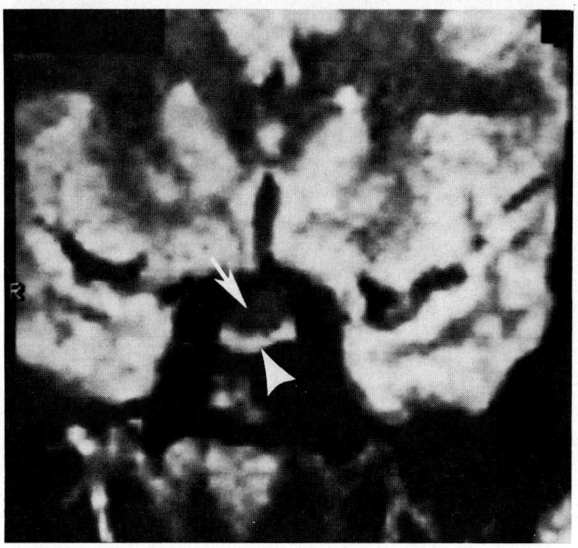

FIGURE 6-20

Empty sella filled with CSF (arrow). Note flattened pituitary gland (arrowhead) inferiorly.

neighboring vascular channels (*i.e.,* the cavernous sinus, carotid artery, and intrasellar blood vessels lateral to the gland).

The pituitary stalk or infundibulum is easily identified as a dot on axial images (Fig. 6-17*A*) or as a line on sagittal (Fig. 6-15) or coronal images (Fig. 6-17*B*). Above the infundibulum can be seen the optic chiasm and tract (Fig. 6-18). These structures may also be seen on sagittal images, as can the oculomotor nerves (Fig. 6-19). Often, CSF is seen to fill the sella and compress or distort the pituitary. An example of such an *empty sella* is shown in Figure 6-20.

The cavernous sinus is located lateral and slightly inferior to the sella turcica and contains the carotid artery and cranial nerves III through VI. The cavernous carotid artery can be seen on axial and coronal images as a tubular structure of low intensity (Fig. 6-21*A* and *C*). The coronal view allows visualization of the pituitary, infundibulum, and cavernous sinuses (Fig. 6-21*C*). Within the cavernous sinus it is possible to distinguish cranial nerve V and sometimes the other nerves as well (Fig. 6-21*B* and *C*).

The Brain Stem

With MR, a large number of brain stem structures that had never been imaged by any other modality are now visualized with MR. Some of these brain stem nuclei, tracts, and structures can be directly imaged, whereas others can only be identified by virtue of their external contours against CSF. These brain stem structures now revealed by MRI are listed in Table 6-3. Additionally, about 6 of the 12 cranial nerves may at times be visualized in an appropriate MR plane. These are listed in Table 6-4.

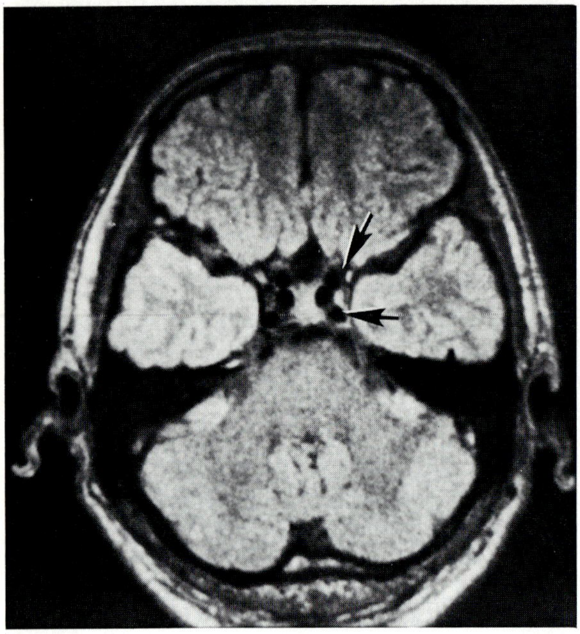

A

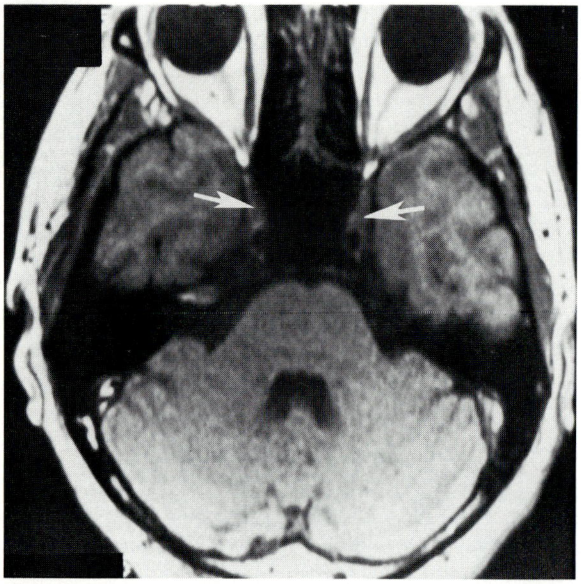

B

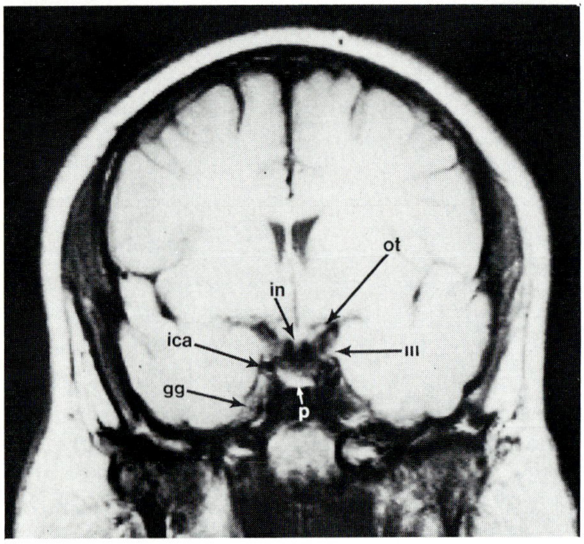

C

FIGURE 6-21

The cavernous sinus. (*A*) Axial section demonstrates the cavernous portion of the internal carotid artery (arrows) flanking the pituitary gland. (*B*) Lower level shows cranial nerve V in the cavernous sinus (arrows). (Figures 6-21*A* and 6-21*B* courtesy of Fonar Corporation, 110 Marcus Drive, Melville, NY 11747). (*C*) Coronal image demonstrates a number of anatomic structures: in = infundibulum; ot = optic tract; III = oculomotor nerve (cranial nerve III); p = pituitary gland; gg = gasserian ganglion; ica = internal carotid artery. (Courtesy of Technicare Corporation; © 1985)

TABLE 6-3

MRI of Brain Stem Nuclei and Tracts

Midbrain	
Corticospinal tract	Seen on ventral surface of midbrain silhouetted against CSF on axial view (Fig. A-12)
Coliculi, superior and inferior	Seen posteriorly on sagittal images; difficult to distinguish superior from inferior colliculi on axial images (Figs. A-7, S-8, S-9, S-10)
Medial lemniscus	Especially well seen on sagittal view; may be identified on axial images (Fig. S-10)
Substantia nigra	Routinely imaged on T2-weighted axial or coronal views (Fig. C-8)
Red nucleus	Low intensity area near substantia nigra (Figs. A-8, C-8, S-10)
Pons	
Cerebellar peduncles (superior and middle)	Best seen on axial or coronal images (Figs. A-9, A-10, C-9, S-4)
Medulla	
Cerebellar peduncle (inferior)	Axial or coronal (Fig. A-11)
Olivary nucleus	Coronal or sagittal (Fig. C-9)
Gracile nucleus	Sagittal images, on posterior medulla silhouetted against CSF (Fig. S-10)

TABLE 6-4

Imaging of Cranial Nerves by MR

I.	Olfactory	Occasionally seen on coronal images only in the olfactory groove. (Fig. C-4)
II.	Optic	Routinely visualized in all planes (Figs. 6-18, A-9, C-2, C-3, S-9)
III.	Oculomotor	Occasionally seen on near midline sagittal images (Fig. 6-19)
IV.	Trochlear	Not visualized
V.	Trigeminal	Trigeminal ganglion often seen in Meckel's cave on axial or coronal (Figs. A-9, A-10, 6-21)
VI.	Abducens	Not visualized
VII.	Facial	Routinely seen on sagittal and coronal images together with cranial nerve VIII in the internal auditory canal (Figs. C-7, S-3)
VIII.	Vestibulocochlear	See VII
IX.	Glossopharyngeal	Not routinely visualized
X.	Vagus	Not routinely visualized
XI.	Spinal accessory	Not routinely visualized
XII.	Hypoglossal	Occasionally seen in hypoglossal canal on axial images through the foramen magnum (Fig. A-13)

ATLAS

Because of the large amount of anatomic detail, the following full-page illustrations are presented as a multiplanar atlas of the human brain. Space does not allow each section of brain to be presented using every type of pulse sequence or combination of imaging parameters. Usually the pulse sequence and parameters that would be most typical or demonstrate anatomy best are presented. Where appropriate, either T1-weighted or T2-weighted images will be shown. Where there is confusion or significant variance between the structures revealed by these techniques, both will be used.

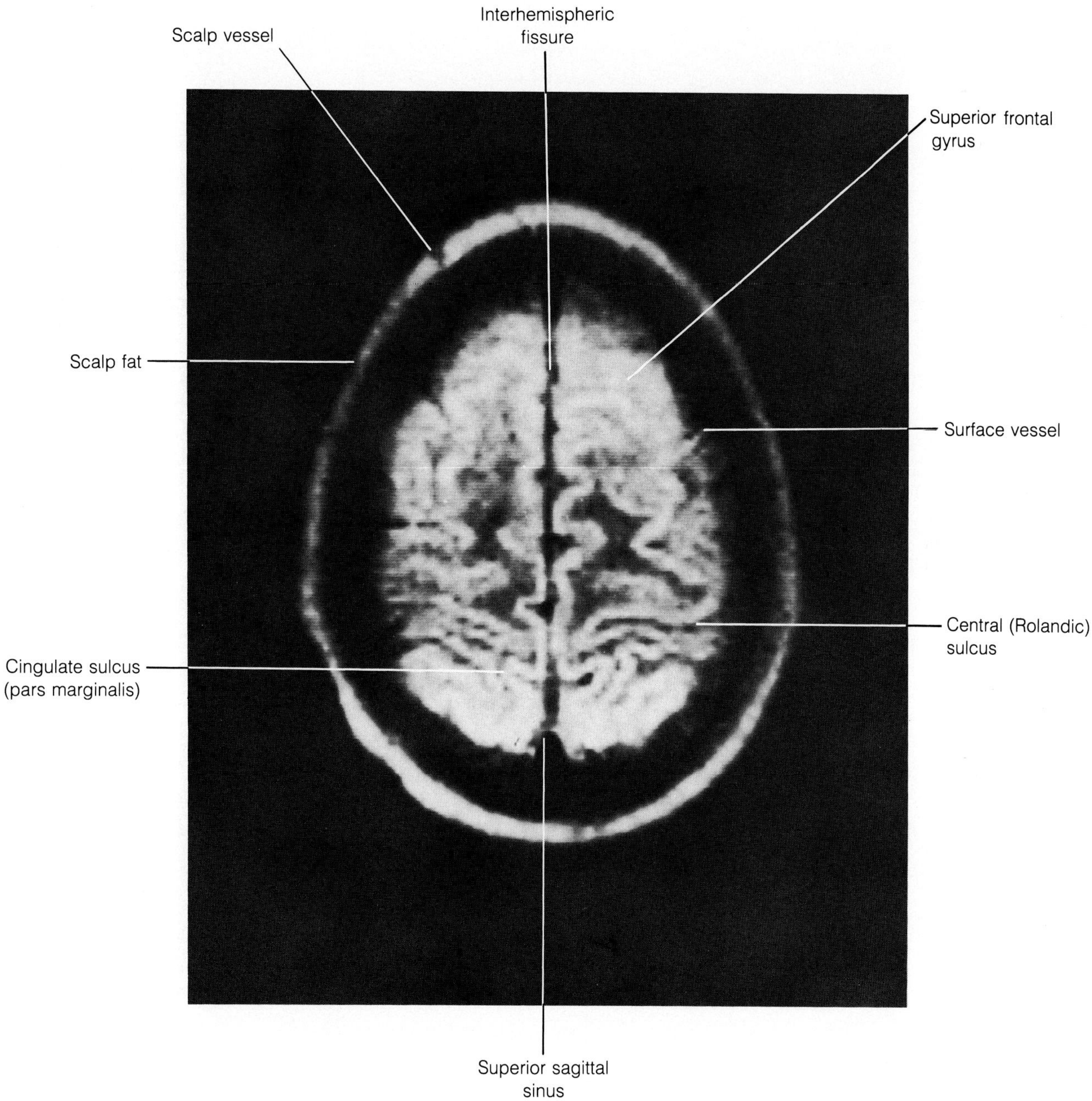

FIGURE A-1

Axial SE 2000/28 image near the skull vertex.

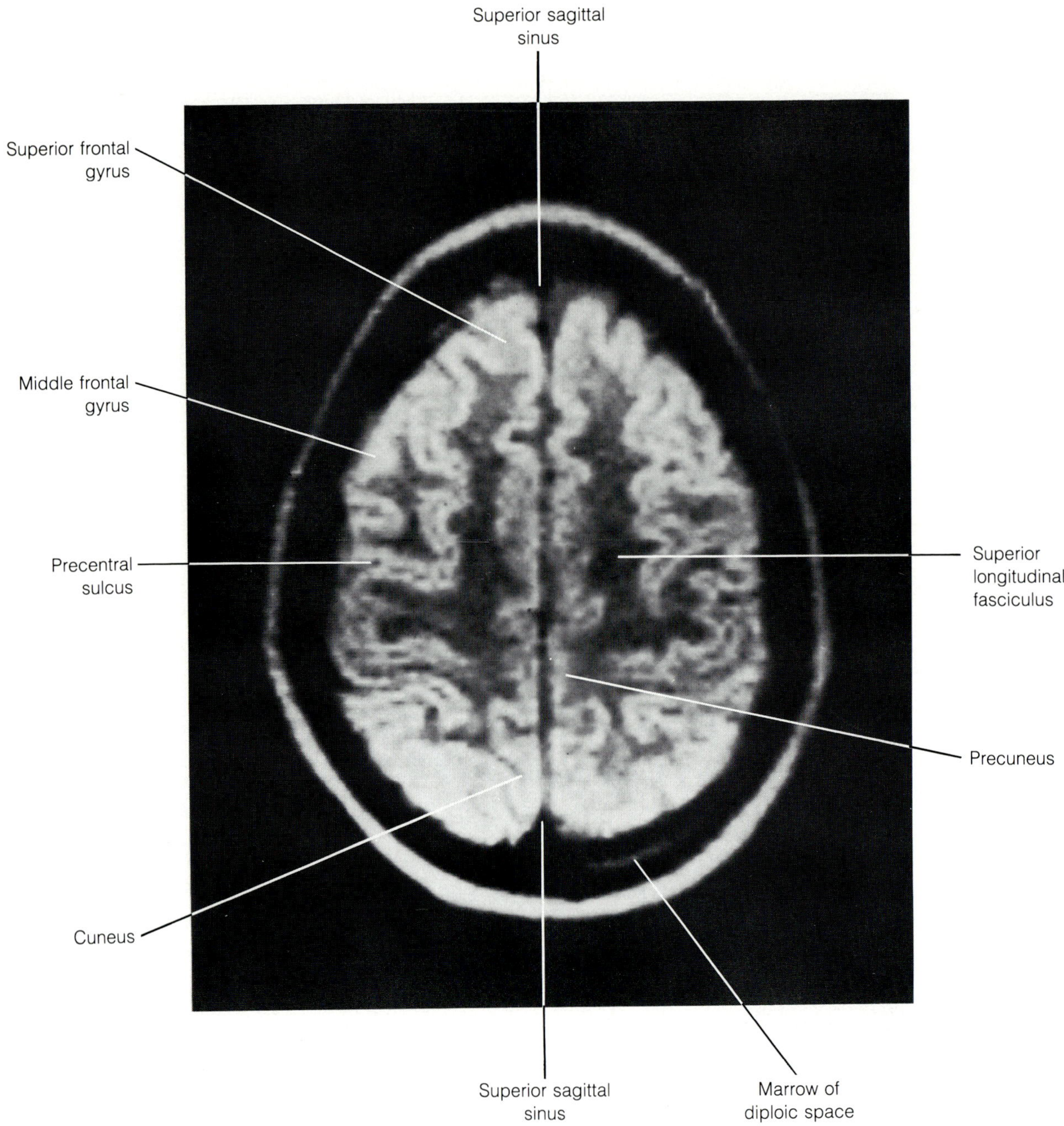

FIGURE A-2

Axial SE 2000/28 image through the upper head 1 cm caudal to Figure A-1.

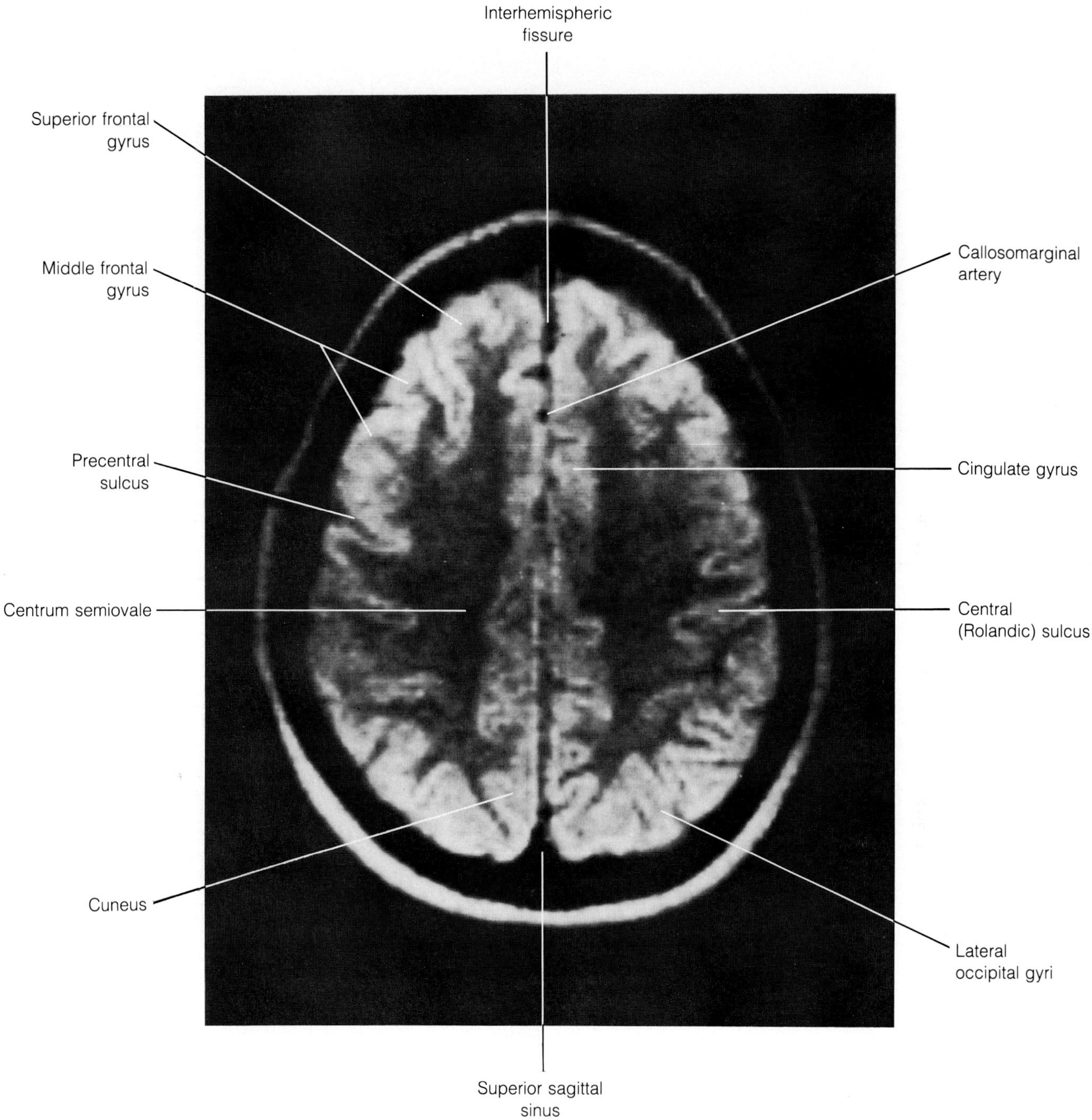

FIGURE A-3

Axial SE 2000/28 image 1 cm caudal to Figure A-2. Note the good differentiation of gray matter and white matter with this technique.

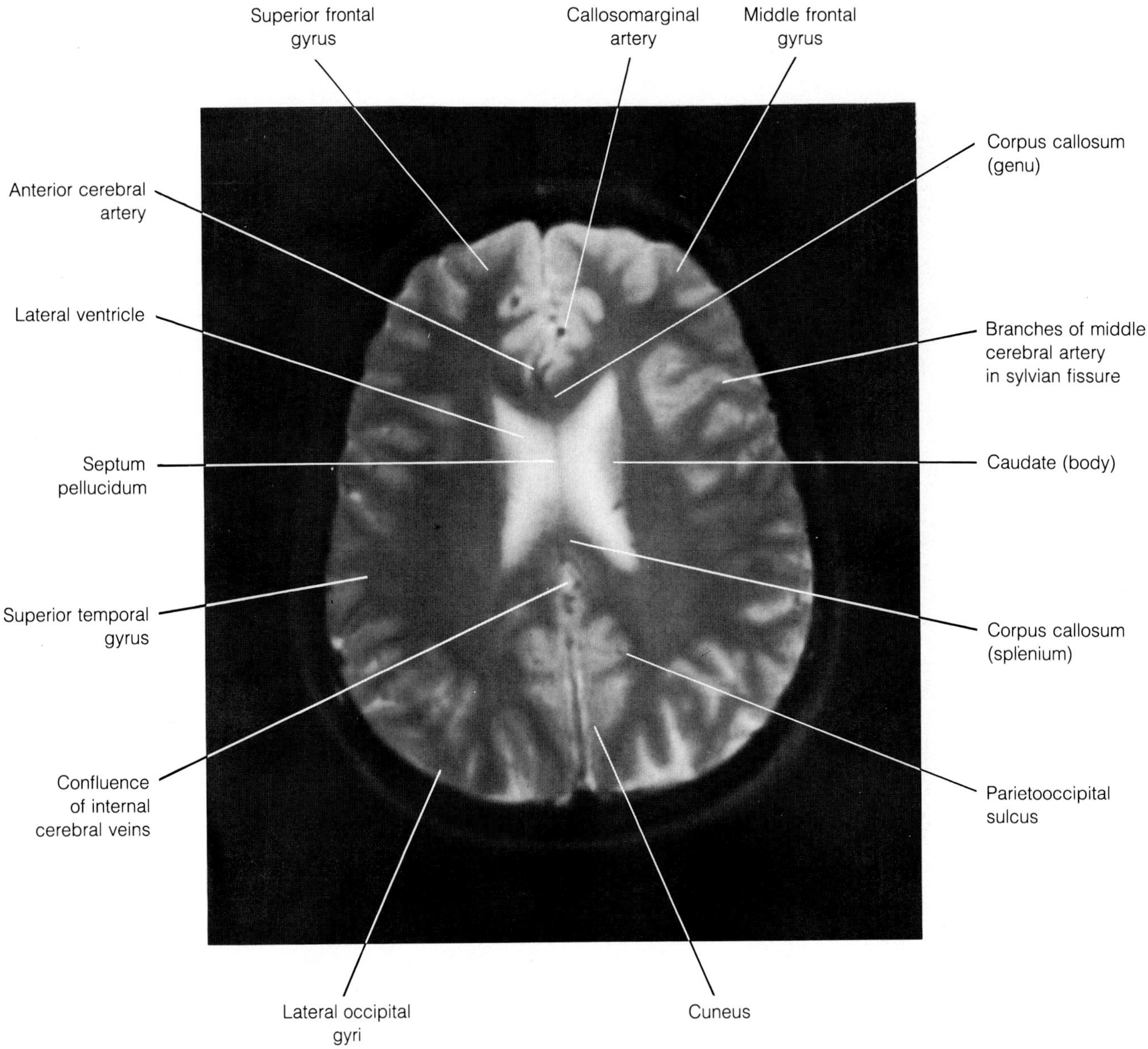

FIGURE A-4

Axial SE 3000/60 produces a heavily T2-weighted image through a plane about 1 cm caudal to Figure A-3. Note intensely white CSF in the sulci and lateral ventricles. (Courtesy of Siemens)

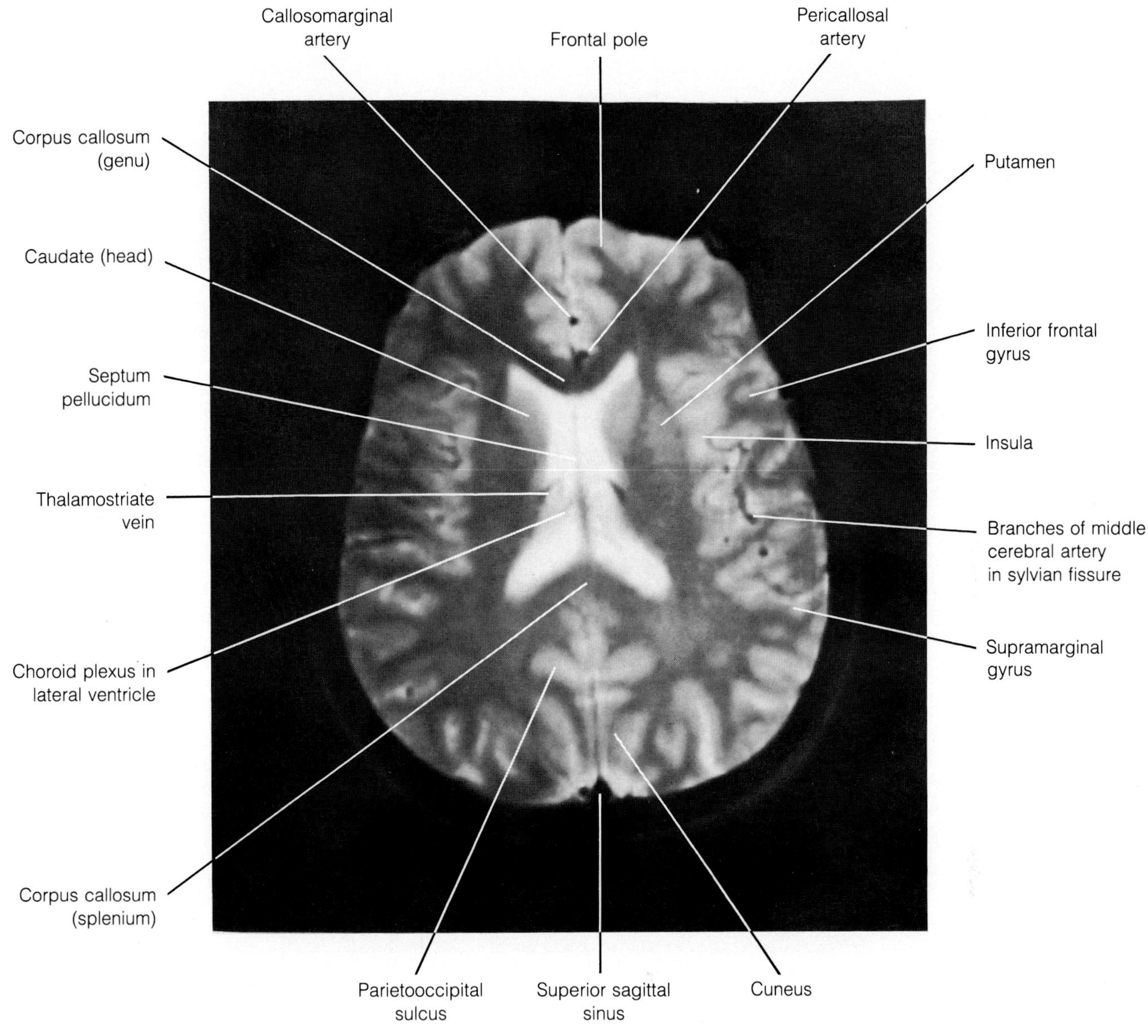

FIGURE A-5

Axial SE 3000/60 image 1 cm caudal to Figure A-4. Blood vessels in the fissures and ventricles are well seen with this technique. (Courtesy of Siemens)

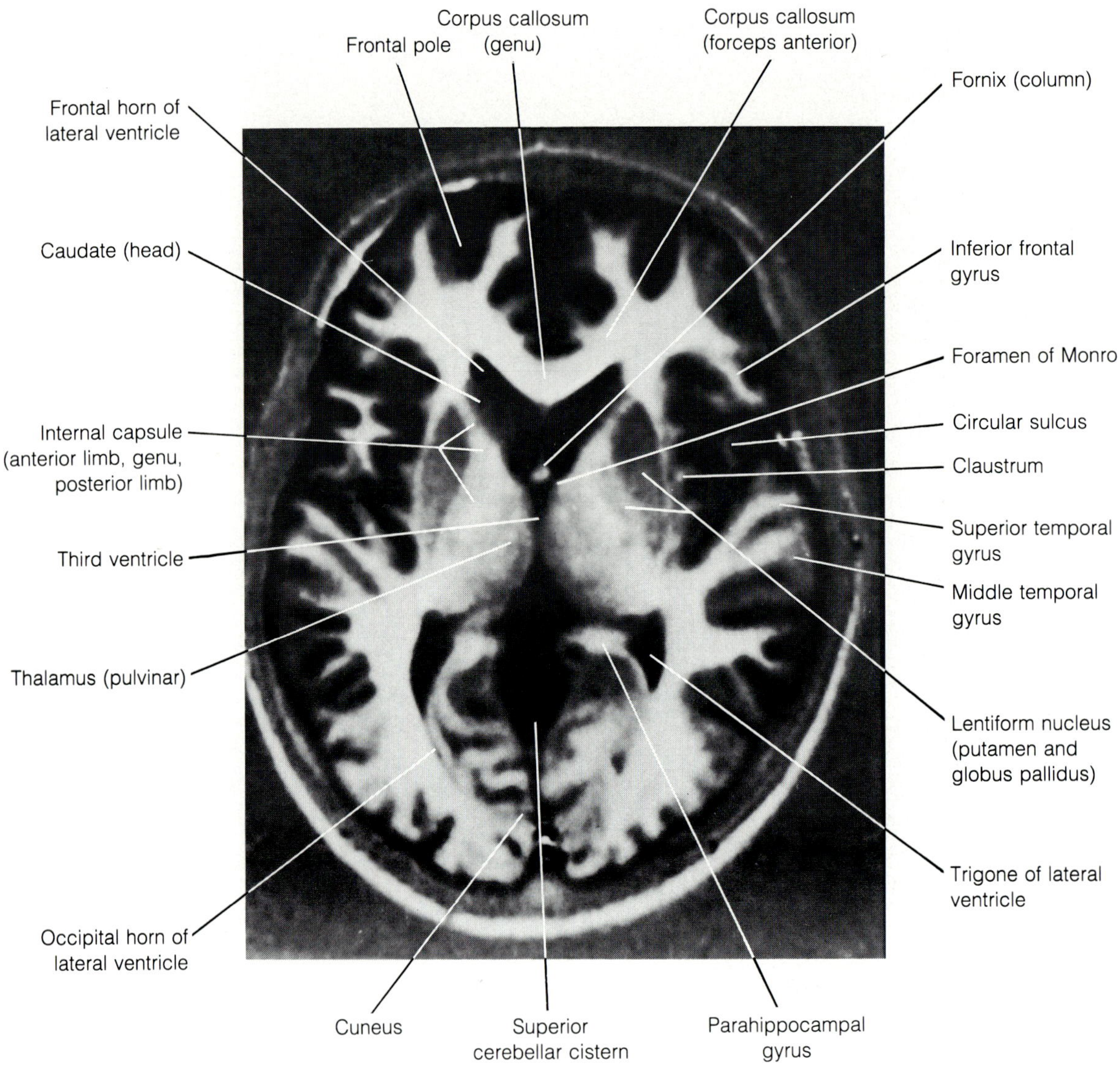

FIGURE A-6

IR 2500/400/43 technique provides superb gray–white differentiation in this axial section at the midthalamic level. (Courtesy of Siemens)

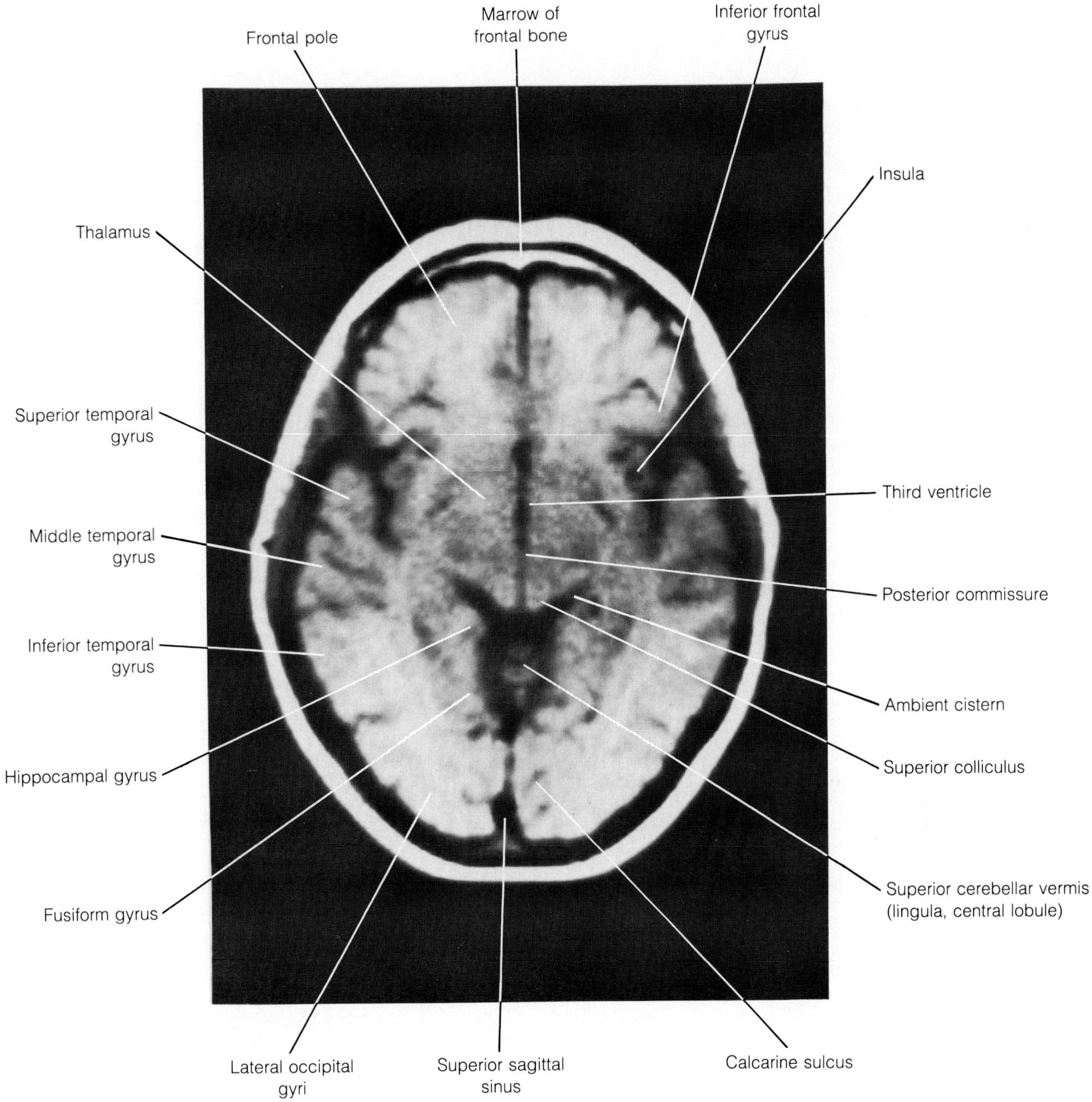

FIGURE A-7

Axial SE 500/28 image through the brain about 1 cm caudal to Figure A-6. With this technique, gray matter–white matter differentiation is lost but good contrast is noted between brain and CSF-containing spaces.

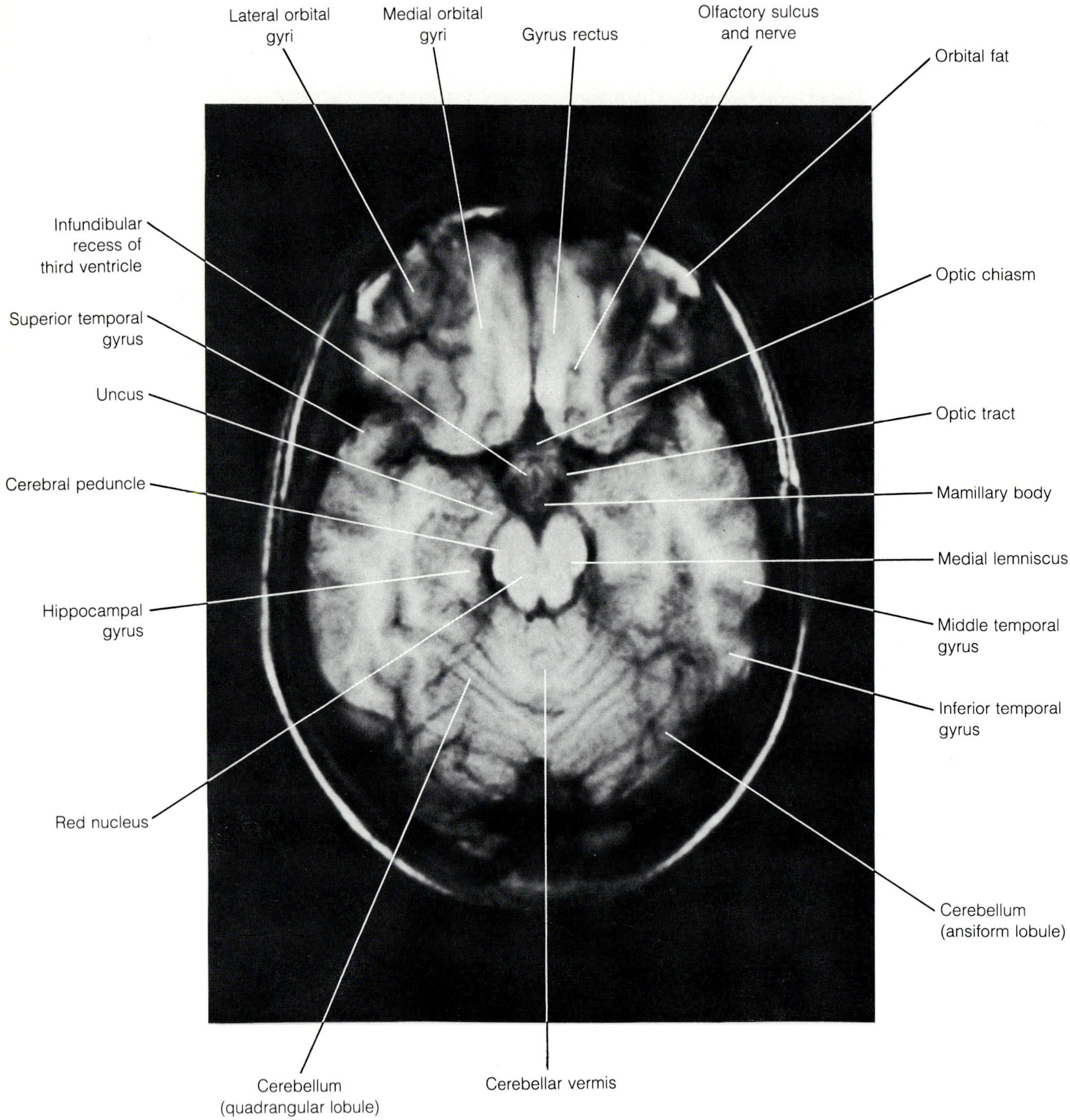

FIGURE A-8

Axial SE 500/40 image 1 cm caudal to Figure A-7 through the lower midbrain. (Courtesy of Picker International, Clinical Sciences Center)

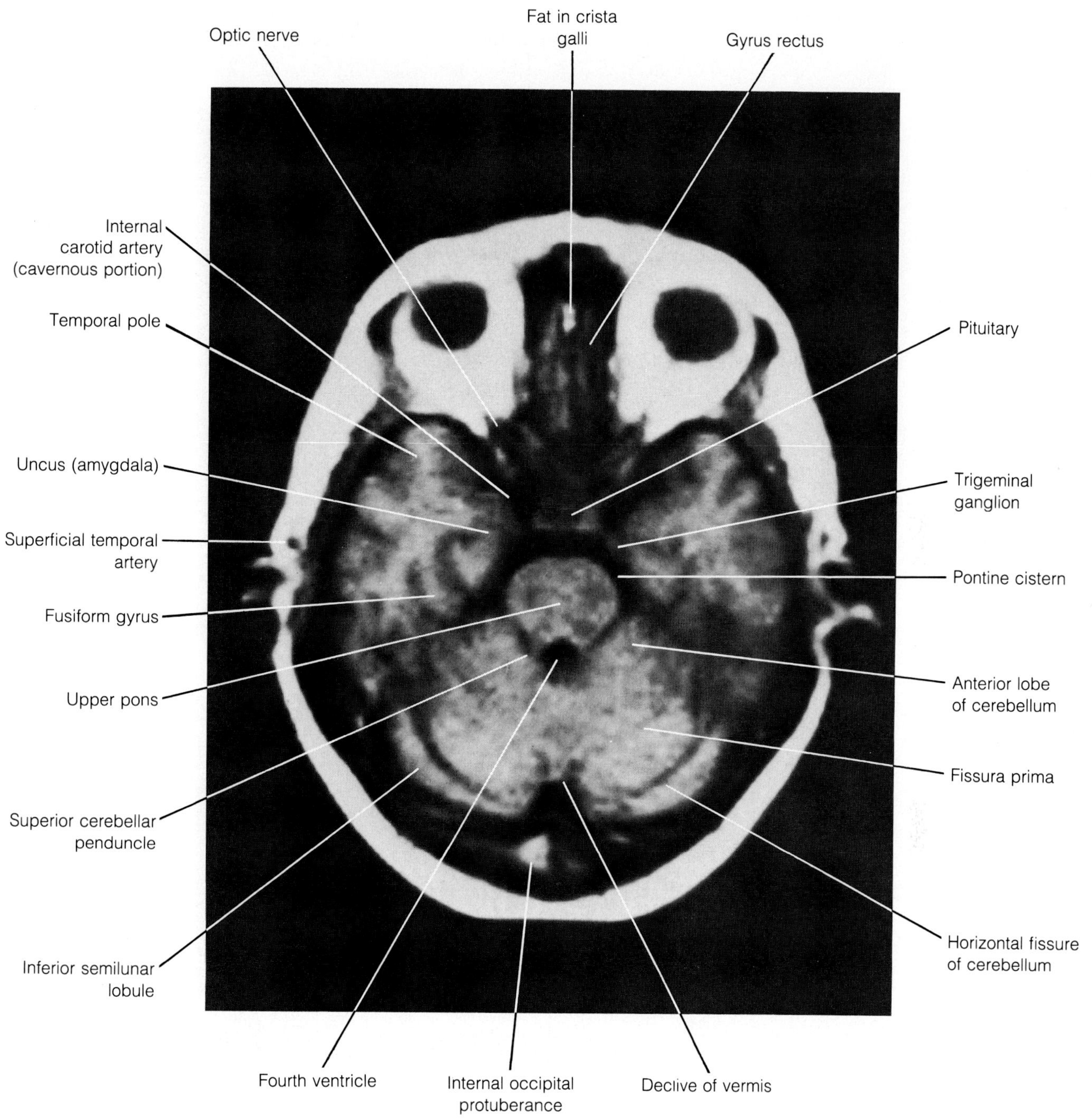

FIGURE A-9

Axial SE 500/28 image 1 cm caudal to Figure A-8. Detailed views of the orbit and optic chiasm appear in Chapter 7.

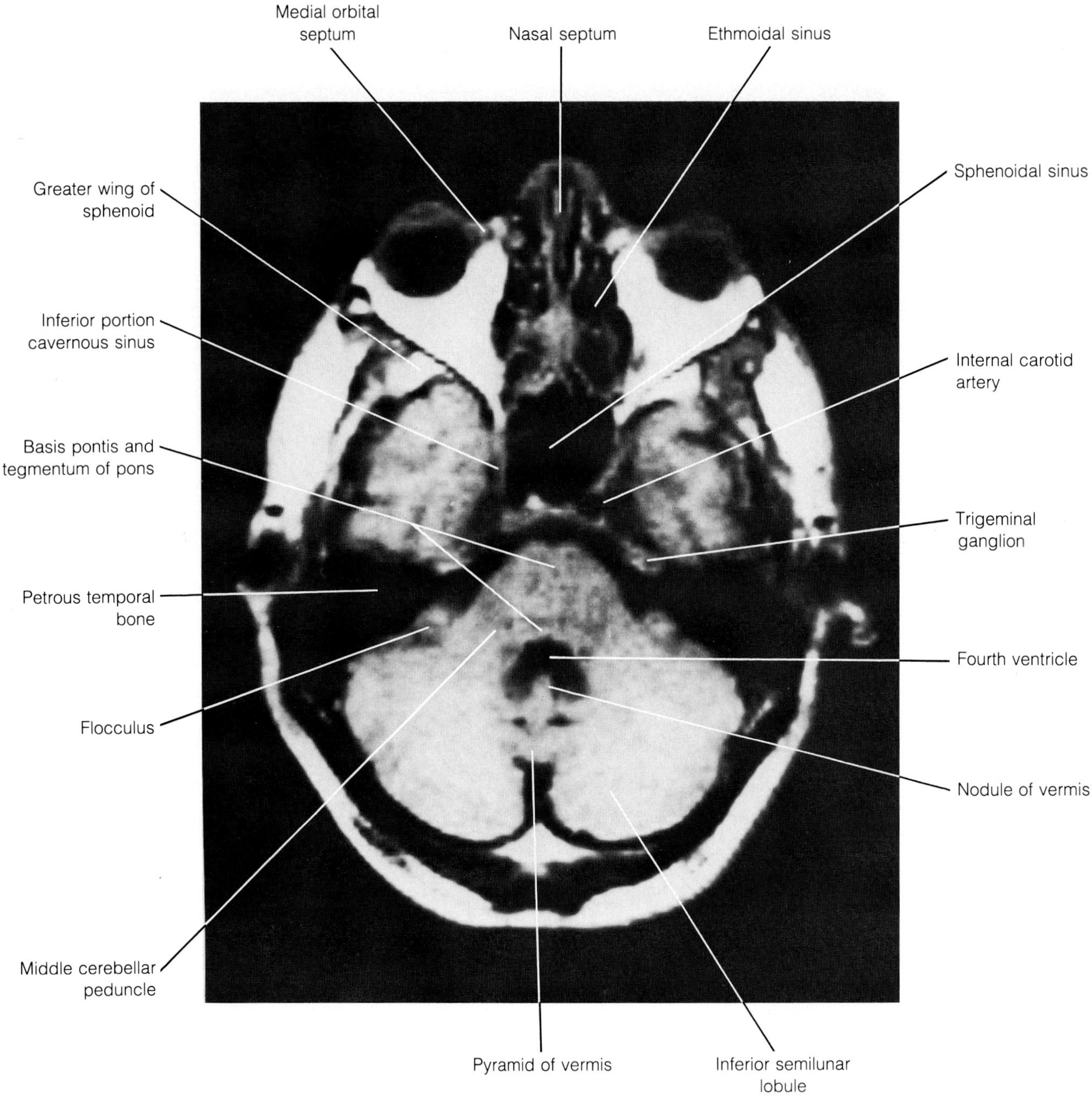

FIGURE A-10

Axial SE 500/28 image 1 cm caudal to Figure A-9.

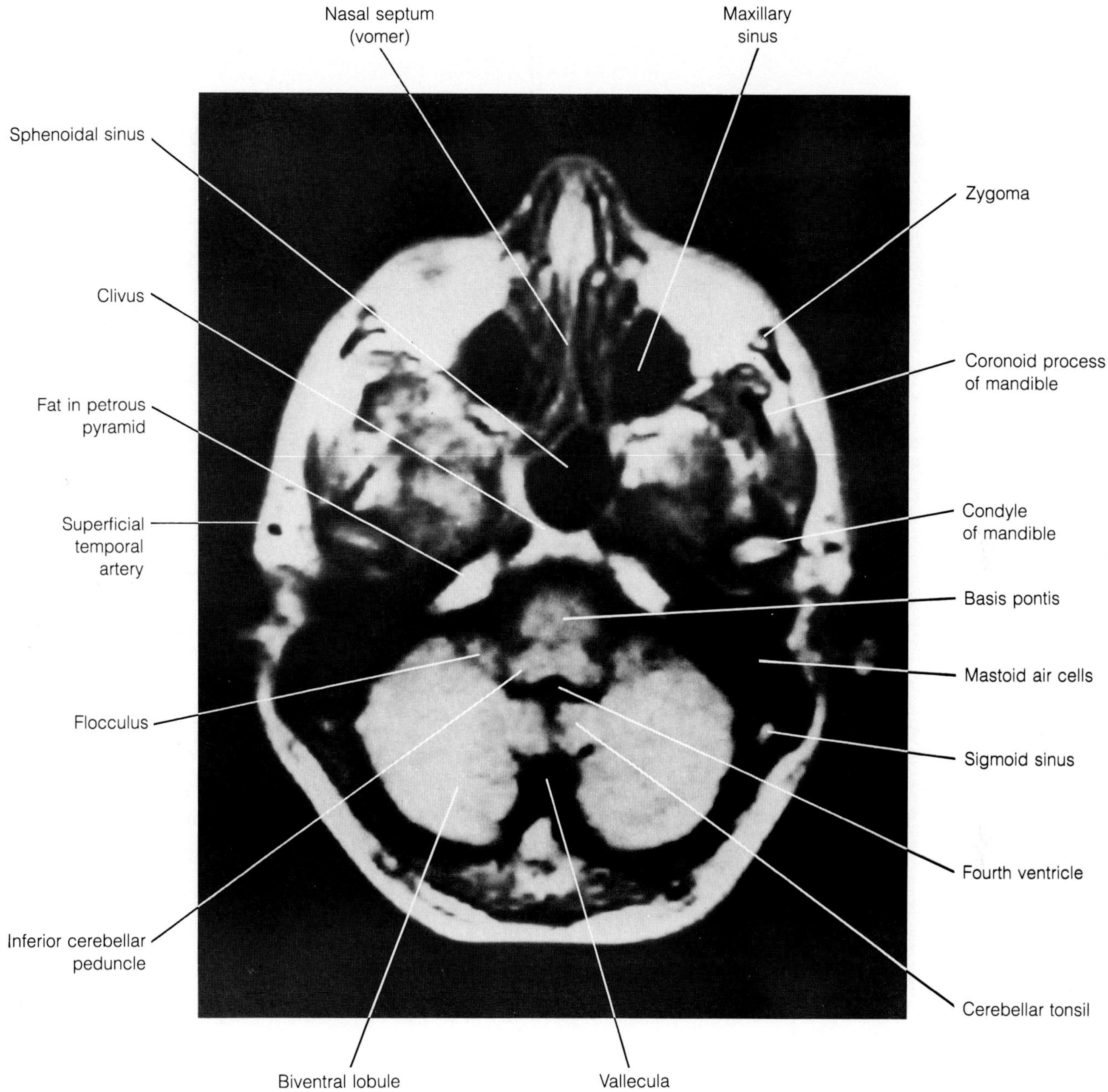

FIGURE A-11

Axial SE 500/28 section 1 cm caudal to Figure A-10. Note good delineation of posterior fossa and brain stem structures.

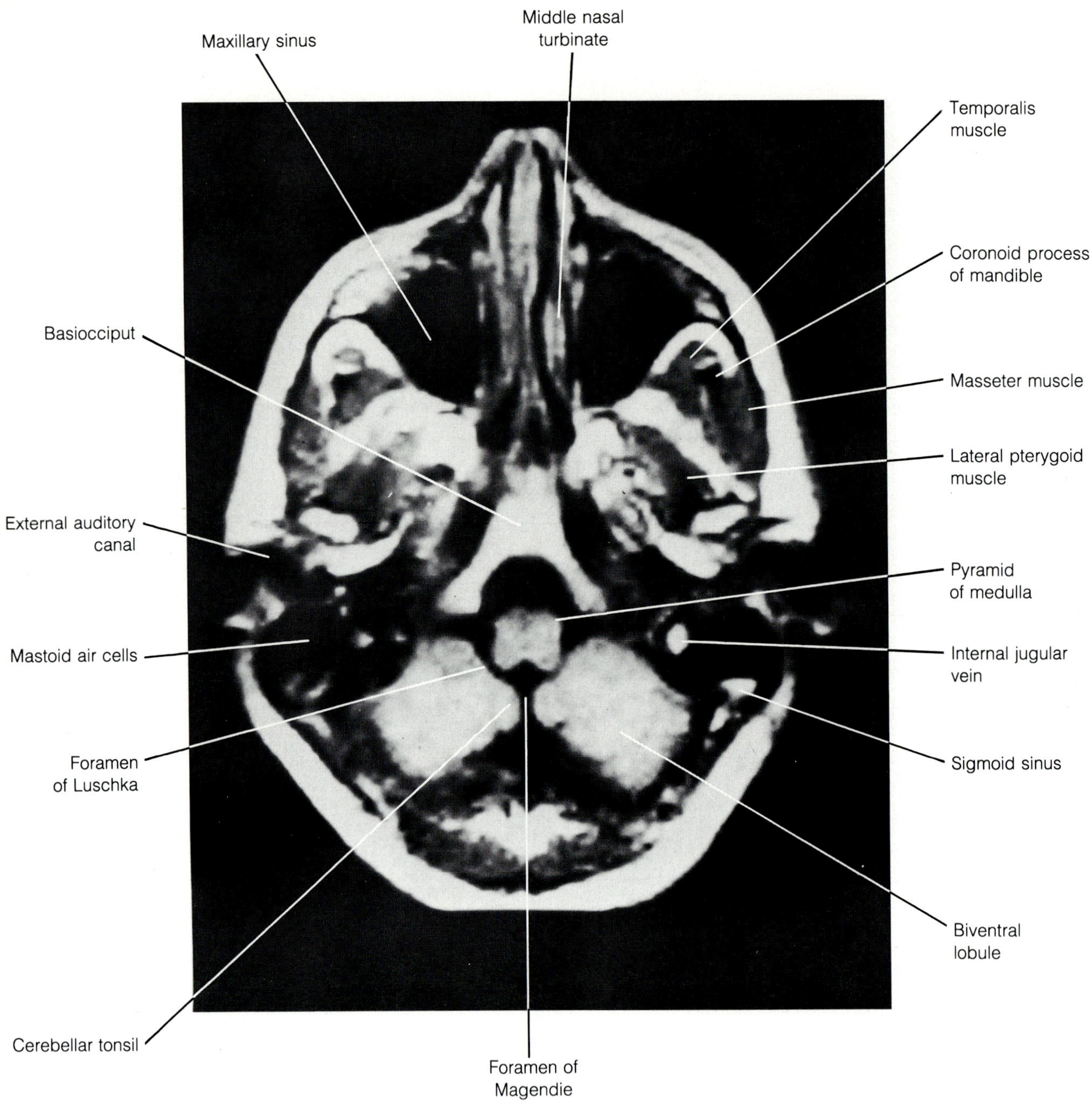

FIGURE A-12

Axial SE 500/28 image through the lower medulla.

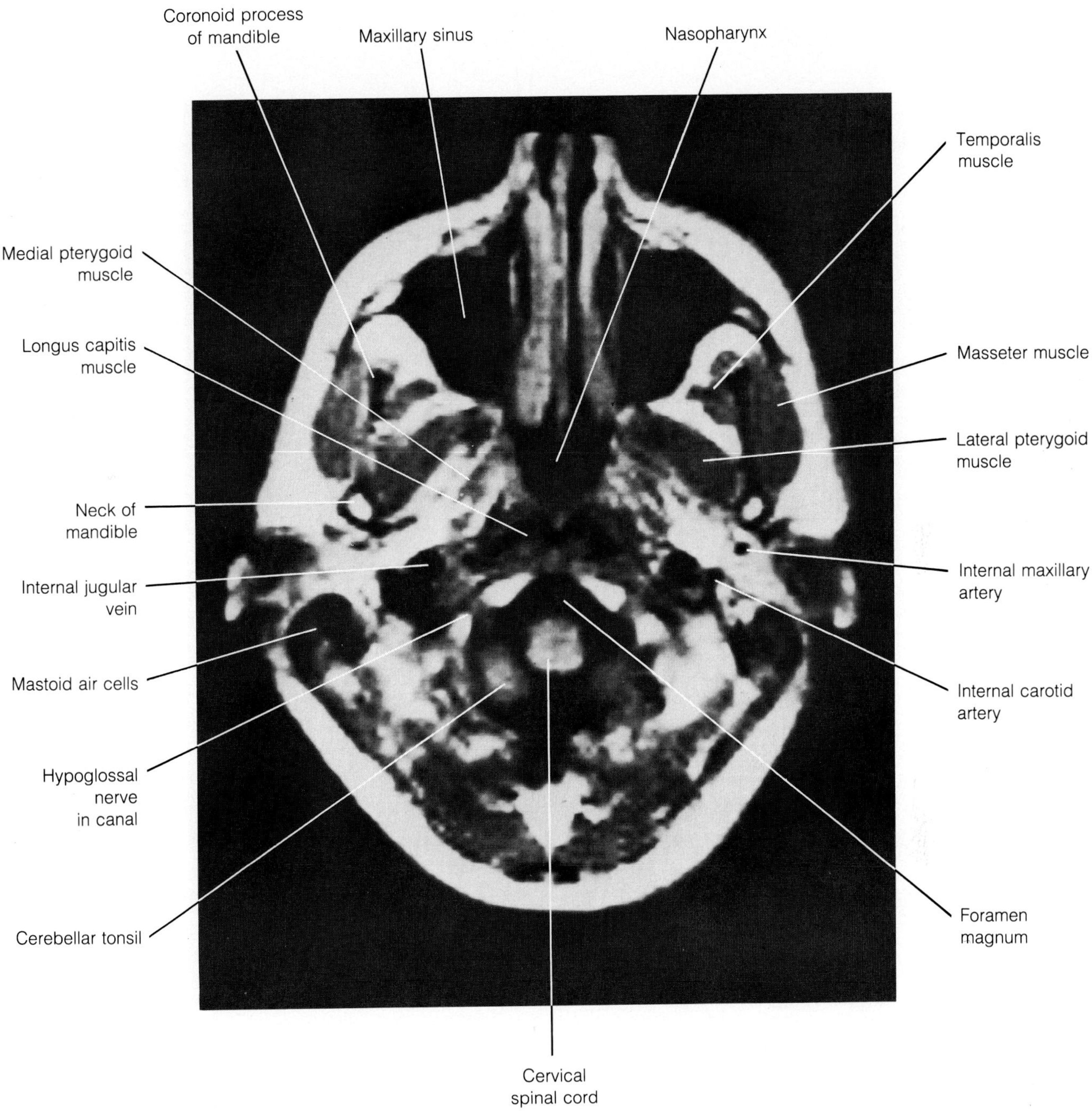

FIGURE A-13

Axial SE 500/28 image 1 cm caudal to Figure A-12 shows cervical cord with cerebellar tonsil tips as the only remaining parts of the CNS now seen.

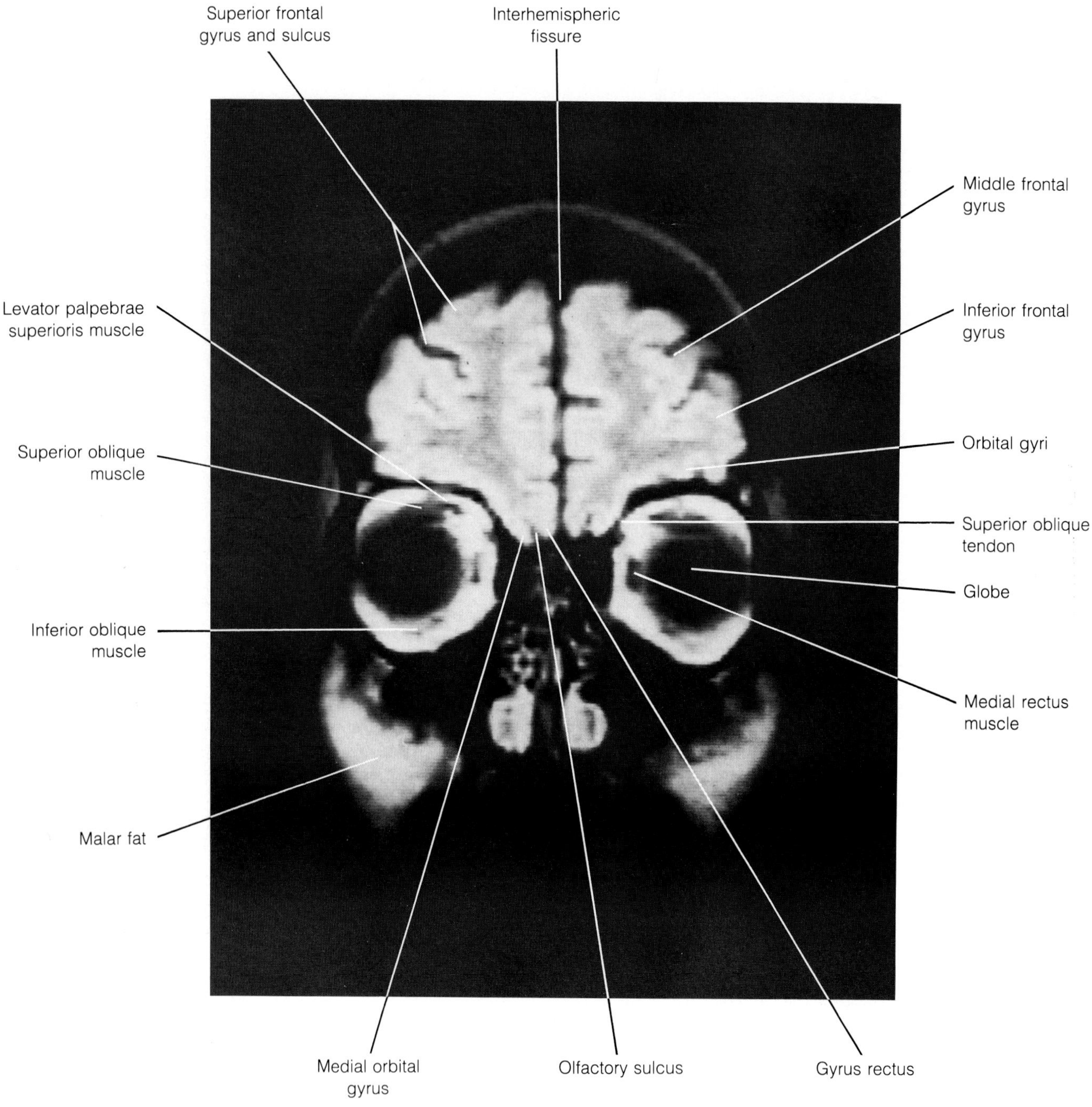

FIGURE C-1

Coronal SE 1500/28 image through the orbits and frontal lobes. Detailed orital anatomy is shown in Chapter 7.

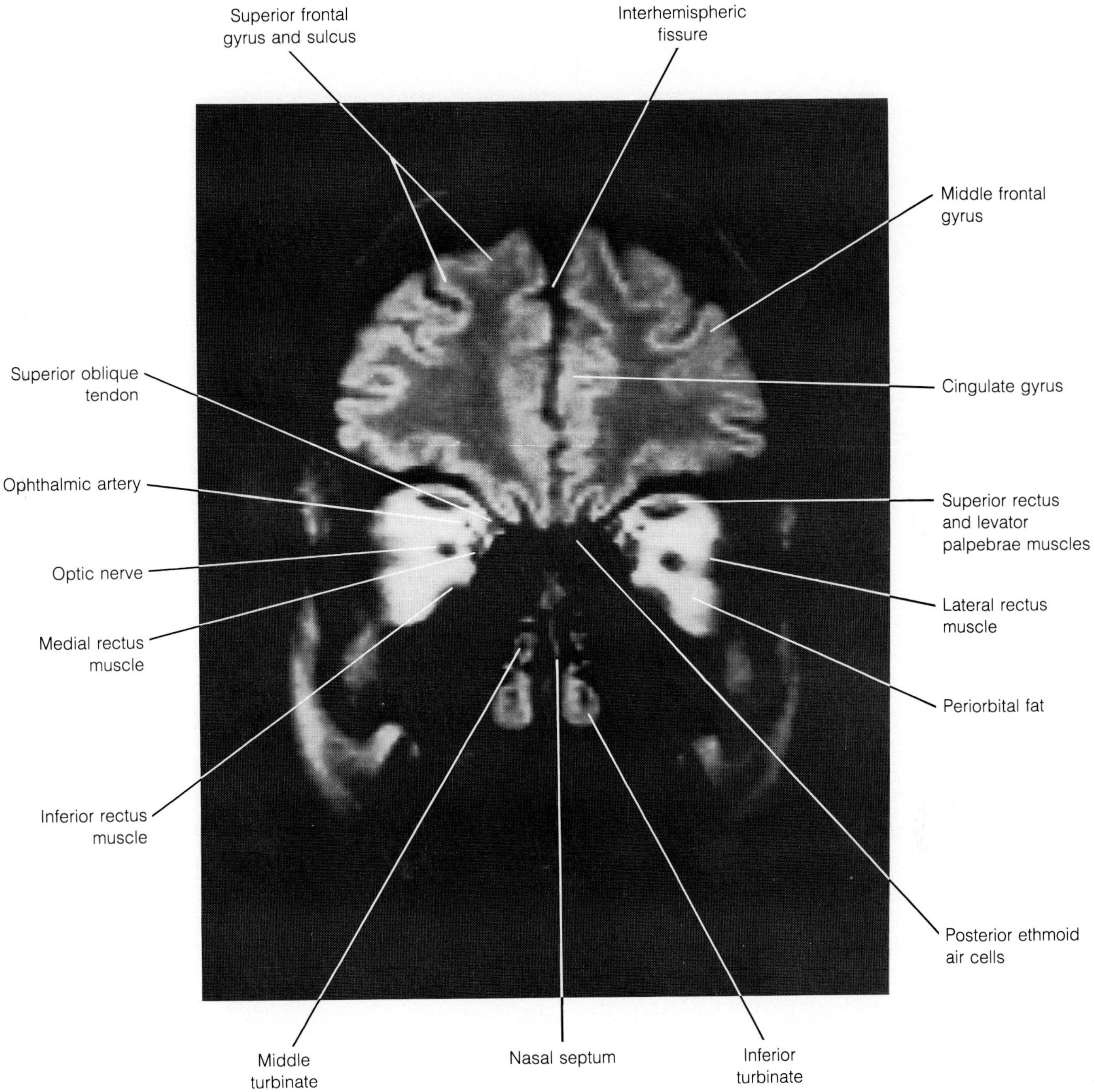

FIGURE C-2

Coronal SE 1500/28 image 1 cm posterior to Figure C-1.

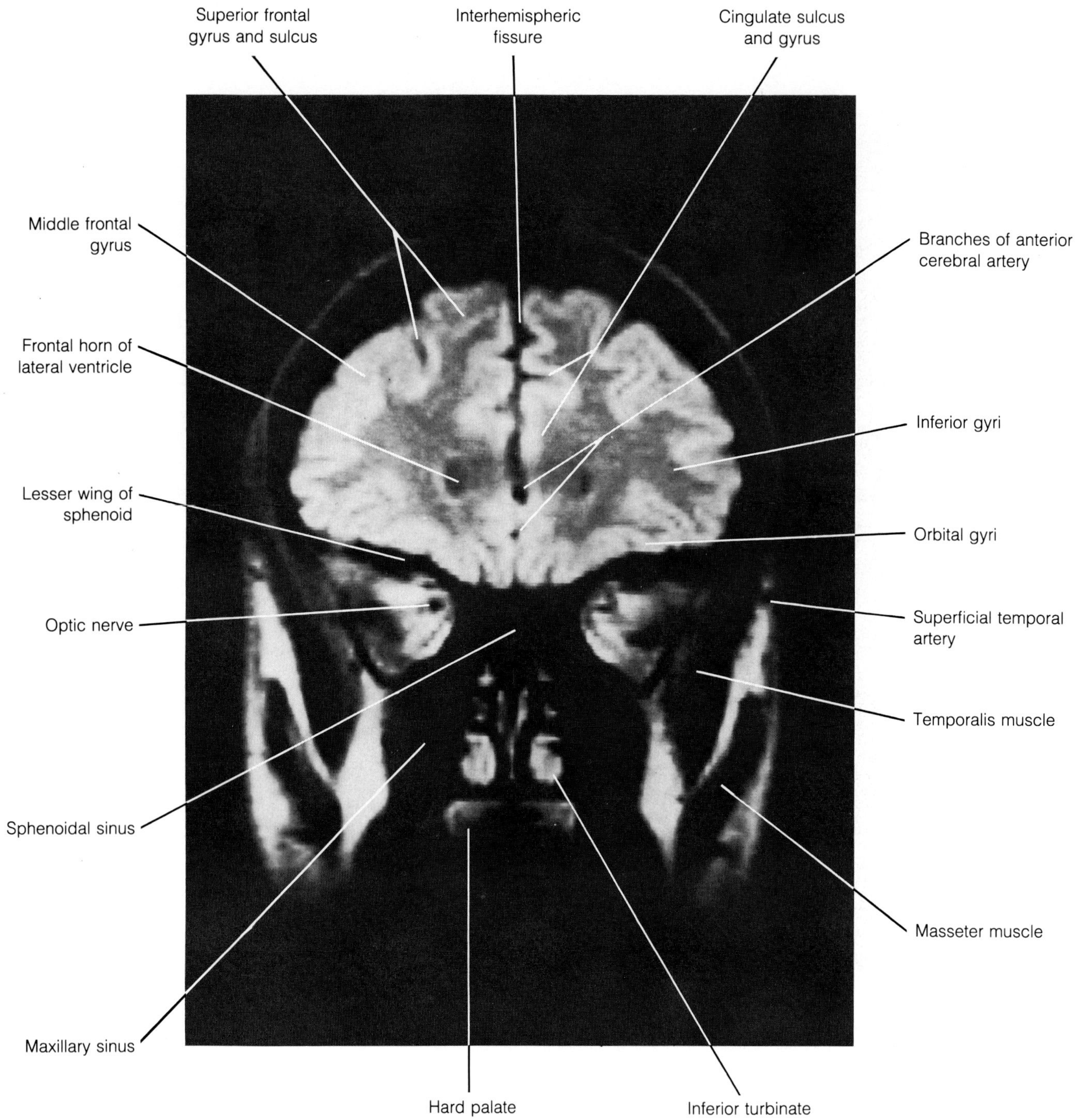

FIGURE C-3

Coronal SE 1500/28 image 1 cm posterior to Figure C-2.

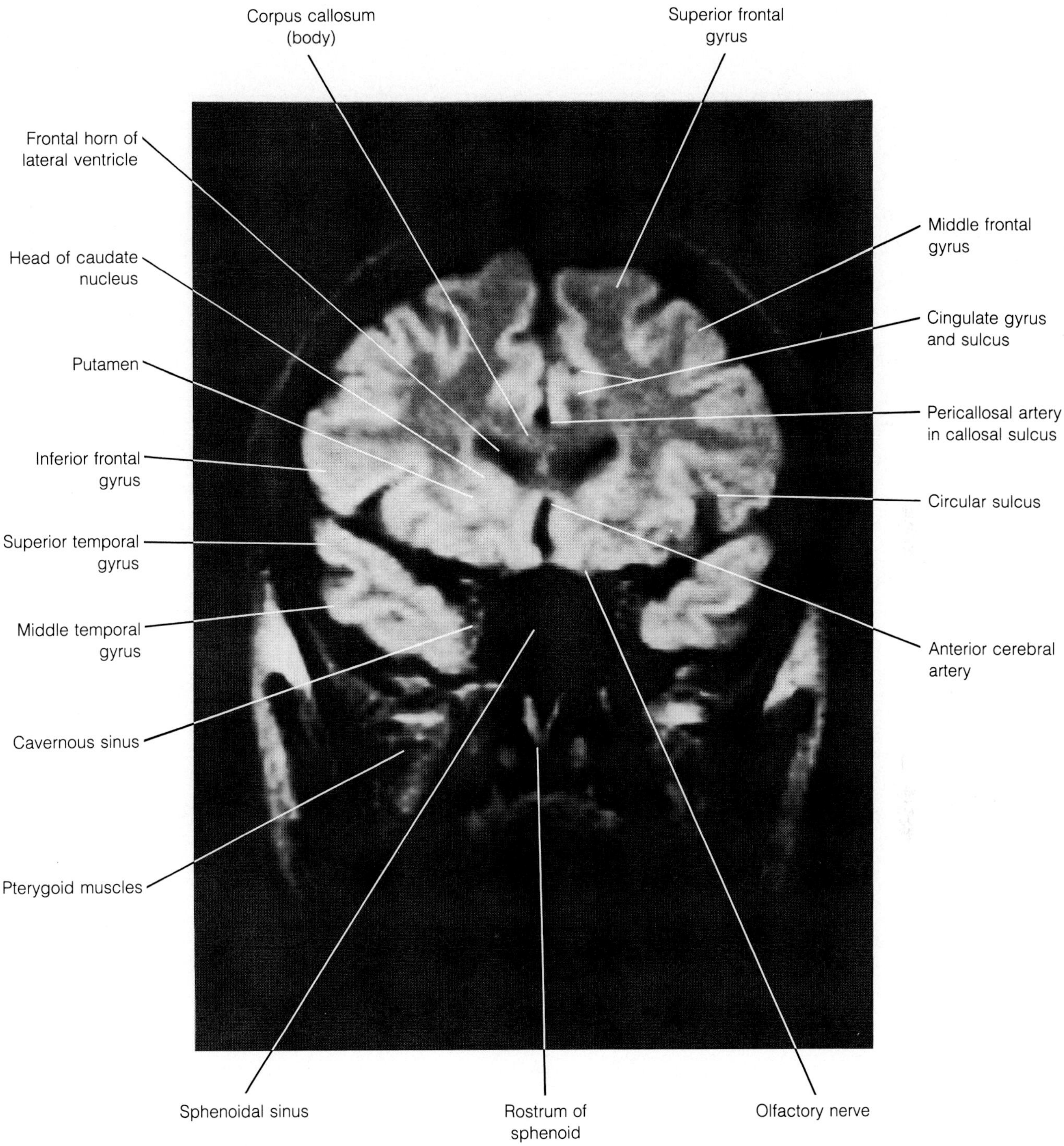

FIGURE C-4

Coronal SE 1500/28 image 1 cm posterior to Figure C-3.

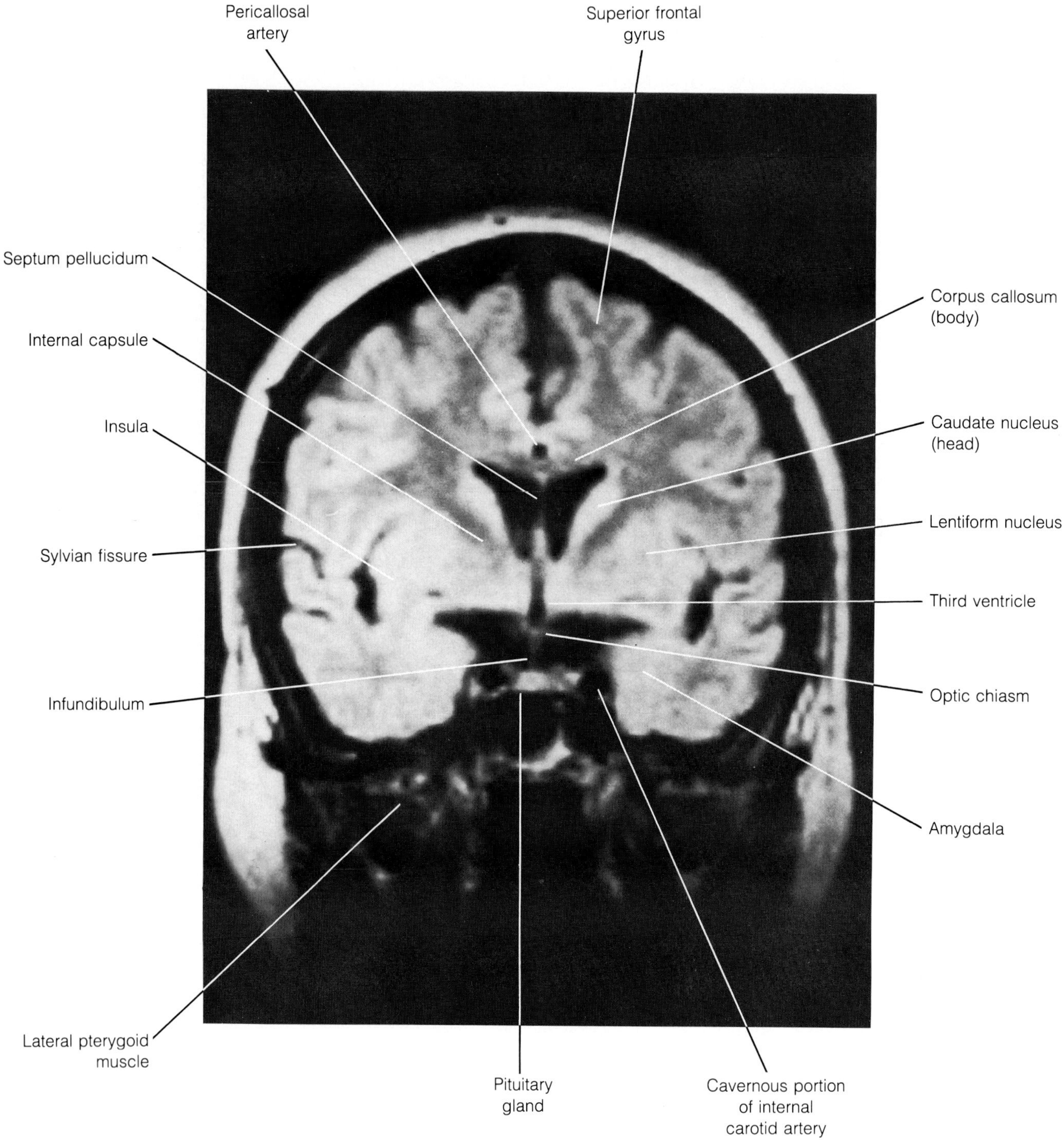

FIGURE C-5

Coronal SE 1500/28 image through the sella. Further details of this region are found earlier in this chapter.

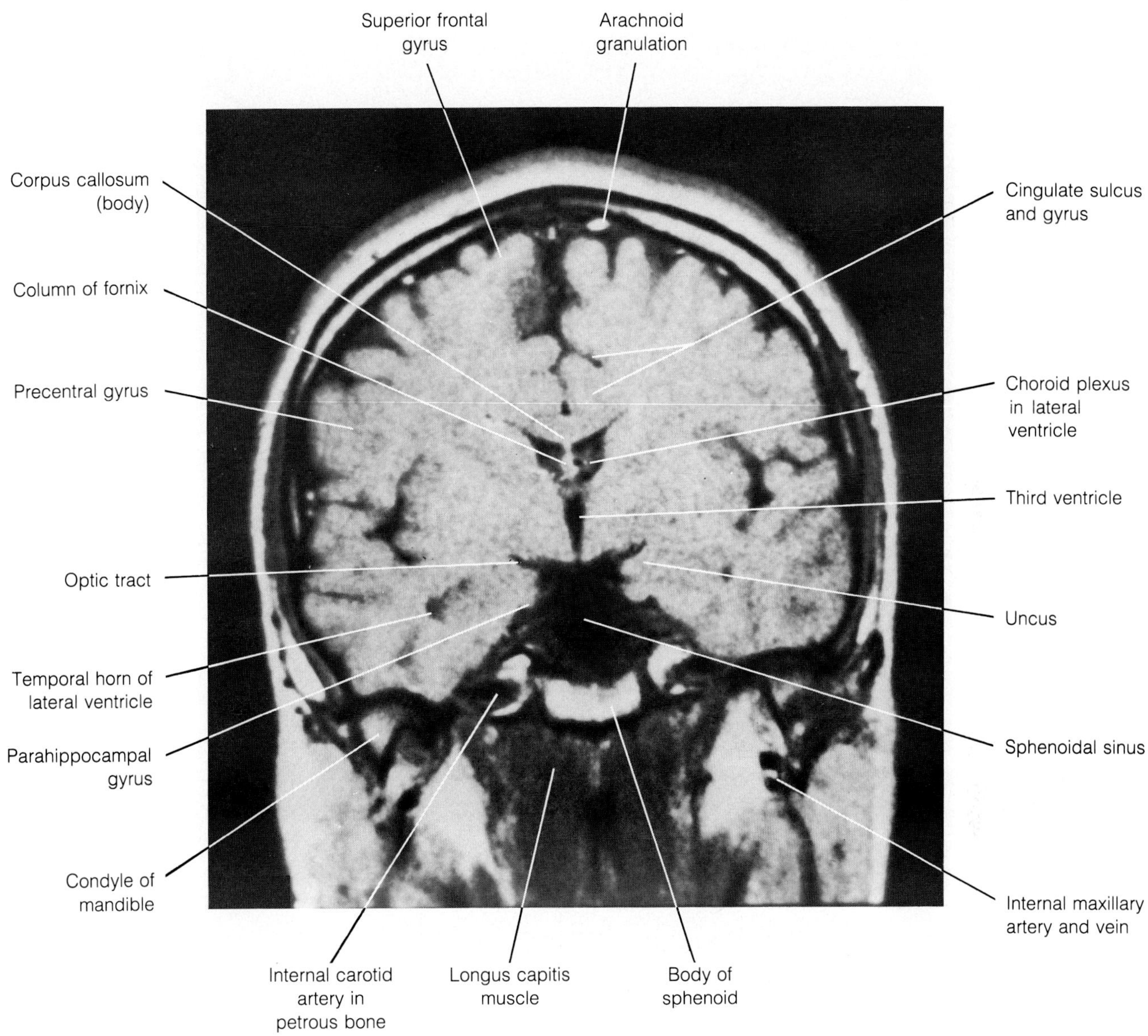

FIGURE C-6

Coronal SE 400/28 image 1 cm posterior to Figure C-5 demonstrates similar anatomy in a T1-weighted format. (Courtesy of Fonar Corp., 110 Marcus Drive, Melville, NY 11747)

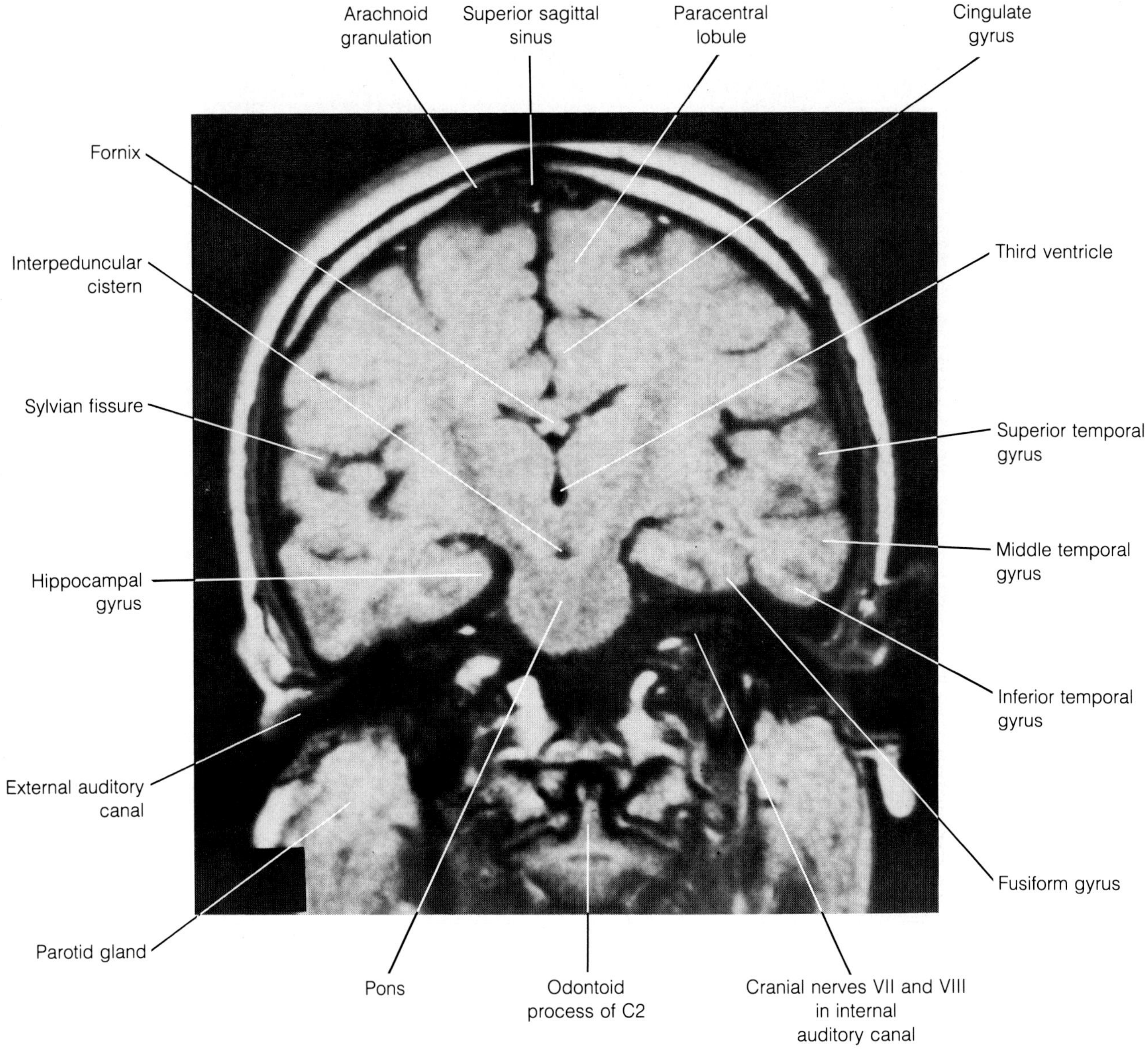

FIGURE C-7

Coronal SE 400/28 image through the midpons, about 1 cm posterior to Figure C-6. (Courtesy of Fonar Corp., 110 Marcus Drive, Melville, NY 11747)

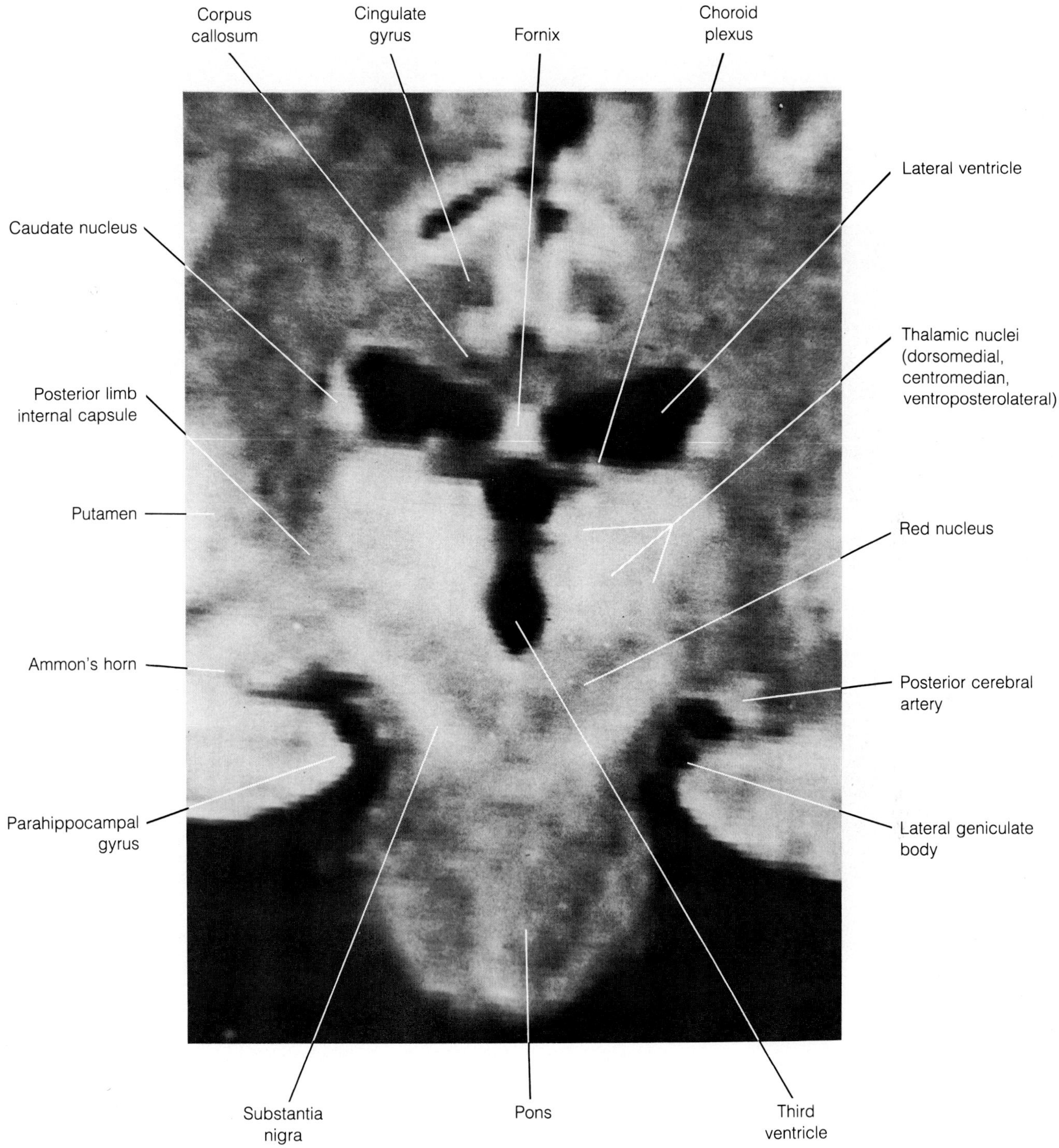

FIGURE C-8

Magnified SE 1500/28 coronal image through the midbrain near the same level shown in Figure C-7.

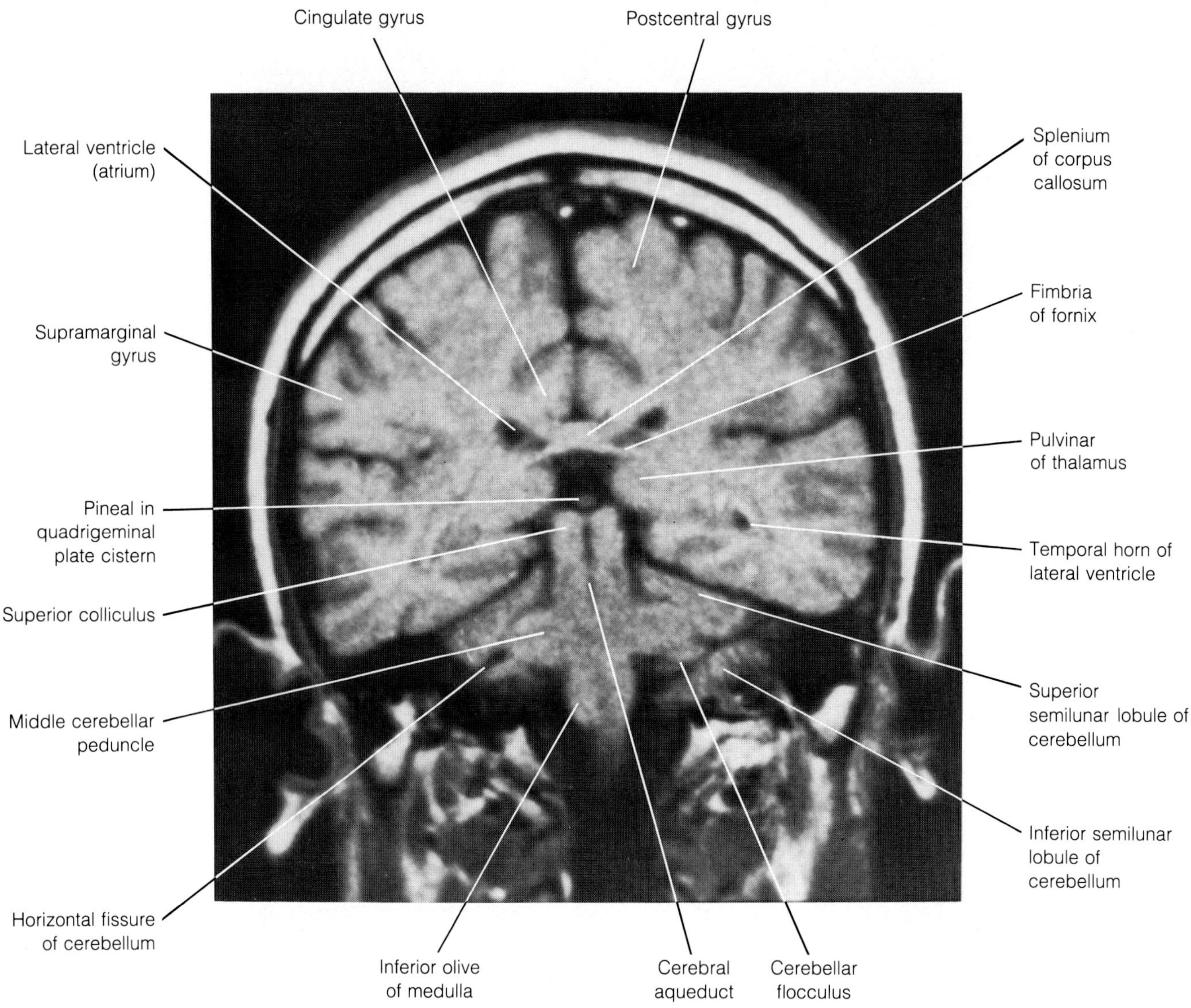

FIGURE C-9

Coronal SE 400/28 section about 1 cm posterior to Figures C-7 and C-8, through the pineal and dorsal brain stem. (Courtesy of Fonar Corp., 110 Marcus Drive, Melville, NY 11747)

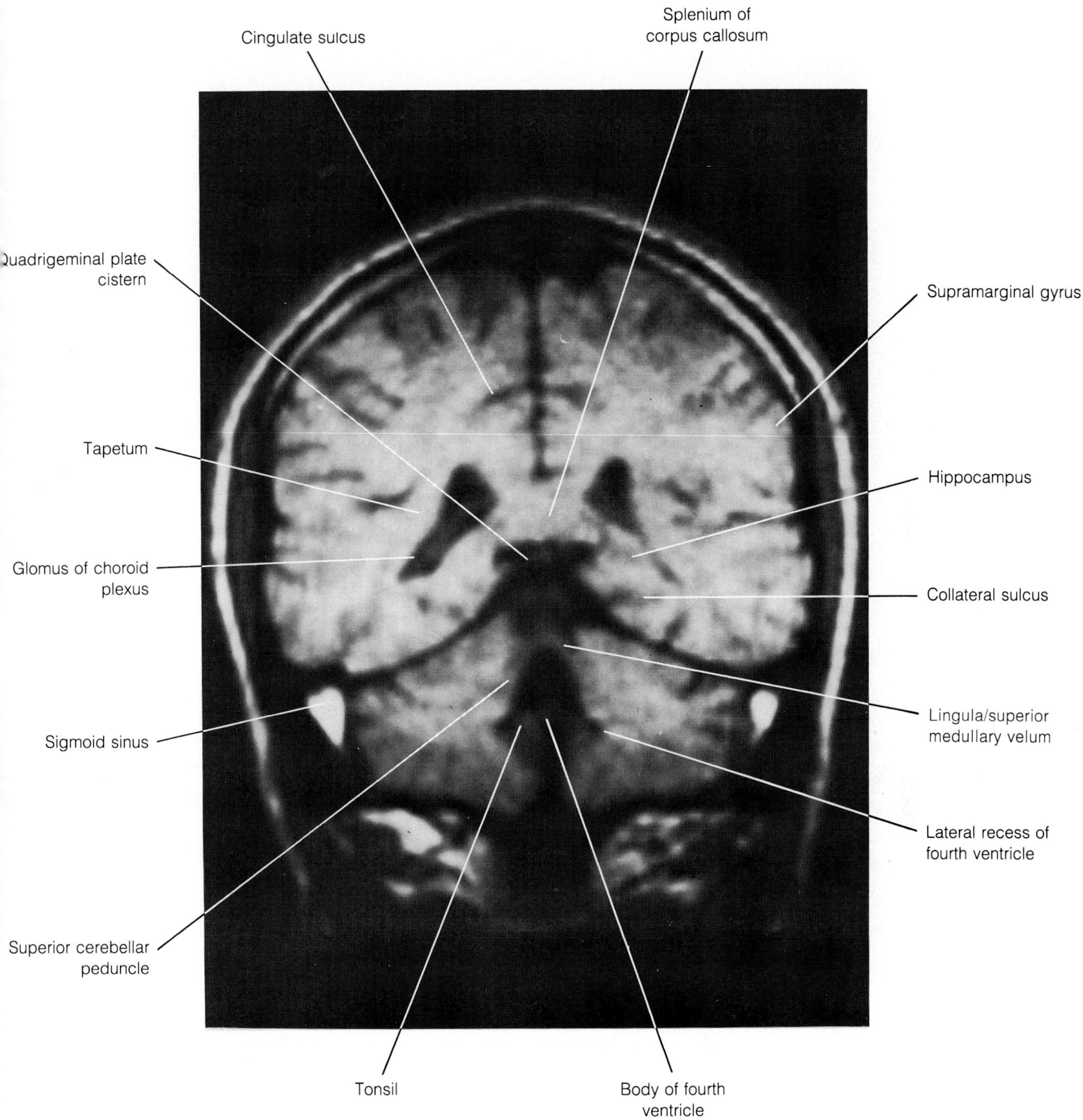

FIGURE C-10

Coronal SE 500/28 image about 1 cm posterior to Figure C-9, through the fourth ventricle.

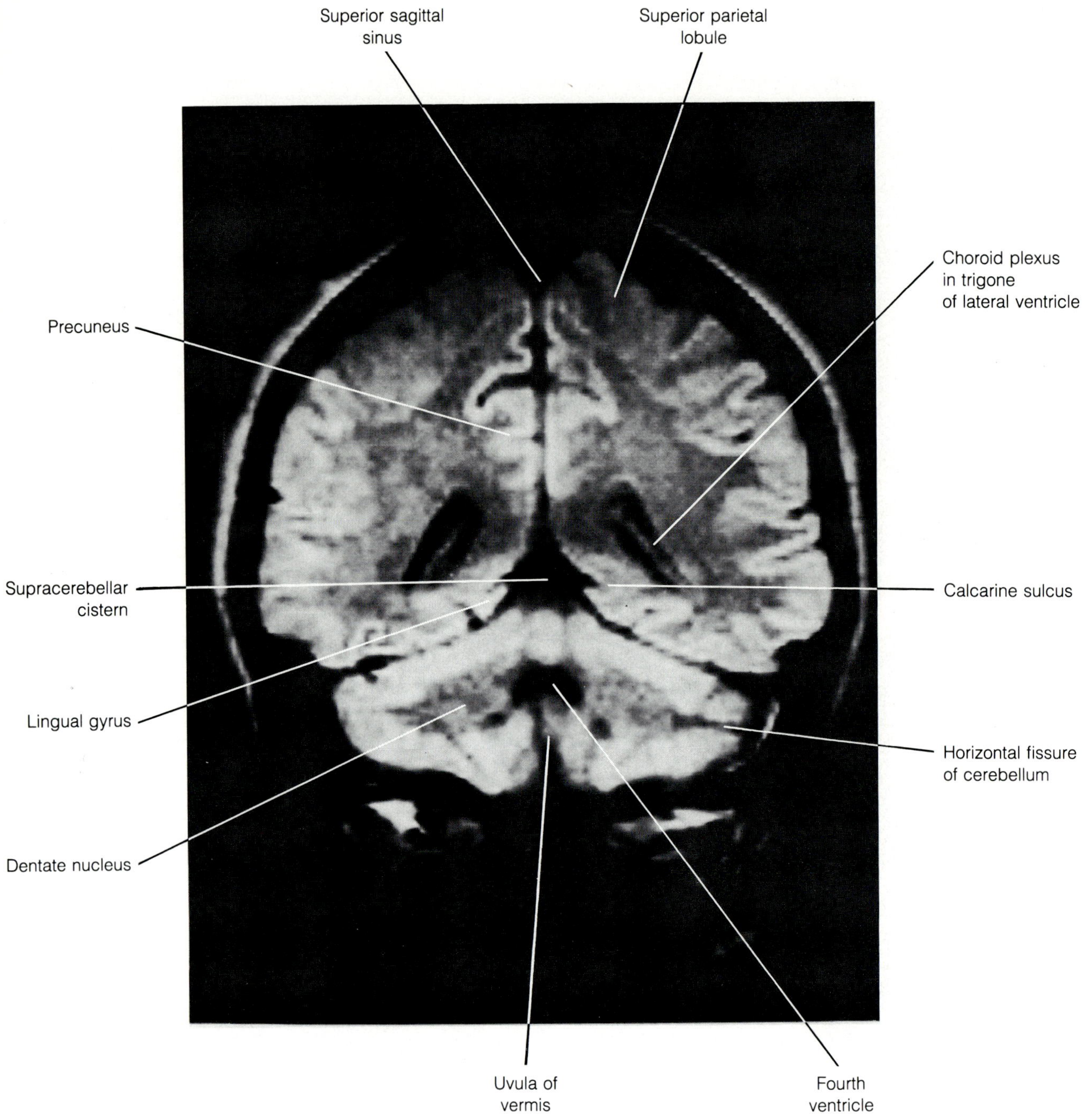

FIGURE C-11

Coronal SE 1500/28 image about 1 cm posterior to Figure C-10.

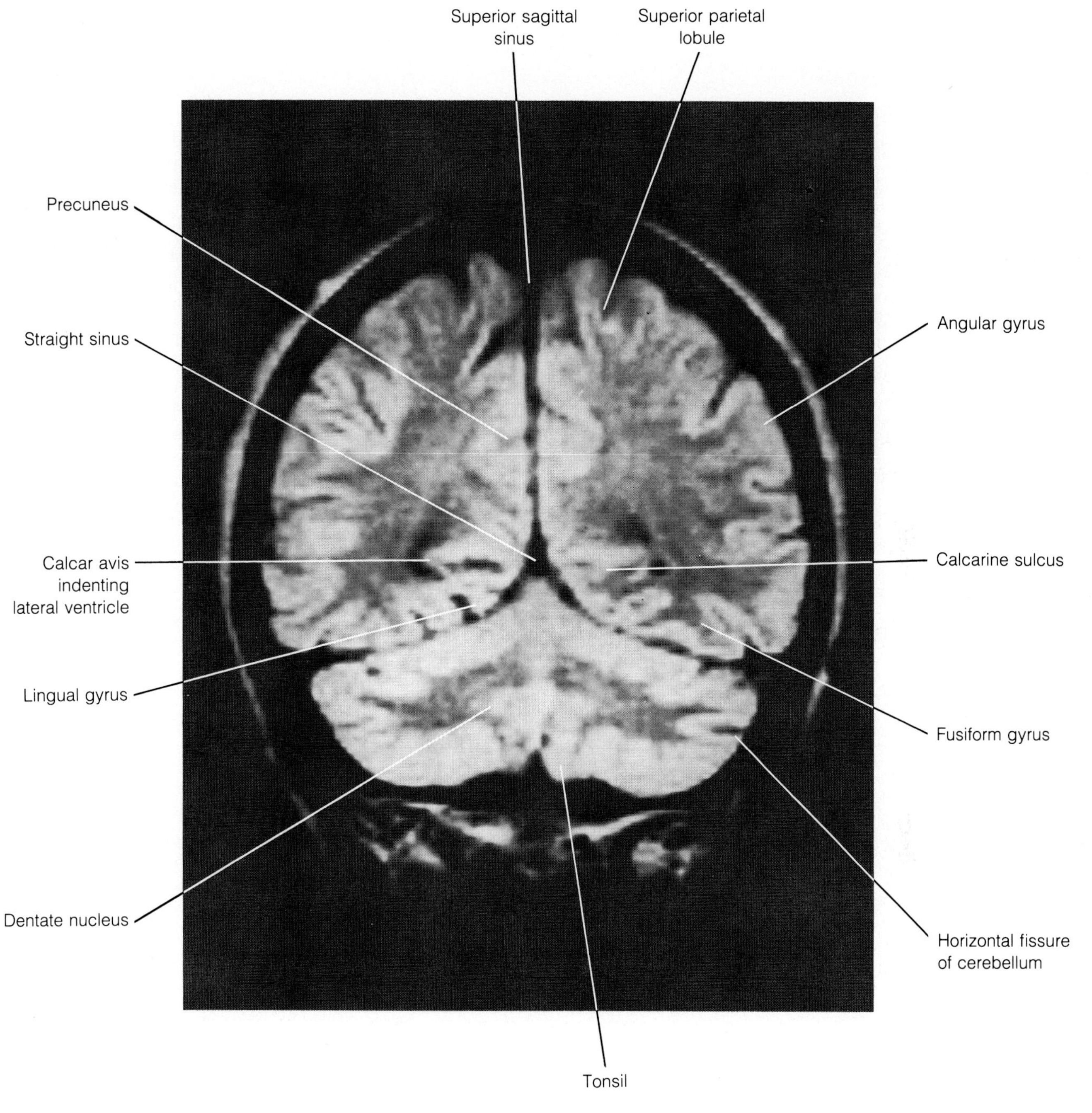

FIGURE C-12

Coronal SE 1500/28 image about 1 cm posterior to Figure C-11.

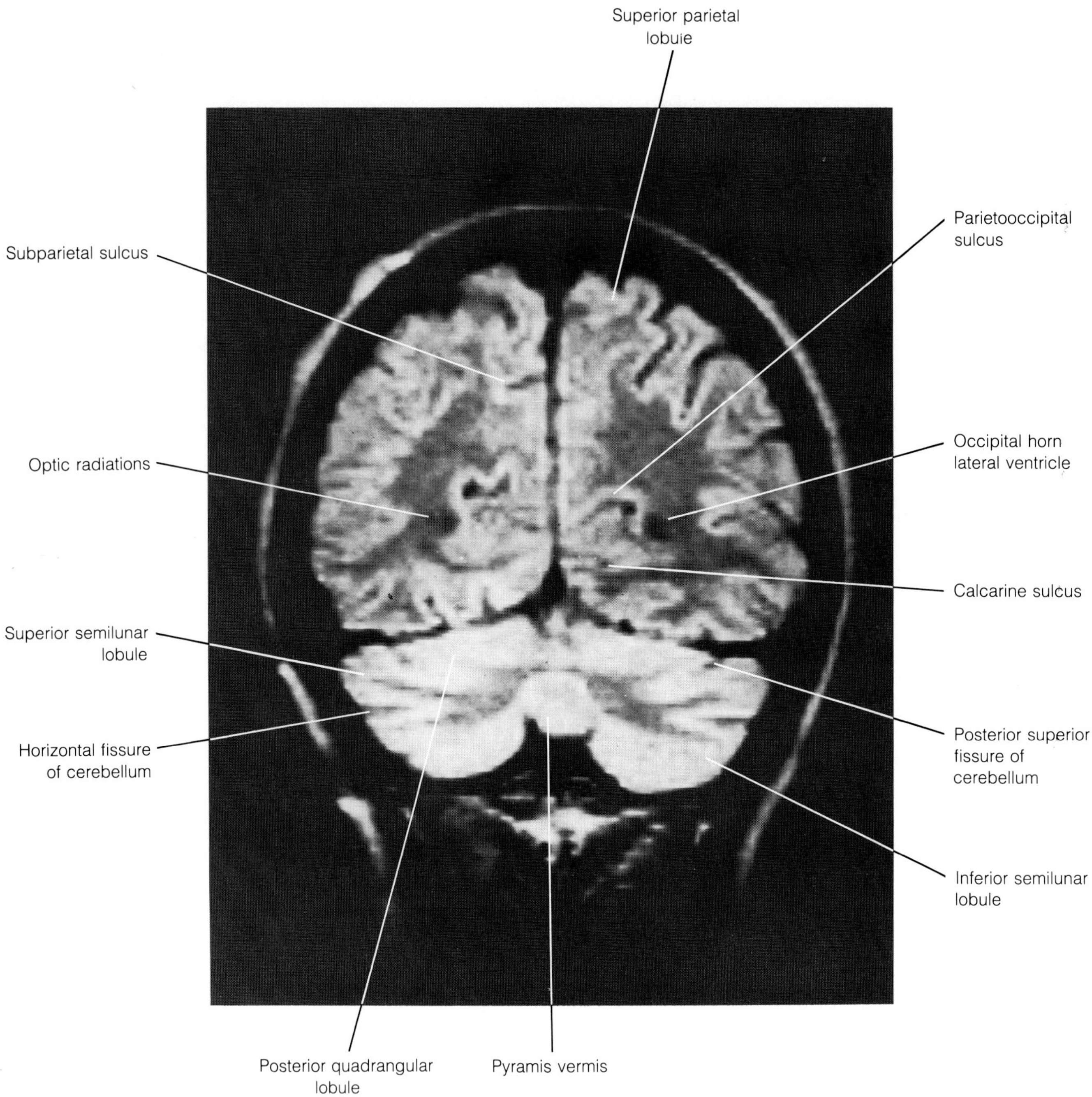

FIGURE C-13

Coronal SE 1500/28 image through the posterior cerebellum and occipital lobes.

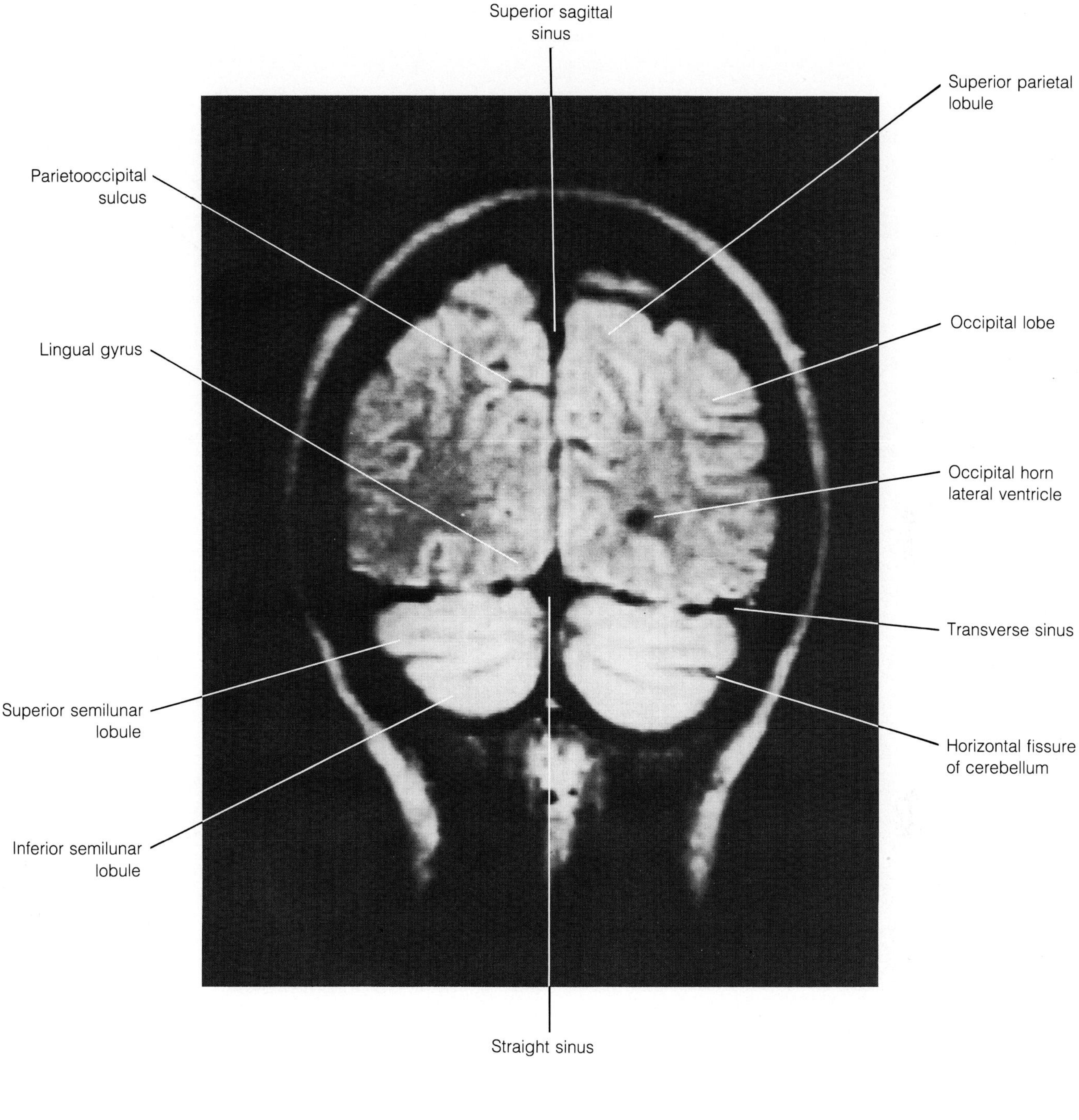

FIGURE C-14

Coronal SE 1500/28 through the occipital lobe, 1 cm posterior to Figure C-13.

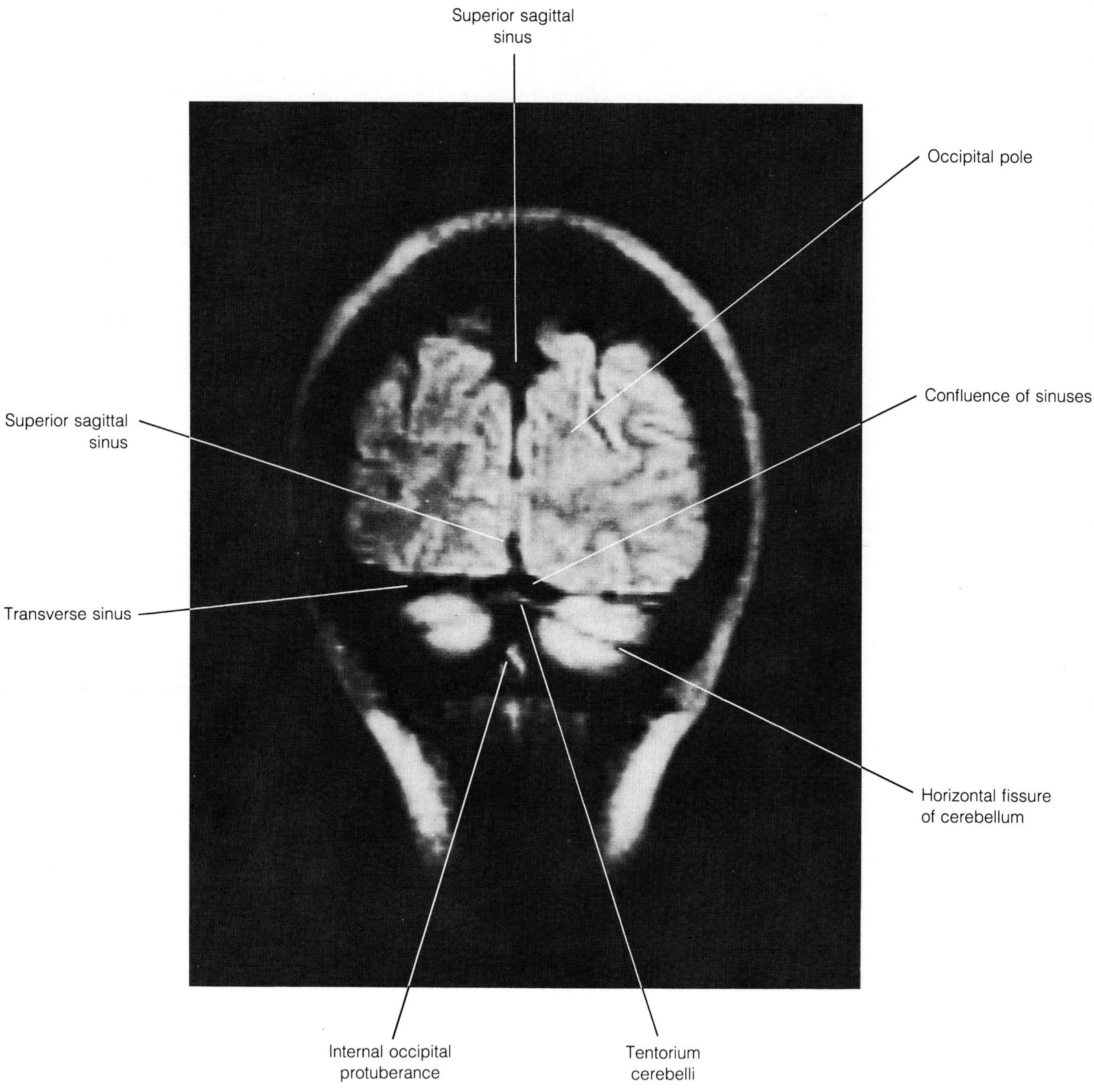

FIGURE C-15

Coronal SE 1500/28 most posterior cut through the cerebellum and occipital lobes.

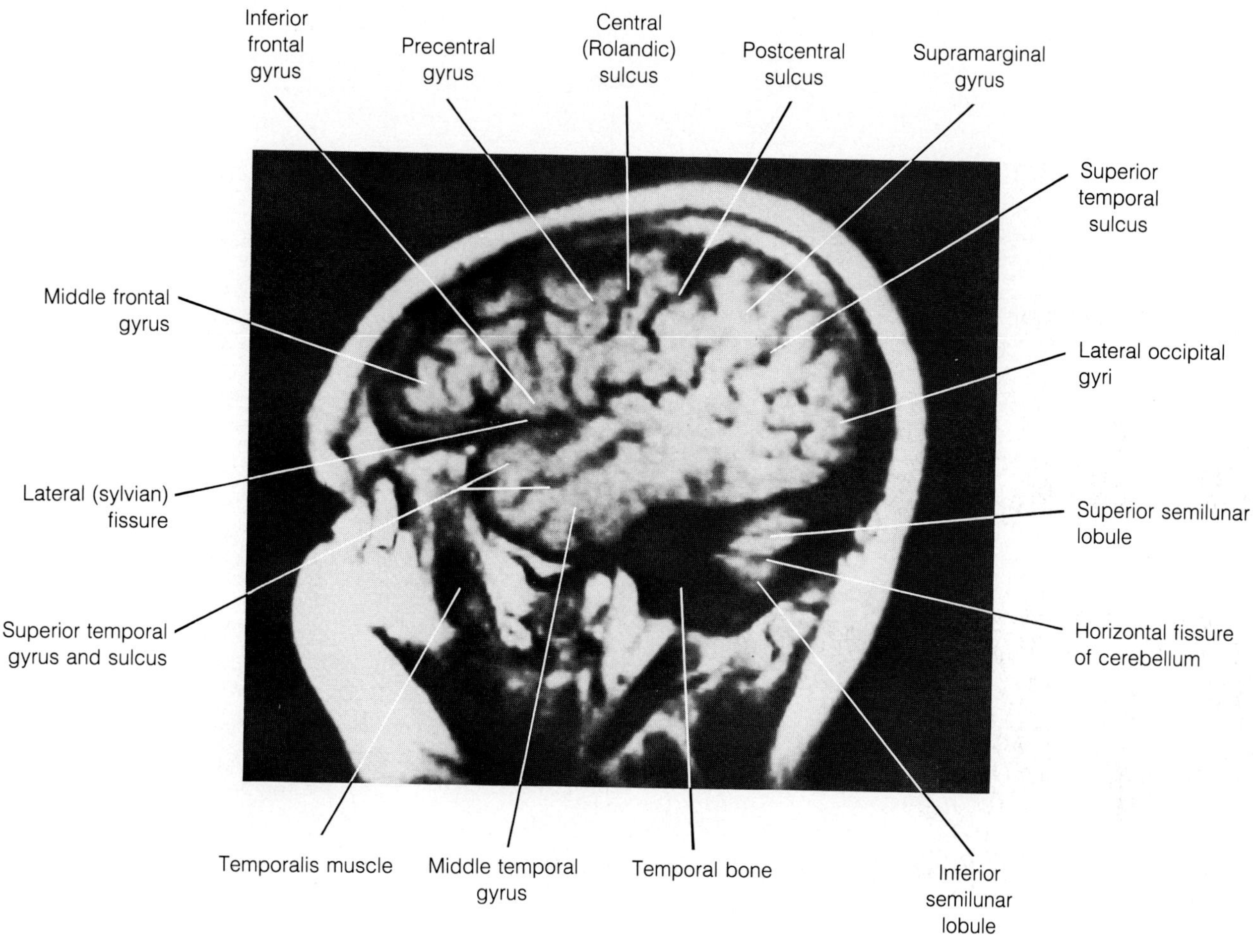

FIGURE S-1

Sagittal SE 500/28 image through the far lateral portion of the brain.

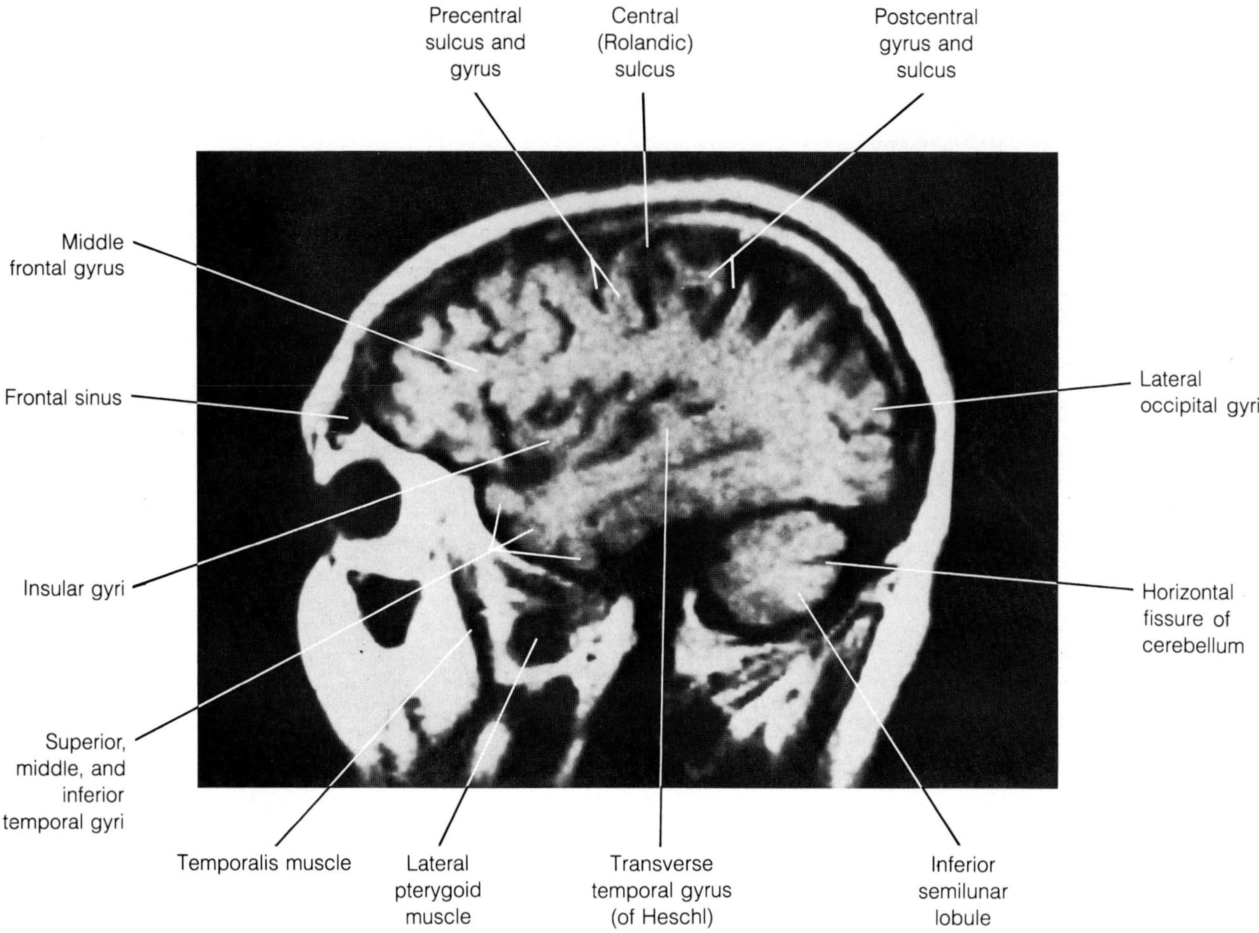

FIGURE S-2

Sagittal SE 500/28 image 1 cm medial to Figure S-1.

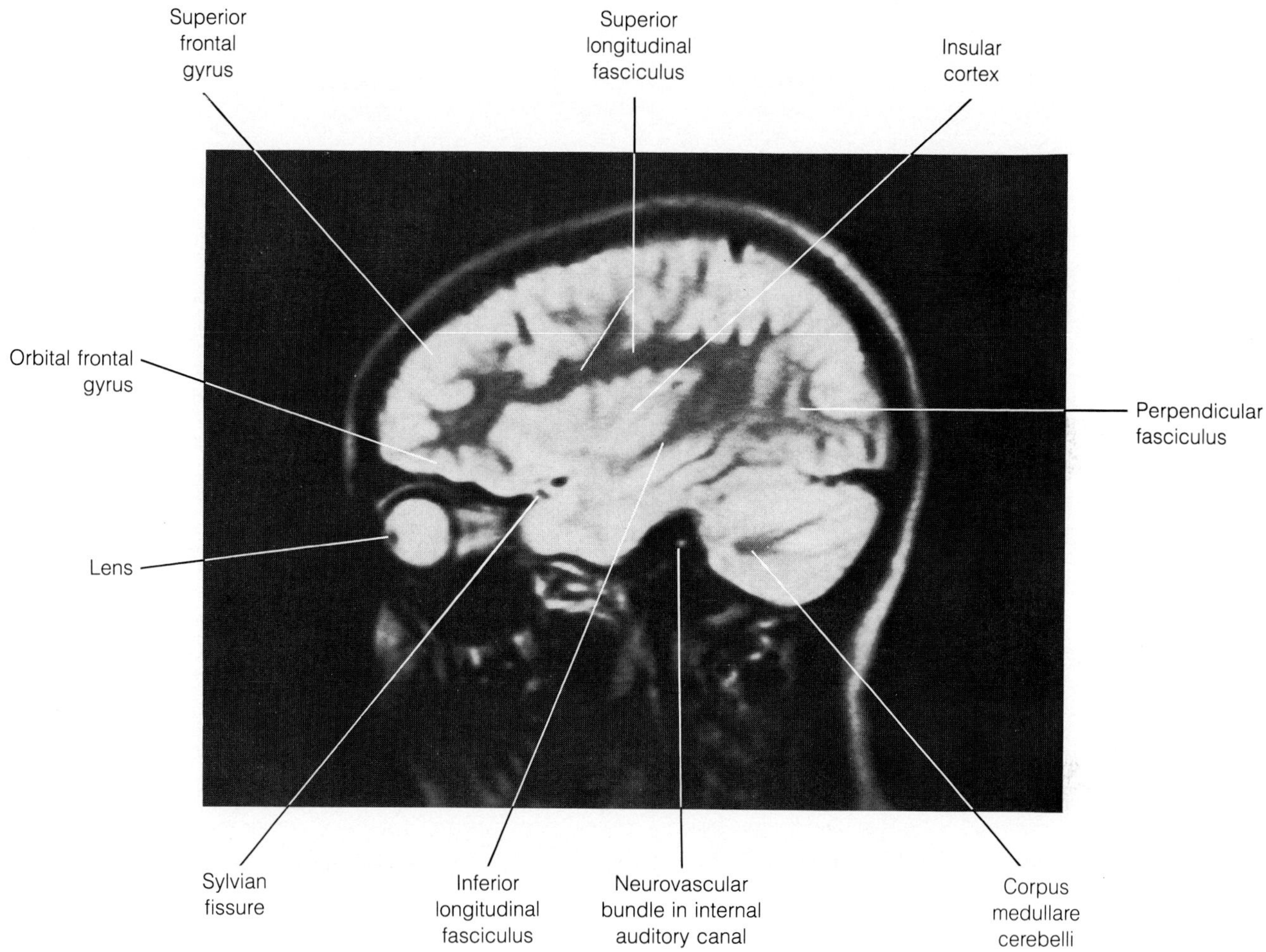

FIGURE S-3

Sagittal SE 2000/100 image about ½ cm medial to Figure S-2, demonstrating white matter tracts in the cerebellum and cerebrum. (Courtesy of Fonar Corp., 110 Marcus Drive, Melville, NY 11747)

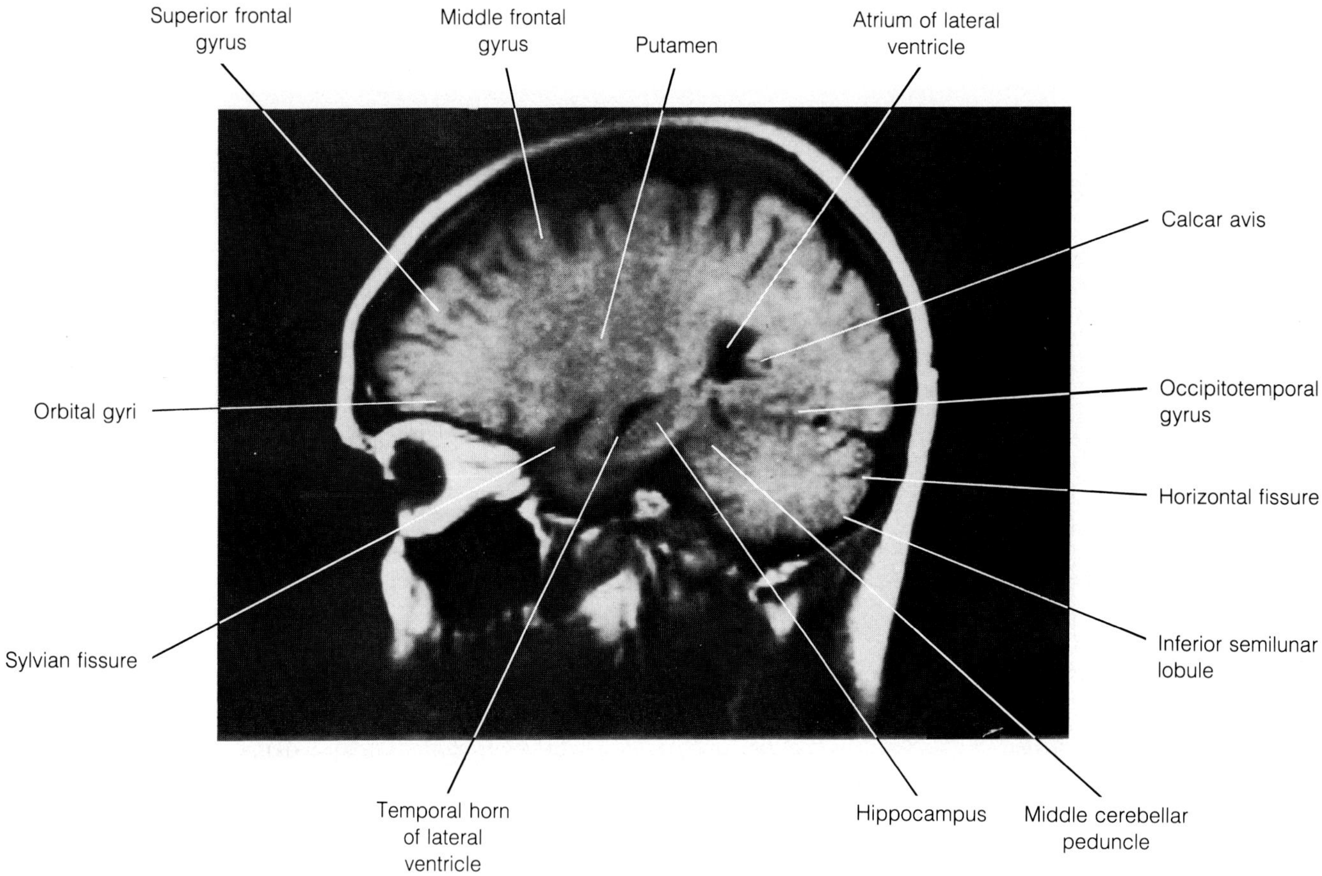

FIGURE S-4

Sagittal SE 500/28 image about 1 cm medial to Figure S-3.

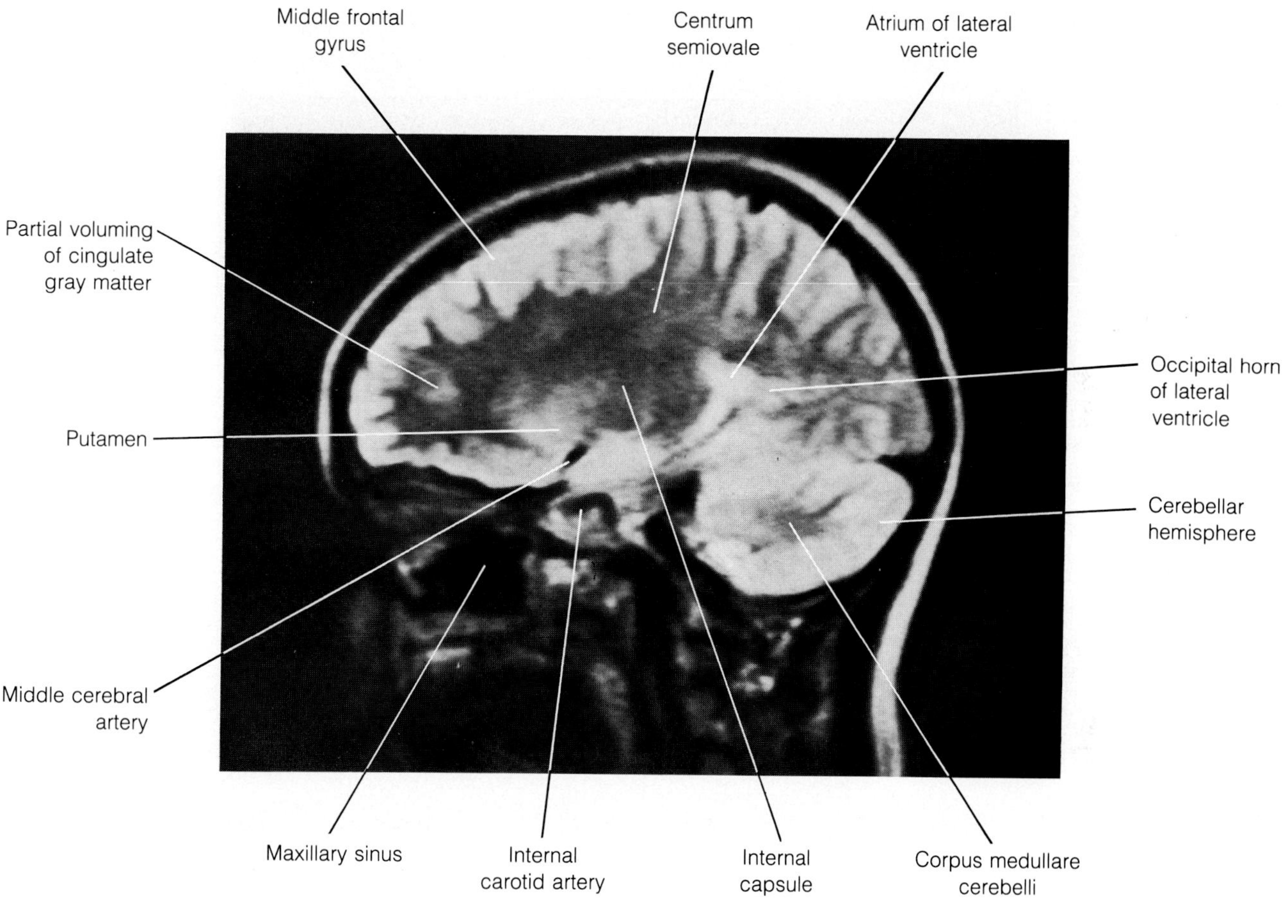

FIGURE S-5

Sagittal SE 2000/100 about ½ cm medial to Figure S-4, showing many of the same anatomic features but in a T2-weighted format. (Courtesy of Fonar Corp., 110 Marcus Drive, Melville, NY 11747)

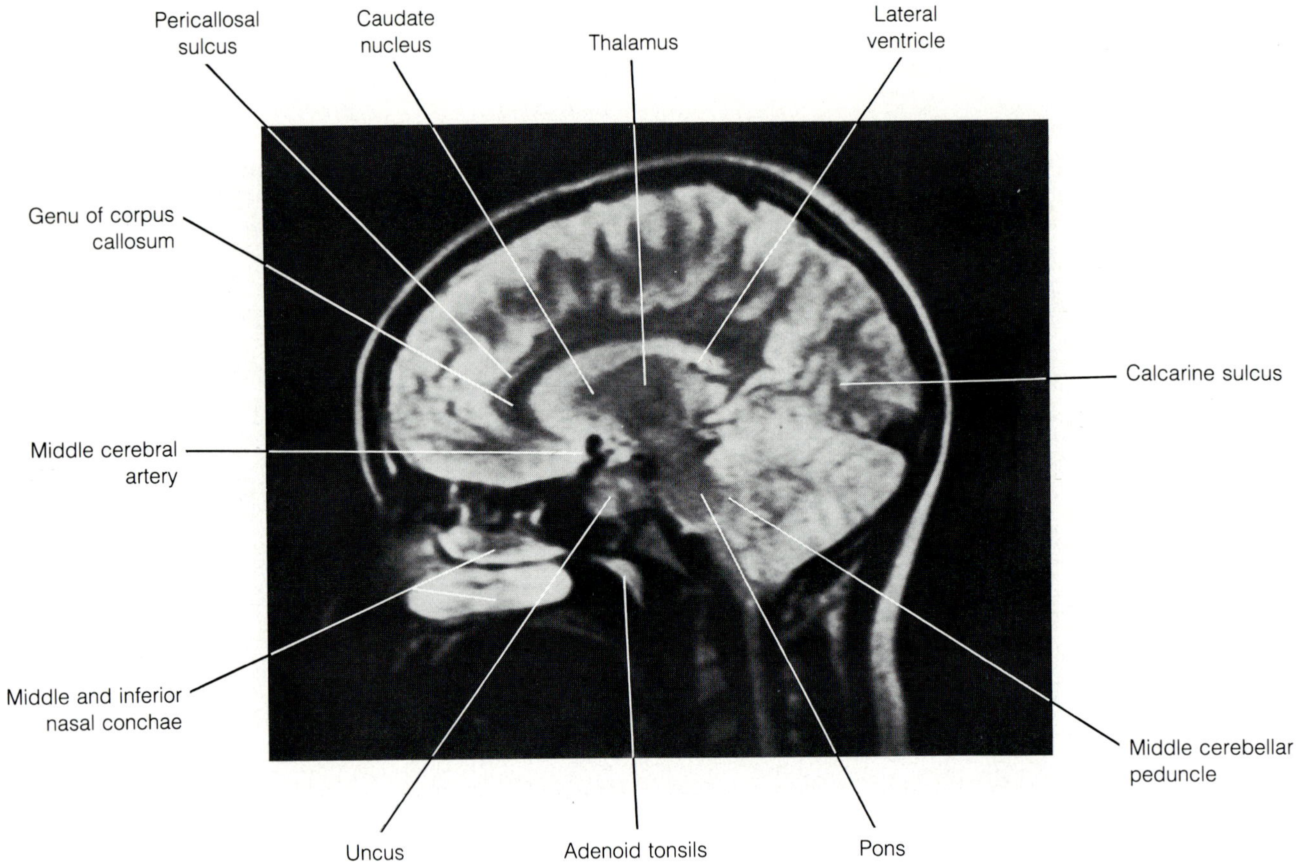

FIGURE S-6

Sagittal SE 2000/100 image about 1 cm medial to Figure S-5. (Courtesy of Fonar Corp., 110 Marcus Drive, Melville, NY 11747)

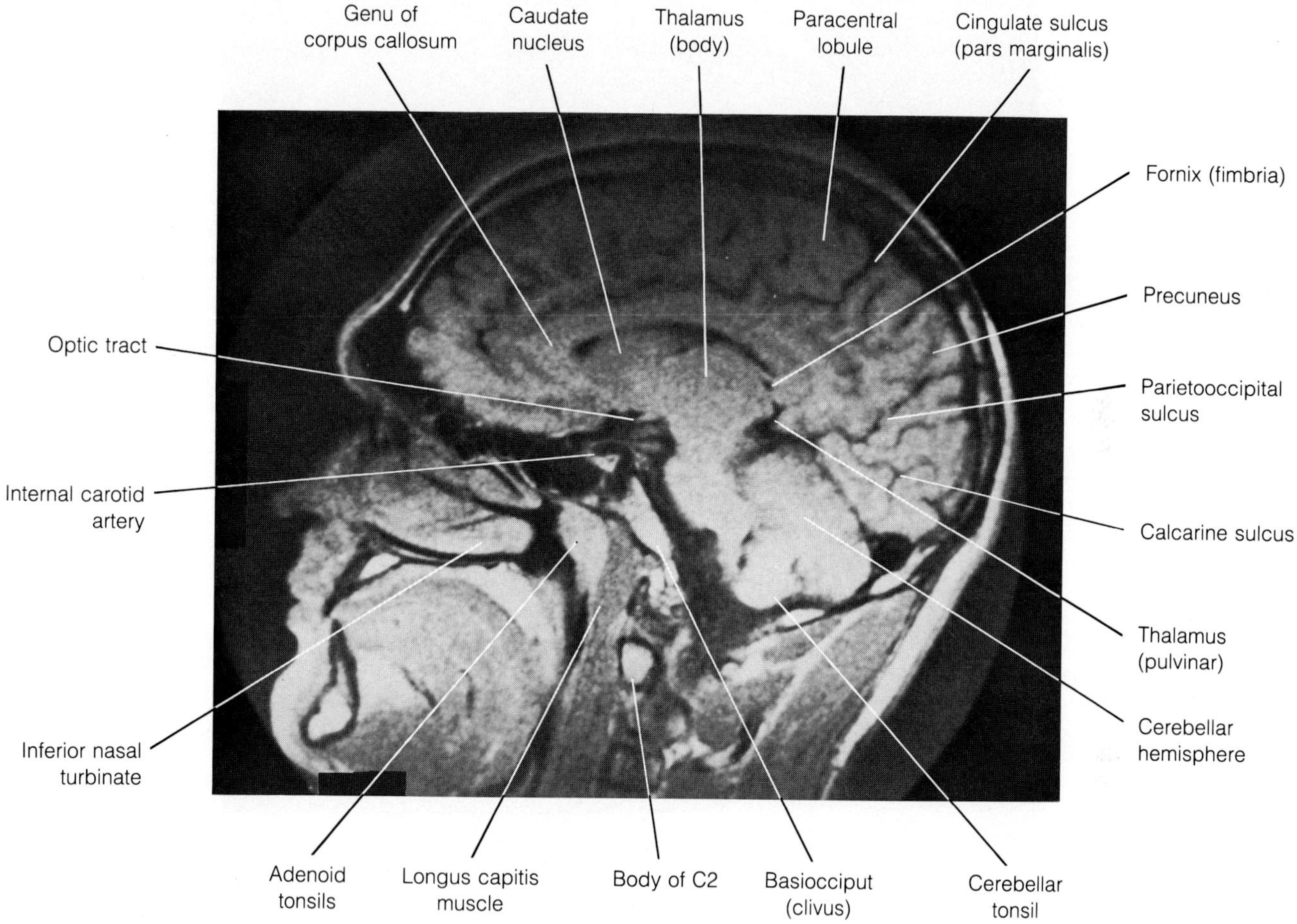

FIGURE S-7

Sagittal SE 400/28 image about ½ cm medial to Figure S-6. (Courtesy of Fonar Corp., 110 Marcus Drive, Melville, NY 11747)

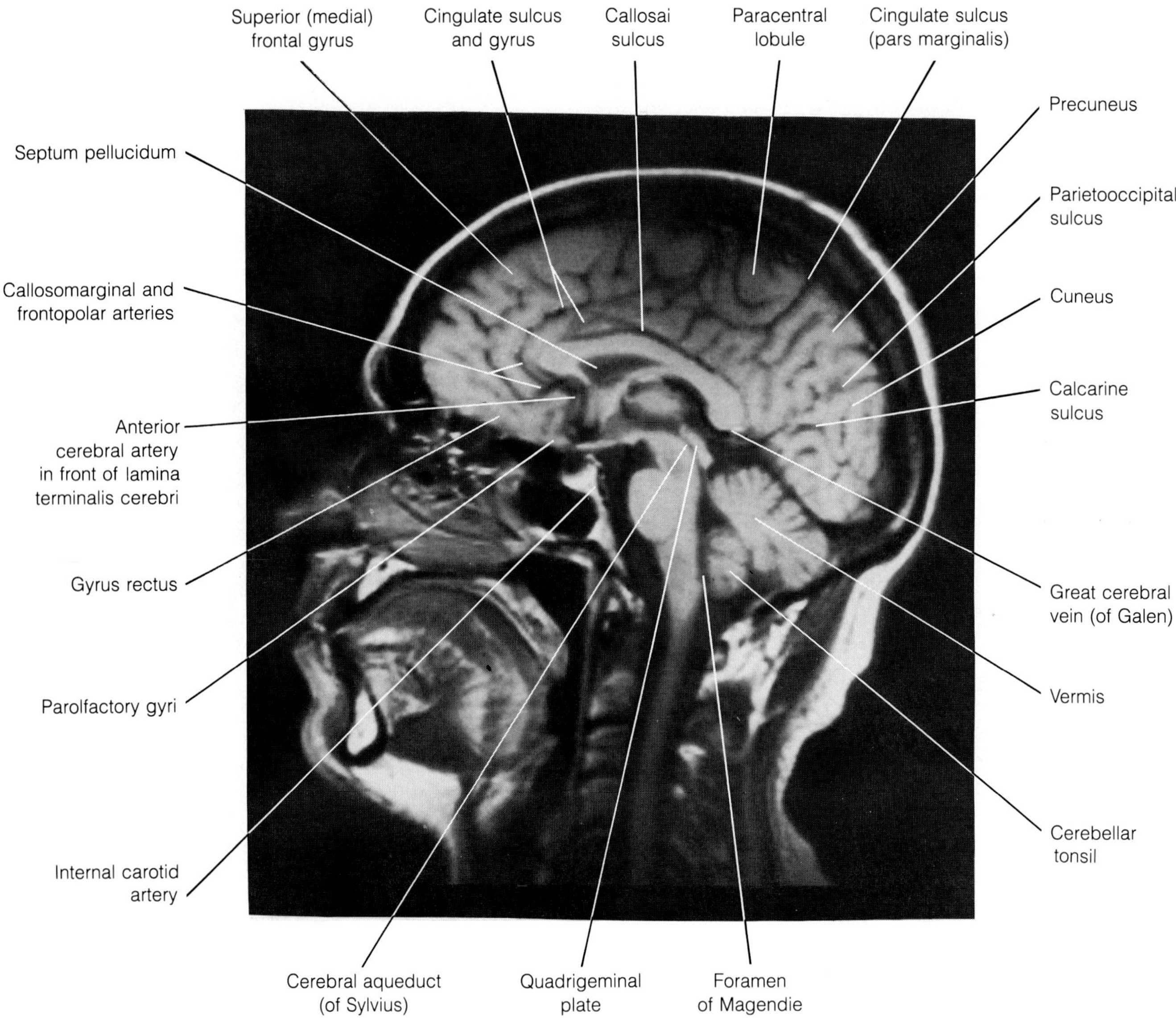

FIGURE S-8

Midline sagittal image SE 600/35 shows superb detail and anatomic relations. (Courtesy of Siemens)

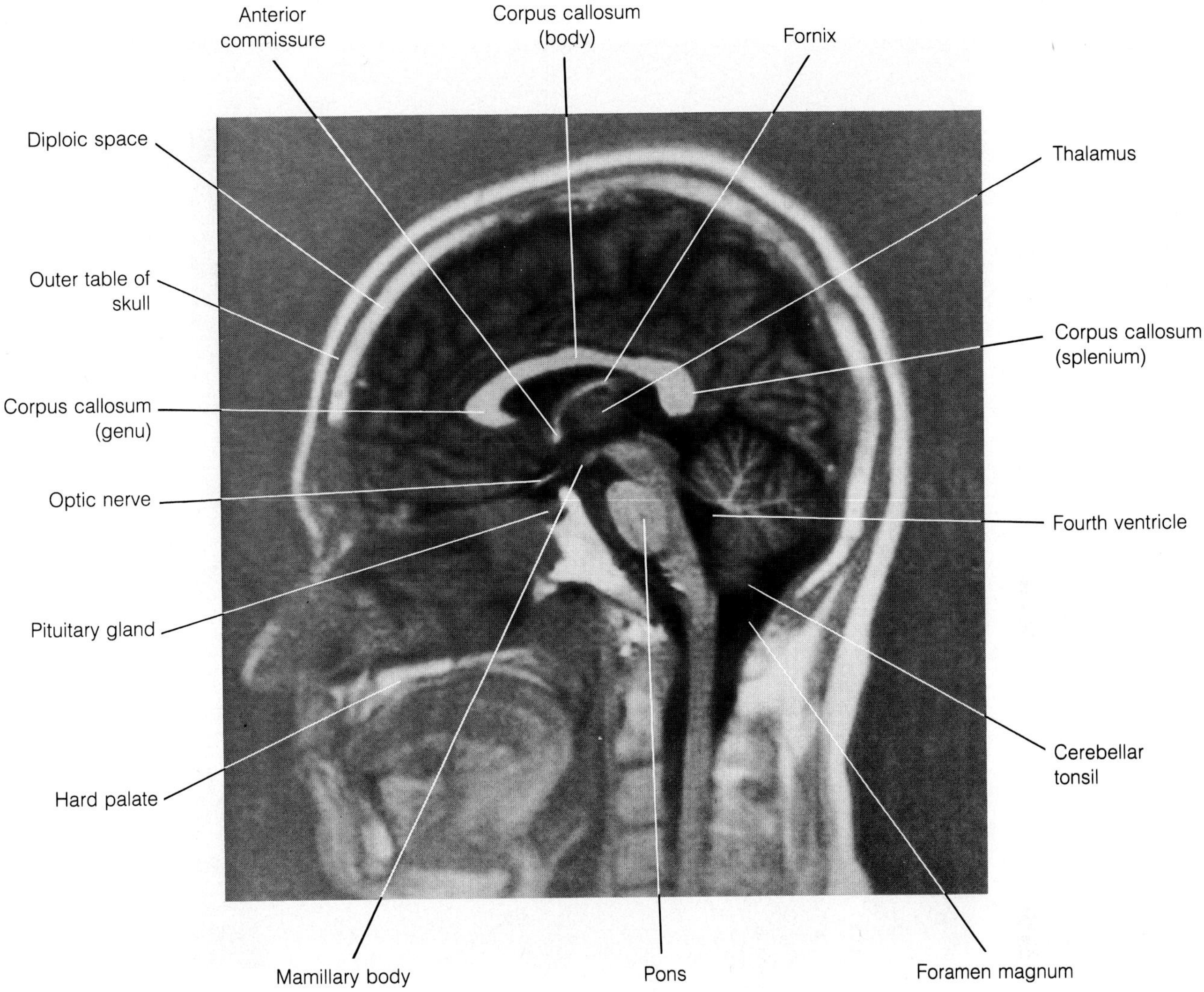

FIGURE S-9

Midline sagittal IR 2500/400/43 image provides excellent gray matter–white matter differentiation. (Courtesy of Siemens)

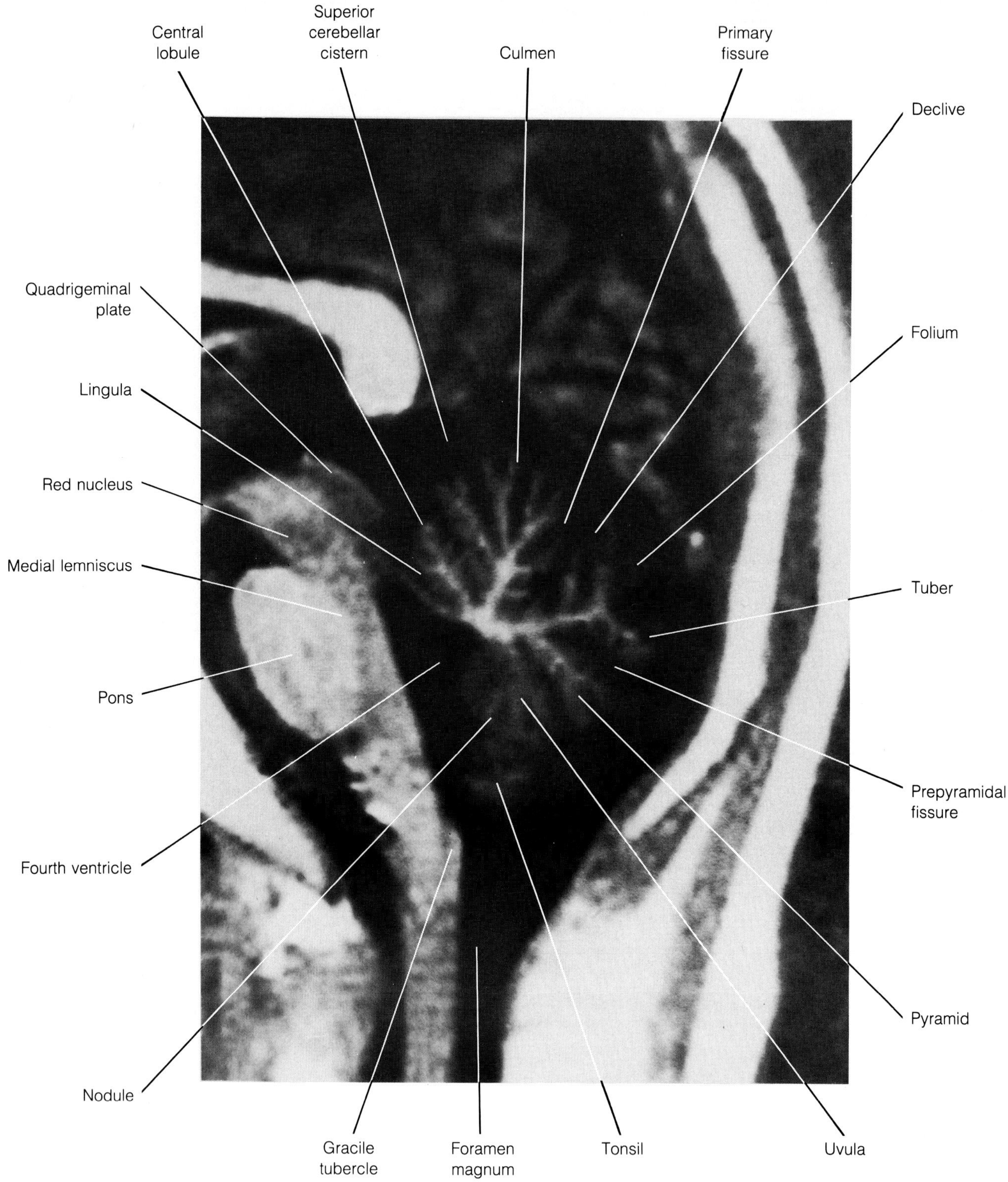

FIGURE S-10

Magnified view of Figure S-9 showing parts of the cerebellar vermis and brain stem. (Courtesy of Siemens)

CHAPTER 7

The Head and Neck
(Excluding Brain)

MR has enjoyed various degrees of success in imaging the extracranial head and neck. This chapter focuses on several different regions of the head and neck (excluding the brain and cervical spine) that are suitable for evaluation by MRI. These areas include the orbit, temporal bone, paranasal sinuses, nasopharynx, oropharynx, and soft tissues of the neck.

The Orbit and Optic Nerves

Techniques

The orbit is well-suited for MRI, although CT still remains the modality of choice in most situations. MR offers the advantages of direct multiplanar imaging and does not require ionizing radiation. MR may play a more important role in the future because it affords better visualization of the intracanalicular portion of the optic nerve and optic tract.

In 1985, most clinical MR facilities were using standard head radio-frequency (RF) coils for imaging the orbit. With the use of thin-section (3 mm to 5 mm) imaging, it is possible to obtain reasonably good evaluations of the orbit and optic nerves using head coils only. Now available commercially are surface coils that facilitate much finer resolution and higher signal-to-noise ratios (Fig. 7-1). The use of such surface coils allows very small imaging volume elements (voxels) to be used, on the order of 0.5 × 0.5 × 3 mm. Most of the images of the orbit in this chapter were made using surface coil techniques.

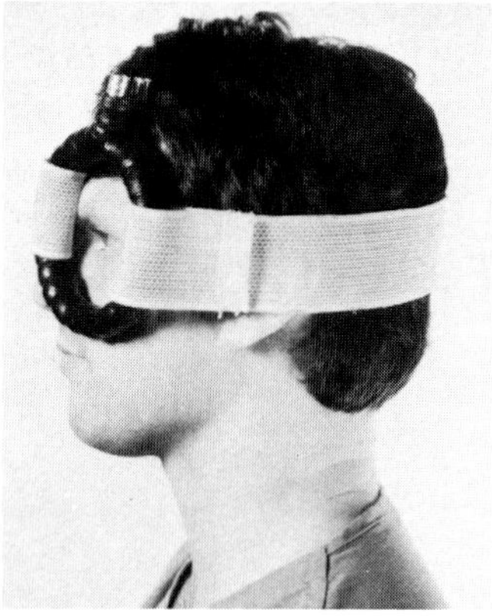

FIGURE 7-1

Surface coils for the orbit allow increased spatial resolution and improved signal-to-noise ratio. (Courtesy of Fonar Corporation, 110 Marcus Drive, Melville, NY 11747)

The ideal imaging sequences for detecting optic lesions are yet to be determined. Routine axial and coronal projections are generally most useful, with sagittal imaging performed only in certain situations (*e.g.,* blowout fractures, tumor extension). As elsewhere in the body, the use of two orthogonal planes often increases one's diagnostic confidence.

Partial saturation sequences such as PS 300 have been said to provide the best spatial resolution. Short spin-echo sequences such as SE 500/28 are also acceptable. The use of a second echo or longer TR will allow tissue T1 or T2 estimates to be made and may be a more sensitive means of imaging certain types of pathological conditions. Spatial resolution will be sacrificed somewhat, however.

Orbital Anatomy

The bones and soft tissues of the orbit are well delineated by MRI because of the inherent natural contrast of T1 and T2 values. The bony orbital walls are largely devoid of fatty marrow, so they appear black on all imaging sequences. The superior and lateral walls may be identified, however, by their contrasting borders with the orbital fat, brain, or adjacent temporalis muscle (Fig. 7-2). The inferior and medial walls of the orbit interface with air in the maxillary and ethmoidal sinuses, respectively. Unless these sinuses are filled with fluid, the inferior and medial orbital walls cannot be visualized (Fig. 7-2).

Orbital fat has a short T1 and hence high signal intensity on PS or SE sequences used to image the orbit. All other structures (globe, muscles, vessels, nerves) are silhouetted against this white background as masses of lower intensity. The high-intensity fat produces a form of spatial blurring akin to bone artifact on CT (Fig. 7-3). Future developments such as image intensity scaling and fat suppression techniques should reduce this problem and increase contrast resolution.

The globe and its internal anatomy may be delineated. The vitreous humor is 99% water and has long T1 and T2 values. The lens is about 65% water and 35% protein; it has a moderately long T1 and a short T2. Accordingly, the lens will be brighter than the vitreous on T1-weighted pulse sequences. For

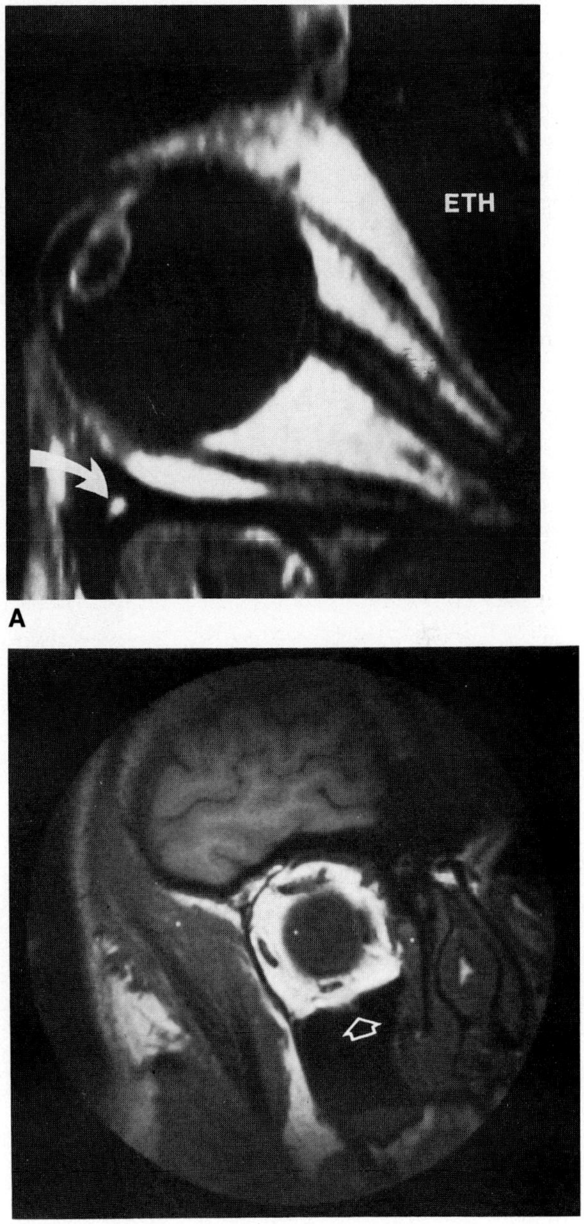

FIGURE 7-2

Orbital walls. (*A*) The bony orbital walls appear black, contrasted by high-intensity orbital fat on one side and brain or muscle on the other. Note fatty marrow (arrow) in the zygoma. Since the medial orbital wall is bounded by air in the ethmoidal sinuses (ETH), its margins cannot be distinguished. (Courtesy of Fonar Corporation, 110 Marcus Drive, Melville, NY 11747). (*B*) Like the medial orbital wall, the orbital floor is adjacent to air in the maxillary sinus and cannot be distinguished. Note the infraorbital nerve in its canal (arrow) coursing within the bony orbital floor. (Reprinted with permission from Schenck JF, Hart HR Jr, Foster TH et al: Improved MR imaging of the orbit at 1.5 T with surface coils. AJR 144:1033, 1985)

T2-weighted sequences, a contrast reversal will occur, the lens appearing darker than the vitreous.

The sclera and choroid/retina may be distinguished reliably in motionless patients using a surface coil technique. The more fibrous sclera has a consistently weaker signal than the more intense choroid and retina. The iris and ciliary body may also be distinguished in motionless patients.

A common artifact that should not be mistaken for normal layers of the retina nor of retinal hemorrhage or detachment is produced by motion of the globe during scanning (Fig. 7-4). These characteristic multiple curvilinear bands situated posteriorly in the globe should be easily recognized.

A number of other anatomic landmarks within the orbit may be identified. These include the lacrimal gland, extraocular muscles, nerves, and blood vessels. Surface coil images of the orbit in axial, coronal, and sagittal planes are shown in Figures 7-5 through 7-7.

(Text continues on p. 134.)

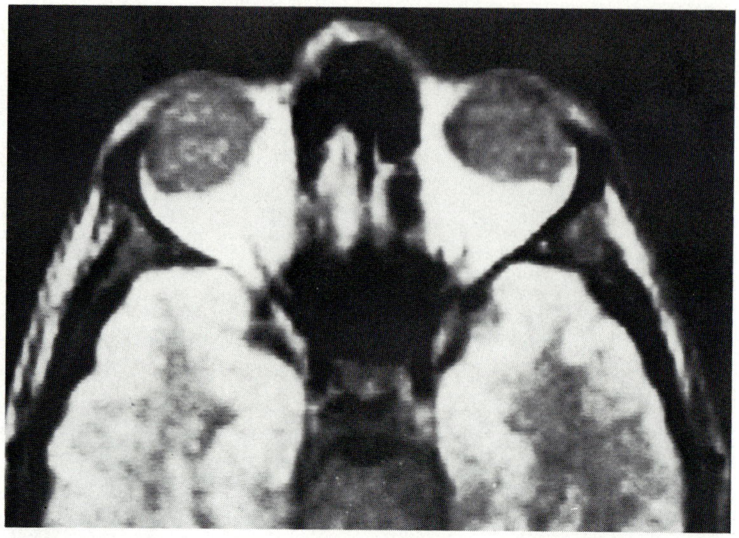

FIGURE 7-3

High-intensity fat causes a spatial blurring artifact akin to bone artifact on CT that "spills over" and partially obscures lower-intensity orbital structures.

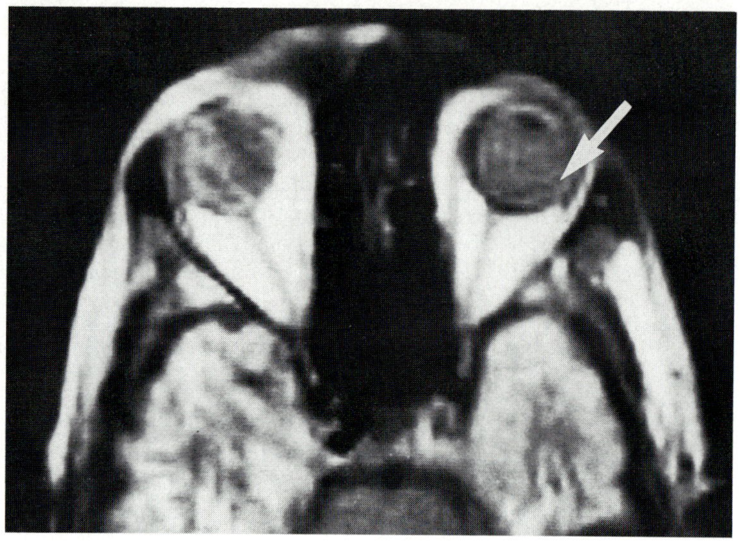

FIGURE 7-4

Motion artifact of the globe produces characteristic curvilinear bands posteriorly (arrow) which should not be misinterpreted as retinal detachment or hemorrhage.

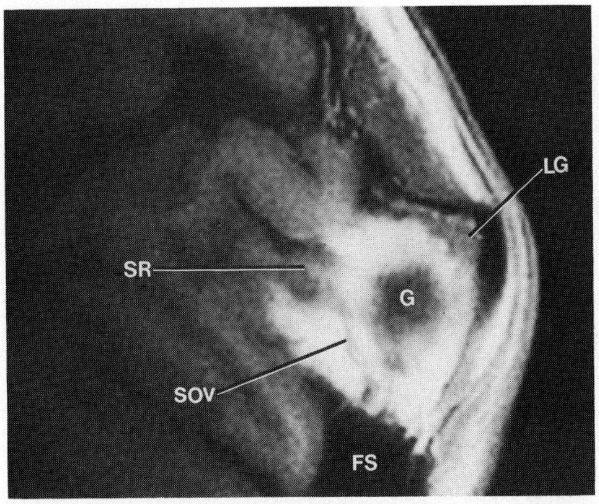

A

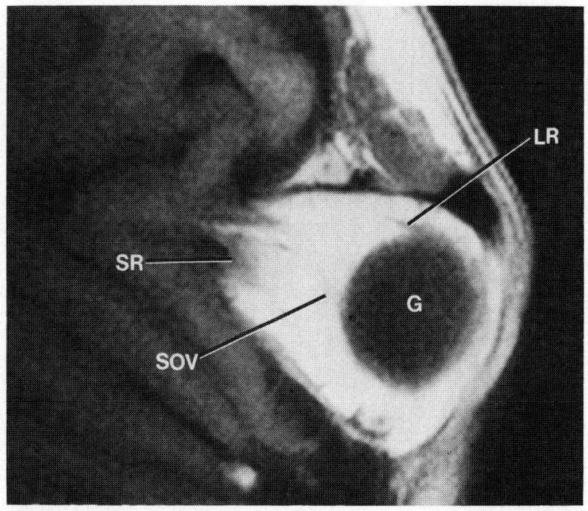

B

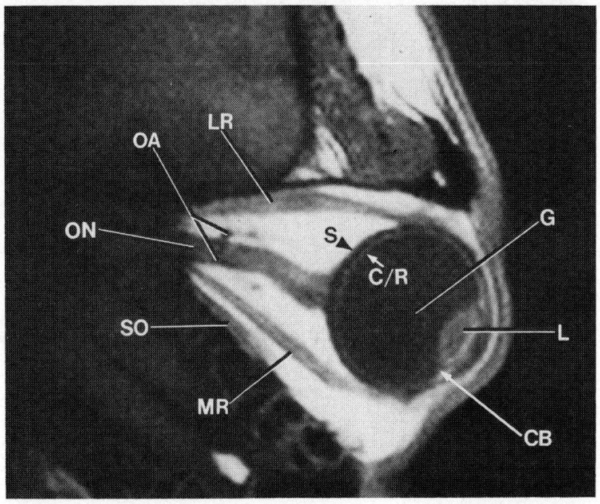

C

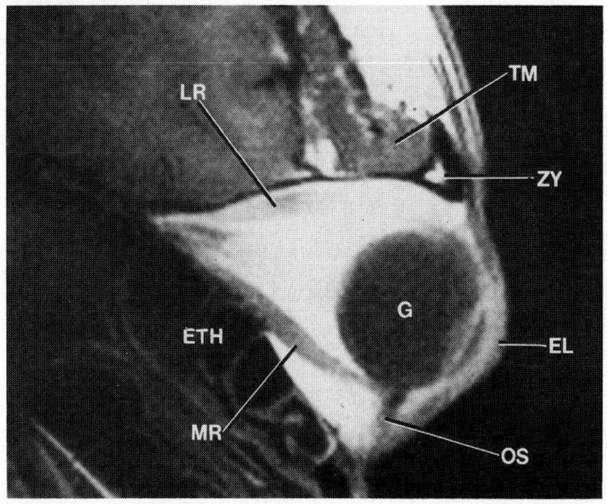

D

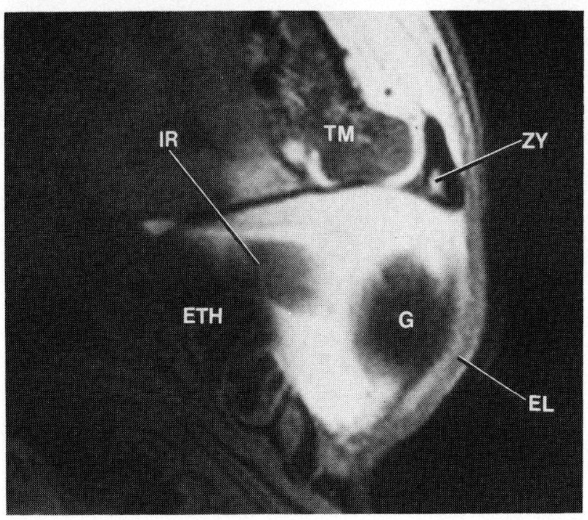

E

CB	ciliary body
C/R	choroid/retina
EL	eyelid
ETH	ethmoidal air cells
FN	frontal nerve
FS	frontal sinus
FV	branch of facial vein
G	globe
IN	infraorbital nerve
IO	inferior oblique muscle
IR	inferior rectus muscle
L	lens
LG	lacrimal gland
LR	lateral rectus muscle
MR	medial rectus muscle
MS	maxillary sinus
OA	ophthalmic artery and ciliary branches
ON	optic nerve
OS	orbital septum
S	sclera
SO	superior oblique muscle
SOV	superior ophthalmic vein
SR	superior rectus/levator palpebrae superioris muscles
TM	temporalis muscle
ZY	zygoma

FIGURE 7-5

Axial surface coil MR images of the orbit using SE 500/30 technique. (Courtesy of Technicare Corporation, Technicare Corp. © 1985)

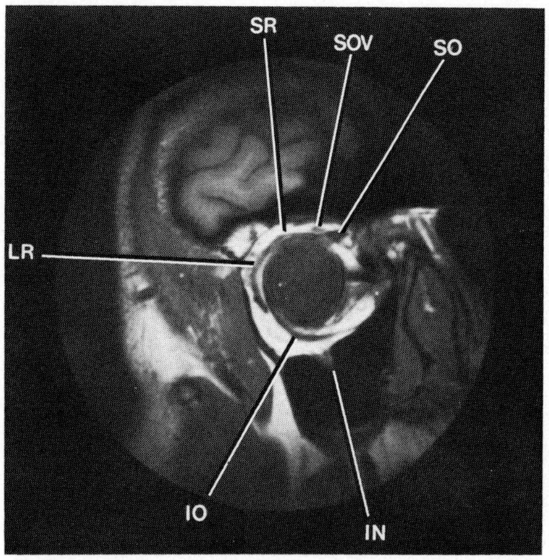

A

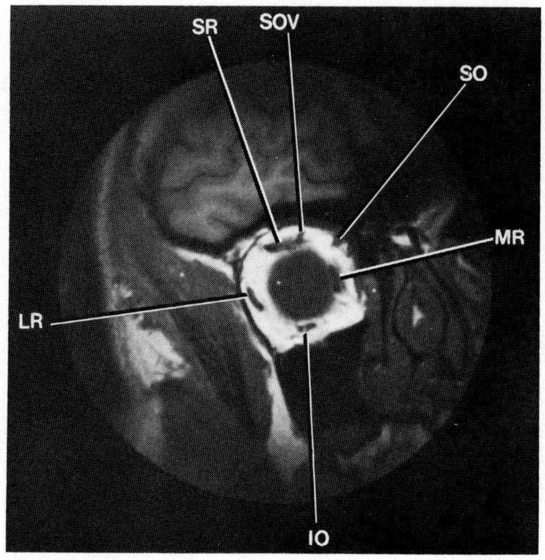

B

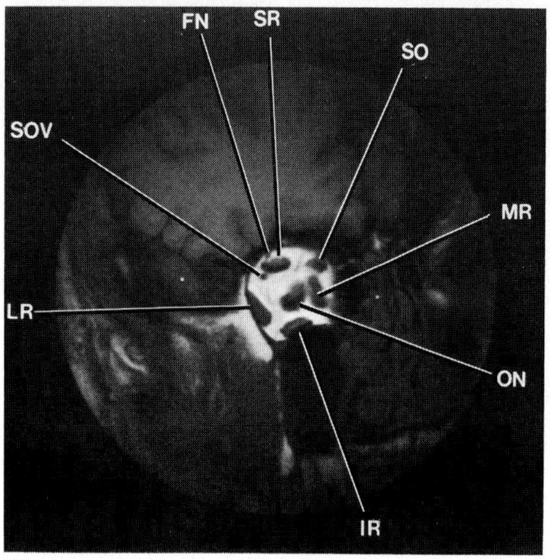

C

FIGURE 7-6

Coronal surface coil images of the orbit from anterior to posterior using PS 400 technique.

CB	ciliary body
C/R	choroid/retina
EL	eyelid
ETH	ethmoidal air cells
FN	frontal nerve
FS	frontal sinus
FV	branch of facial vein
G	globe
IN	infraorbital nerve
IO	inferior oblique muscle
IR	inferior rectus muscle
L	lens
LG	lacrimal gland
LR	lateral rectus muscle
MR	medial rectus muscle
MS	maxillary sinus
OA	ophthalmic artery and ciliary branches
ON	optic nerve
OS	orbital septum
S	sclera
SO	superior oblique muscle
SOV	superior ophthalmic vein
SR	superior rectus/levator palpebrae superioris muscles
TM	temporalis muscle
ZY	zygoma

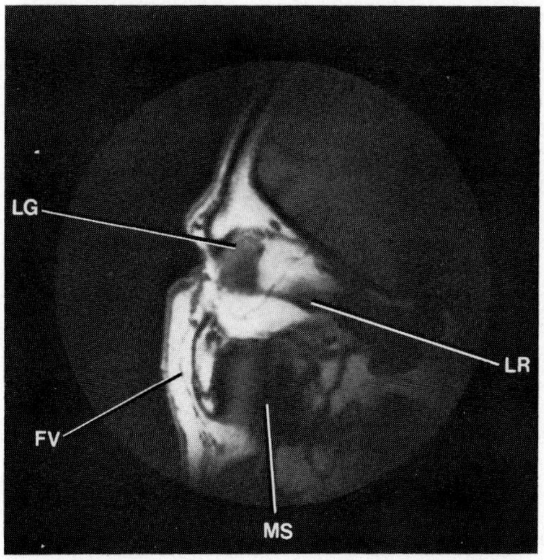

A

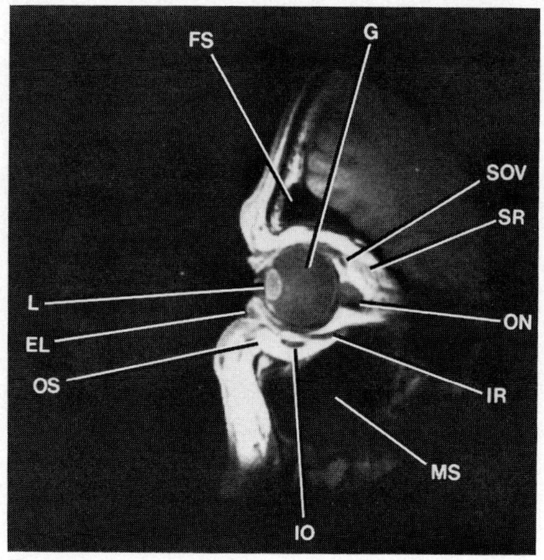

B

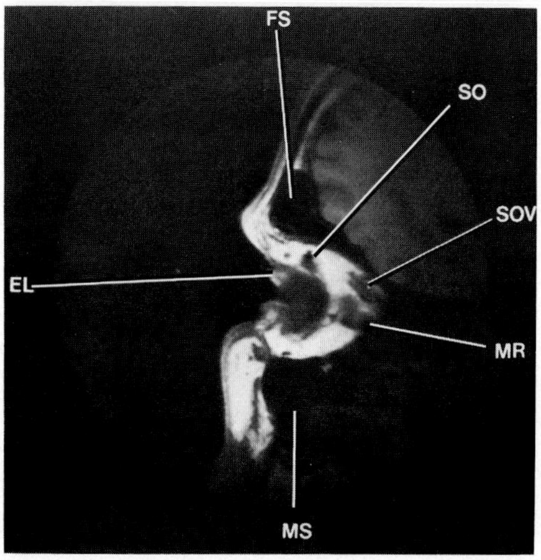

C

FIGURE 7-7

Sagittal surface coil images of the orbit from lateral to medial using PS 400 technique. (Figures 7-6 and 7-7 provided courtesy of Dr. John Schenck and General Electric Medical Systems Inc. Reprinted with permission from Schenck JF, Hart HR Jr, Foster TH et al: Improved MR imaging of the orbit at 1.5 T with surface coils. AJR 144:1033, 1985)

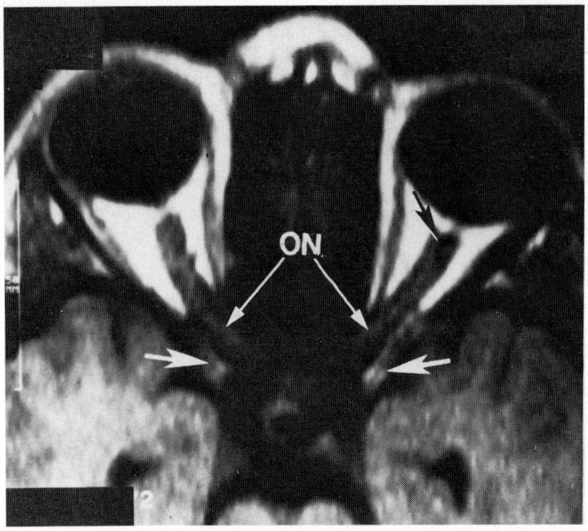

FIGURE 7-8

The ophthalmic artery (black arrow) may be seen adjacent to the optic nerve (ON). Note high-intensity signal from fat in the anterior clinoid processes (white arrows). (Courtesy of Fonar Corporation, 110 Marcus Drive, Melville NY 11747)

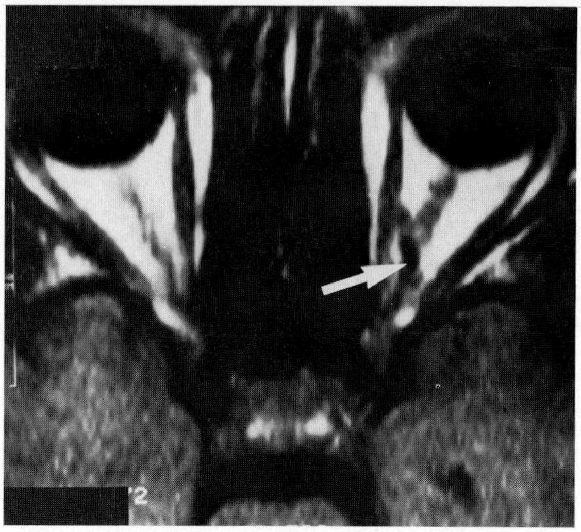

FIGURE 7-9

The superior ophthalmic vein (arrow) seen as a low-intensity tubular structure crossing obliquely in the orbit. (Courtesy of Fonar Corporation, 110 Marcus Drive, Melville, NY 11747)

Optic Nerves and Chiasm

The optic nerves are usually well-visualized in their course from the globe to the chiasm. The optic nerve has a signal intensity similar to that of cerebral white matter. The ophthalmic artery may also be seen coursing along with the nerve as a low-intensity structure (Fig. 7-8). More superiorly, the superior ophthalmic vein may also be seen crossing above the optic nerve (Fig. 7-9). The low intensity from either vessel may at times be volume averaged with the optic nerve. This may mask a high-intensity pathological lesion within the nerve.

The optic nerves and ophthalmic arteries may be followed through the approximately 7-mm-long optic canals. No fat is present alongside the nerve in the optic canal. Tissue contrast for visualization of the nerve is a result of the fact that it is surrounded by dense cortical bone, which produces no signal. Occasionally, fat in the anterior clinoid processes may be seen adjacent to the nerve in this region (Fig. 7-8). Clinoid signal should be recognized by virtue of its location and usual symmetry and should not be confused with an intensifying mass in or near the optic nerve.

A second problem in evaluating the optic nerve in the optic canal may arise when fluid exists in the posterior ethmoidal sinuses. Adjacent intensity in these sinuses may give a misleading appearance of mass or enlargement of the optic nerve medially. Usually the use of coronal images in addition to axial images will clarify this situation.

The optic chiasm may be visualized anterior to the infundibulum and superior to the pituitary gland proper. This is shown on axial and sagittal views in Figure 7-10. The optic tract may be followed back into the brain, as shown in Figure 7-11. Other relationships of the optic nerves and parasellar structures are illustrated in Chapter 6. A possible protocol for imaging the orbit and optic nerves is presented in Table 7-1.

TABLE 7-1

Possible Protocol for MRI of the Orbit and Optic Nerves

1. Use surface coils when available and thin (<3-mm) slices
2. Remove mascara before scanning, since certain brands containing iron oxides produce artifacts
3. Coronal PS 300 or SE 500/30
4. Axial PS 300 or SE 500/30
5. Axial SE 1500/30,60
6. Sagittal SE 1000/30,60 useful for optic nerves near the chiasma

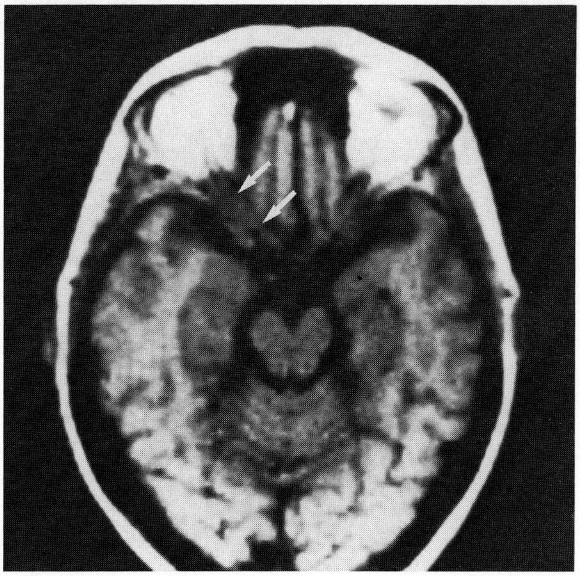

A

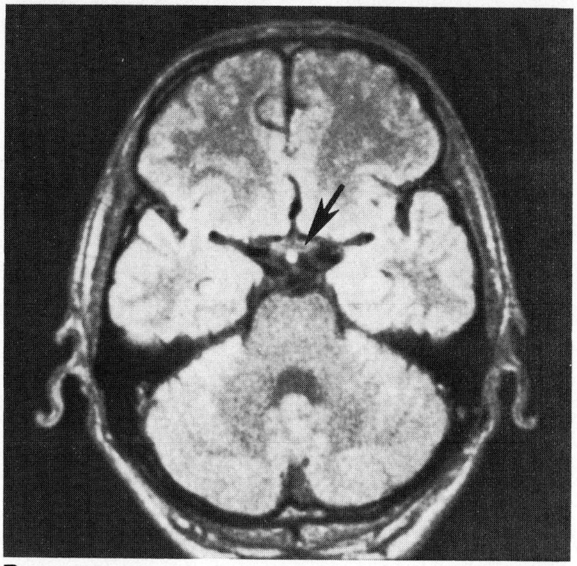

B

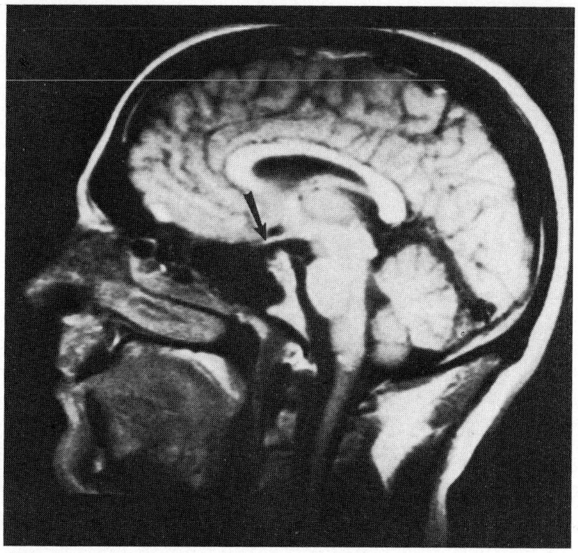

C

FIGURE 7-10

The optic nerves and chiasm. (*A*) The optic nerves (arrows) can be followed posteriorly on axial images. (*B*) The optic chiasm is seen on axial image (arrow) just anterior to the pituitary stalk (white dot). (Courtesy of Fonar Corporation, 110 Marcus Drive, Melville, NY 11747). (*C*) The optic chiasm can also be seen on sagittal midline images (arrow).

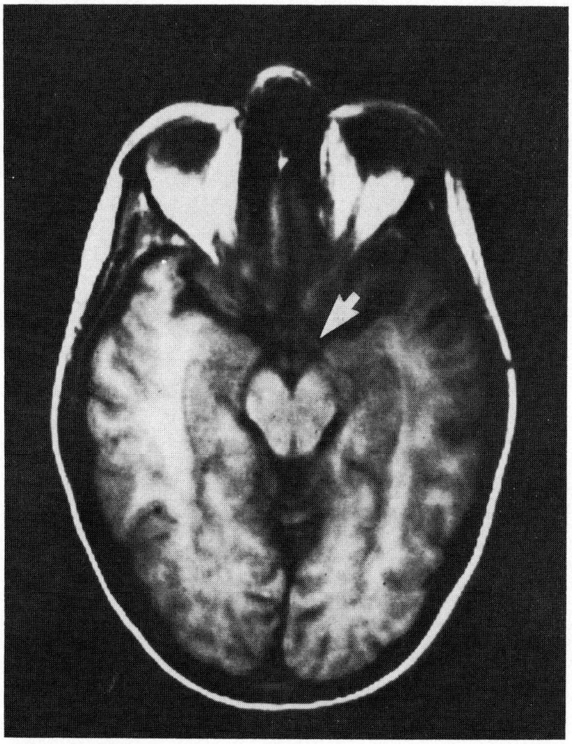

FIGURE 7-11

The optic tract (arrow) may be followed posteriorly into the brain on axial images such as this PS 400. (Courtesy of General Electric)

The Temporal Bone

As discussed in Chapter 6, the petrous portion of the temporal bone is largely devoid of MR signal because it is composed mostly of dense cortical bone and air cells. Pathological processes in the temporal bone may be recognized with a high degree of sensitivity as relatively high-intensity foci against this black background. As for the orbit, surface coils are needed to delineate accurately the minute neurovascular structures within the temporal bone (Fig. 7-12).

Routine MR scans using larger head coils can normally detect several signals from within the petrous temporal bone. The tips of the petrous pyramids often contain a large component of fatty marrow and may appear quite intense on T1-weighted sequences (Fig. 7-13). The neurovascular bundle of the internal auditory canal is commonly imaged on routine head MR scans, particularly by T2-weighted sequences. These structures appear linear on axial or coronal views (Fig. 7-14A) and as a dot on sagittal views (Fig. 7-14B). Slowly flowing blood in the jugular bulb may occasionally produce a high-intensity signal in the petrous bone. This is best seen on second echo axial images in a characteristic location (Fig. 7-15).

The origin of the facial and vestibulocochlear nerves from the brain stem are best seen using T1-weighted techniques (*e.g.,* PS 300 or SE 500/28). The dimensions of these nerves in the internal auditory canal can be most accurately estimated on T1-weighted sequences. The separation of nerves in the internal auditory canal is sometimes possible on coronal T1-weighted images (Fig. 7-16).

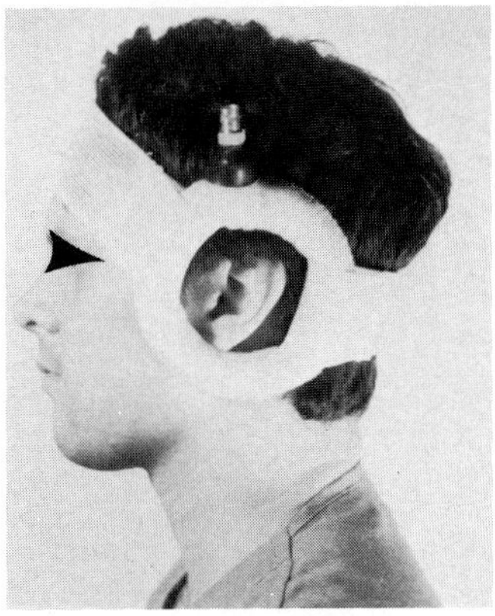

FIGURE 7-12

Surface coils similar to those used for the orbit may be applied to the temporal bone. (Courtesy of Fonar Corporation, 110 Marcus Drive, Melville, NY 11747)

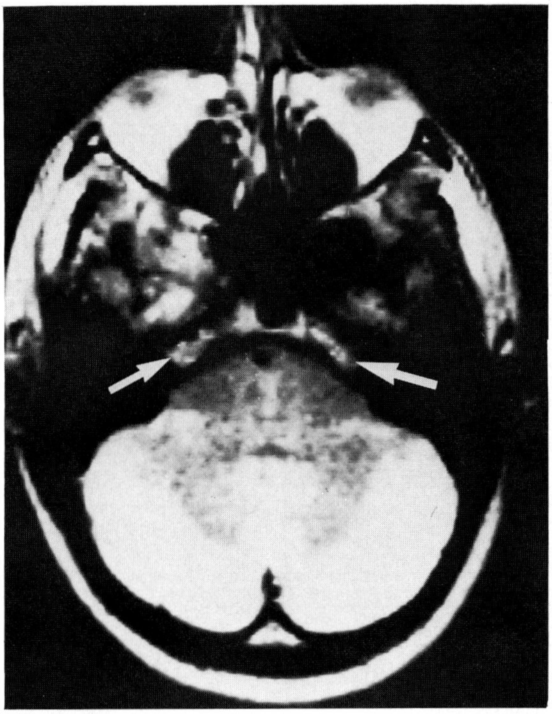

FIGURE 7-13

Fat in the tips of the petrous pyramids (arrows) may produce high-intensity signals from the temporal bone.

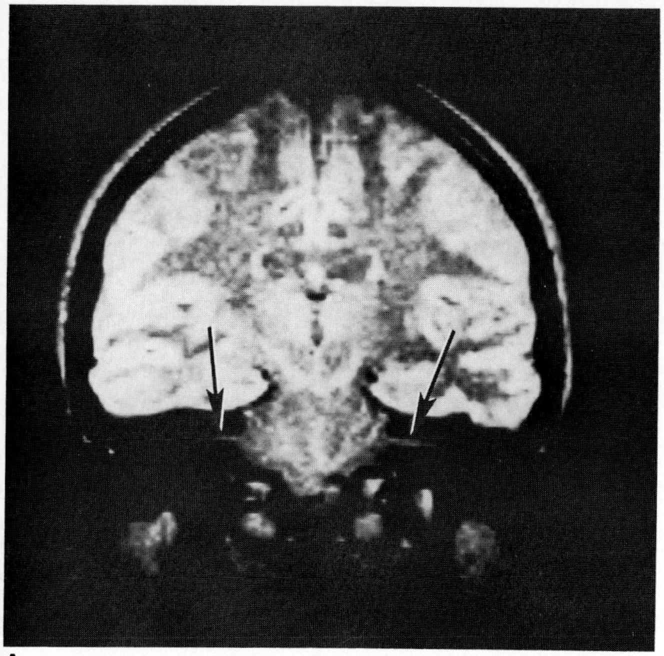

A

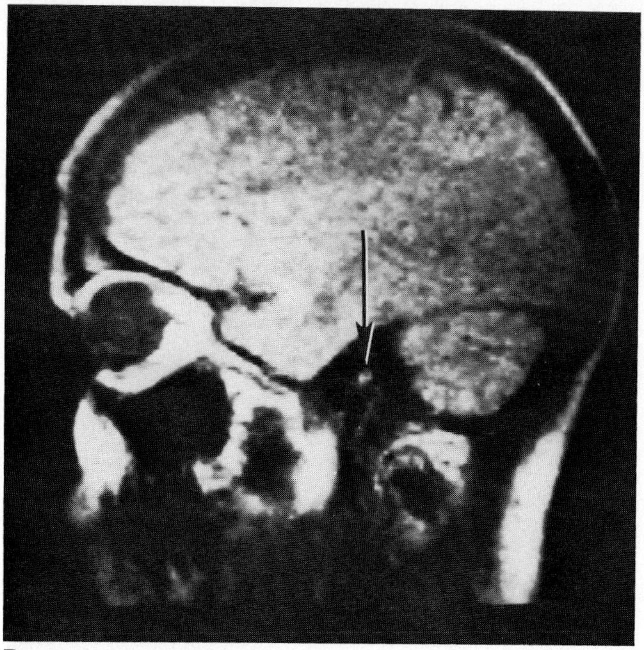

B

FIGURE 7-14

Neurovascular bundle in the internal auditory canal appears as a line on axial or coronal images (*A*) or as a dot on sagittal images (*B*).

FIGURE 7-15

Slowly flowing blood in the jugular bulb (arrow) may produce a bright signal, particularly on even echo images.

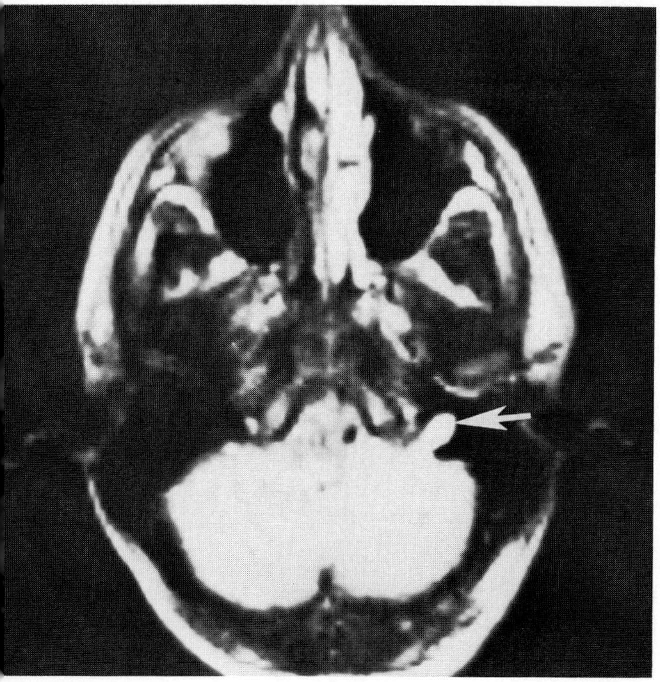

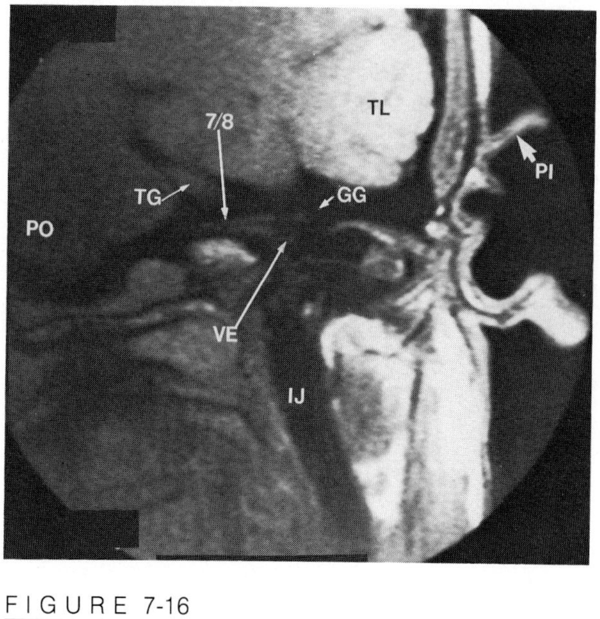

FIGURE 7-16

Coronal SE 500/28 surface coil image of the temporal bone demonstrates distinction of the seventh and eighth cranial nerves in the internal auditory canal (7/8). The geniculate ganglion (GG) of the facial nerve is seen. Also noted pons (PO), trigeminal nerve (TG), internal jugular vein (IJ), vestibule (VE), temporal lobe (TL), and pinna (PI). (Courtesy of Fonar Corporation, 110 Marcus Drive, Melville, NY 11747)

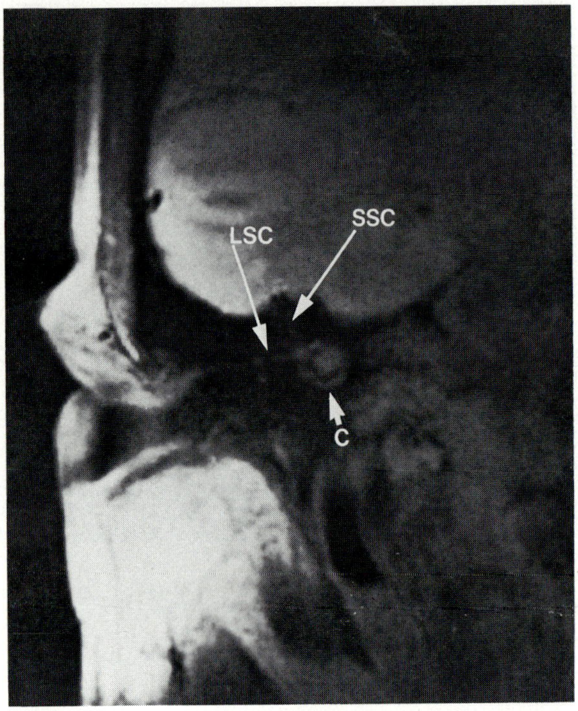

FIGURE 7-17

T2-weighted image (SE 1200/60) demonstrates fluid-filled cochlea (*C*), superior semicircular canal (SSC), and lateral semicircular canal (LSC). (Image obtained on Magniscan 5000, Thomson-CGR MR system)

For optimally demonstrating the cochlea and vestibular apparatus, more heavily T2-weighted sequences are recommended. This will allow the fluids (endolymph and perilymph) to generate a strong MR signal corresponding to long T1 and T2 relaxation times. An example of the cochlea and semicircular canals seen on a T2-weighted image is shown in Figure 7-17. Note that heavily T2-weighted sequences obscure accurate measurement of the intracanalicular neurovascular components, since high intensity from surrounding cerebrospinal fluid (CSF) blurs the individual margins.

Axial, coronal, and sagittal surface coil images of the temporal bone are presented in Figures 7-18 through 7-20. These were all performed with short spin-echo techniques (SE 500/28 or SE 500/30). The coronal and axial views appear to be the most satisfactory for displaying normal anatomy and pathological processes. The sagittal projection is useful to see the course of the vertical portion of the facial nerve but is otherwise somewhat limited. Note that the middle ear ossicles are not visualized, nor are other important bony landmarks used in CT diagnosis. Thus it seems likely that the future role of MR will be to supplement, not to replace, CT in the evaluation of the temporal bone. A possible protocol for imaging the internal auditory canal and temporal bone is presented in Table 7-2.

TABLE 7-2

Possible Protocol for MRI of the Temporal Bone

1. Use surface coils when available and thin (<3-mm) slices
2. Axial PS 300 or SE 500/25 (best for medial portions of internal auditory canals and proximal cranial nerves VII and VIII)
3. Axial SE 1500/60,120 (SE 1500/60 best for lateral portions of internal auditory canals; SE 1500/120 best for cochlea and semicircular canals)
4. Coronal PS 300 or SE 500/25
5. Sagittal SE 500/25 or PS 300 for descending limb of facial nerve and external auditory canal lesions

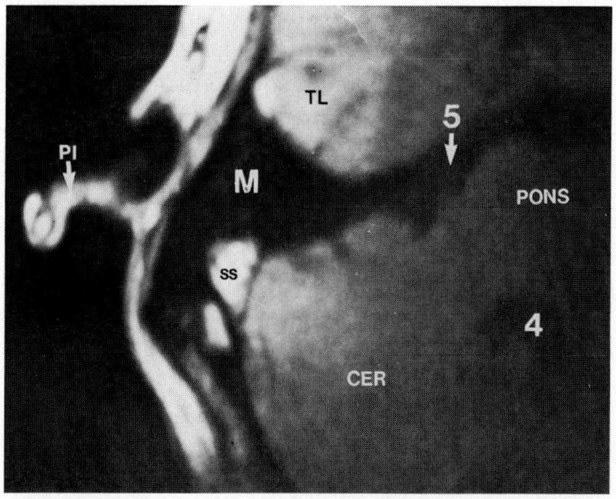

A

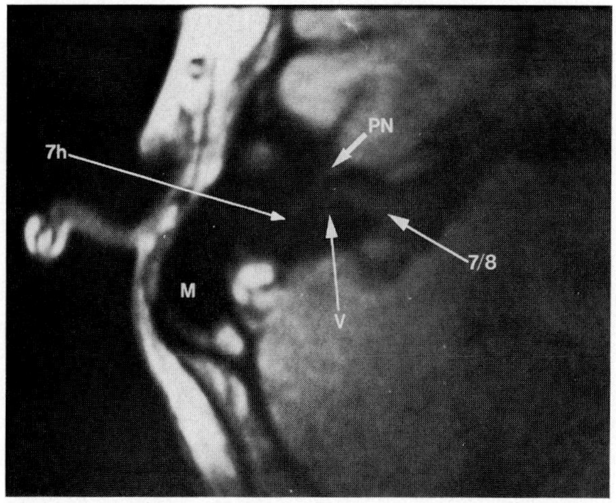

B

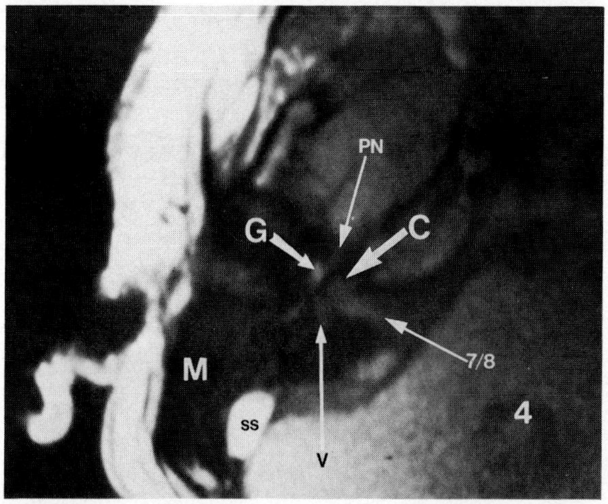

C

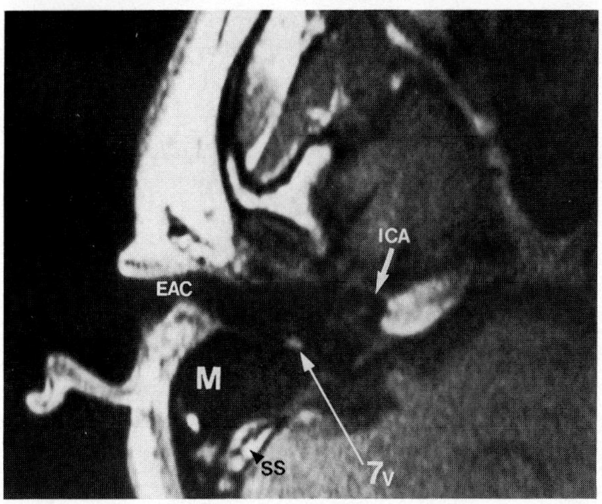

D

FIGURE 7-18

Axial SE 500/28 surface coil images of the temporal bone from superior to inferior. (Courtesy of Fonar Corporation, 110 Marcus Drive, Melville, NY 11747)

4	fourth ventricle
5	trigeminal nerve
7	facial nerve
7h	horizontal segment facial nerve
7v	vertical segment facial nerve
8	vestibulocochlear nerve
C	cochlea
CER	cerebellum
EAC	external auditory canal
F	flocculus
G	geniculate ganglion
ICA	internal carotid artery
IJ	internal jugular vein
IV	inferior vestibular nerve
JT	jugular tubercle
LP	lateral pterygoid muscle
M	mastoid air cells
MP	mastoid process
PI	pinna
PN	greater superficial petrosal nerve
SMF	stylomastoid foramen
SS	sigmoid sinus
SV	superior vestibular nerve
TC	tympanic cavity
TL	temporal lobe
TM	temporalis muscle
V	vestibule

The Temporomandibular Joint

Imaging of the temporomandibular joint (TMJ) is a natural extension of temporal bone MR imaging. The same surface coil and T1-weighted pulse techniques used for the temporal bone proper may be used to image the TMJ. Very little research has been published concerning the use of MR in imaging diseases of the TMJ.

Imaging of the TMJ should be performed using surface coils in the sagittal plane. T1-weighted sequences provide the best anatomic detail. A single set of images may be performed with the mouth partially open. Alternatively, two sets of sagittal images with both open- and closed-mouth views may be employed, particularly when meniscal dislocation is suspected. Visualized anatomic structures include the mandibular condyle, condylar articular cartilages, meniscus, and the insertion of the lateral pterygoid into the meniscus and neck of the condyle (Fig. 7-21A).

Direct coronal imaging demonstrates the relationships of the mandibular condyle, TMJ, and parotid gland (Fig. 7-21B). The coronal plane may be helpful in evaluating the extension of parotid tumors. It is only occasionally useful for assessing the TMJ, however. A possible protocol for imaging the TMJ is presented in Table 7-3.

TABLE 7-3

Possible Protocol for MRI of the TMJ

1. Use surface coils and thin slices (<3 mm)
2. Sagittal SE 600/30 or SE 1000/25
3. Open- and closed-mouth images

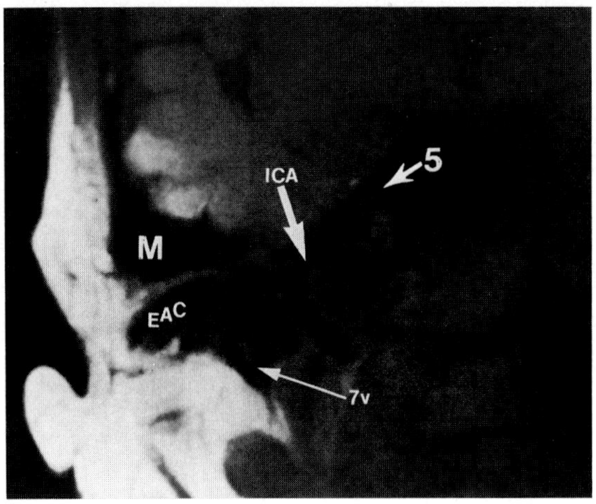

A

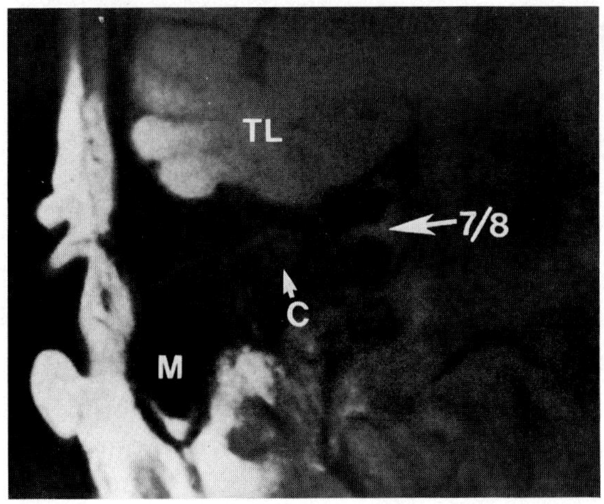

B

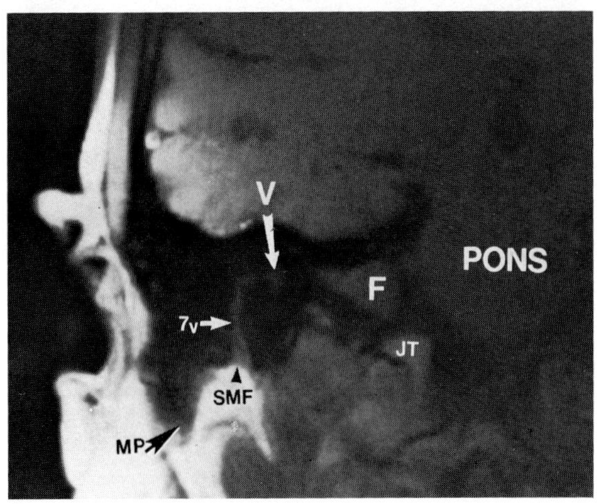

C

FIGURE 7-19

Coronal SE 500/30 surface coil images of the temporal bone from anterior to posterior. (Images obtained on Magniscan 5000, Thomson-CRG MR system)

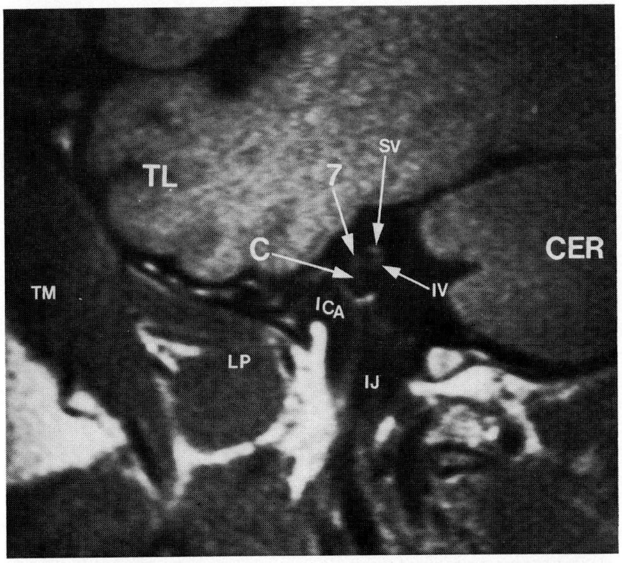

A

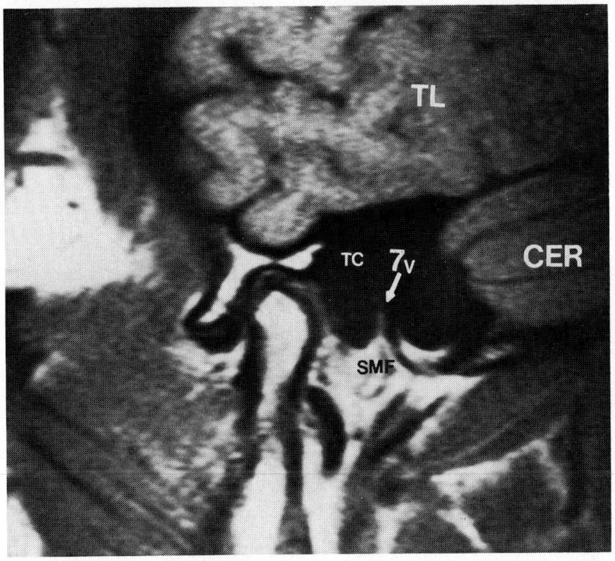

B

FIGURE 7-20

Sagittal SE 500/28 surface coil images of the temporal bone from medial to lateral. (Courtesy of Fonar Corporation, 110 Marcus Drive, Melville, NY 11747)

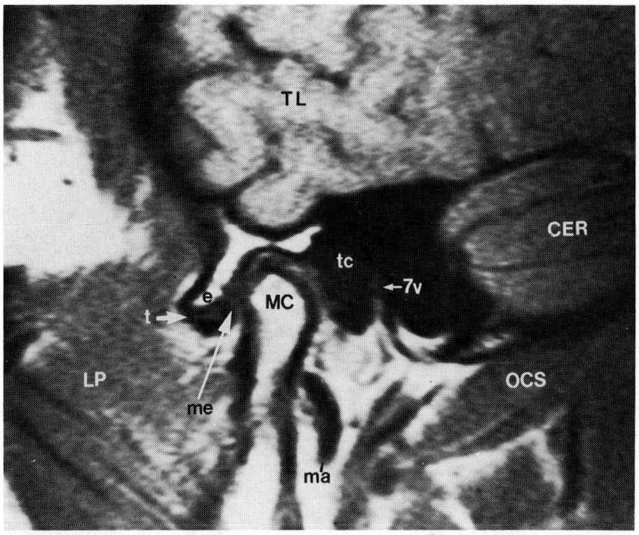

A

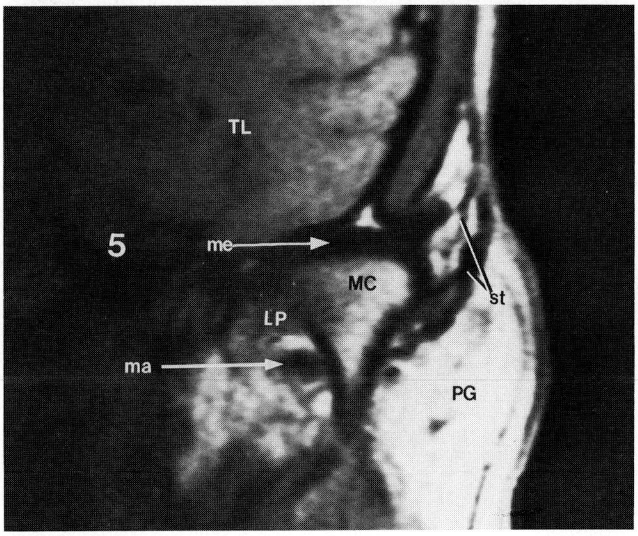

B

FIGURE 7-21

Axial (*A*) and coronal (*B*) views of the TMJ performed using surface coil SE 500/28 technique. Abbreviations are the same as for Figures 7-18 to 7-20 plus: mandibular condyle (MC), meniscus (me), internal maxillary artery (ma), eminence (e), tendon of lateral pterygoid (t), parotid gland (PG), oblique capitis superioris muscle (OCS), and superficial temporal vessels (st). (Courtesy of Fonar Corporation, 110 Marcus Drive, Melville, NY 11747)

The Nose and Paranasal Sinuses

The nose and paranasal sinuses are predominantly air-filled chambers bounded by dense bone. Neither air nor cortical bone contains a high density of hydrogen protons to generate an MR signal. Accordingly, MR has not yet proved as reliable as CT in evaluating lesions confined to the nose or paranasal sinuses. MR does offer, however, a high index of sensitivity for detection of pathological processes in

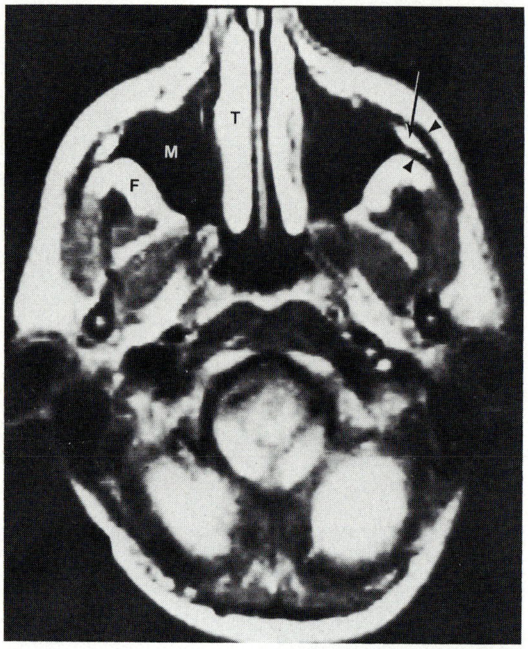

A

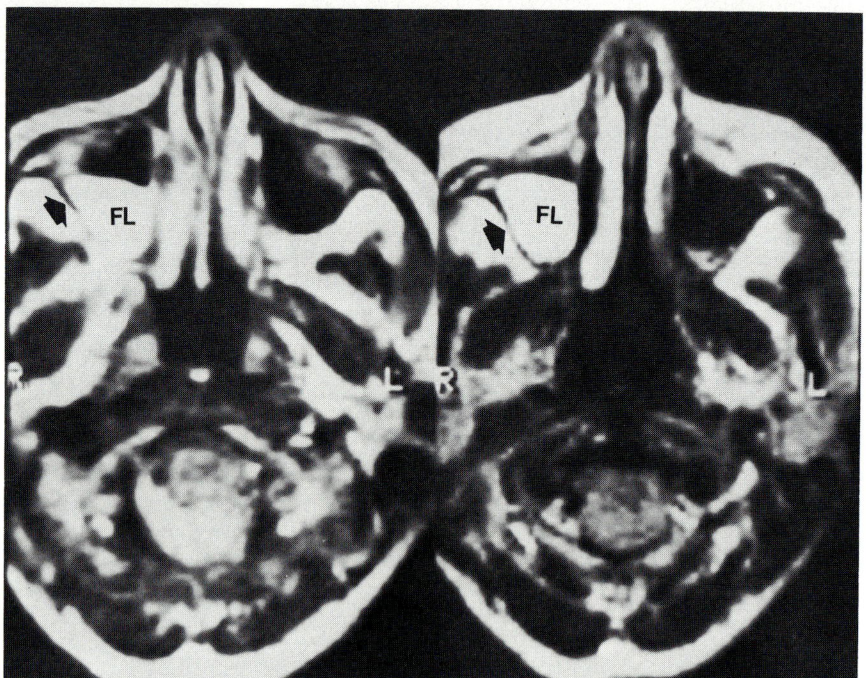

B

FIGURE 7-22

(*A*) The maxillary antrum (M) is seen on an axial SE 500/28 image. The posterior bony wall of the antrum cannot normally be seen, but rather an interface of this wall with retroantral fat (F). Laterally, fatty marrow (arrow) may be seen in the zygomatic process of the maxilla, defining anterior and posterior cortices. Note also the high-intensity signal from the nasal turbinate (T). (*B*) When fluid (FL) fills a maxillary sinus, its posterior wall may be clearly identified (arrows).

these areas. Moreover, when tumors or infections of the nose or paranasal sinuses extend into the nasopharynx or skull base, MR may prove very useful for quantitating this extension.

The walls of the paranasal sinuses are difficult to delineate precisely, because they represent an interface of cortical bone and air. What appears to be the posterior limit of the maxillary sinus, for example, is the edge of retroantral fat that lies external to the cortex of the posterior sinus wall (Fig. 7-22A). When fluid or mass fills the sinus, its true wall can be identified (Fig. 7-22B). Likewise, where a margin of the sinus is bordered by marrow-containing bone, the high-intensity marrow will delineate the true margin of the sinus (Fig. 7-22A).

The nasal turbinates are covered by a layer of lipid and water-rich cells and mucus. They are well delineated on most imaging sequences and produce a relatively intense signal (Fig. 7-22A). Commonly, one turbinate may appear much more intense than another, possibly, because of allergic inflammation or rhinitis. This is often seen so frequently in the absense of symptoms as to be considered a "normal" variant. Recesses and meatuses into which the sinuses empty may be seen on appropriate MR images (Fig. 7-23).

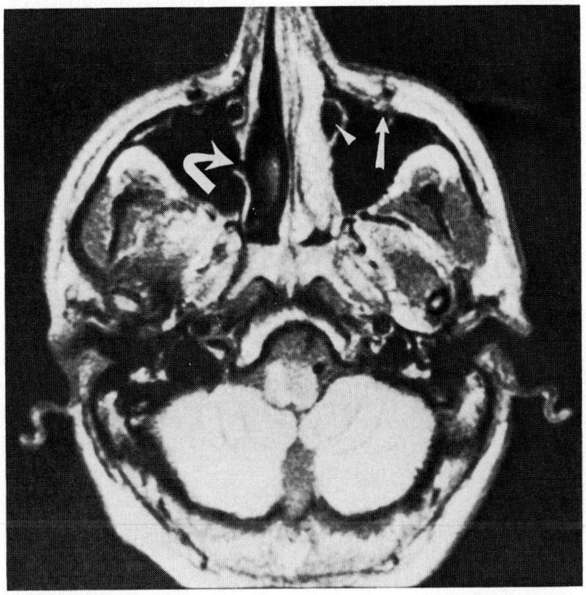

FIGURE 7-23

Landmarks adjacent to the maxillary antra. Curved arrow = ostium of maxillary sinus; straight arrow = canal for infraorbital nerve; arrowhead = nasolacrimal duct. (Courtesy of Fonar Corporation, 110 Marcus Drive, Melville, NY 11747)

Nasopharynx

MR is capable of demonstrating normal nasopharyngeal anatomy better than CT in most instances, and without the need for intravenous contrast. Vascular structures may be easily distinguished from lymph nodes on single slices by MR imaging. MR can be superior to CT in demonstrating the extent and margins of nasopharyngeal tumor, as well as associated adenopathy. If denervation of nasopharyngeal musculature occurs secondary to tumor or central nervous system (CNS) disease, fatty change in the denervated muscles may be recognized by MR as a very early sign. The ability to image directly in coronal and sagittal planes is an advantage of MR in the nasopharynx as it is in other areas of the body.

Only a few reports have appeared in the MR literature concerning imaging strategies for the nasopharynx. Table 7-1 provides a suggested protocol. As elsewhere in the body, both T1- and T2-weighted sequences are recommended for maximal detection and characterization of pathological processes. In general, T2-weighted sequences demonstrate normal anatomy and pathological masses. The T1-weighted sequences are more useful in defining the extent of certain tumors and in identifying lymph node metastases in the fatty spaces of the neck.

The axial plane remains singularly the most reliable for evaluating the entire nasopharynx and neck. Direct coronal and sagittal images are useful in a number of situations. They are probably required in evaluating possible tumor extension into the base of the skull because, like with CT, axial images alone may prove unreliable. Sagittal or coronal images are also sometimes helpful in evaluating the spread of infection or tumor along vertically oriented tissue planes in the neck.

The superficial landmarks of the nasopharynx are well delineated by their covering with high-intensity mucous membrane and lymphatic tissue. In young patients, high-intensity adenoidal tissue may be seen in a characteristic location (Fig. 7-24A,B). The distinction between this tissue, the mucous membrane, and the underlying pharyngeal musculature is well seen. In older patients, adenoidal tissue is not usually prominent (Fig. 7-24C). Likewise, the contrast between mucous membrane and underlying musculature may be lost, possibly as a result of an age-related involution of mucous glands, adenoidal tissue, and musculature.

The torus tubarius, pharyngeal recess (fossa of Rosenmüller), and eustachian tube orifice are well seen (Fig. 7-25). As with CT, symmetry is an important clue to the presence or absence of disease. The mastoid air cells should be inspected and are normally air filled (low signal intensity). Blockage or dysfunction of the eustachian tube may be an early sign of nasopharyngeal tumor or pathological process. In these situations, the presence of high-intensity fluid in the mastoid air cells should direct closer inspection of the nasopharynx.

Fat in the parapharyngeal spaces should be triangular and symmetrical lateral to the nasopharynx. Within these spaces, branches of the external carotid artery and pharyngeal veins may be visualized as low-intensity round and tubular structures. Laterally and posteriorly, the parapharyngeal space borders the deep lobe of the parotid gland (Fig. 7-26A). This gland is of lower intensity (shorter T2) than fat on long spin-echo images. Its relation to the external carotid artery and maxillary artery may be recognized.

The carotid sheath is seen posteriorly and contains the carotid artery, jugular vein, nerves, and lymphatics (Fig. 7-26A). Normally, because of rapidly flowing blood, the artery and vein have no MR signal and appear dark. Occasionally, particularly on even echo images, slow or turbulent flow in a small internal jugular vein may produce a signal. The syloid process, which lies anterolateral to the vascular bundle, may often be seen (Fig. 7-26B). If it contains fatty marrow, it may produce an intense signal; otherwise, it appears dark.

A possible protocol for imaging the face, paranasal sinuses, oropharynx, and nasopharynx is presented in Table 7-4. Axial, coronal, and sagittal images of these regions are presented in Figures 7-27, 7-28, and 7-29, respectively.

TABLE 7-4

Possible Protocol for MRI of the Face, Sinuses, Oropharynx, and Nasopharynx

1. Axial plane, SE 500/30
2. Axial plane, SE 2000/30,60
3. Coronal Plane, SE 1500/30,60 (to clarify extent of tumors and possible base of skull invasion)

(Text continues on p. 158.)

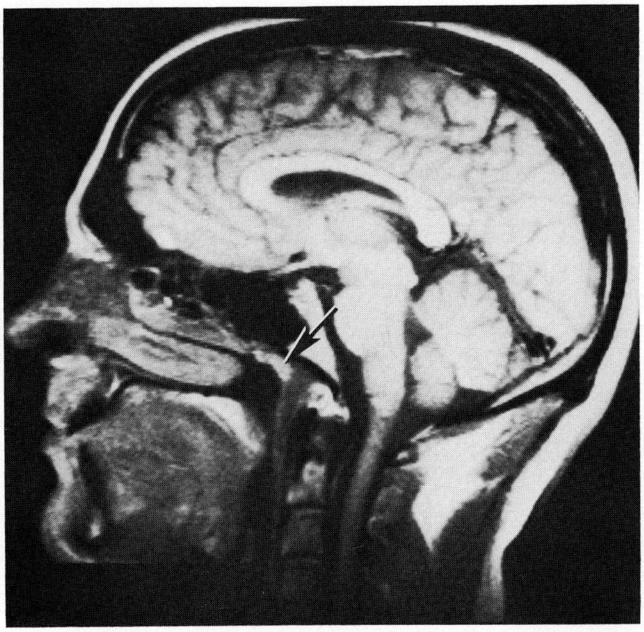

A

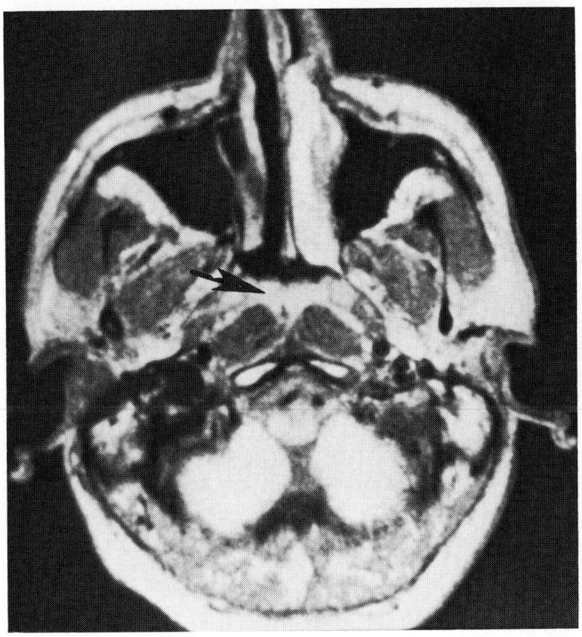

B

FIGURE 7-24

Normal adenoidal tissue (arrows) in axial (*A*) and sagittal (*B*) planes. In an older patient (*C*), this adenoidal tissue is less prominent. (Figure 7-24*A* courtesy of Fonar Corporation, 110 Marcus Drive, Melville, NY 11747, Figure 7-24*B* courtesy of Technicare Corporation © 1985, Figure 7-24*C* courtesy of General Electric Medical Systems)

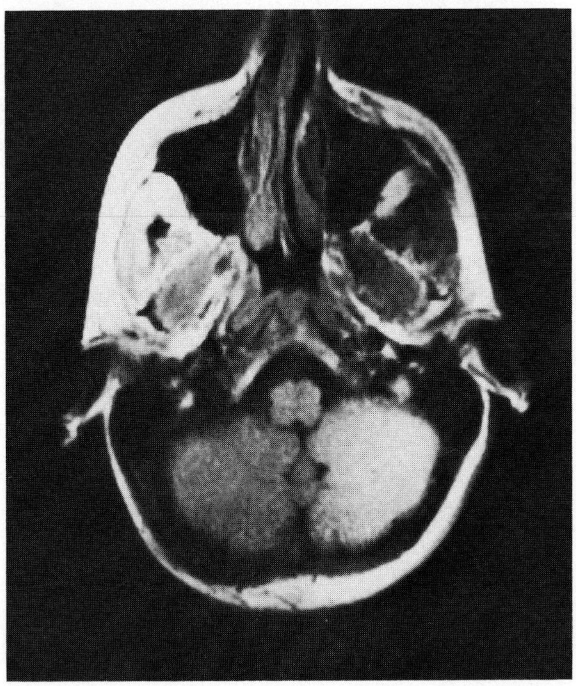

C

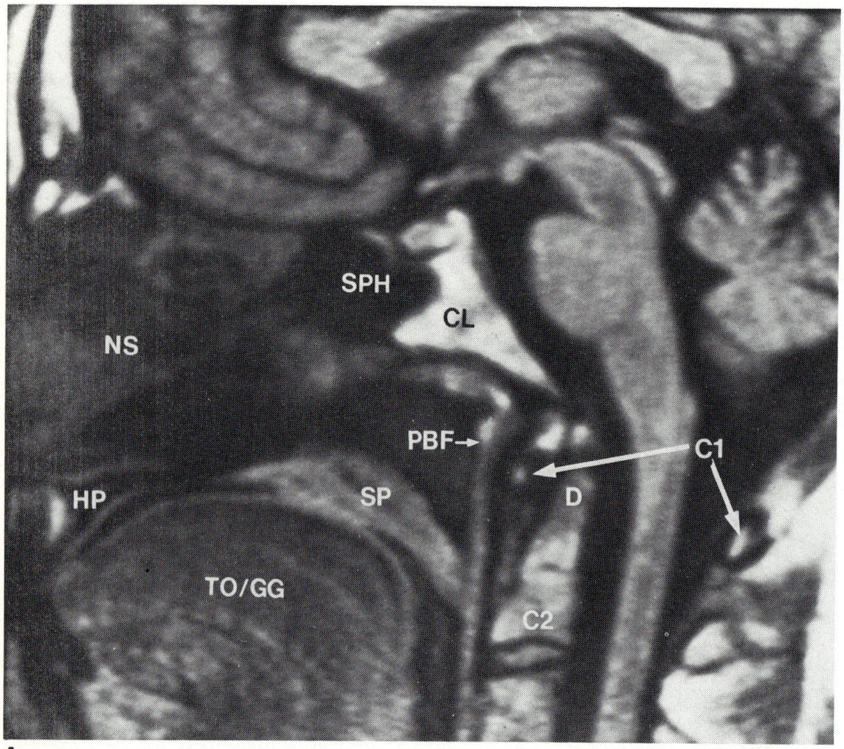

A

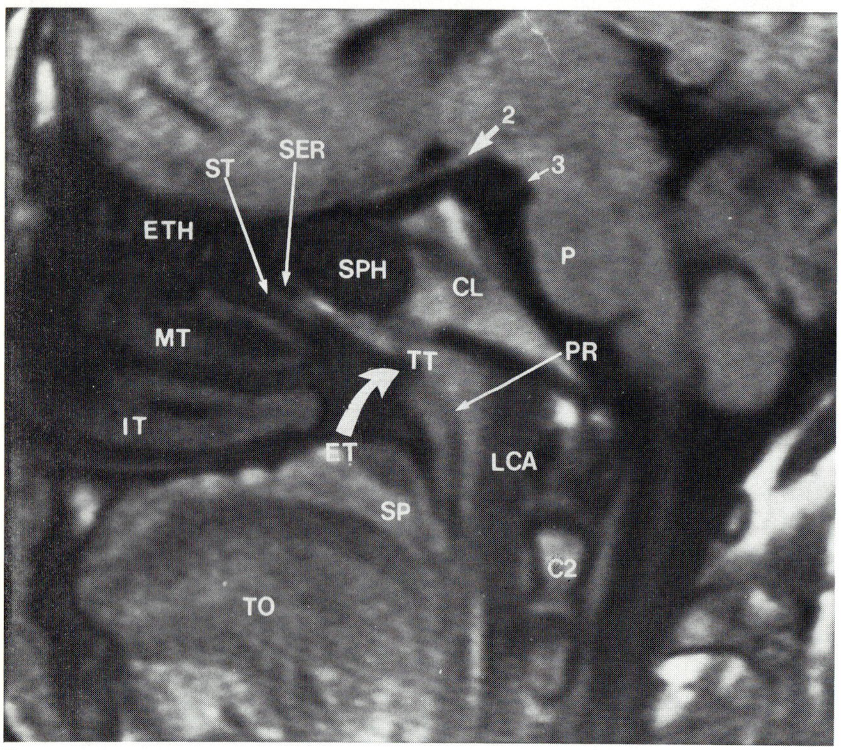

B

FIGURE 7-25

Midline and parasagittal SE 400/28 images of the nasopharynx. (Courtesy of Fonar Corporation, 110 Marcus Drive, Melville, NY 11747)

2	optic nerve (cranial nerve II)
3	oculomotor nerve (cranial nerve) III)
C1, C2	first and second cervical vertebrae
CL	clivus
D	dens
ETH	ethmoidal sinus
HP	hard palate
IT	inferior turbinate
LCA	longus capitis muscle
MT	middle turbinate
NS	nasal septum
P	pons
PBF	pharyngobasilar fascia
PR	pharyngeal recess (fossa of Rosenmüller)
SER	sphenoethmoidal recess
SP	soft palate
SPH	sphenoidal sinus
ST	superior turbinate
TT	torus tubarius
TO/GG	tongue/genioglossus

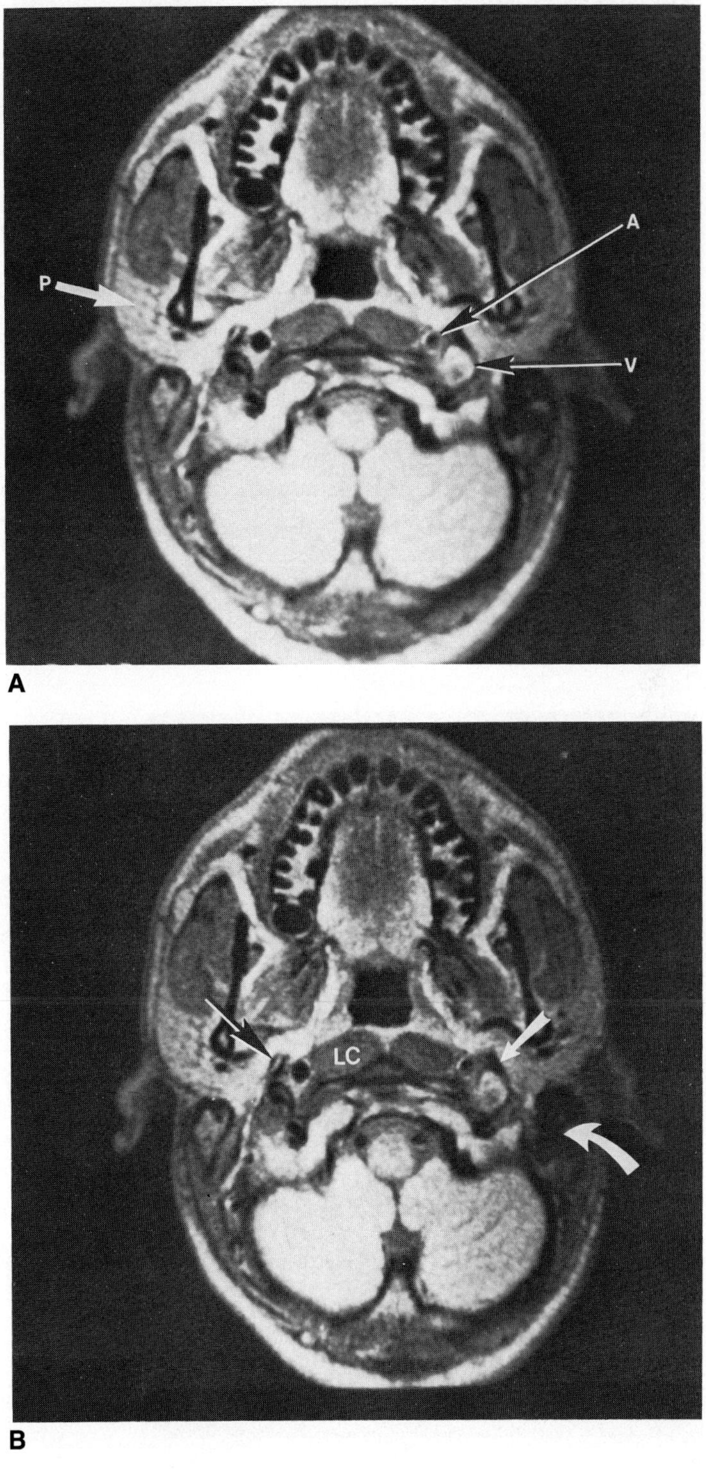

FIGURE 7-26

(*A*) Parapharyngeal spaces are filled with symmetrical fat. A = internal carotid artery; V = internal jugular vein; P = parotid gland. (*B*) Styloid process is anterolateral to the vascular bundle and may be filled with fatty marrow (black arrow) or have low signal as cortical bone (white arrow). Note also air-filled mastoid cells (curved arrow). (Courtesy of Fonar Corporation, 110 Marcus Drive, Melville, NY 11747)

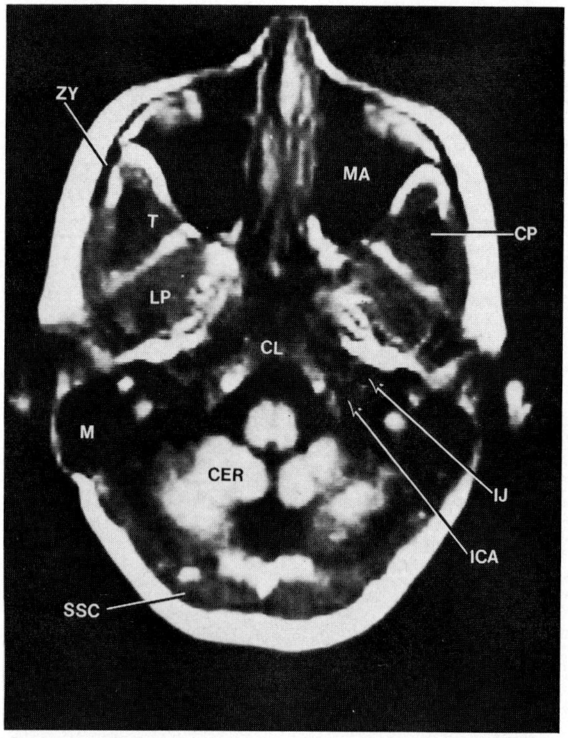

A

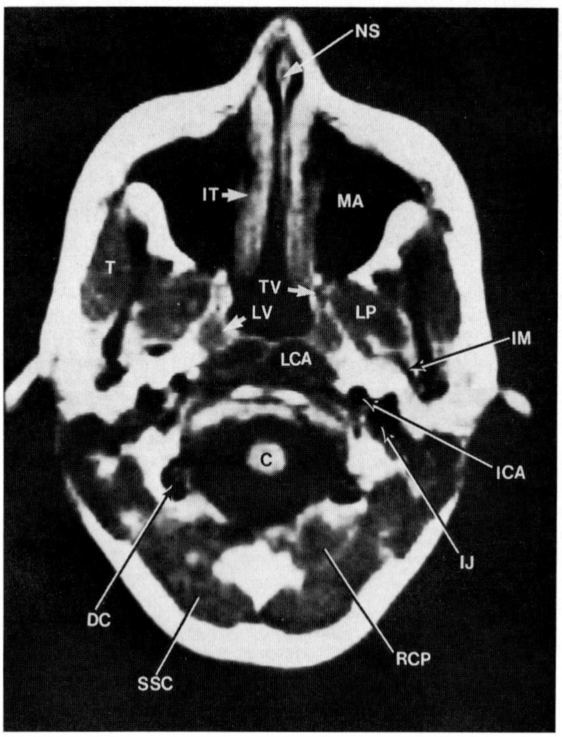

B

FIGURE 7-27

Axial SE 500/28 images of the head from the level of the orbital floor (*A*) to the bottom of the mandible.

7/8	7th and 8th cranial nerves in internal auditory canal
AT	atrium
BM	body of mandible
BU	buccinator muscle
C	spinal cord
C1, C2, C3, C4	cervical vertebrae 1, 2, 3, 4
CER	cerebellum
CL	clivus
CO	pharyngeal constrictor
CP	coronoid process of mandible
D	dens
DC	deep cervical vein
DI	digastric muscle (posterior belly)
E	esophagus
EAC	external auditory canal
EC	external carotid artery
EJ	external jugular vein
ETH	ethmoid sinus
EU	eustachian tube orifice
F	facial artery
FS	frontal sinus
G	globe
GG	genioglossus muscle
GH	geniohyoid muscle
GWS	greater wing of sphenoid
HP	hard palate
ICA	internal carotid artery
IJ	internal jugular vein
IM	internal maxillary artery
IT	inferior turbinate
LC	longus colli muscle
LCA	longus capitis muscle
LEP	levator palati muscle
LG	lacrimal gland
LP	lateral pterygoid muscle
LS	levator scapulae muscle
LV	levator veli palatini muscle
M	mastoid air cells
MA	maxillary antrum
MB	mandibular body
MC	mandibular condyle
MH	myohyoid muscle
MM	masseter muscle
MP	medial pterygoid muscle
MR	medial rectus muscle
MT	middle turbinate
NP	nasopharynx
NS	nasal septum
OC	occipital condyle
OCI	obliquus capitis inferior muscle
ON	optic nerve
OP	oropharynx
OR	orbital rim
PG	parotid gland
RA	median raphe (septum) of tongue
RCP	rectus capitis posterior muscle
RM	ramus of mandible
SCM	sternocleidomastoid muscle
SMG	submandibular gland
SP	soft palate
SPH	sphenoid sinus
SPL	splenius capitis muscle
SR	superior rectus muscle
SS	sigmoid sinus
SSC	semispinalis capitis muscle
ST	superior nasal turbinate
T	temporalis muscle
TE	teeth
TO	tongue
TR	trapezius muscle
TT	torus tubarius
TV	tensor veli palatini
TVS	transversospinalis muscle
U	uvula
V	vallecula
VA	vertebral artery
VE	vestibule
ZP	zygomatic process of maxilla
ZY	zygomatic arch

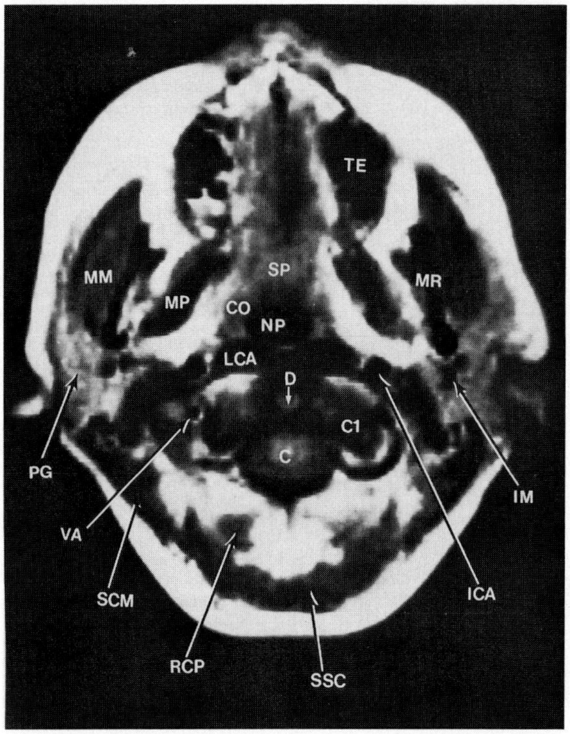
TE
SP
MM
MP
CO
NP
MR
LCA
D
C1
C
PG
VA
SCM
RCP
SSC
ICA
IM

C

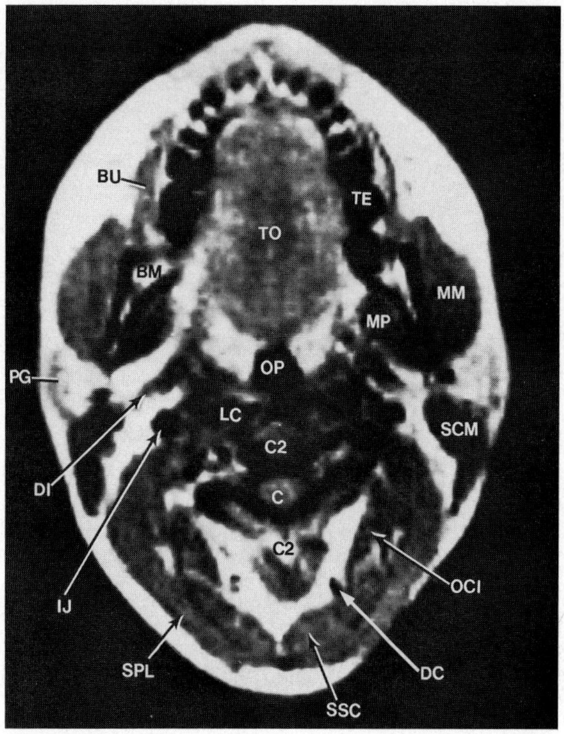
BU
TE
TO
BM
MM
MP
OP
PG
LC
C2
SCM
C
DI
C2
OCI
IJ
SPL
DC
SSC

D

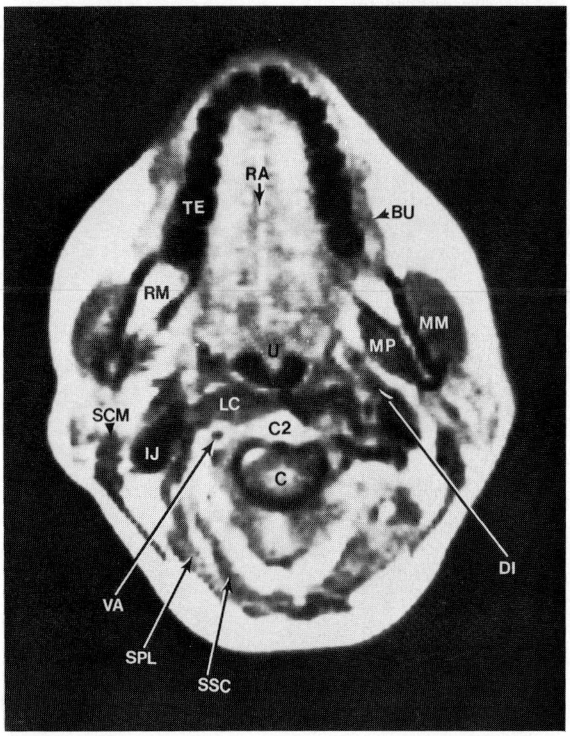
RA
TE
BU
RM
MM
MP
U
LC
SCM
C2
IJ
C
DI
VA
SPL
SSC

E

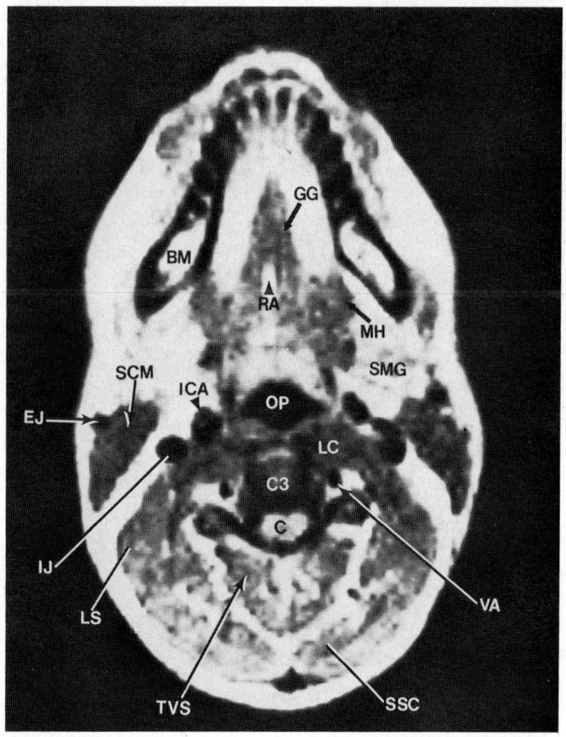
GG
BM
RA
MH
SCM
SMG
ICA
EJ
OP
LC
C3
C
IJ
VA
LS
TVS
SSC

F

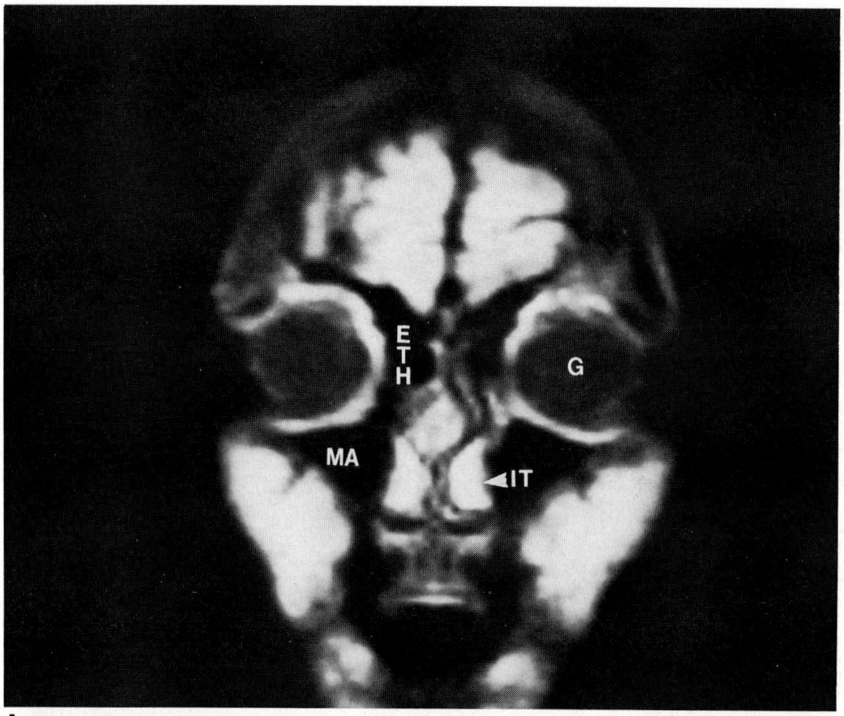

A

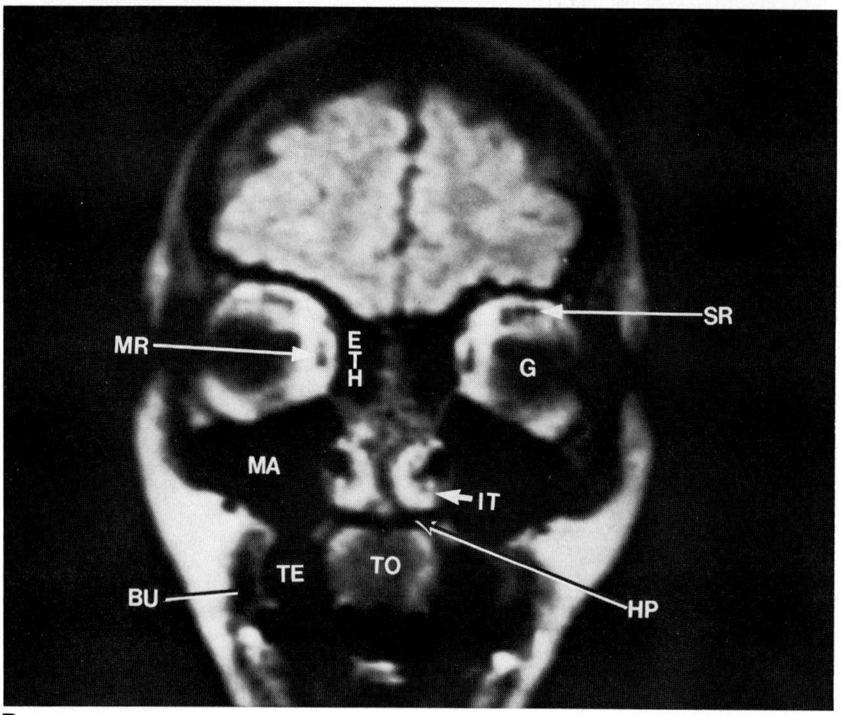

B

FIGURE 7-28

Coronal SE 1000/28 images of the head in successive 1-cm slices from anterior to posterior.

7/8	7th and 8th cranial nerves in internal auditory canal
AT	atrium
BM	body of mandible
BU	buccinator muscle
C	spinal cord
C1, C2, C3, C4	cervical vertebrae 1, 2, 3, 4
CER	cerebellum
CL	clivus
CO	pharyngeal constrictor
CP	coronoid process of mandible
D	dens
DC	deep cervical vein
DI	digastric muscle (posterior belly)
E	esophagus
EAC	external auditory canal
EC	external carotid artery
EJ	external jugular vein
ETH	ethmoid sinus
EU	eustachian tube orifice
F	facial artery
FS	frontal sinus
G	globe
GG	genioglossus muscle
GH	geniohyoid muscle
GWS	greater wing of sphenoid
HP	hard palate
ICA	internal carotid artery
IJ	internal jugular vein
IM	internal maxillary artery
IT	inferior turbinate
LC	longus colli muscle
LCA	longus capitis muscle
LEP	levator palati muscle
LG	lacrimal gland
LP	lateral pterygoid muscle
LS	levator scapulae muscle
LV	levator veli palatini muscle
M	mastoid air cells
MA	maxillary antrum

MB	mandibular body
MC	mandibular condyle
MH	myohyoid muscle
MM	masseter muscle
MP	medial pterygoid muscle
MR	medial rectus muscle
MT	middle turbinate
NP	nasopharynx
NS	nasal septum
OC	occipital condyle
OCI	obliquus capitis inferior muscle
ON	optic nerve
OP	oropharynx
OR	orbital rim
PG	parotid gland
RA	median raphe (septum) of tongue
RCP	rectus capitis posterior muscle
RM	ramus of mandible
SCM	sternocleidomastoid muscle
SMG	submandibular gland
SP	soft palate
SPH	sphenoid sinus
SPL	splenius capitis muscle
SR	superior rectus muscle
SS	sigmoid sinus
SSC	semispinalis capitis muscle
ST	superior nasal turbinate
T	temporalis muscle
TE	teeth
TO	tongue
TR	trapezius muscle
TT	torus tubarius
TV	tensor veli palatini
TVS	transversospinalis muscle
U	uvula
V	vallecula
VA	vertebral artery
VE	vestibule
ZP	zygomatic process of maxilla
ZY	zygomatic arch

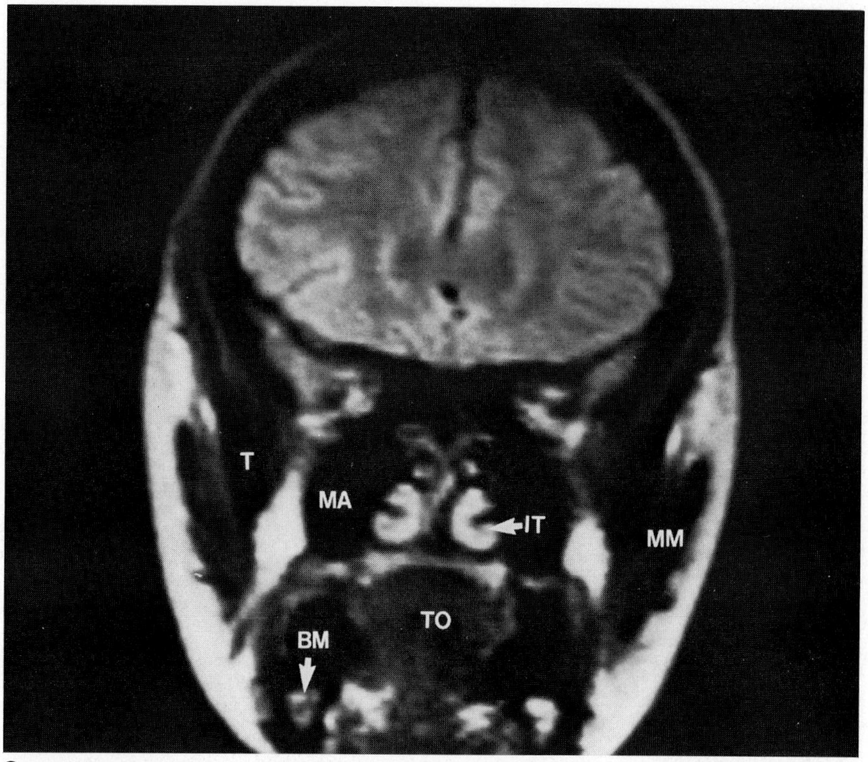

C

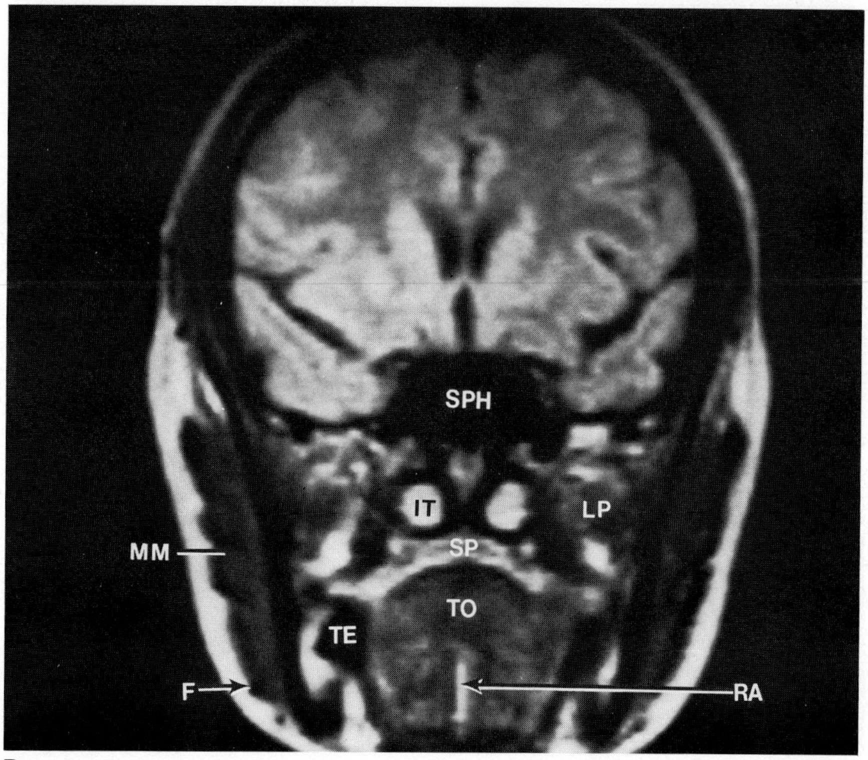

D

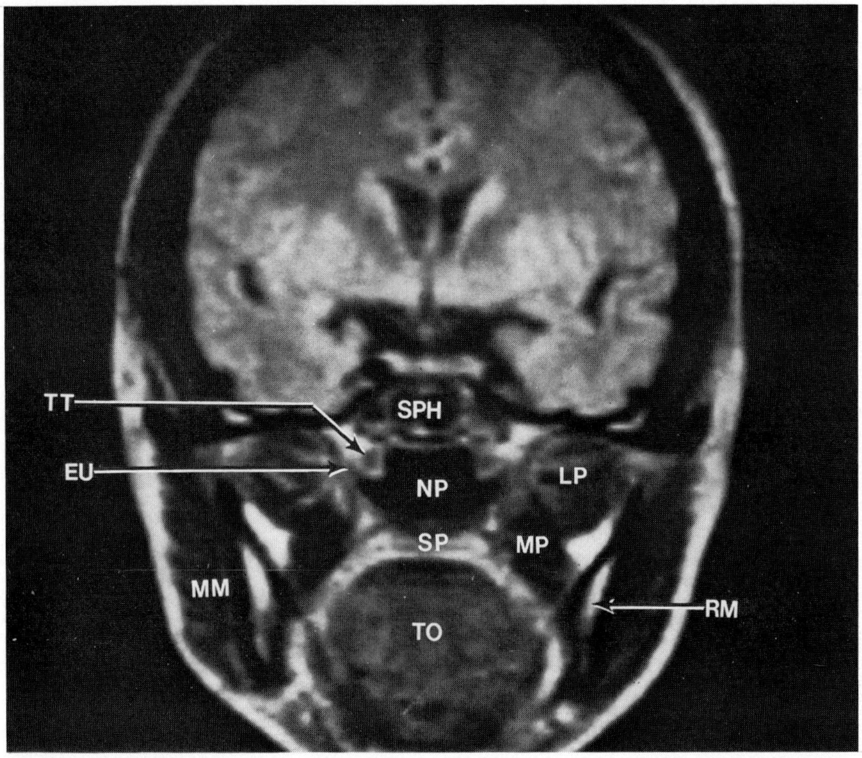

E

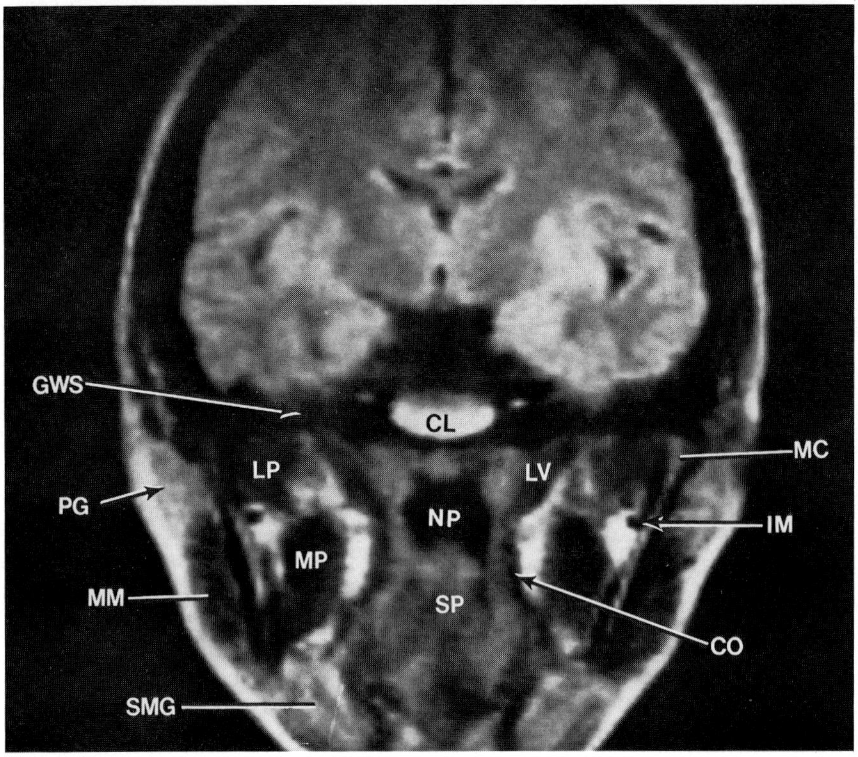

F

FIGURE 7-28 *(cont.)*

Coronal SE 1000/28 images of the head in successive 1-cm slices from anterior to posterior.

7/8	7th and 8th cranial nerves in internal auditory canal
AT	atrium
BM	body of mandible
BU	buccinator muscle
C	spinal cord
C1, C2, C3, C4	cervical vertebrae 1, 2, 3, 4
CER	cerebellum
CL	clivus
CO	pharyngeal constrictor
CP	coronoid process of mandible
D	dens
DC	deep cervical vein
DI	digastric muscle (posterior belly)
E	esophagus
EAC	external auditory canal
EC	external carotid artery
EJ	external jugular vein
ETH	ethmoid sinus
EU	eustachian tube orifice
F	facial artery
FS	frontal sinus
G	globe
GG	genioglossus muscle
GH	geniohyoid muscle
GWS	greater wing of sphenoid
HP	hard palate
ICA	internal carotid artery
IJ	internal jugular vein
IM	internal maxillary artery
IT	inferior turbinate
LC	longus colli muscle
LCA	longus capitis muscle
LEP	levator palati muscle
LG	lacrimal gland
LP	lateral pterygoid muscle
LS	levator scapulae muscle
LV	levator veli palatini muscle
M	mastoid air cells
MA	maxillary antrum

MB	mandibular body
MC	mandibular condyle
MH	myohyoid muscle
MM	masseter muscle
MP	medial pterygoid muscle
MR	medial rectus muscle
MT	middle turbinate
NP	nasopharynx
NS	nasal septum
OC	occipital condyle
OCI	obliquus capitis inferior muscle
ON	optic nerve
OP	oropharynx
OR	orbital rim
PG	parotid gland
RA	median raphe (septum) of tongue
RCP	rectus capitis posterior muscle
RM	ramus of mandible
SCM	sternocleidomastoid muscle
SMG	submandibular gland
SP	soft palate
SPH	sphenoid sinus
SPL	splenius capitis muscle
SR	superior rectus muscle
SS	sigmoid sinus
SSC	semispinalis capitis muscle
ST	superior nasal turbinate
T	temporalis muscle
TE	teeth
TO	tongue
TR	trapezius muscle
TT	torus tubarius
TV	tensor veli palatini
TVS	transversospinalis muscle
U	uvula
V	vallecula
VA	vertebral artery
VE	vestibule
ZP	zygomatic process of maxilla
ZY	zygomatic arch

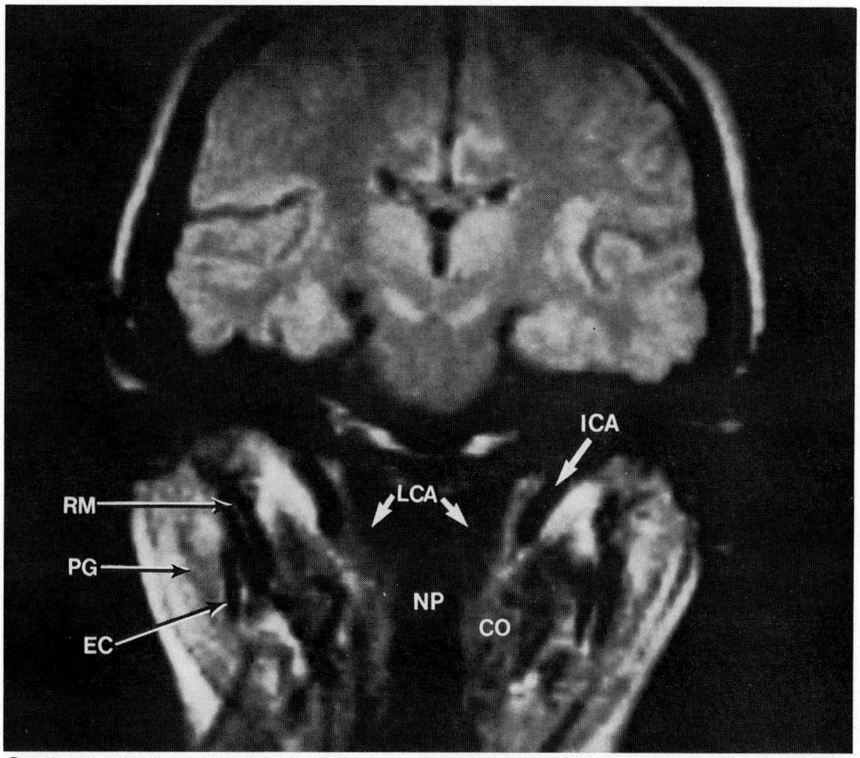

G

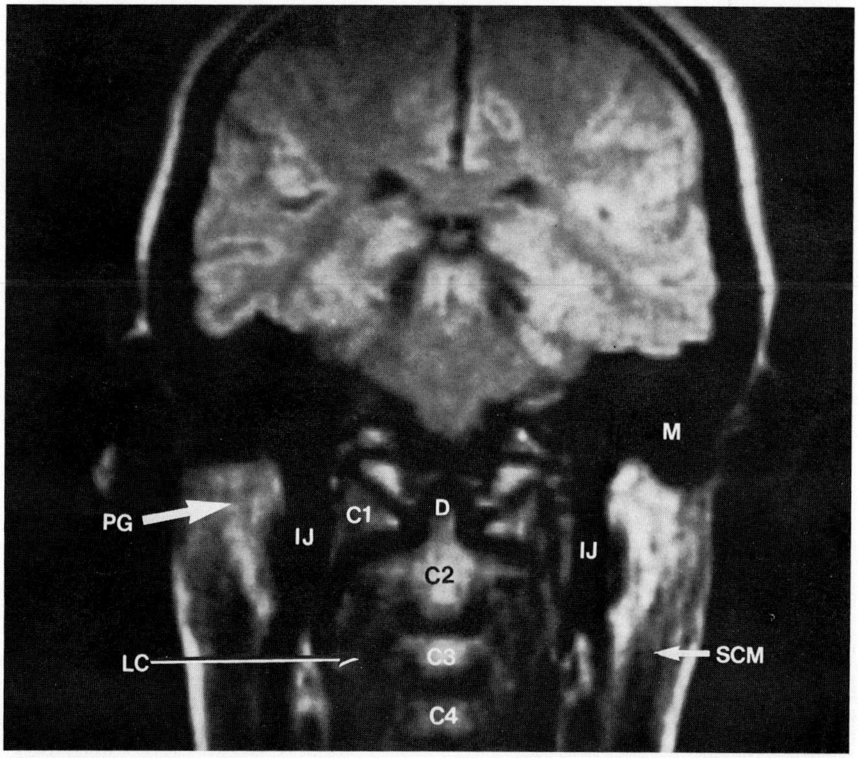

H

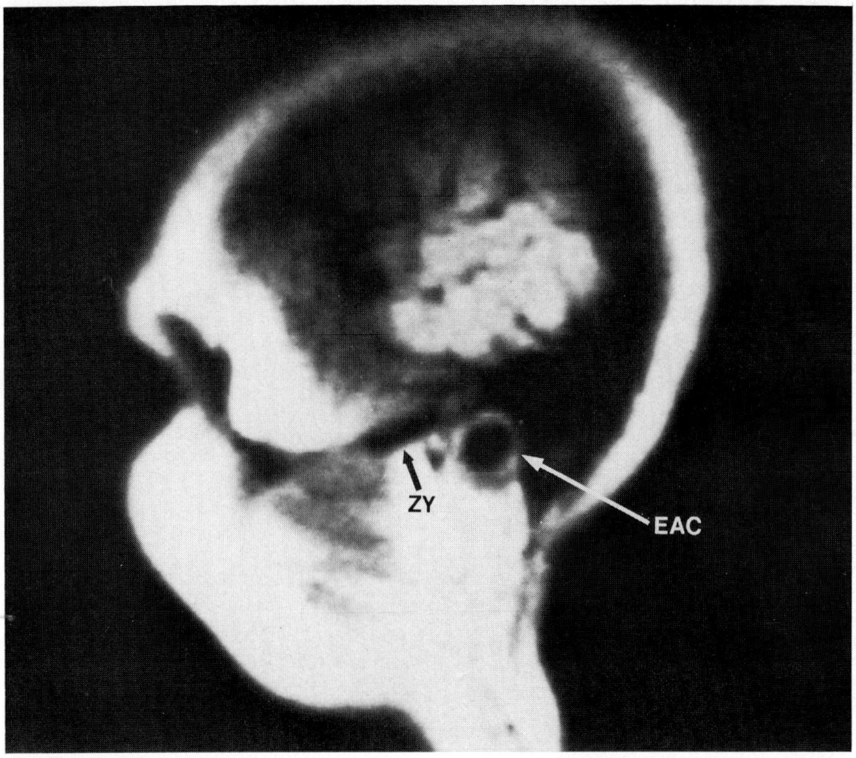

A

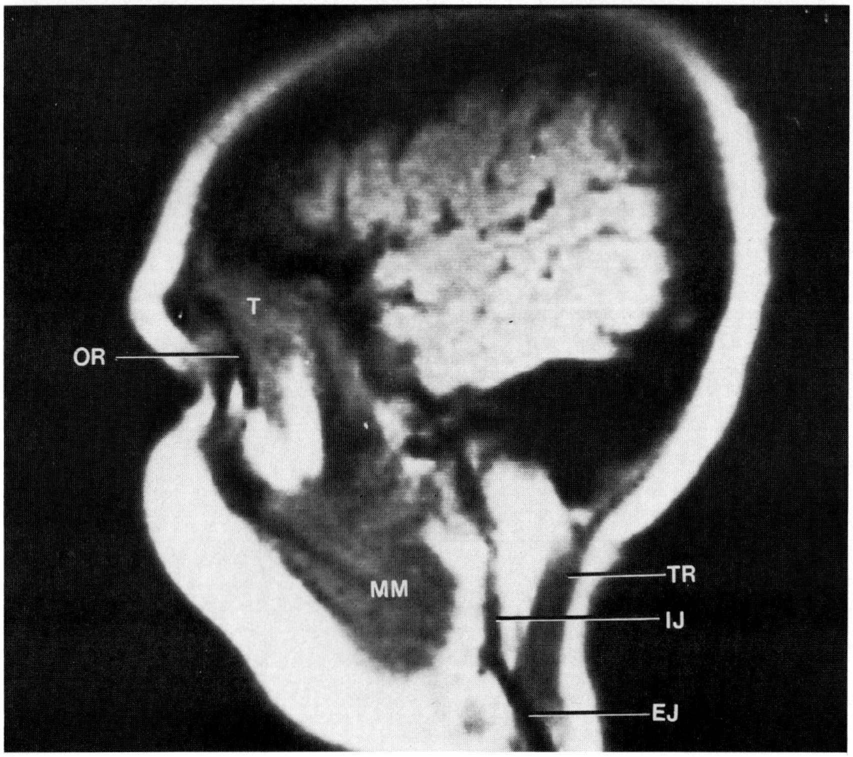

B

FIGURE 7-29

Sagittal SE 1000/28 images of the head from lateral to midline in successive 1-cm slices.

7/8	7th and 8th cranial nerves in internal auditory canal
AT	atrium
BM	body of mandible
BU	buccinator muscle
C	spinal cord
C1, C2, C3, C4	cervical vertebrae 1, 2, 3, 4
CER	cerebellum
CL	clivus
CO	pharyngeal constrictor
CP	coronoid process of mandible
D	dens
DC	deep cervical vein
DI	digastric muscle (posterior belly)
E	esophagus
EAC	external auditory canal
EC	external carotid artery
EJ	external jugular vein
ETH	ethmoid sinus
EU	eustachian tube orifice
F	facial artery
FS	frontal sinus
G	globe
GG	genioglossus muscle
GH	geniohyoid muscle
GWS	greater wing of sphenoid
HP	hard palate
ICA	internal carotid artery
IJ	internal jugular vein
IM	internal maxillary artery
IT	inferior turbinate
LC	longus colli muscle
LCA	longus capitis muscle
LEP	levator palati muscle
LG	lacrimal gland
LP	lateral pterygoid muscle
LS	levator scapulae muscle
LV	levator veli palatini muscle
M	mastoid air cells
MA	maxillary antrum

MB	mandibular body
MC	mandibular condyle
MH	myohyoid muscle
MM	masseter muscle
MP	medial pterygoid muscle
MR	medial rectus muscle
MT	middle turbinate
NP	nasopharynx
NS	nasal septum
OC	occipital condyle
OCI	obliquus capitis inferior muscle
ON	optic nerve
OP	oropharynx
OR	orbital rim
PG	parotid gland
RA	median raphe (septum) of tongue
RCP	rectus capitis posterior muscle
RM	ramus of mandible
SCM	sternocleidomastoid muscle
SMG	submandibular gland
SP	soft palate
SPH	sphenoid sinus
SPL	splenius capitis muscle
SR	superior rectus muscle
SS	sigmoid sinus
SSC	semispinalis capitis muscle
ST	superior nasal turbinate
T	temporalis muscle
TE	teeth
TO	tongue
TR	trapezius muscle
TT	torus tubarius
TV	tensor veli palatini
TVS	transversospinalis muscle
U	uvula
V	vallecula
VA	vertebral artery
VE	vestibule
ZP	zygomatic process of maxilla
ZY	zygomatic arch

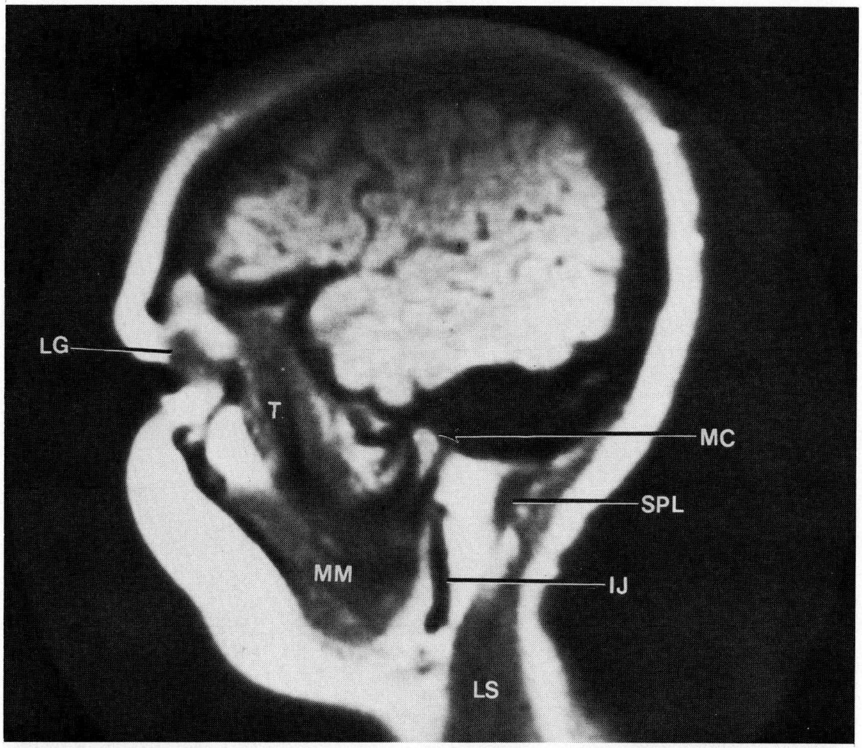

C

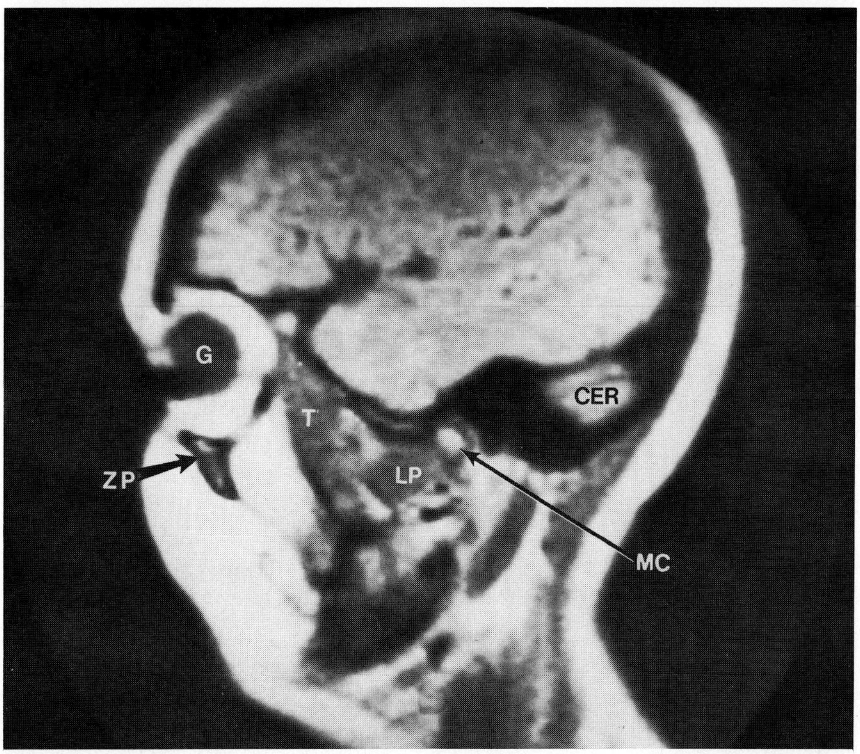

D

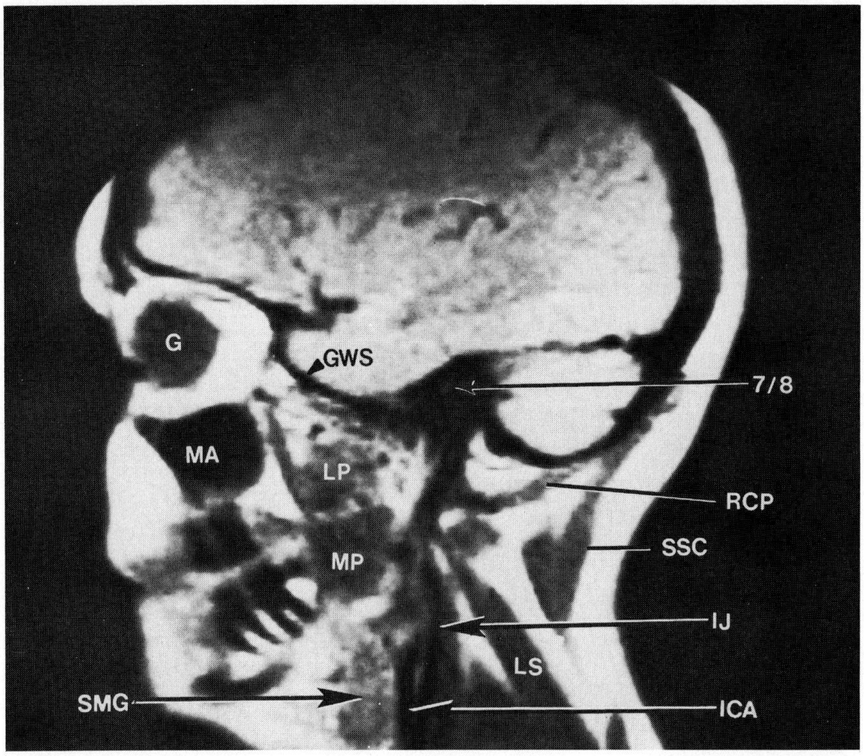

E

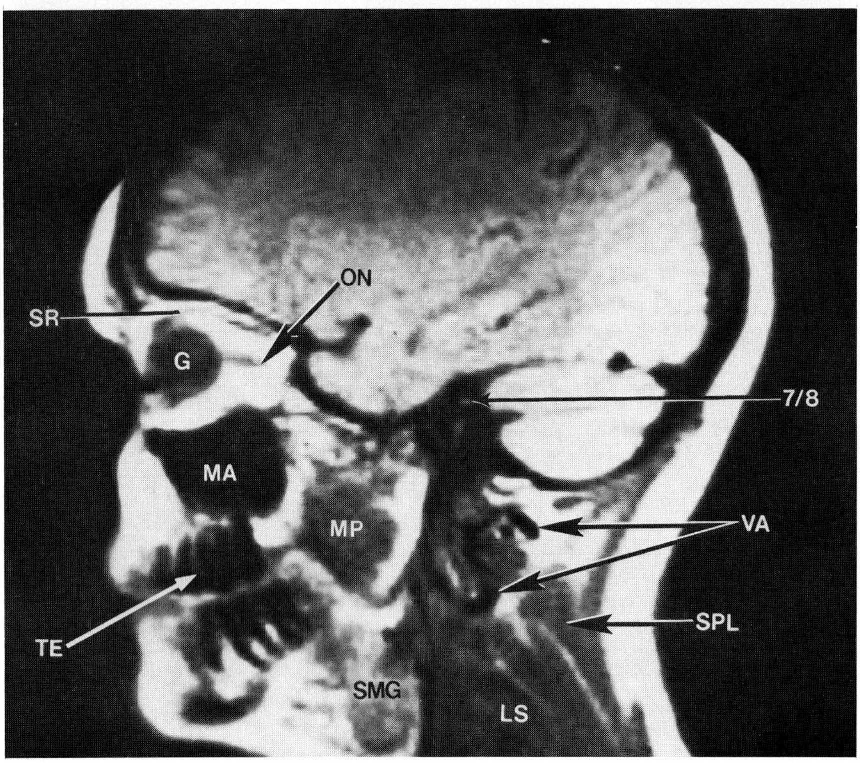

F

FIGURE 7-29 *(cont.)*

Sagittal SE 1000/28 images of the head from lateral to midline in successive 1-cm slices.

7/8	7th and 8th cranial nerves in internal auditory canal
AT	atrium
BM	body of mandible
BU	buccinator muscle
C	spinal cord
C1, C2, C3, C4	cervical vertebrae 1, 2, 3, 4
CER	cerebellum
CL	clivus
CO	pharyngeal constrictor
CP	coronoid process of mandible
D	dens
DC	deep cervical vein
DI	digastric muscle (posterior belly)
E	esophagus
EAC	external auditory canal
EC	external carotid artery
EJ	external jugular vein
ETH	ethmoid sinus
EU	eustachian tube orifice
F	facial artery
FS	frontal sinus
G	globe
GG	genioglossus muscle
GH	geniohyoid muscle
GWS	greater wing of sphenoid
HP	hard palate
ICA	internal carotid artery
IJ	internal jugular vein
IM	internal maxillary artery
IT	inferior turbinate
LC	longus colli muscle
LCA	longus capitis muscle
LEP	levator palati muscle
LG	lacrimal gland
LP	lateral pterygoid muscle
LS	levator scapulae muscle
LV	levator veli palatini muscle
M	mastoid air cells
MA	maxillary antrum

MB	mandibular body
MC	mandibular condyle
MH	myohyoid muscle
MM	masseter muscle
MP	medial pterygoid muscle
MR	medial rectus muscle
MT	middle turbinate
NP	nasopharynx
NS	nasal septum
OC	occipital condyle
OCI	obliquus capitis inferior muscle
ON	optic nerve
OP	oropharynx
OR	orbital rim
PG	parotid gland
RA	median raphe (septum) of tongue
RCP	rectus capitis posterior muscle
RM	ramus of mandible
SCM	sternocleidomastoid muscle
SMG	submandibular gland
SP	soft palate
SPH	sphenoid sinus
SPL	splenius capitis muscle
SR	superior rectus muscle
SS	sigmoid sinus
SSC	semispinalis capitis muscle
ST	superior nasal turbinate
T	temporalis muscle
TE	teeth
TO	tongue
TR	trapezius muscle
TT	torus tubarius
TV	tensor veli palatini
TVS	transversospinalis muscle
U	uvula
V	vallecula
VA	vertebral artery
VE	vestibule
ZP	zygomatic process of maxilla
ZY	zygomatic arch

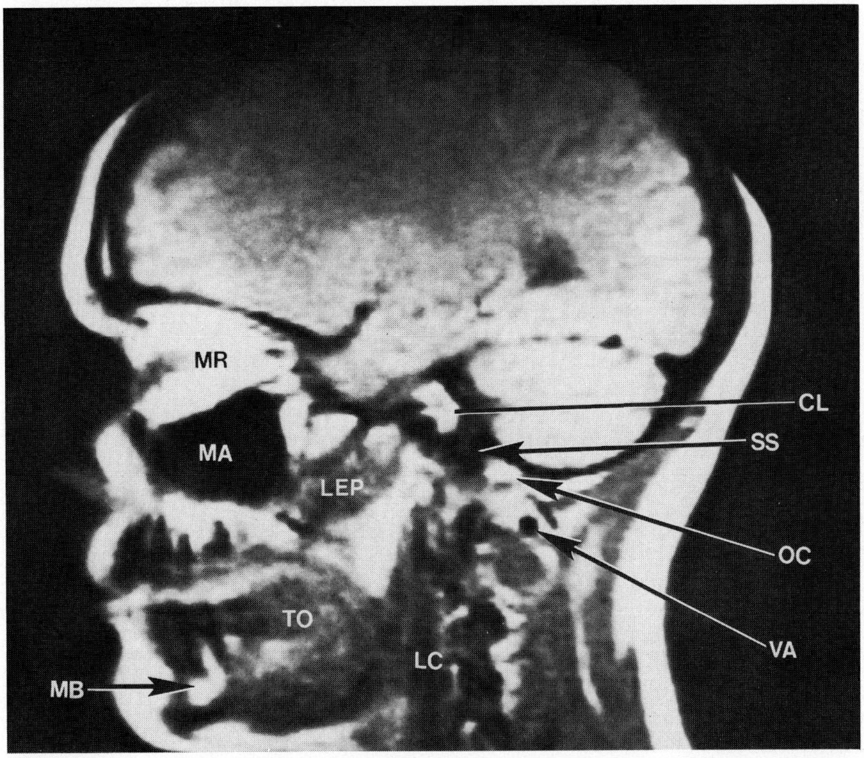

G

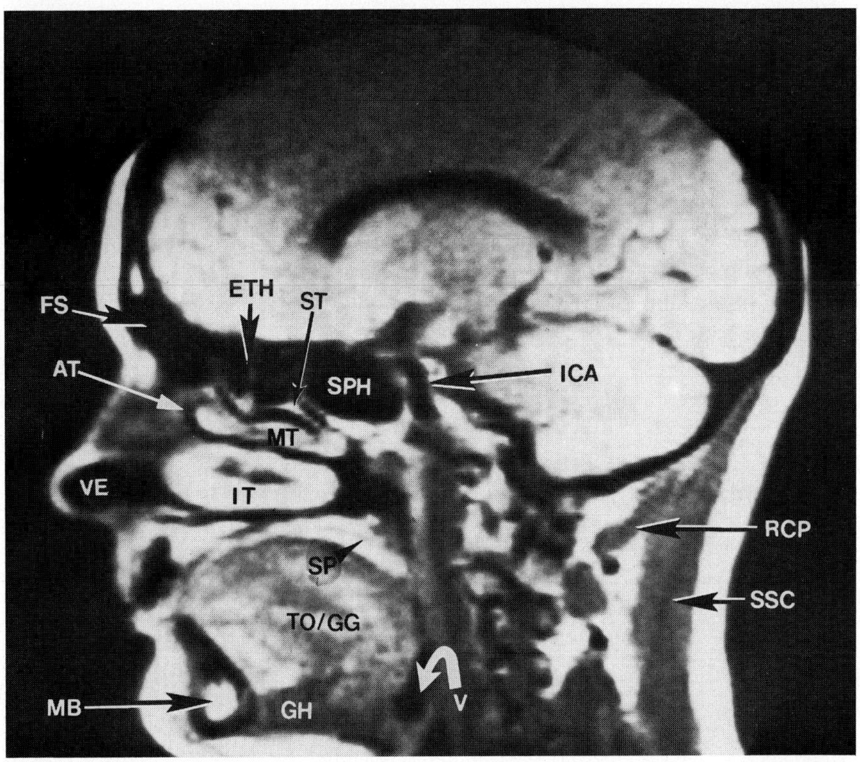

H

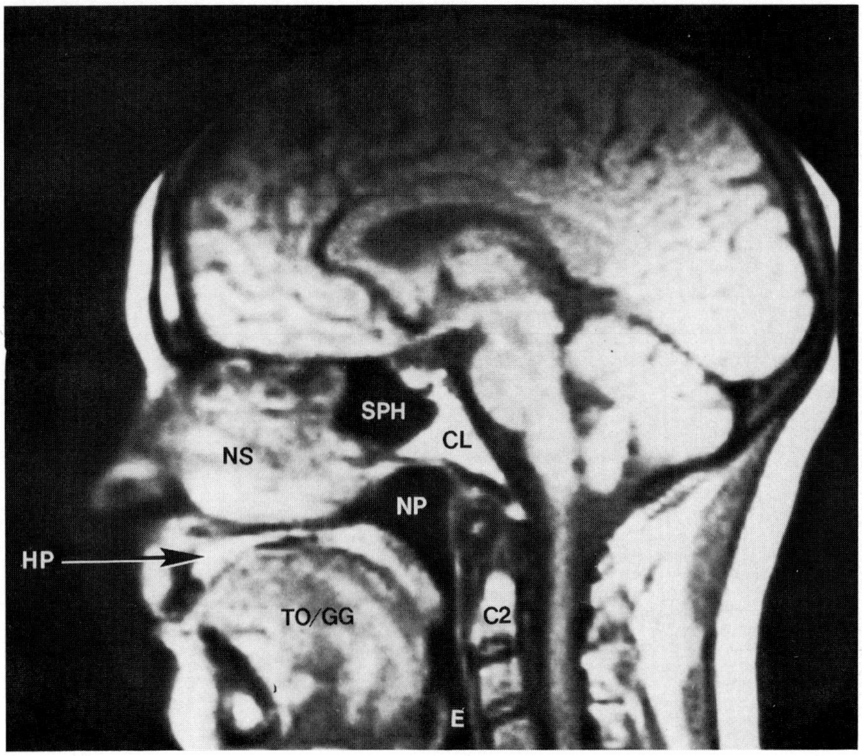

I

FIGURE 7-29 *(cont.)*

Sagittal SE 1000/28 images of the head from lateral to midline in successive 1-cm slices.

C2	cervical vertebrae 2
Cl	clivus
E	esophagus
HP	hard plate
NP	masopharynx
NS	nasal septum
SPH	sphenoid sinus
TO/GG	tongue and genioglossus muscle

Neck

MR is well suited for imaging the soft tissues of the neck because it incorporates many of the advantages of CT without the need for intravenous contrast or ionizing radiation. Additionally, multiplanar visualization of the neck structures is possible directly without the errors and difficulties of reformatting encountered with CT.

TABLE 7-5

Representative T1 and T2 Relaxation Times of Neck Tissues at 0.3 T

Tissue	T1 (msec)	T2 (msec)
Fat	300	55
Thymus	460	70
Thyroid	620	45
Muscle	690	30
Lymph node	820	55

Table 7-5 lists the T1 and T2 values of the normal tissues of the neck computed at 0.3. Using this table or an equivalent T1–T2 graph, it is possible to predict the various signal intensities of different neck tissues depending on imaging sequence. In the neck as a whole, contrast resolution for masses and nodes is probably best attained using a technique such as SE 2000/28. For the larynx, however, best anatomic detail for evaluation of tumor spread is seen with T1-weighted sequences, such as SE 500/30. When available, surface coils markedly increase spatial resolution. This may be particularly important in MR imaging of the larynx.

The *axial plane* remains the mainstay for evaluation of the neck because of the familiar anatomy it presents, as well as the facility for comparing each side for symmetry. The paralaryngeal spaces and anterior margins of the pyriform sinuses are best seen axially. Fatty areolar tissue in the pre-epiglottic space is also well evaluated. Vertical extension of lesions is probably better evaluated in coronal or sagittal planes, however. Sequential axial images of the neck appear in Figure 7-30.

(Text continues on p. 162.)

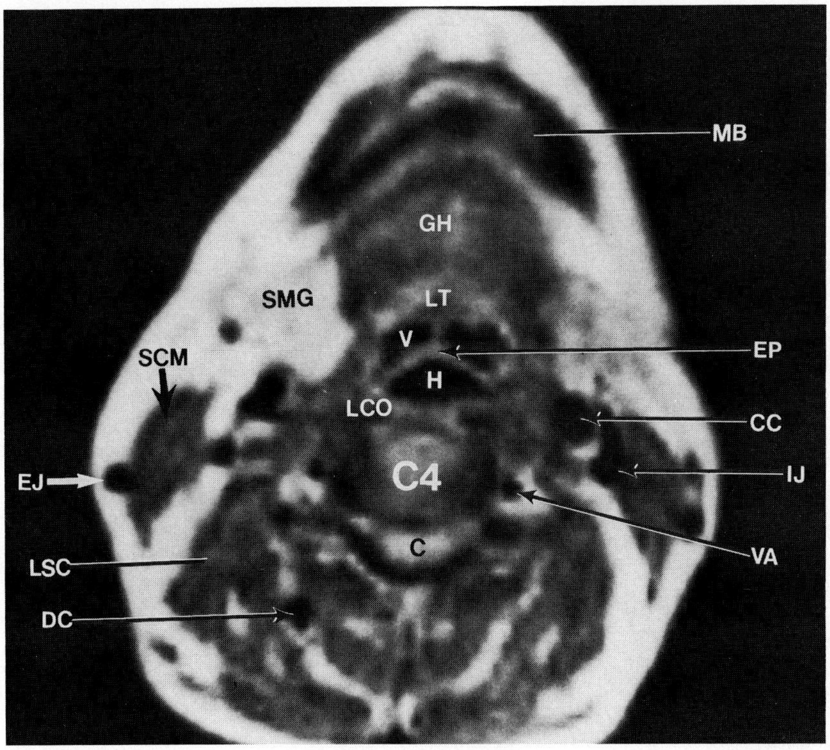

A

FIGURE 7-30

Axial SE 2000/28 images of the neck from the inferior margin of the mandible to the thoracic inlet in successive 1-cm slices.

A	artifact from dental bridgework
AE	arytenoepiglottic fold
AR	arytenoid cartilage
AS	anterior scalene muscle
BP	brachial plexus
C	spinal cord
C1 to C7	cervical vertebrae 1 to 7
CA	posterior cricoarytenoid muscle
CC	common carotid artery
CL	clavicle
CRI	cricoid cartilage
CT	cricothyroid muscle
DC	deep cervical vein
DI	intervertebral disc
E	esophagus
EJ	external jugular vein
EP	epiglottis
ES	erector spinae muscle
F	false cord
GG	genioglossus
GH	geniohyoid
H	hypopharynx
HP	hard palate
HY	hyoid bone
IA	innominate artery
ICA	internal carotid artery
IJ	internal jugular vein
IVF	intervertebral foramen
LBV	left brachiocephalic vein
LCA	longus capitis muscle
LCO	longus colli muscle
LP	lateral pterygoid muscle
LSC	levator scapulae muscle
LSCA	left subclavian artery
LSCV	left subclavian vein
LT	lingual tonsil
LV	laryngeal ventricle
M	masseter muscle
MA	maxillary antrum
MB	mandibular body
MH	myohyoid muscle
MP	medial pterygoid muscle
MR	mandibular ramus
NP	nasopharynx
O	oropharynx
OCI	oblique capitis inferior muscle
PG	parotid gland
PRE	pre-epiglottic fat
PYR	pyriform sinus
R1	rib 1
R2	rib 2
RCP	rectus capitis posterior muscles
RS	rostrum of sphenoid
RSCA, RSCV	right subclavian artery, vein
SA	anterior scalene muscle
SC	splenius capitis muscle
SCM	sternocleidomastoid muscle
SCP	posterior scalene muscle
SME	scalenus medius muscle
SMG	submandibular gland
SP	soft palate
SPL	splenius muscle
SPP	spinous process
SSC	semispinalis capitis muscle
ST	sternothyroid muscle
STR	strap muscles
SU	supraspinatus muscle
T	trachea
T1	thoracic vertebra 1
TC	thyroid cartilage
THY	thyroid gland
TP	transverse process
TR	trapezius muscle
TT	torus tubarius
TVS	transversospinalis muscle
U	uvula
V	vallecula
VA	vertebral artery
VE	vestibule
VF	vocal fold (true cord)

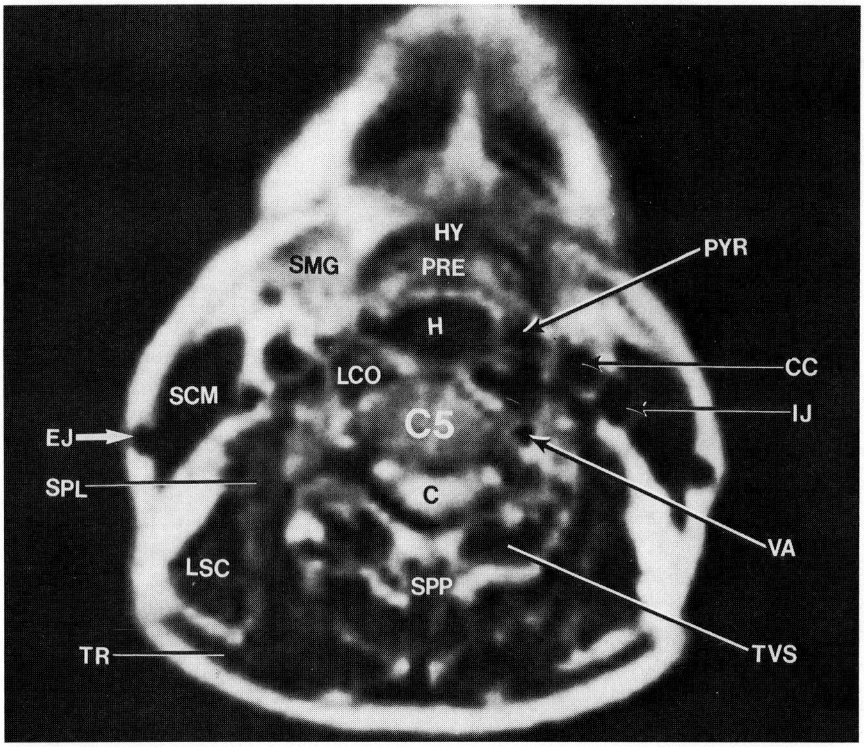

B

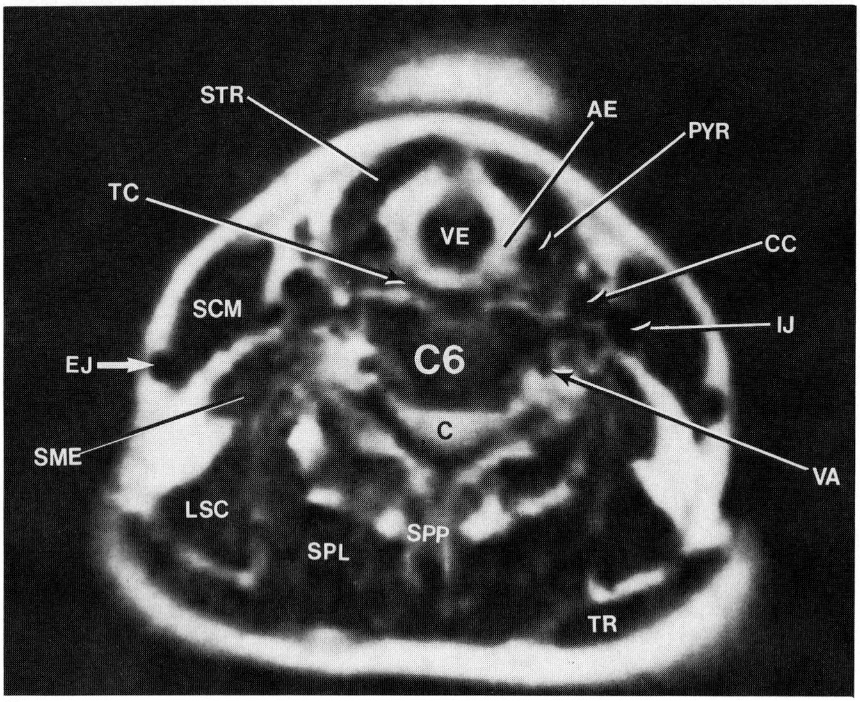

C

FIGURE 7-30 *(cont.)*

Axial SE 2000/28 images of the neck from the inferior margin of the mandible to the thoracic inlet in successive 1-cm slices.

A	artifact from dental bridgework
AE	arytenoepiglottic fold
AR	arytenoid cartilage
AS	anterior scalene muscle
BP	brachial plexus
C	spinal cord
C1 to C7	cervical vertebrae 1 to 7
CA	posterior cricoarytenoid muscle
CC	common carotid artery
CL	clavicle
CRI	cricoid cartilage
CT	cricothyroid muscle
DC	deep cervical vein
DI	intervertebral disc
E	esophagus
EJ	external jugular vein
EP	epiglottis
ES	erector spinae muscle
F	false cord
GG	genioglossus
GH	geniohyoid
H	hypopharynx
HP	hard palate
HY	hyoid bone
IA	innominate artery
ICA	internal carotid artery
IJ	internal jugular vein
IVF	intervertebral foramen
LBV	left brachiocephalic vein
LCA	longus capitis muscle
LCO	longus colli muscle
LP	lateral pterygoid muscle
LSC	levator scapulae muscle
LSCA	left subclavian artery
LSCV	left subclavian vein
LT	lingual tonsil
LV	laryngeal ventricle
M	masseter muscle
MA	maxillary antrum
MB	mandibular body
MH	myohyoid muscle
MP	medial pterygoid muscle

MR	mandibular ramus
NP	nasopharynx
O	oropharynx
OCI	oblique capitis inferior muscle
PG	parotid gland
PRE	pre-epiglottic fat
PYR	pyriform sinus
R1	rib 1
R2	rib 2
RCP	rectus capitis posterior muscles
RS	rostrum of sphenoid
RSCA, RSCV	right subclavian artery, vein
SA	anterior scalene muscle
SC	splenius capitis muscle
SCM	sternocleidomastoid muscle
SCP	posterior scalene muscle
SME	scalenus medius muscle
SMG	submandibular gland
SP	soft palate
SPL	splenius muscle
SPP	spinous process
SSC	semispinalis capitis muscle
ST	sternothyroid muscle
STR	strap muscles
SU	supraspinatus muscle
T	trachea
T1	thoracic vertebra 1
TC	thyroid cartilage
THY	thyroid gland
TP	transverse process
TR	trapezius muscle
TT	torus tubarius
TVS	transversospinalis muscle
U	uvula
V	vallecula
VA	vertebral artery
VE	vestibule
VF	vocal fold (true cord)

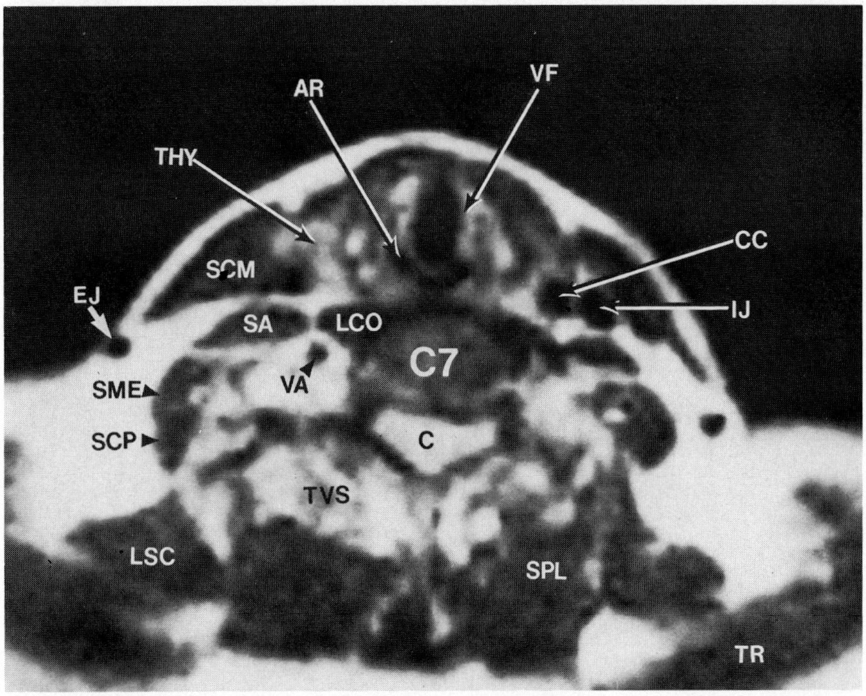

D

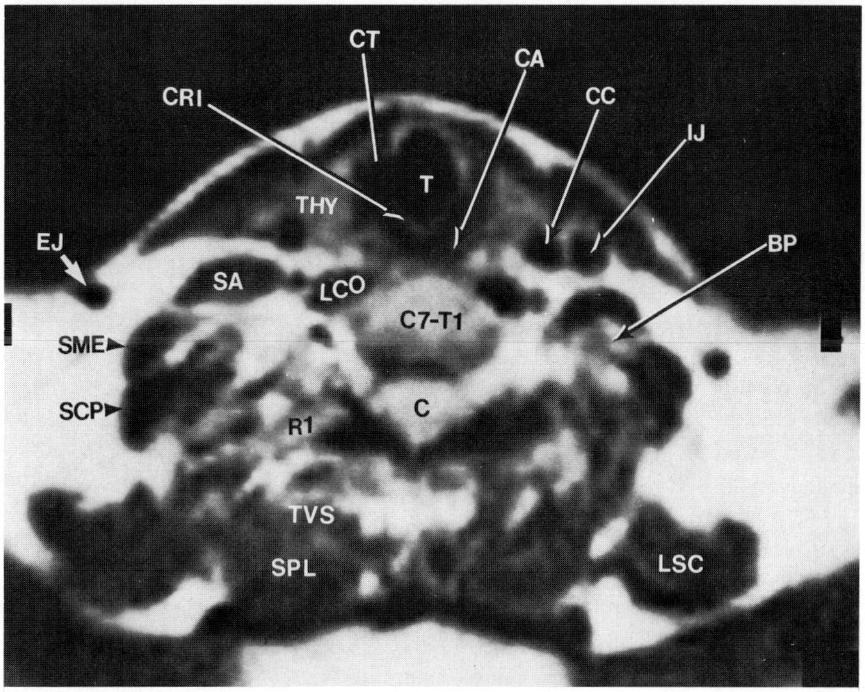

E

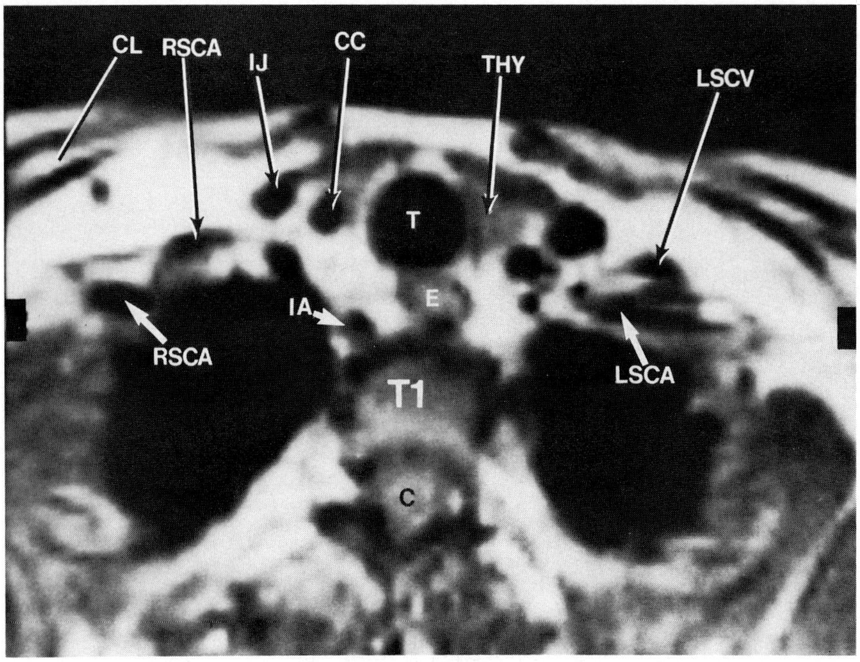

F

FIGURE 7-30 *(cont.)*

Axial SE 2000/28 images of the neck from the inferior margin of the mandible to the thoracic inlet in successive 1-cm slices.

The *coronal plane* demonstrates a number of elegant relationships of the aerodigestive tract. The spread of tumors and other diseases between the oropharynx and hypopharynx is well appreciated. Unfortunately, the larynx has been somewhat difficult to evaluate in the coronal plane by MR imaging. The degree of abduction of the true and false cords is variable, and they may be difficult to distinguish. The false cords contain more fatty connective tissue and mucous glands and will appear brighter than the true cords on most imaging sequences. Best anatomic delineation of laryngeal musculature is obtained by short spin-echo sequences (*e.g.,* SE 500/28). Coronal SE 1000/28 images of the neck appear in Figure 7-31.

The *sagittal plane* is useful in several situations. The brachial plexus may be followed as it emerges between the scalene muscles far laterally. The entire course of the internal jugular vein and internal jugular lymph node chain may be observed. Near the thoracic inlet, the branching of subclavian and common carotid arteries is well defined.

Perhaps the best use for the sagittal plane is in evaluation of the aerodigestive pathway, including the tongue, valleculae, epiglottis, hyoid, vocal folds, and trachea. The evaluation of cephalocaudal extension of tumor is critical prior to surgery and for radiotherapy. Off-midline sagittal sections of the larynx can become confusing, and at present, lateral extension of tumor is best evaluated using axial images. Serial sagittal images through the neck are presented in Figure 7-32. A possible protocol for MR imaging of the soft tissues of the neck is presented in Table 7-6.

TABLE 7-6

Possible Protocol for MRI of the Neck (Excluding Cervical Spine)

1. Surface coil or speciality neck coil if available
2. Axial SE 2000/30,60
3. Coronal SE 1000/30,60. Use coronal plane when diseases of larynx or pyriform sinuses are suspected.
4. Sagittal 500/30. Use when tumors or diseases of supraglottic larynx, epiglottis, vallecula, or base of tongue are suspected. Also helpful in establishing extent of retropharyngeal abscesses and masses. May visualize disease of the carotid arteries in this projection.

FIGURE 7-31

Coronal SE 1500/28 images of the neck and cervical spine in 1-cm slices from anterior to posterior.

A	artifact from dental bridgework
C	spinal cord
CC	common carotid artery
CL	clavicle
E	esophagus
F	false cord
GG	genioglossus
IA	innominate artery
IJ	internal jugular vein
LSCA	left subclavian artery
LSCV	left subclavian vein
LV	laryngeal ventricle
M	masseter muscle
MA	maxillary antrum
MB	mandibular body
MH	myohyoid muscle
RSCA	right subclavian
SCM	sternocleidomastoid muscle
STR	strap muscles
T	trachea
T1	thoracic vertebra 1
THY	thyroid gland
VE	vestibule
VF	vocal fold (true cord)

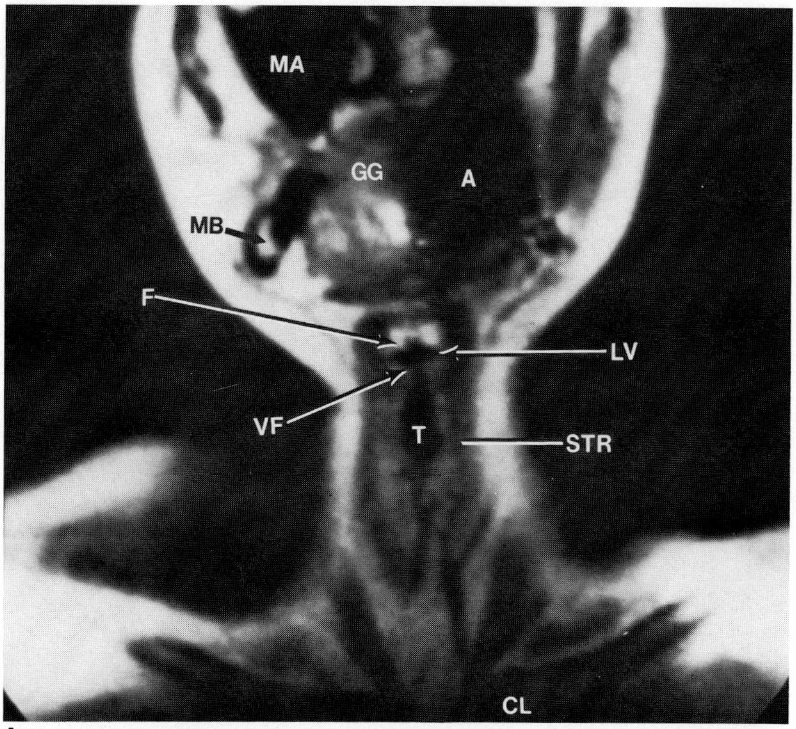

A

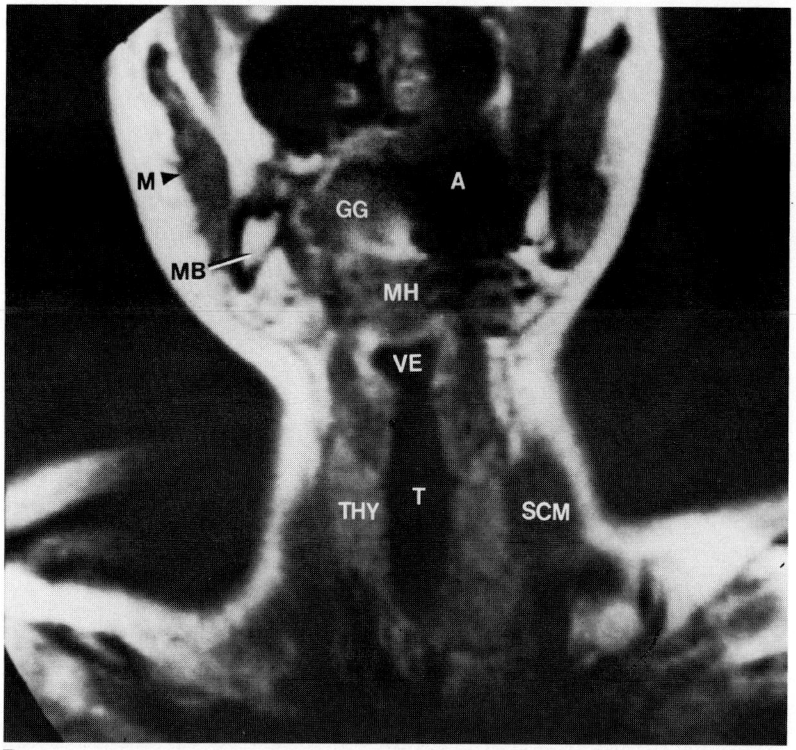

B

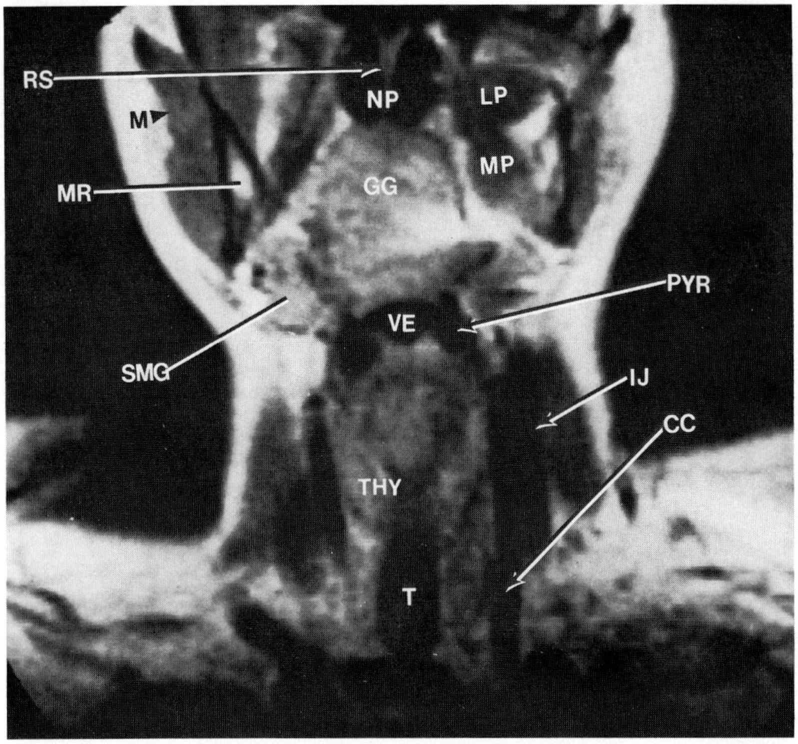

C

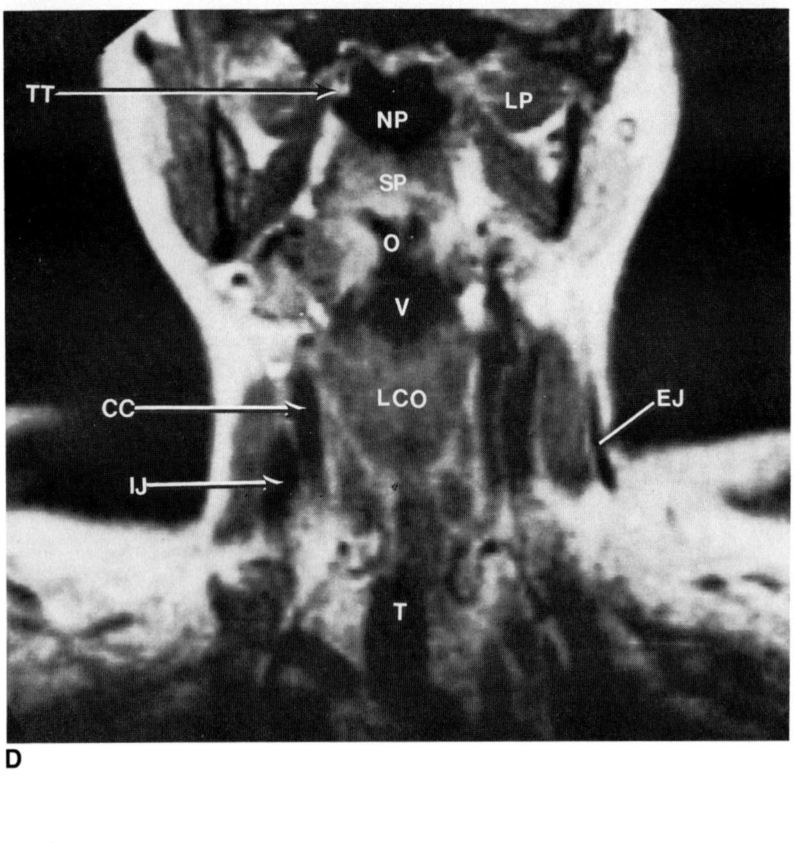

D

FIGURE 7-31 *(cont.)*

Coronal SE 1500/28 images of the neck and cervical spine in 1-cm slices from anterior to posterior.

A	artifact from dental bridgework
AE	arytenoepiglottic fold
AR	arytenoid cartilage
AS	anterior scalene muscle
BP	brachial plexus
C	spinal cord
C1 to C7	cervical vertebrae 1 to 7
CA	posterior cricoarytenoid muscle
CC	common carotid artery
CL	clavicle
CRI	cricoid cartilage
CT	cricothyroid muscle
DC	deep cervical vein
DI	intervertebral disc
E	esophagus
EJ	external jugular vein
EP	epiglottis
ES	erector spinae muscle
F	false cord
GG	genioglossus
GH	geniohyoid
H	hypopharynx
HP	hard palate
HY	hyoid bone
IA	innominate artery
ICA	internal carotid artery
IJ	internal jugular vein
IVF	intervertebral foramen
LBV	left brachiocephalic vein
LCA	longus capitis muscle
LCO	longus colli muscle
LP	lateral pterygoid muscle
LSC	levator scapulae muscle
LSCA	left subclavian artery
LSCV	left subclavian vein
LT	lingual tonsil
LV	laryngeal ventricle
M	masseter muscle
MA	maxillary antrum
MB	mandibular body
MH	myohyoid muscle
MP	medial pterygoid muscle

MR	mandibular ramus
NP	nasopharynx
O	oropharynx
OCI	oblique capitis inferior muscle
PG	parotid gland
PRE	pre-epiglottic fat
PYR	pyriform sinus
R1	rib 1
R2	rib 2
RCP	rectus capitis posterior muscles
RS	rostrum of sphenoid
RSCA, RSCV	right subclavian artery, vein
SA	anterior scalene muscle
SC	splenius capitis muscle
SCM	sternocleidomastoid muscle
SCP	posterior scalene muscle
SME	scalenus medius muscle
SMG	submandibular gland
SP	soft palate
SPL	splenius muscle
SPP	spinous process
SSC	semispinalis capitis muscle
ST	sternothyroid muscle
STR	strap muscles
SU	supraspinatus muscle
T	trachea
T1	thoracic vertebra 1
TC	thyroid cartilage
THY	thyroid gland
TP	transverse process
TR	trapezius muscle
TT	torus tubarius
TVS	transversospinalis muscle
U	uvula
V	vallecula
VA	vertebral artery
VE	vestibule
VF	vocal fold (true cord)

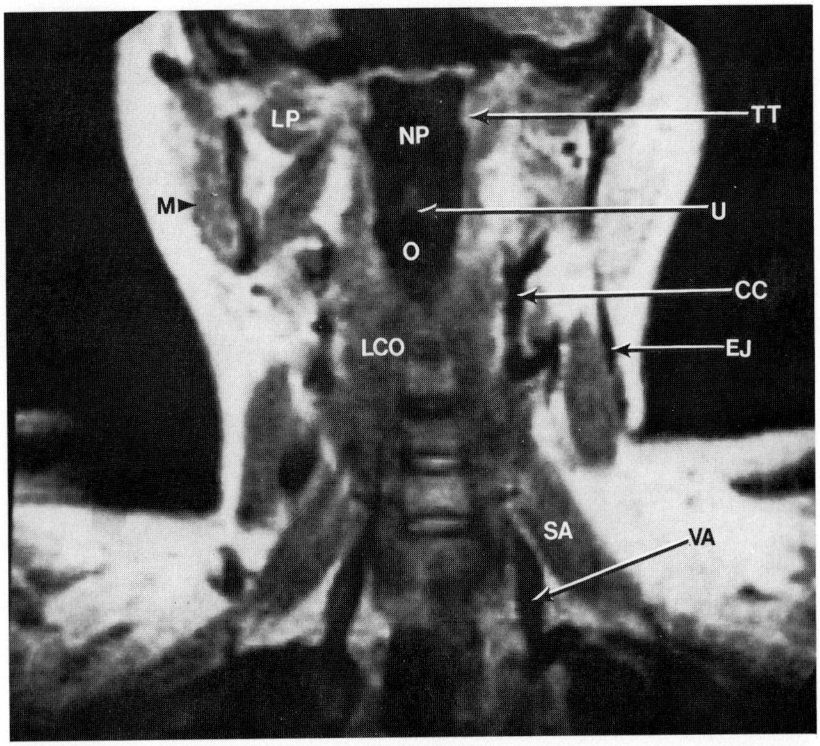

E

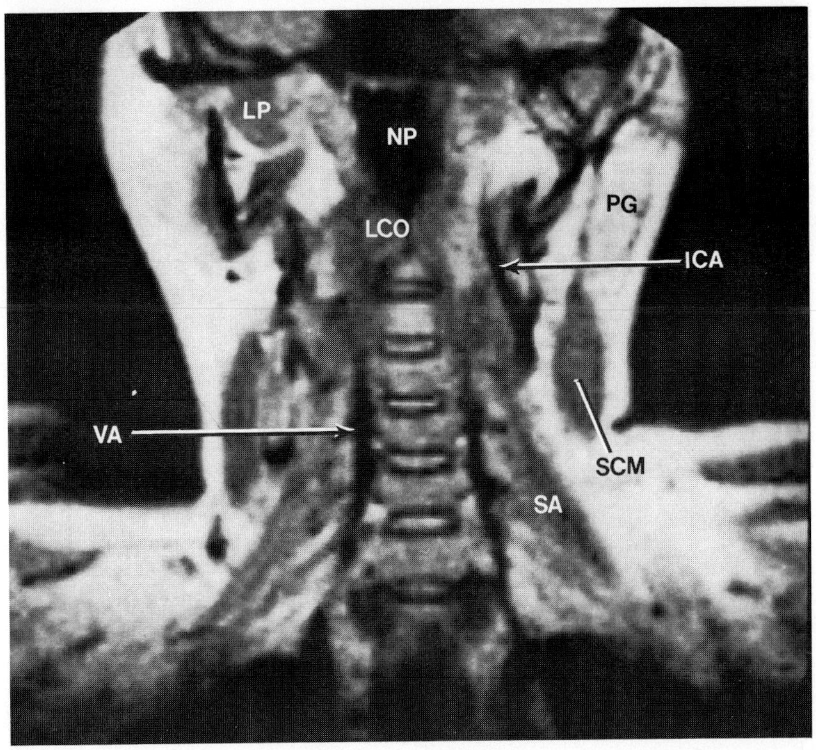

F

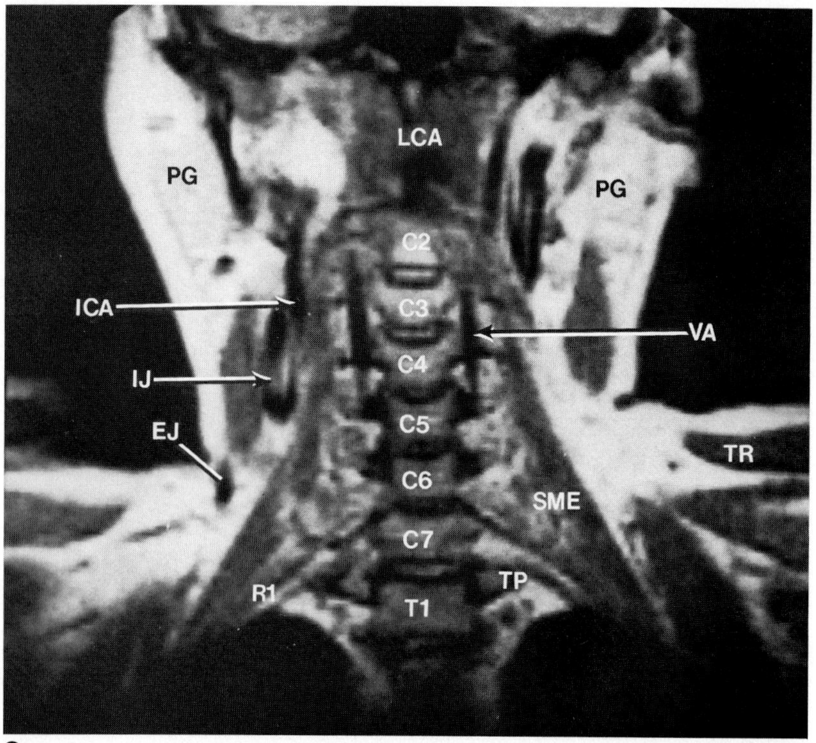

G

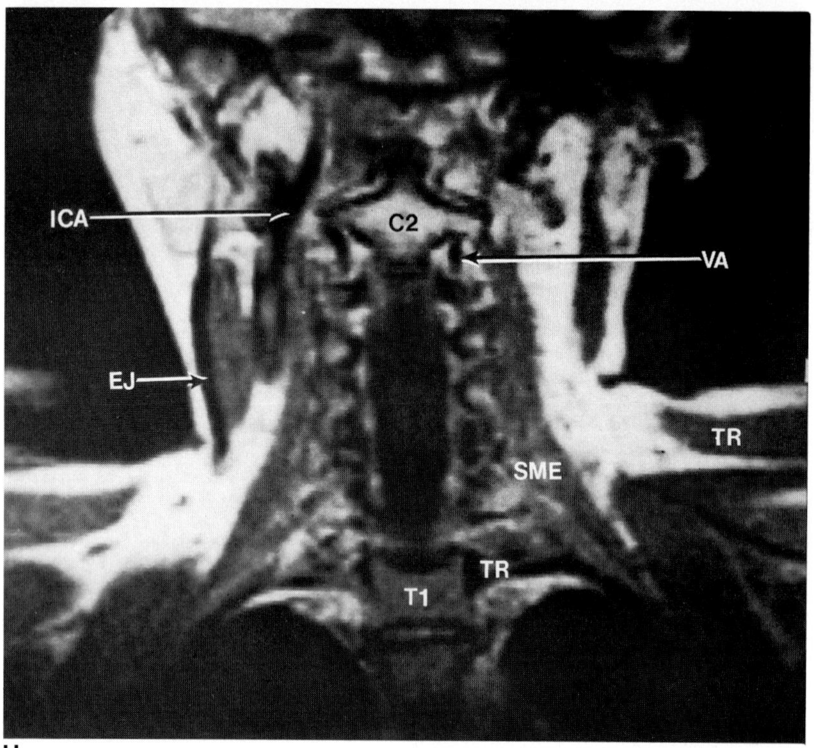

H

FIGURE 7-31 *(cont.)*

Coronal SE 1500/28 images of the neck and cervical spine in 1-cm slices from anterior to posterior.

A	artifact from dental bridgework
AE	arytenoepiglottic fold
AR	arytenoid cartilage
AS	anterior scalene muscle
BP	brachial plexus
C	spinal cord
C1 to C7	cervical vertebrae 1 to 7
CA	posterior cricoarytenoid muscle
CC	common carotid artery
CL	clavicle
CRI	cricoid cartilage
CT	cricothyroid muscle
DC	deep cervical vein
DI	intervertebral disc
E	esophagus
EJ	external jugular vein
EP	epiglottis
ES	erector spinae muscle
F	false cord
GG	genioglossus
GH	geniohyoid
H	hypopharynx
HP	hard palate
HY	hyoid bone
IA	innominate artery
ICA	internal carotid artery
IJ	internal jugular vein
IVF	intervertebral foramen
LBV	left brachiocephalic vein
LCA	longus capitis muscle
LCO	longus colli muscle
LP	lateral pterygoid muscle
LSC	levator scapulae muscle
LSCA	left subclavian artery
LSCV	left subclavian vein
LT	lingual tonsil
LV	laryngeal ventricle
M	masseter muscle
MA	maxillary antrum
MB	mandibular body
MH	myohyoid muscle
MP	medial pterygoid muscle

MR	mandibular ramus
NP	nasopharynx
O	oropharynx
OCI	oblique capitis inferior muscle
PG	parotid gland
PRE	pre-epiglottic fat
PYR	pyriform sinus
R1	rib 1
R2	rib 2
RCP	rectus capitis posterior muscles
RS	rostrum of sphenoid
RSCA, RSCV	right subclavian artery, vein
SA	anterior scalene muscle
SC	splenius capitis muscle
SCM	sternocleidomastoid muscle
SCP	posterior scalene muscle
SME	scalenus medius muscle
SMG	submandibular gland
SP	soft palate
SPL	splenius muscle
SPP	spinous process
SSC	semispinalis capitis muscle
ST	sternothyroid muscle
STR	strap muscles
SU	supraspinatus muscle
T	trachea
T1	thoracic vertebra 1
TC	thyroid cartilage
THY	thyroid gland
TP	transverse process
TR	trapezius muscle
TT	torus tubarius
TVS	transversospinalis muscle
U	uvula
V	vallecula
VA	vertebral artery
VE	vestibule
VF	vocal fold (true cord)

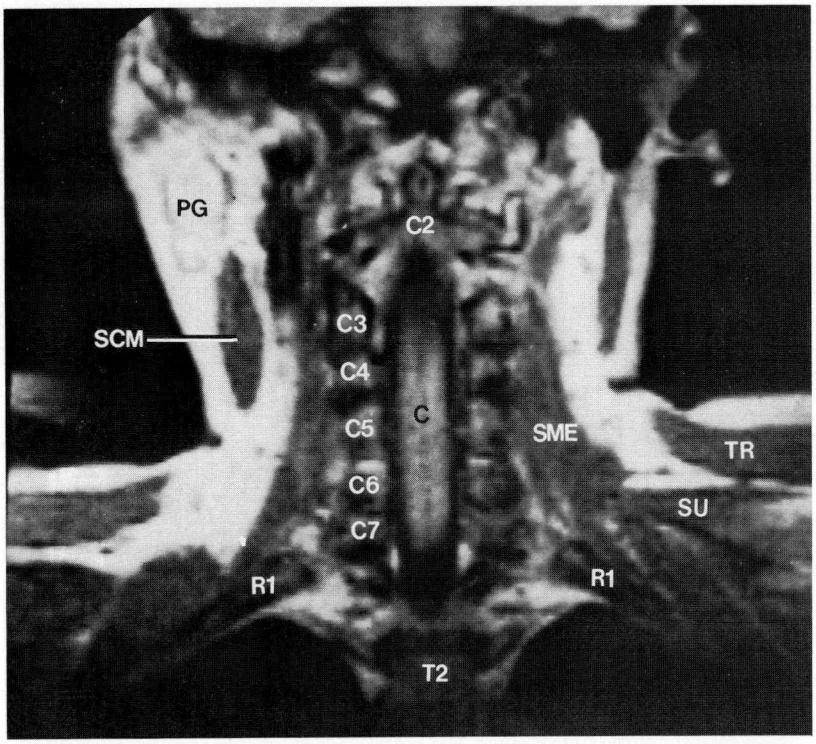

I

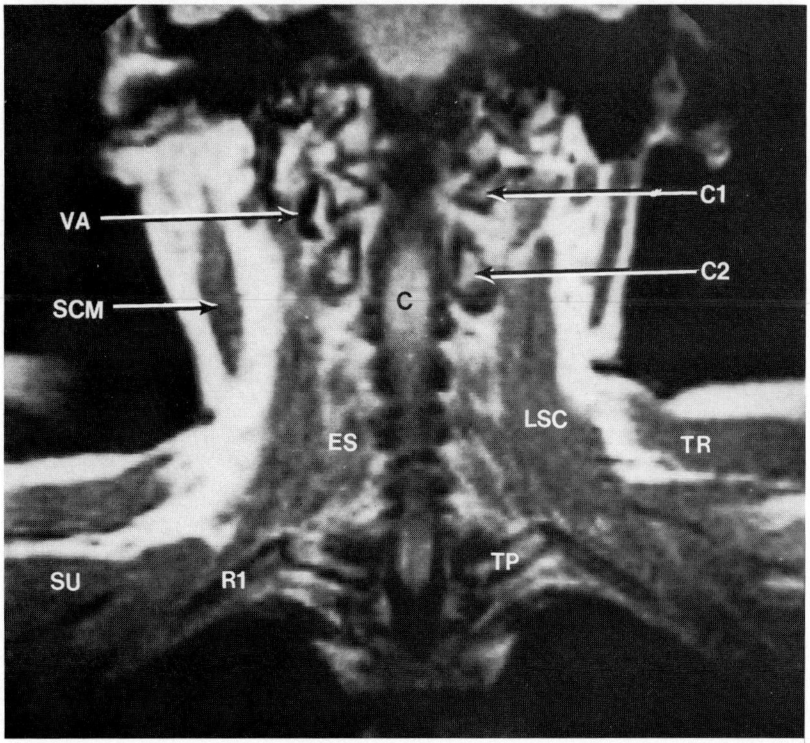

J

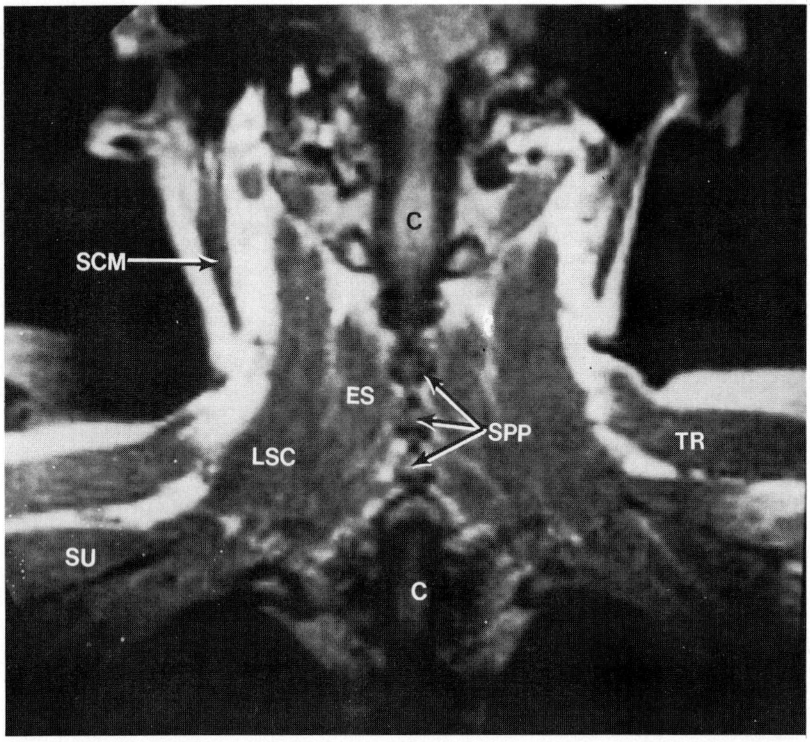

K

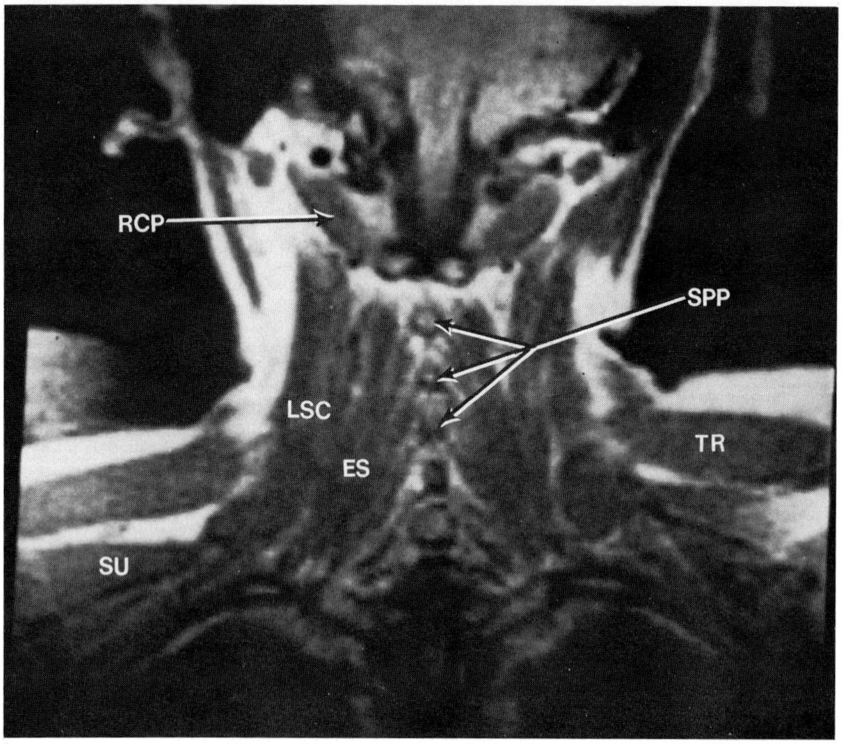

L

FIGURE 7-31 *(cont.)*

Coronal SE 1500/28 images of the neck and cervical spine in 1-cm slices from anterior to posterior.

A	artifact from dental bridgework
AE	arytenoepiglottic fold
AR	arytenoid cartilage
AS	anterior scalene muscle
BP	brachial plexus
C	spinal cord
C1 to C7	cervical vertebrae 1 to 7
CA	posterior cricoarytenoid muscle
CC	common carotid artery
CL	clavicle
CRI	cricoid cartilage
CT	cricothyroid muscle
DC	deep cervical vein
DI	intervertebral disc
E	esophagus
EJ	external jugular vein
EP	epiglottis
ES	erector spinae muscle
F	false cord
GG	genioglossus
GH	geniohyoid
H	hypopharynx
HP	hard palate
HY	hyoid bone
IA	innominate artery
ICA	internal carotid artery
IJ	internal jugular vein
IVF	intervertebral foramen
LBV	left brachiocephalic vein
LCA	longus capitis muscle
LCO	longus colli muscle
LP	lateral pterygoid muscle
LSC	levator scapulae muscle
LSCA	left subclavian artery
LSCV	left subclavian vein
LT	lingual tonsil
LV	laryngeal ventricle
M	masseter muscle
MA	maxillary antrum
MB	mandibular body
MH	myohyoid muscle
MP	medial pterygoid muscle

MR	mandibular ramus
NP	nasopharynx
O	oropharynx
OCI	oblique capitis inferior muscle
PG	parotid gland
PRE	pre-epiglottic fat
PYR	pyriform sinus
R1	rib 1
R2	rib 2
RCP	rectus capitis posterior muscles
RS	rostrum of sphenoid
RSCA, RSCV	right subclavian artery, vein
SA	anterior scalene muscle
SC	splenius capitis muscle
SCM	sternocleidomastoid muscle
SCP	posterior scalene muscle
SME	scalenus medius muscle
SMG	submandibular gland
SP	soft palate
SPL	splenius muscle
SPP	spinous process
SSC	semispinalis capitis muscle
ST	sternothyroid muscle
STR	strap muscles
SU	supraspinatus muscle
T	trachea
T1	thoracic vertebra 1
TC	thyroid cartilage
THY	thyroid gland
TP	transverse process
TR	trapezius muscle
TT	torus tubarius
TVS	transversospinalis muscle
U	uvula
V	vallecula
VA	vertebral artery
VE	vestibule
VF	vocal fold (true cord)

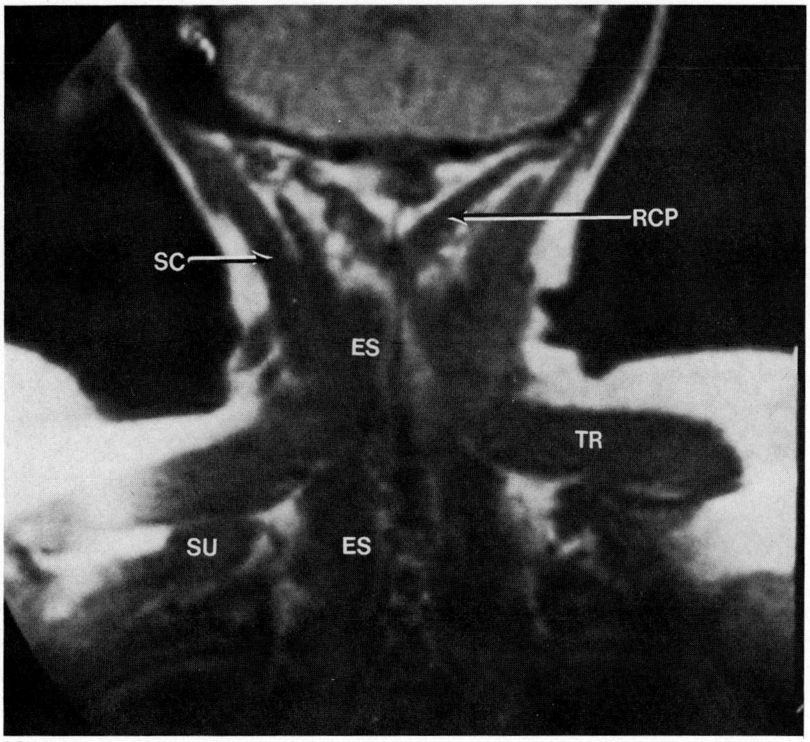

M

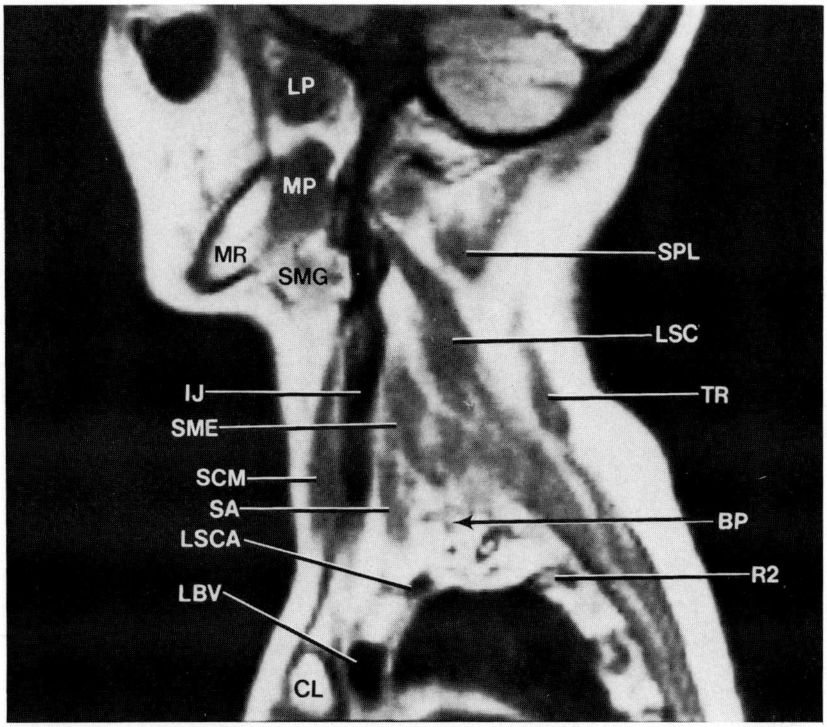

A

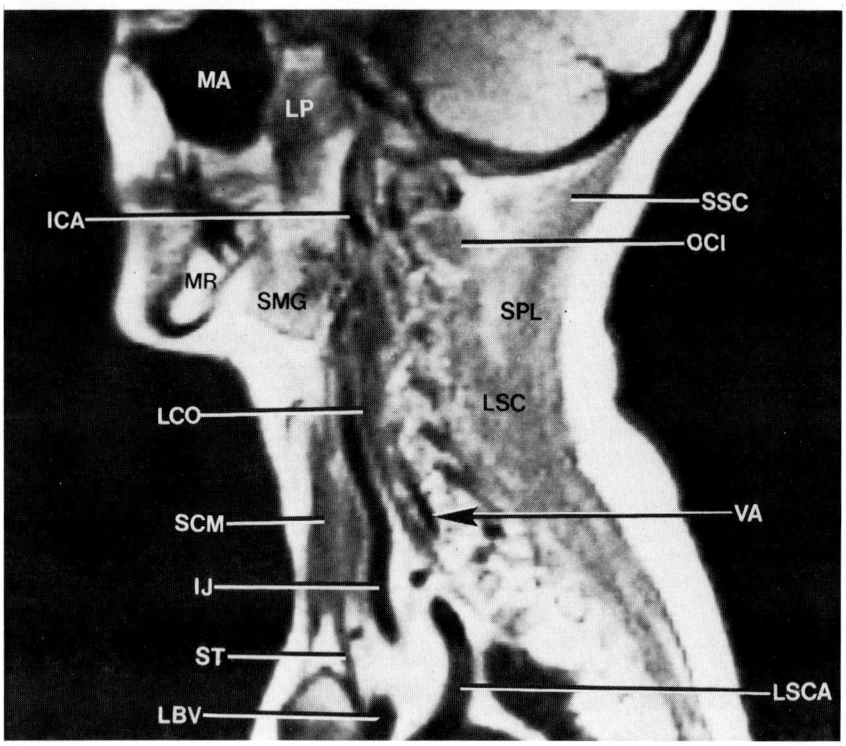

B

FIGURE 7-32

Sagittal SE 1000/28 images of the neck and cervical spine from lateral to medial.

A	artifact from dental bridgework
AE	arytenoepiglottic fold
AR	arytenoid cartilage
AS	anterior scalene muscle
BP	brachial plexus
C	spinal cord
C1 to C7	cervical vertebrae 1 to 7
CA	posterior cricoarytenoid muscle
CC	common carotid artery
CL	clavicle
CRI	cricoid cartilage
CT	cricothyroid muscle
DC	deep cervical vein
DI	intervertebral disc
E	esophagus
EJ	external jugular vein
EP	epiglottis
ES	erector spinae muscle
F	false cord
GG	genioglossus
GH	geniohyoid
H	hypopharynx
HP	hard palate
HY	hyoid bone
IA	innominate artery
ICA	internal carotid artery
IJ	internal jugular vein
IVF	intervertebral foramen
LBV	left brachiocephalic vein
LCA	longus capitis muscle
LCO	longus colli muscle
LP	lateral pterygoid muscle
LSC	levator scapulae muscle
LSCA	left subclavian artery
LSCV	left subclavian vein
LT	lingual tonsil
LV	laryngeal ventricle
M	masseter muscle
MA	maxillary antrum
MB	mandibular body
MH	myohyoid muscle
MP	medial pterygoid muscle

MR	mandibular ramus
NP	nasopharynx
O	oropharynx
OCI	oblique capitis inferior muscle
PG	parotid gland
PRE	pre-epiglottic fat
PYR	pyriform sinus
R1	rib 1
R2	rib 2
RCP	rectus capitis posterior muscles
RS	rostrum of sphenoid
RSCA,	right subclavian
RSCV	artery, vein
SA	anterior scalene muscle
SC	splenius capitis muscle
SCM	sternocleidomastoid muscle
SCP	posterior scalene muscle
SME	scalenus medius muscle
SMG	submandibular gland
SP	soft palate
SPL	splenius muscle
SPP	spinous process
SSC	semispinalis capitis muscle
ST	sternothyroid muscle
STR	strap muscles
SU	supraspinatus muscle
T	trachea
T1	thoracic vertebra 1
TC	thyroid cartilage
THY	thyroid gland
TP	transverse process
TR	trapezius muscle
TT	torus tubarius
TVS	transversospinalis muscle
U	uvula
V	vallecula
VA	vertebral artery
VE	vestibule
VF	vocal fold (true cord)

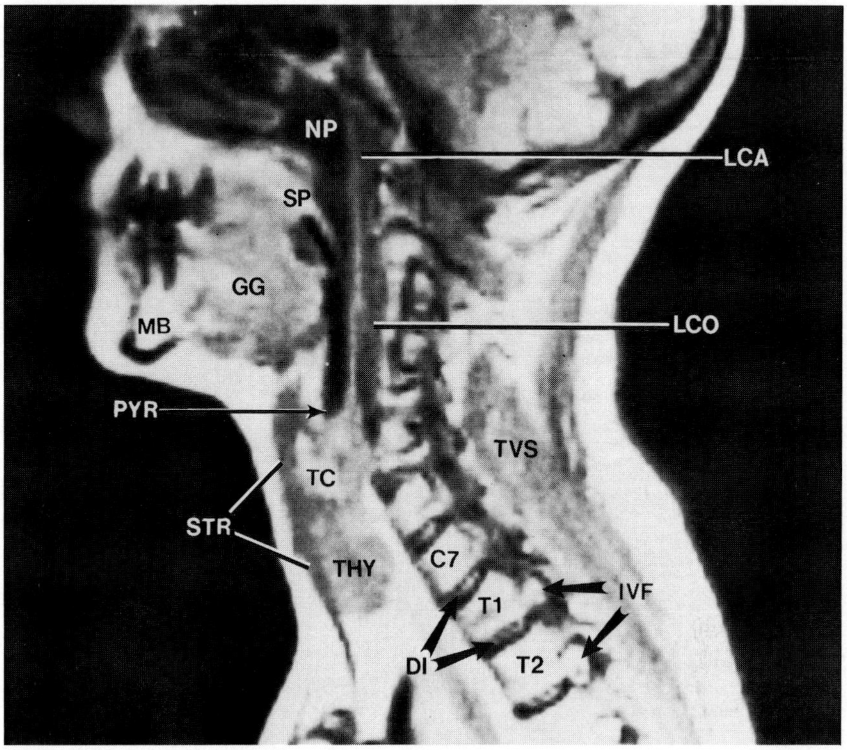

C

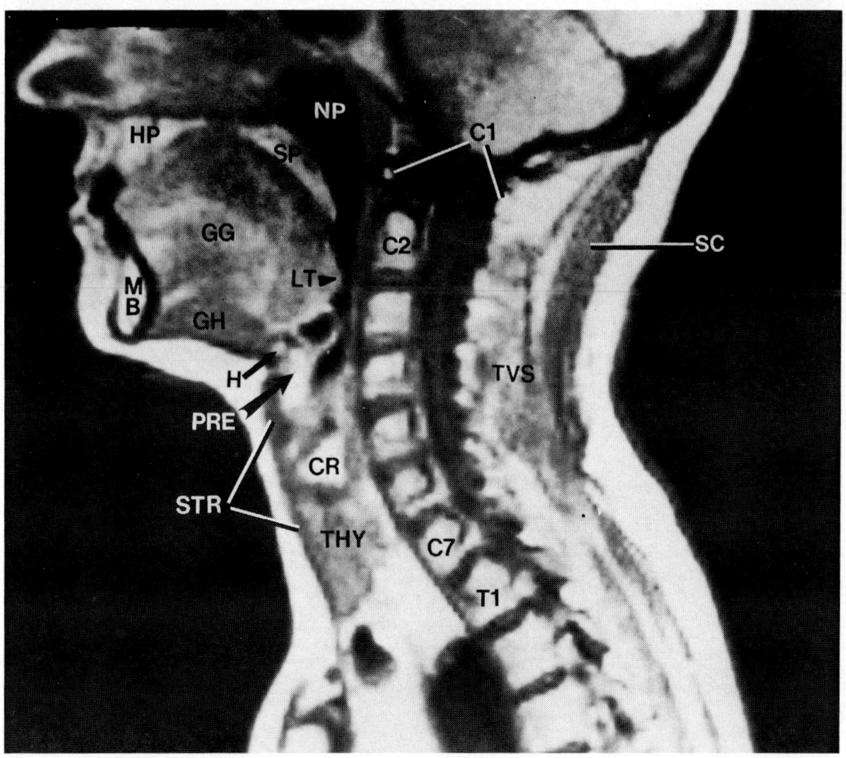

D

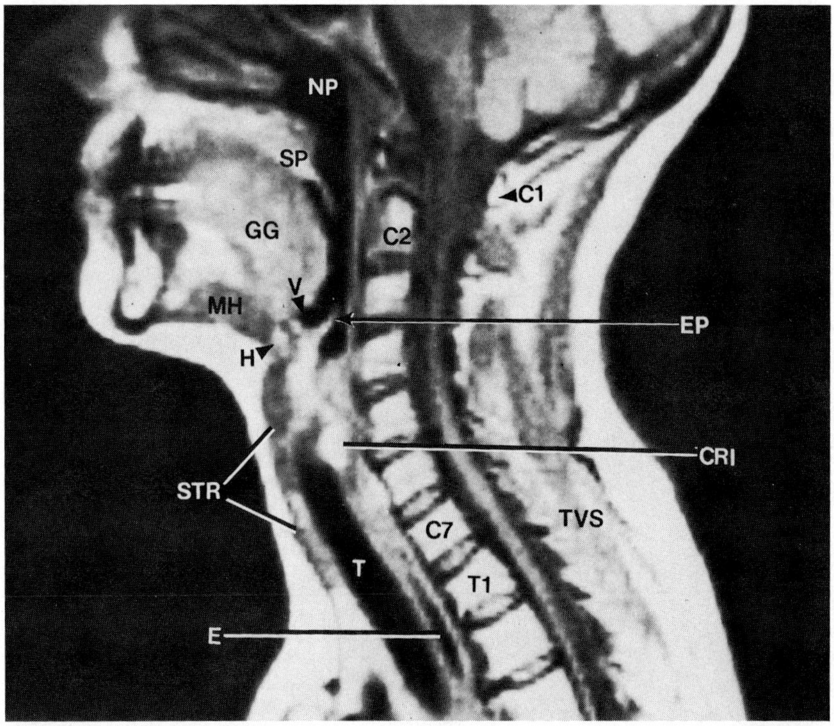

E

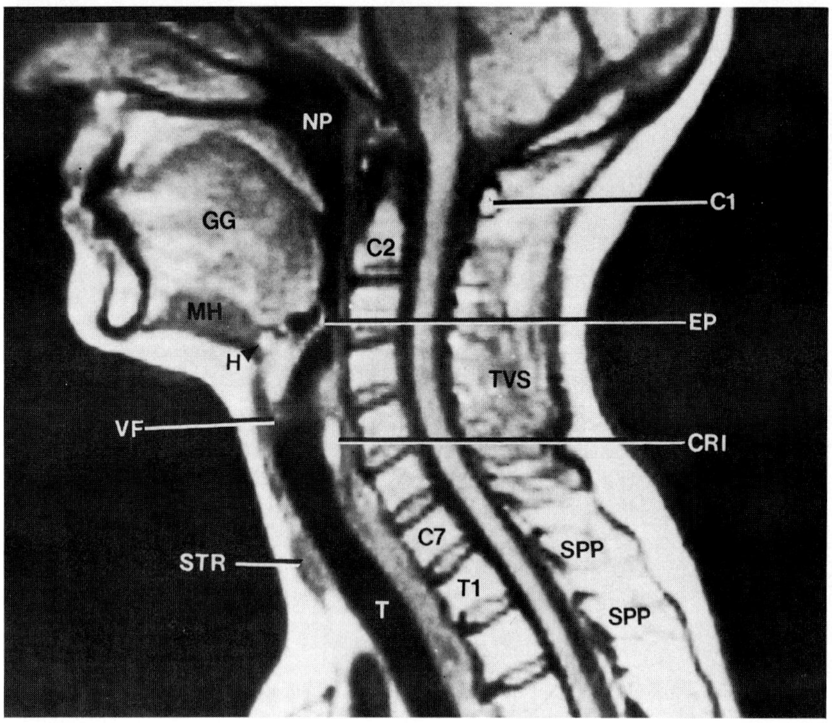

F

FIGURE 7-32 *(cont.)*

Sagittal SE 1000/28 images of the neck and cervical spine from lateral to medial.

C1 to C7	cervical vertebrae 1 to 7
CRI	cricoid cartilage
E	esophagus
EP	epiglottis
GG	genioglossus
H	hypopharynx
MH	myohyoid muscle
NP	nasopharynx
SP	soft palate
SPP	spinous process
STR	strap muscles
T	trachea
T1	thoracic vertebra 1
TVS	transversospinalis muscle
V	vallecula
VF	vocal fold (true cord)

CHAPTER 8

The Chest

MR holds promise for becoming a major imaging modality for diseases of the chest. As in other areas of the body, MR is able to provide direct images in multiple planes through the thorax, a capability that may be useful in defining the relationships of hilar or mediastinal masses and normal structures. Perhaps the greatest advantage of MRI of the chest lies in its ability to distinguish vascular structures from solid masses without the use of intravenous contrast. Since vascular structures contain flowing blood, their signal strength is low. Solid masses, on the other hand, virtually always have more signal than vessels. It may be possible, for example, to decide easily whether a hilar mass represents adenopathy or a large pulmonary vessel.

MR also may one day become a primary modality for imaging the heart itself. By means of *gating* MR signal acquisition at various times in the electrocardiogram (ECG), it is possible to obtain stop-action images through the heart at various times during its cycle. Although the widespread use of many such techniques is still experimental to a large degree, it has been possible to diagnose ventricular aneurysms, clot, hypertrophy, and various congenital abnormalities. It is also possible, by careful measurements, to compute chamber size, stroke volume, cardiac index, and ejection fraction. As will be demonstrated, much internal cardiac architecture can be directly visualized without the need for intravenous contrast.

Despite these advantages, the applications of MR in the chest are still limited for several reasons. First, techniques of respiratory gating are not yet sufficiently refined for consistent use in the evaluation of small pulmonary nodules or masses. Second, MR is unable to detect the presence of calcium in such nodules, an important radiographic feature for distinguishing benign from malignant masses. Third, the spatial resolution of MR in the chest still lags slightly behind the best CT, and imaging time is longer. Finally, patients with cardiac pacemakers are excluded from study, since MR fields might induce pacemaker dysfunction, leading to fatal arrhythmias.

Selection of Planes for Chest MRI

MR offers the potential for imaging the chest in multiple planes—axially, coronally, sagittally, and obliquely. In view of these many options, it may be a little disappointing to learn that the *axial plane* still remains the best single direction for imaging most intrathoracic structures. It is the belief of many investigators including the author that *every* MR scan of the chest should begin with a set of axial images. Of course it is permissible to supplement axial information with that from additional planes, but axial imaging should probably always be done. The axial plane is particularly well suited for evaluating the paratracheal spaces, the anterior mediastinum, and the hila. The sagittal, coronal, and oblique planes can be unsatisfactory at times in evaluating these critical areas. Nevertheless, these other planes can be very useful in a number of situations.

The *coronal plane* can be helpful in three areas: the thoracic inlet, the aorticopulmonary window, and the lung bases. Masses at the lung apex or lung base may be difficult to define using axial images alone. The relationship of these masses to the major vascular trunks or to the diaphragm is aided by coronal views. Similarly, the region of the aorticopulmonary window, where the transverse aorta, left pulmonary artery, and mediastinal lymph nodes are closely apposed, can present a difficult problem in axial imaging when these structures are volume averaged together. Coronal MR imaging may be helpful in defining masses in this region.

Coronal imaging is also well suited for visualization of structures whose longitudinal axes lie in or near the coronal plane. These structures include the vena cava, trachea, mainstem bronchi, subclavian arteries, posterior azygous vein, and the pulmonary arteries. Laterally situated hilar masses are well seen, but anterior or posterior hilar masses are better evaluated from axial sections.

Sagittally oriented images may be useful in a number of situations. Like the coronal plane, the sagittal plane shows to good advantage the lung apices, thoracic inlet, and the lung bases. The characteristics of masses and fluid collections near the diaphragm may be better defined. The aortic arch and origins of the great vessels are well seen. The sagittal view should probably be used routinely when aortic disease (*e.g.*, aneurysm, dissection, coarctation) is considered. Finally, sagittal images have been shown to be useful in evaluating the extent of subcarinal masses and their relationship to the left atrium.

The coronal and sagittal planes hold one advantage over the axial plane that has nothing to do with their powers for diagnosis, but rather by the format in which they display disease for clinicians. One must remember that most clinicians outside of diagnostic imaging are not very familiar with the axial anatomy of the chest. They are much more accustomed to thinking of the chest in coronal and sagittal planes, as they would view posteroanterior and lateral chest radiographs. Accordingly, coronal and sagittal MR images may convey much more meaning to clinicians about the extent and location of a patient's disease than would axial images of the same patient.

Several investigators have recently stressed the need for *oblique planes* in chest imaging. These oblique planes may be especially useful in visualizing the heart and major vessels. Oblique imaging may be most advantageous when accurate measurements of cardiac wall motion or myocardial thickness are needed. Further discussion of the use of oblique planes will be included in the section entitled Cardiac MRI.

In summary, therefore, the axial plane remains the most reliable single plane for chest imaging. Coronal and sagittal imaging may be useful in certain areas like the thoracic inlet, lung base, or aorticopulmonary window. Oblique planes may be helpful for evaluating the heart or aorta. The advantages and disadvantages of each plane for thoracic imaging are presented in Table 8-1.

TABLE 8-1

Advantages and Disadvantages of Various Planes for Thoracic Imaging

Axial Plane
- Single best plane for imaging mediastinum and hila
- Good for chest wall lesions
- Acceptable for heart, pericardium
- Less useful at lung apices and at juxtadiaphragmatic regions

Coronal Plane
- Confirmation of equivocal findings in axial plane
- Good for aorticopulmonary window, lung apices, thoracic inlet, major vessels of superior mediastinum
- Good for laterally situated perihilar masses but poor for anteriorly or posteriorly situated perihilar masses
- Good for juxtadiaphragmatic masses, fluid collections
- Easy for clinicians who are accustomed to posteroanterior chest radiographs to understand the anatomic relationships of the disease processes imaged

Sagittal Plane
- Confirmation of equivocal findings in axial plane
- Good for thoracic inlet, demonstrating extension of disease processes into the neck
- Good for lung apices and juxtadiaphragmatic areas
- Good for aortic arch
- Fair for pretracheal and postracheal disease, but partial voluming limits value for lateral peritracheal masses
- Good for evaluating relationship of subcarinal masses to the left atrium

Oblique Planes
- Best for accurate measurements of cardiac wall motion, myocardial thickness, and dynamics
- May be helpful for certain diseases of the aortic arch (*e.g.*, long dissections)
- Problems with patient positioning and motion; reformation techniques still largely experimental

Gating Techniques

The superior mediastinum and upper chest wall move relatively little with cardiac or respiratory motion. MR scanning of these regions may be performed employing routine techniques used elsewhere in the body.

MR imaging of the heart, lungs, and diaphragm, when performed with routine technique, is plagued by artifacts from the motion of these structures. A variety of *gating* methods have been developed to correct for cardiac and respiratory motion artifacts. Gating techniques synchronize MR signal acquisition with certain phases of the cardiac or respiratory cycle. At the present, gating techniques may be classified into three categories: (1) cardiac gating alone, (2) respiratory gating alone, and (3) combined gating.

Cardiac gating involves the synchronization of MR signal acquisition to the cardiac cycle, usually by recording the ECG. Three standard electrodes with nonmagnetic lead wires are attached to the patient's chest and upper abdomen. A trigger device detects the rising edge of the R wave and produces an electronic signal to begin data acquisition. By inserting an appropriate delay after R-wave detection, the operator can obtain an image at any time in the cardiac cycle. A special circuit is also required to prevent gradient pulses from the magnetic field from being recorded and misinterpreted as R waves.

Using cardiac gating, it is not possible to choose the pulse sequence repetition time, TR, independently. Instead, TR depends on the heart rate. For example, a heart rate of 60 beats/minute corresponds to a TR of 1.0 second. A heart rate of 100 beats/minute corresponds to a TR of 0.6 seconds. It is possible to sample every second or third heartbeat by means of electronic circuitry. This results in a lengthening of TR by the appropriate factor.

When cardiac gating is used, certain MR scanners have restrictions on the number of simultaneous slices or interleaving processes that normally speed up image acquisition. The use of cardiac gating, therefore, may lengthen the time of the examination. In the event that an irregular cardiac rhythm occurs, cardiac gating becomes unreliable or impossible.

The appearance of the chest, using MR with and without cardiac gating, is shown in Figure 8-1A,B.

Respiratory Gating

Cardiac gating alone is capable of significantly improving MR image quality in the thorax. Even further improvement can be obtained with the use of respiratory gating. Several techniques are available for eliminating the artifacts induced by respiratory motion.

The characteristic artifact induced by respiratory motion is the ghost-image artifact (Fig. 8-1B). This artifact is especially prominent at short values of TR (<0.5 sec). The artifact is less well seen at longer TR values, but it still may affect image quality. An interesting feature of respiratory motion ghosting is that such ghosting is not confined to only body parts in motion. Respiratory motion may also produce ghosting in stationary objects, such as nearby phantoms attached to the table and not touching the patient. This illustrates the complex nature of the artifact phenomenon of ghosting, which displaces the image along the phase-encoding axis.

One technique to correct for respiratory movement is to place a tight cinch around the patient's upper abdomen. The patient is thus converted from an "abdominal breather" (primary motion of the diaphragm) to a "chest breather" (primary motion of the chest wall, with limited diaphragmatic motion). This may be entirely satisfactory for many clinical applications, such as imaging the liver. It is unlikely to be satisfactory for evaluating small pulmonary lesions or lesions near the chest wall, however.

A better but more complicated and time-consuming technique involves actual gating of MR signal acquisition to the respiratory cycle. A belt device containing a strain sensor may be placed around the patient's chest or upper abdomen to detect respiratory motion. A second method using electrodes (impedance plethysmography) may also be employed to detect respiratory motion based on variation in transthoracic electric resistance with changes in lung volume.

A certain time penalty must be paid for the improved image quality obtained by respiratory gating. If uncontrolled tidal breathing is allowed, gated studies may take two to four times longer than nongated studies. If the patient is instructed to lengthen the time between breaths, and if a special data acquisition mode called *spin-conditioning* is used, the time penalty can be reduced to only an additional 30% to 50%. An example of a chest image using respiratory gating alone is shown in Figure 8-1C.

Several experimental techniques are being developed to help eliminate respiratory motion artifacts without time penalty. Rapid scanning using *echo-planar* or *steady-state free precession* methods may allow acquisition of images during a few seconds of breath holding. *Ordered phase encoding* techniques (such as General Electric's "Exorcist" and Picker's "COPE") eliminate many artifacts by destroying the effective periodicity of respiratory motion. By matching phase encoding amplitudes to the respiratory pattern, ghosts can be effectively filtered or focused outside the field of view.

Combined Respiratory and Cardiac Gating

Combined respiratory and cardiac gating is superior to either technique alone, although the incremental improvement in image quality may not be as great as might be expected. Better internal cardiac detail can be noted in the axial plane when combined gating is compared with cardiac gating alone. The improvement in the coronal and sagittal planes is less impressive. Combined gating definitely delineates the diaphragm and lung bases better than does either gating method alone. This improvement is especially noted in the sagittal and coronal planes.

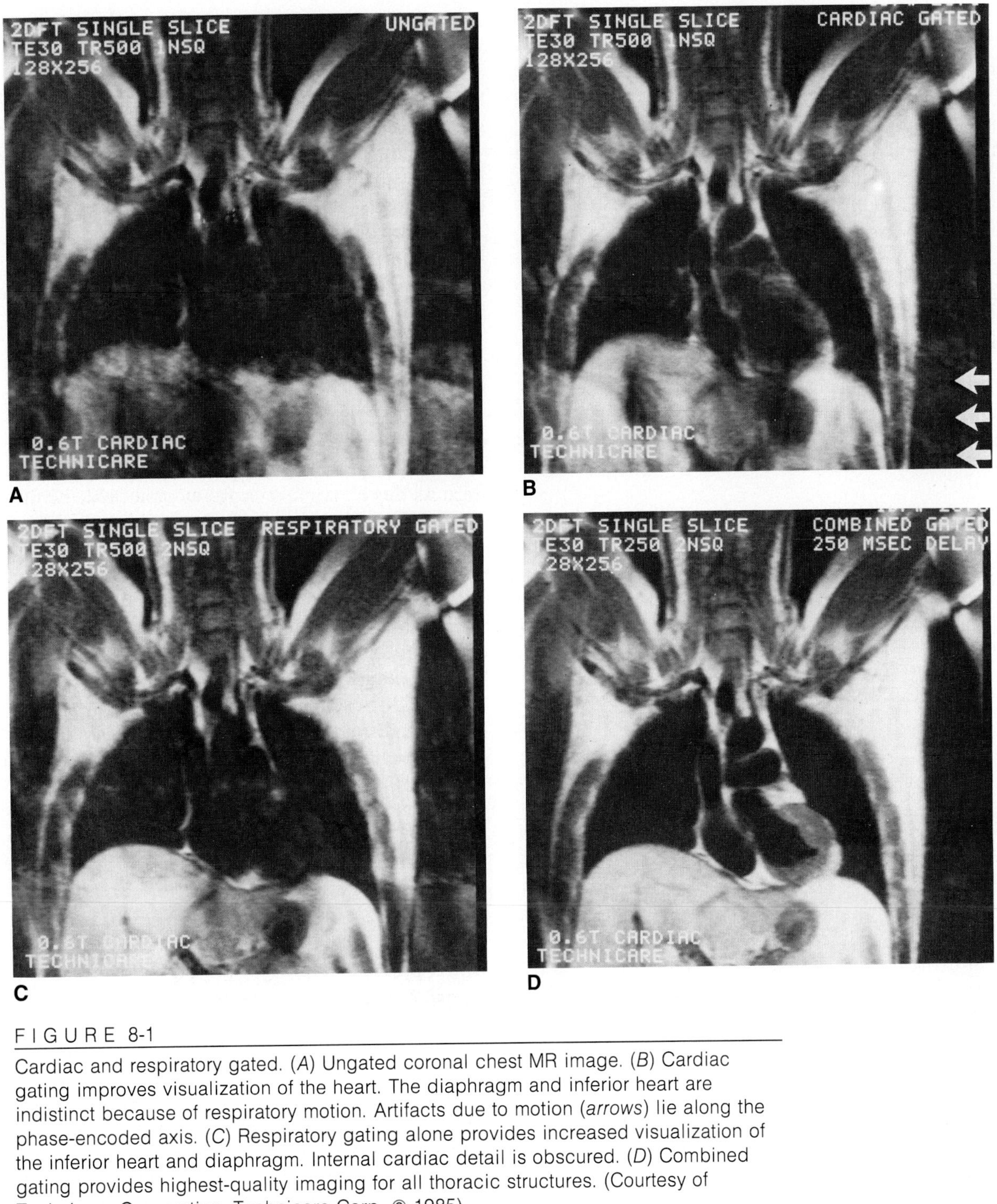

FIGURE 8-1

Cardiac and respiratory gated. (*A*) Ungated coronal chest MR image. (*B*) Cardiac gating improves visualization of the heart. The diaphragm and inferior heart are indistinct because of respiratory motion. Artifacts due to motion (*arrows*) lie along the phase-encoded axis. (*C*) Respiratory gating alone provides increased visualization of the inferior heart and diaphragm. Internal cardiac detail is obscured. (*D*) Combined gating provides highest-quality imaging for all thoracic structures. (Courtesy of Technicare Corporation, Technicare Corp. © 1985)

Combined gating requires more sophisticated electronics than does either method alone. Cardiac-gated signal acquisition is only allowed to take place at appropriate times in the respiratory cycle, as determined by the respiratory system. The time penalty for combined gating is the same as that for respiratory gating alone, with TR equal to the cardiac period. An example of combined gating is shown in Figure 8-1D.

Pulse Sequences and Parameters for Chest Imaging

The spin-echo technique has been found to be most useful for both the demonstration of normal anatomy and for the detection of pathological processes in the chest. In general, both T1- and T2-weighted sequences should be performed for maximum sensitivity. Echo times (TE) of 25 msec to 60 msec combined with TR of 0.5 and 2.0 seconds have been employed with good success.

In the mediastinum, the T1 values of tumor and fat are usually distinct, whereas T2 values have shown significant overlap. Thus, when attempting to evaluate mediastinal masses, T1-weighted images are most helpful. In these images, mediastinal fat will appear bright, whereas tumors and adenopathy are usually of lower intensity.

T2-weighted images (with a long TR) will provide the best image quality and higher signal-to-noise ratios, increasing resolving power and signal strength and making smaller hilar and lung lesions easier to detect. These advantages may be offset somewhat by artifacts from patient motion occurring during longer TR intervals. In uncomfortable or uncooperative patients, it may be more sensible to use shorter TR times for better-quality images.

By comparing signal intensities between short and long TE sequences, T2 values may be estimated. Since fluids have long T2 values, they may be detected on T2-weighted images. As elsewhere in the body, prolonged T2 is nonspecific and may be seen in fluid-filled cysts, liquefied abscesses, loculated effusions, and necrotic tumors. Sample protocols for chest MR imaging are presented in Table 8.2.

TABLE 8-2

Possible Protocols for Chest MR Imaging

Evaluation of Mediastinal Masses or Nodes

Protocol:
1. Respiratory or cardiac gating is probably not necessary, although image quality will be improved somewhat
2. Axial, SE 500/30
3. Axial, SE 2000/60
4. If lesion is near the thoracic inlet or is a questionable mass in the aorticopulmonary window, do coronal, SE 1500/40,80

"Routine" Cardiac Imaging

Protocol:
1. Use cardiac gating to each beat or every other beat so that TR is about 1000 msec
2. For evaluation of wall motion or intracardiac thrombus, use cycled gating if available
3. For precise wall measurements, use oblique long- and short-axis views
4. Axial SE (TR)/30,60 with modifications as above

Cardiac Imaging for Ischemia or Infarction

Protocol:
1. Use intravenous Gd-DTPA contrast (when available)
2. Use cardiac gating as above
3. Axial SE (TR)/30,60
4. Sagittal SE (TR)/30,60
5. With questionable inferior infarction or aneurysm, do coronal SE (TR)/30,60. May also require respiratory gating

Normal Anatomy of the Mediastinum

Axial images of the mediastinum present a pattern of anatomy easily recognizable to those familiar with CT. As previously noted, the rapidly flowing blood in major mediastinal vessels makes them appear dark. Where these vessels contact the lung, their walls may be seen as a stripe slightly less intense than fat. The air-containing trachea and brochi will likewise cast no signal, except from their walls. They cannot be distinguished from vessels except by location. A nondistended mid-esophagus can be hard to see. Occasionally, an anterior vertebral osteophyte may be confused with an air-filled esophagus. Figure 8-2 demonstrates the normal MR transverse anatomy of the upper chest and mediastinum using SE 1000/28. Transverse anatomy of the heart using cardiac gating is shown in Figure 8-3.

Coronal images of the chest (Fig. 8-4 and 8-5)

(Text continues on p. 187.)

FIGURE 8-2

Axial SE 1000/28 images of the upper chest.

A	aortic arch
AA	ascending aorta
AJL	anterior junction line
APM	anterior papillary muscle
AR	aortic root
AXA	axillary artery
AZ	azygous vein
BCA	brachiocephalic artery
C	coronary sinus
CL	clavicle
CX	left circumflex coronary artery
D	diaphragm
DA	descending aorta
E	esophagus
ES	erector spinae muscle
H	humeral shaft
HH	humeral head
HI	hilum
IS	infraspinatus muscle
ITV	internal thoracic vein
IVC	inferior vena cava
IVS	interventricular septum
L	liver
LA	left atrium
LBV	left brachiocephalic vein
LCC	left common carotid artery
LD	latissimus dorsi muscle
LIJ	left internal jugular vein
LMB	left mainstem bronchus
LPA	left pulmonary artery
LPV	left pulmonary vein
LSCA	left subclavian artery
LSV	left superior pulmonary vein
LV	left ventricle
LVOT	left ventricular outflow tract
MHV	middle hepatic vein
MPA	main pulmonary artery
PC	pericardium
PF	pericardial fat
PMI	pectoralis minor muscle
PMJ	pectoralis major muscle
PV	portal vein
RA	right atrium
RCA	right coronary artery
RCC	right common carotid artery
RH	rhomboid muscles
RIJ	right internal jugular vein
RIJ	right internal jugular vein
RMB	right mainstem bronchus
RPA	right pulmonary artery
RPV	right superior pulmonary vein
RSCA	right subclavian artery
RV	right ventricle
SA	serratus anterior muscle
SAM	scalene anterior muscle
SCM	sternocleidomastoid muscle
SM	scalene medius muscle
SP	spinal cord
St	sternum
ST	stomach
SU	supraspinatus muscle
SVC	superior vena cava
T	trachea
TC	transverse colon
TH	thyroid
TR	trapezius muscle
TV	tricuspid valve

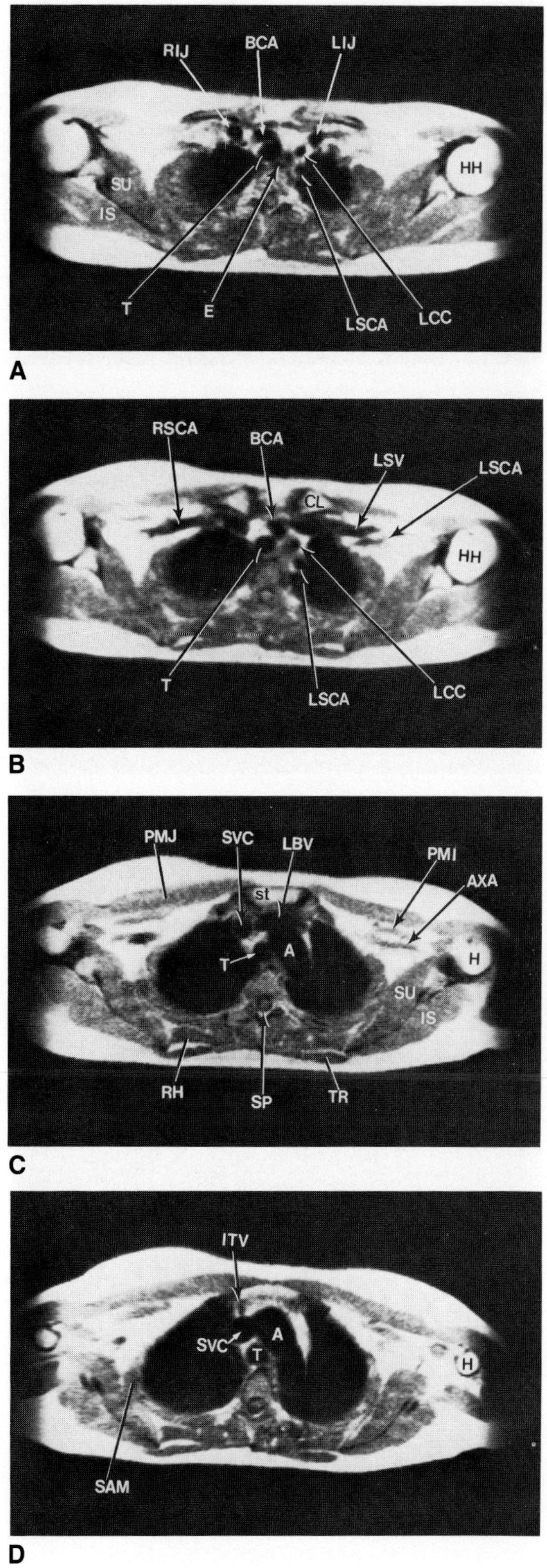

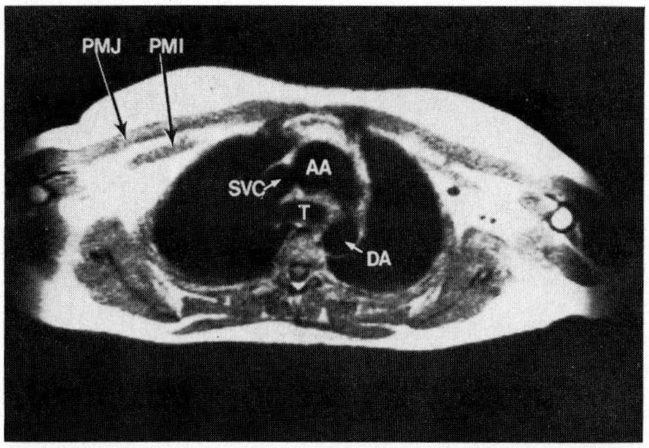

E

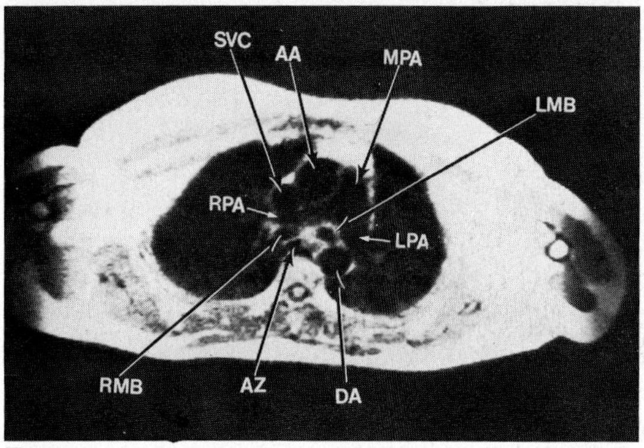

F

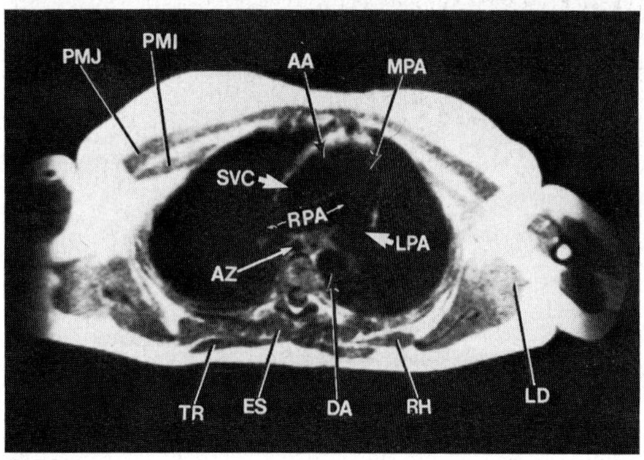

G

FIGURE 8-2 *(cont.)*

Axial SE 1000/28 images of the upper chest.

A	aortic arch
AA	ascending aorta
AJL	anterior junction line
APM	anterior papillary muscle
AR	aortic root
AXA	axillary artery
AZ	azygous vein
BCA	brachiocephalic artery
C	coronary sinus
CL	clavicle
CX	left circumflex coronary artery
D	diaphragm
DA	descending aorta
E	esophagus
ES	erector spinae muscle
H	humeral shaft
HH	humeral head
HI	hilum
IS	infraspinatus muscle
ITV	internal thoracic vein
IVC	inferior vena cava
IVS	interventricular septum
L	liver
LA	left atrium
LBV	left brachiocephalic vein
LCC	left common carotid artery
LD	latissimus dorsi muscle
LIJ	left internal jugular vein
LMB	left mainstem bronchus
LPA	left pulmonary artery
LPV	left pulmonary vein
LSCA	left subclavian artery
LSV	left superior pulmonary vein
LV	left ventricle
LVOT	left ventricular outflow tract
MHV	middle hepatic vein
MPA	main pulmonary artery
PC	pericardium
PF	pericardial fat
PMI	pectoralis minor muscle
PMJ	pectoralis major muscle
PV	portal vein
RA	right atrium
RCA	right coronary artery
RCC	right common carotid artery
RH	rhomboid muscles
RIJ	right internal jugular vein
RIJ	right internal jugular vein
RMB	right mainstem bronchus
RPA	right pulmonary artery
RPV	right superior pulmonary vein
RSCA	right subclavian artery
RV	right ventricle
SA	serratus anterior muscle
SAM	scalene anterior muscle
SCM	sternocleidomastoid muscle
SM	scalene medius muscle
SP	spinal cord
St	sternum
ST	stomach
SU	supraspinatus muscle
SVC	superior vena cava
T	trachea
TC	transverse colon
TH	thyroid
TR	trapezius muscle
TV	tricuspid valve

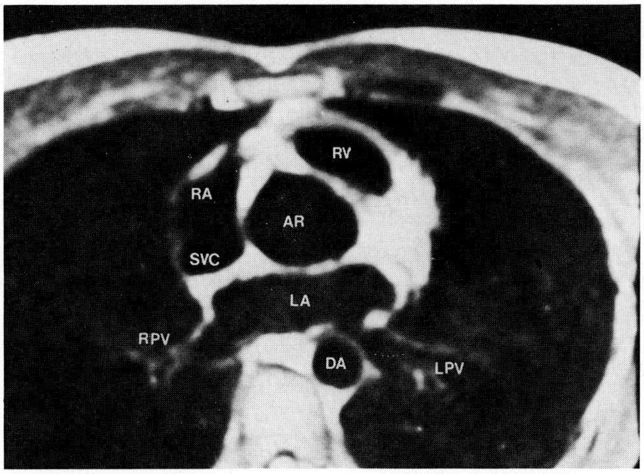

A

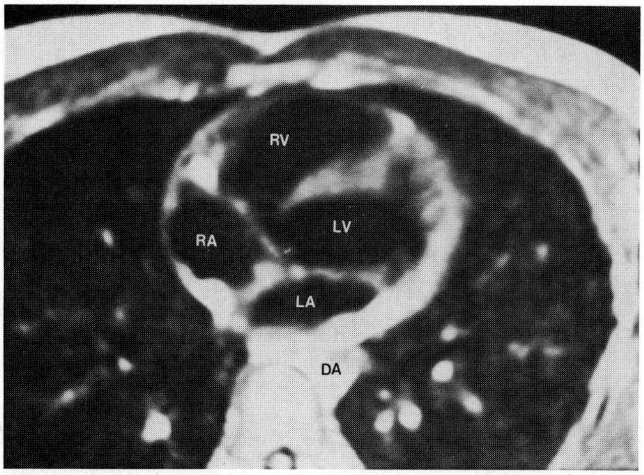

B

FIGURE 8-3

Axial cardiac-gated SE images of the lower chest and heart. (Courtesy of Fonar Corporation, 110 Marcus Drive, Melville, NY 11747)

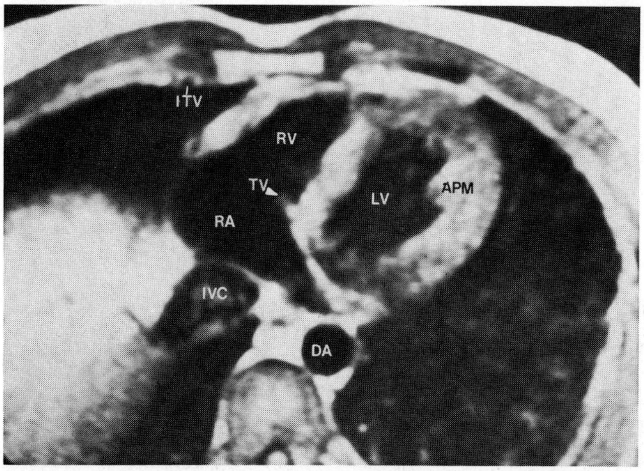

C

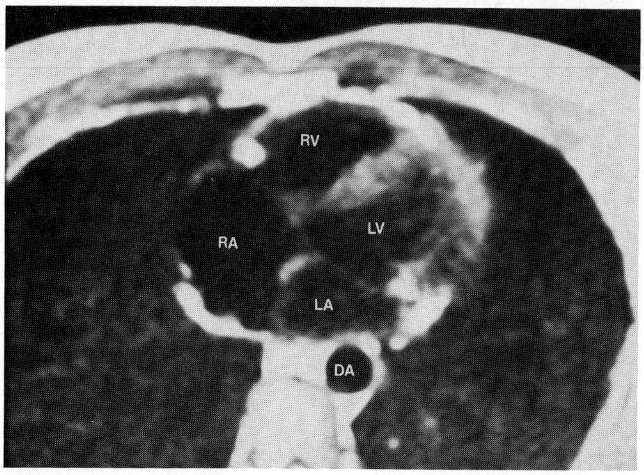

D

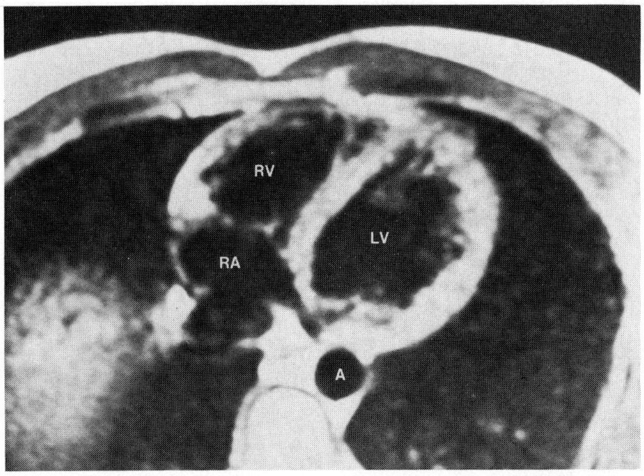

E

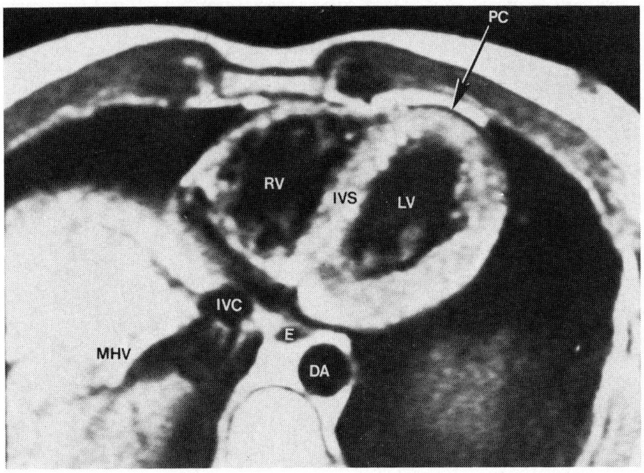

F

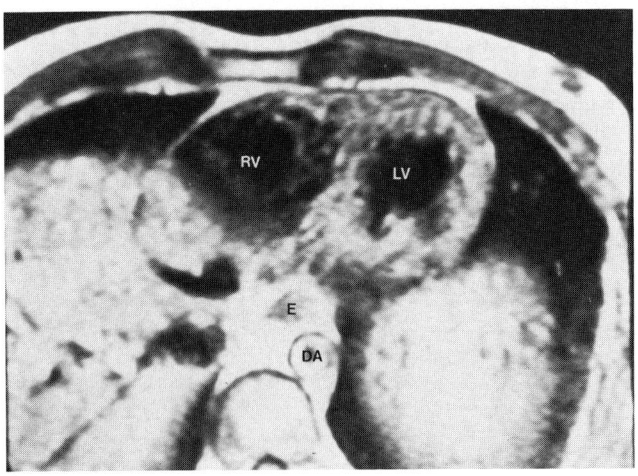

G

FIGURE 8-3 *(cont.)*

Axial cardiac-gated SE images of the lower chest and heart. (Courtesy of Fonar Corporation, 110 Marcus Drive, Melville, NY 11747)

A	aortic arch
AA	ascending aorta
AJL	anterior junction line
APM	anterior papillary muscle
AR	aortic root
AXA	axillary artery
AZ	azygous vein
BCA	brachiocephalic artery
C	coronary sinus
CL	clavicle
CX	left circumflex coronary artery
D	diaphragm
DA	descending aorta
E	esophagus
ES	erector spinae muscle
H	humeral shaft
HH	humeral head
HI	hilum
IS	infraspinatus muscle
ITV	internal thoracic vein
IVC	inferior vena cava
IVS	interventricular septum
L	liver
LA	left atrium
LBV	left brachiocephalic vein
LCC	left common carotid artery
LD	latissimus dorsi muscle
LIJ	left internal jugular vein
LMB	left mainstem bronchus
LPA	left pulmonary artery
LPV	left pulmonary vein
LSCA	left subclavian artery
LSV	left superior pulmonary vein
LV	left ventricle
LVOT	left ventricular outflow tract
MHV	middle hepatic vein
MPA	main pulmonary artery
PC	pericardium
PF	pericardial fat
PMI	pectoralis minor muscle
PMJ	pectoralis major muscle
PV	portal vein
RA	right atrium
RCA	right coronary artery
RCC	right common carotid artery
RH	rhomboid muscles
RIJ	right internal jugular vein
RIJ	right internal jugular vein
RMB	right mainstem bronchus
RPA	right pulmonary artery
RPV	right superior pulmonary vein
RSCA	right subclavian artery
RV	right ventricle
SA	serratus anterior muscle
SAM	scalene anterior muscle
SCM	sternocleidomastoid muscle
SM	scalene medius muscle
SP	spinal cord
St	sternum
ST	stomach
SU	supraspinatus muscle
SVC	superior vena cava
T	trachea
TC	transverse colon
TH	thyroid
TR	trapezius muscle
TV	tricuspid valve

FIGURE 8-4

Coronal cardiac-gated SE images of the chest. (Courtesy of Siemens)

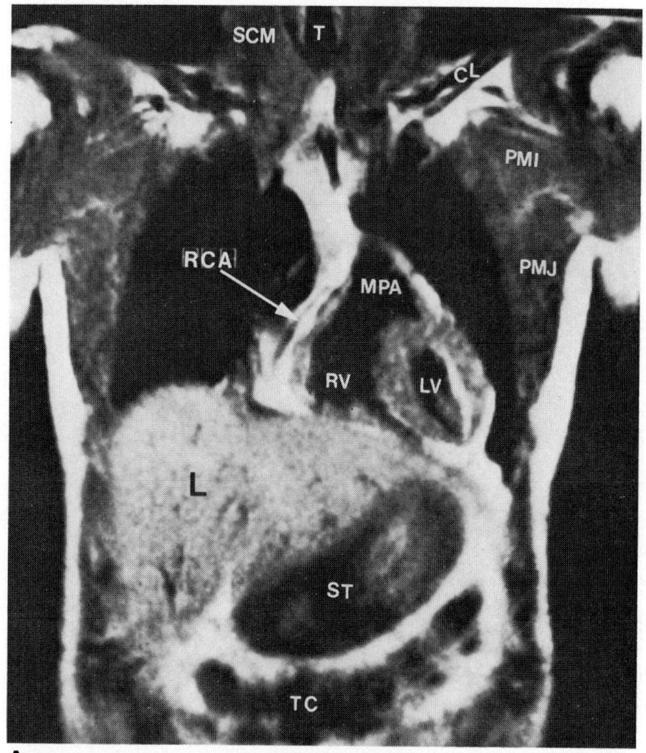

A

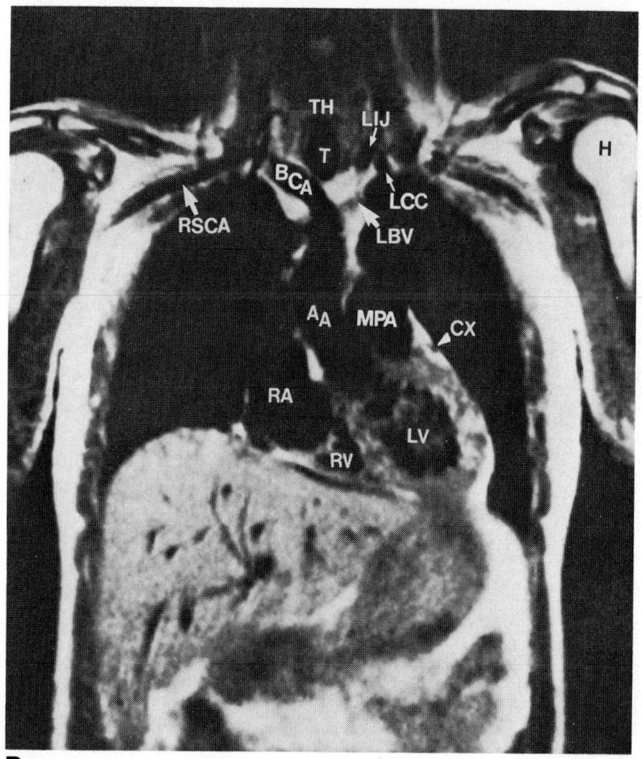

B

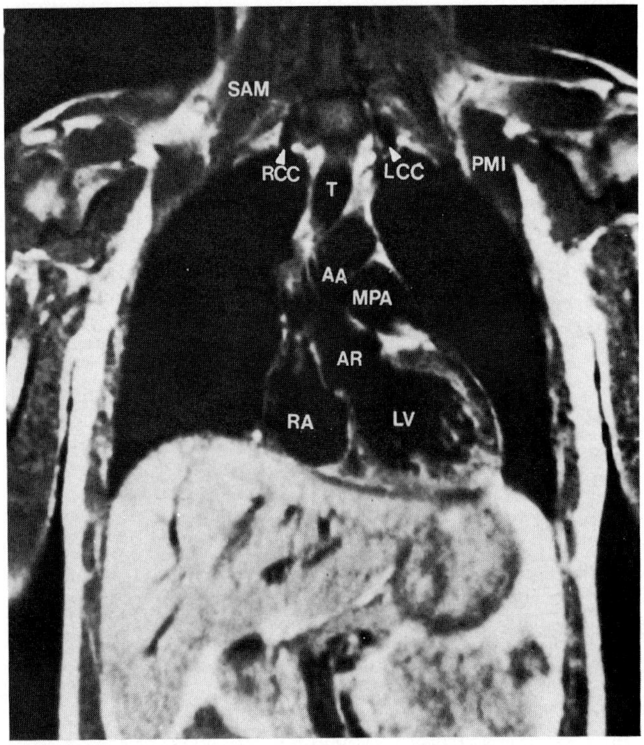

C

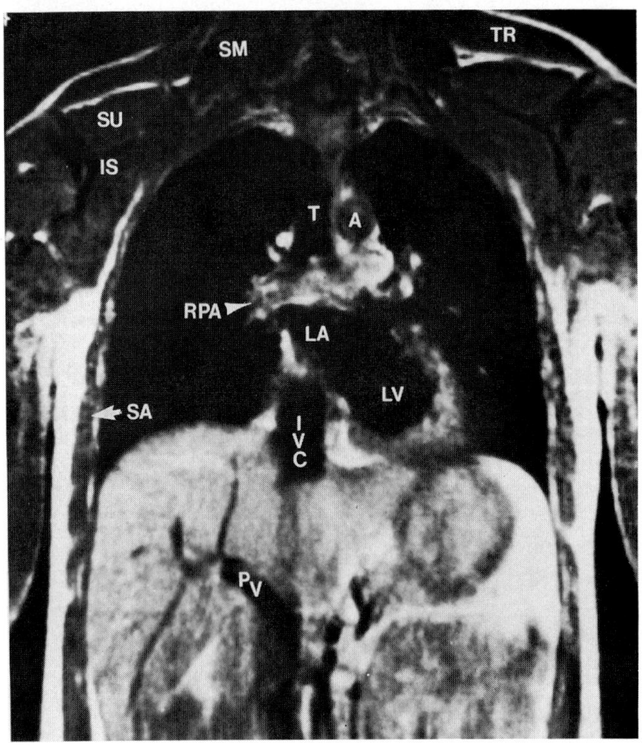

D

FIGURE 8-4 *(cont.)*

Coronal cardiac-gated SE images of the chest. (Courtesy of Siemens)

FIGURE 8-5

Coronal cardiac-gated SE images of the heart. (Courtesy of Fonar Corporation, 110 Marcus Drive, Melville, NY 11747)

A aortic arch
AA ascending aorta
AJL anterior junction line
APM anterior papillary muscle
AR aortic root
AXA axillary artery
AZ azygous vein
BCA brachiocephalic artery
C coronary sinus
CL clavicle
CX left circumflex coronary artery
D diaphragm
DA descending aorta
E esophagus
ES erector spinae muscle
H humeral shaft
HH humeral head
HI hilum
IS infraspinatus muscle
ITV internal thoracic vein
IVC inferior vena cava
IVS interventricular septum
L liver
LA left atrium
LBV left brachiocephalic vein
LCC left common carotid artery
LD latissimus dorsi muscle
LIJ left internal jugular vein
LMB left mainstem bronchus
LPA left pulmonary artery
LPV left pulmonary vein
LSCA left subclavian artery
LSV left superior pulmonary vein
LV left ventricle
LVOT left ventricular outflow tract
MHV middle hepatic vein
MPA main pulmonary artery
PC pericardium
PF pericardial fat
PMI pectoralis minor muscle
PMJ pectoralis major muscle
PV portal vein
RA right atrium
RCA right coronary artery
RCC right common carotid artery
RH rhomboid muscles
RIJ right internal jugular vein
RIJ right internal jugular vein
RMB right mainstem bronchus
RPA right pulmonary artery
RPV right superior pulmonary vein
RSCA right subclavian artery
RV right ventricle
SA serratus anterior muscle
SAM scalene anterior muscle
SCM sternocleidomastoid muscle
SM scalene medius muscle
SP spinal cord
St sternum
ST stomach
SU supraspinatus muscle
SVC superior vena cava
T trachea
TC transverse colon
TH thyroid
TR trapezius muscle
TV tricuspid valve

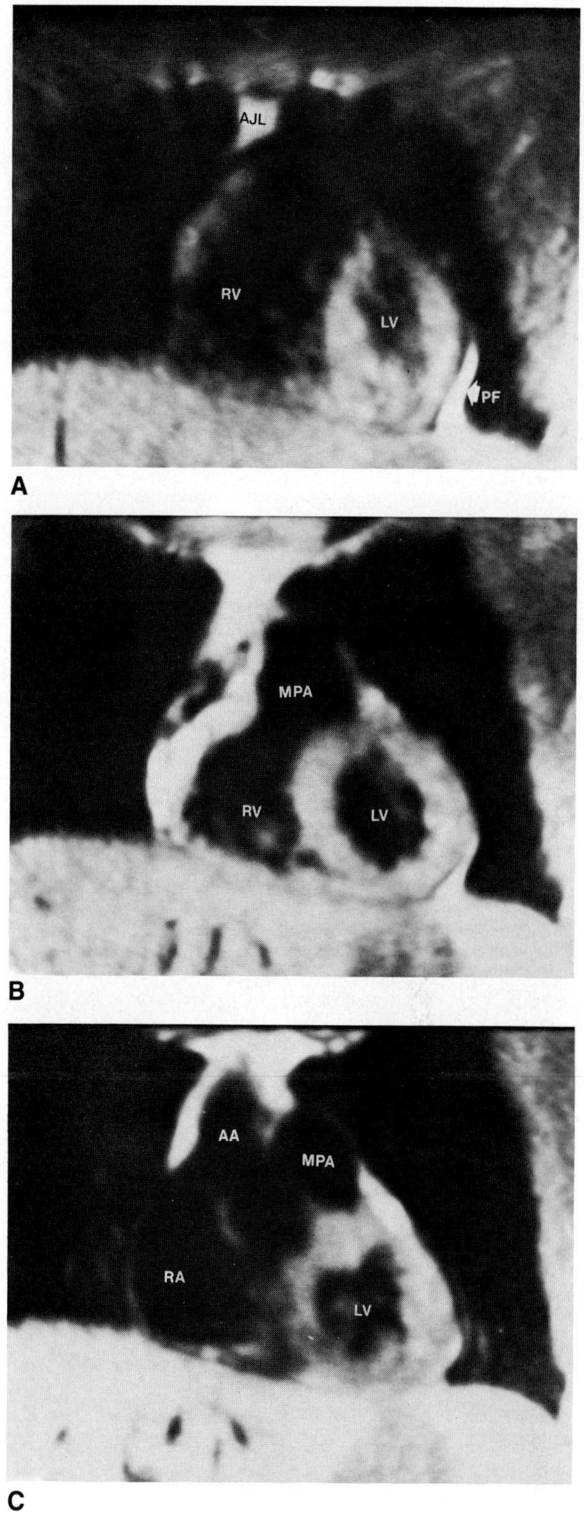

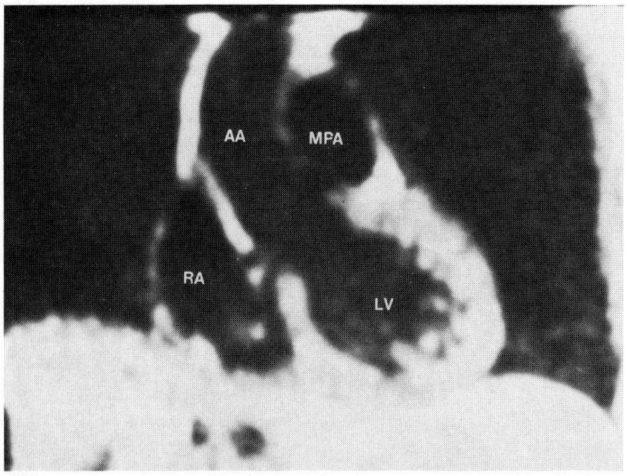

D

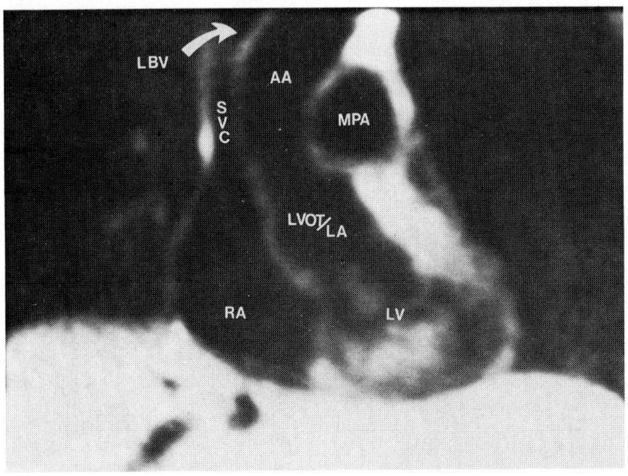

E

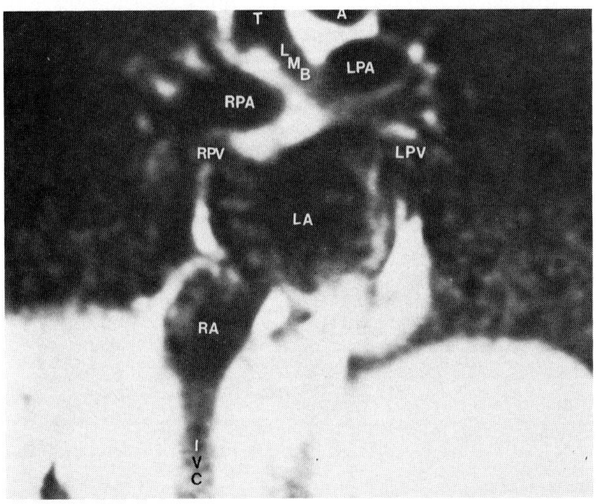

F

FIGURE 8-5 *(cont.)*

Coronal cardiac-gated SE images of the heart. (Courtesy of Fonar Corporation, 110 Marcus Drive, Melville, NY 11747)

A	aortic arch
AA	ascending aorta
AJL	anterior junction line
APM	anterior papillary muscle
AR	aortic root
AXA	axillary artery
AZ	azygous vein
BCA	brachiocephalic artery
C	coronary sinus
CL	clavicle
CX	left circumflex coronary artery
D	diaphragm
DA	descending aorta
E	esophagus
ES	erector spinae muscle
H	humeral shaft
HH	humeral head
HI	hilum
IS	infraspinatus muscle
ITV	internal thoracic vein
IVC	inferior vena cava
IVS	interventricular septum
L	liver
LA	left atrium
LBV	left brachiocephalic vein
LCC	left common carotid artery
LD	latissimus dorsi muscle
LIJ	left internal jugular vein
LMB	left mainstem bronchus
LPA	left pulmonary artery
LPV	left pulmonary vein
LSCA	left subclavian artery
LSV	left superior pulmonary vein
LV	left ventricle
LVOT	left ventricular outflow tract
MHV	middle hepatic vein
MPA	main pulmonary artery
PC	pericardium
PF	pericardial fat
PMI	pectoralis minor muscle
PMJ	pectoralis major muscle
PV	portal vein
RA	right atrium
RCA	right coronary artery
RCC	right common carotid artery
RH	rhomboid muscles
RIJ	right internal jugular vein
RIJ	right internal jugular vein
RMB	right mainstem bronchus
RPA	right pulmonary artery
RPV	right superior pulmonary vein
RSCA	right subclavian artery
RV	right ventricle
SA	serratus anterior muscle
SAM	scalene anterior muscle
SCM	sternocleidomastoid muscle
SM	scalene medius muscle
SP	spinal cord
St	sternum
ST	stomach
SU	supraspinatus muscle
SVC	superior vena cava
T	trachea
TC	transverse colon
TH	thyroid
TR	trapezius muscle
TV	tricuspid valve

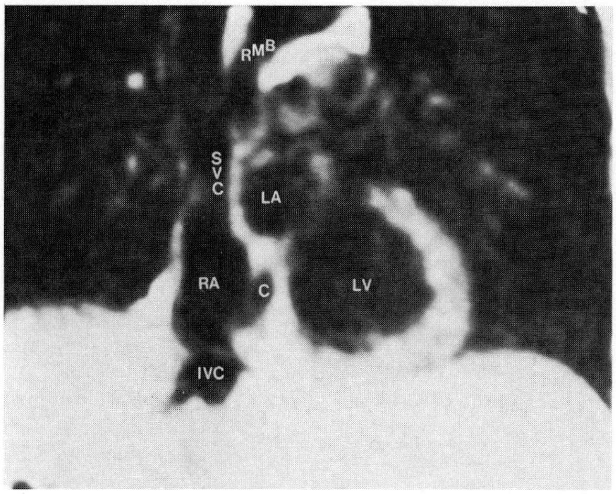

G

FIGURE 8-5 *(cont.)*

Coronal cardiac-gated SE images of the heart. (Courtesy of Fonar Corporation, 110 Marcus Drive, Melville, NY 11747)

present a different but easily recognized pattern of anatomy. Anteriorly, fat is seen between pleural membranes in the retromanubrial space; this represents the anterior junction line. The entire trachea is not usually seen on a single coronal slice because of its posterior inclination. Usually three or four slices will be required to depict it. Pretracheal and posttracheal masses may be difficult to detect because of partial volume effects with the air-filled trachea in the coronal section. Laterally situated paratracheal masses are easily and reliably identified, however.

Most of the mediastinal systemic veins can be consistently visualized in the coronal plane. The left brachiocephalic vein, right brachiocephalic vein, and jugular veins are usually identified on one or two consecutive coronal slices. The superior vena cava is seen on the one or two coronal slices more posteriorly. Posteriorly, the azygous vein may be seen in its characteristic paraspinous location. Occasionally the left-sided hemiazygous vein may also be seen. Sometimes several smaller mediastinal veins are visible, including the internal mammary veins, left superior intercostal vein, and the other intercostal veins.

The aorta and its branches are always visible in coronal section. The origins of each arch vessel are not consistently demonstrated, however. Coronal imaging allows one to follow some of these vessels (like the carotid arteries) along their course out of the thorax and into the neck.

The main pulmonary artery and its branches are nearly always identified. The left and right superior pulmonary veins may be seen in at least half of normal patients. The inferior veins are less well seen.

The aorticopulmonary window region is well evaluated on coronal MR images, and it should have a flat or concave lateral border. The amount of fat in the subcarinal region varies between patients. Fat is usually seen inferior to each main bronchus, traveling farther along the right bronchus than the left. Fat may also be seen surrounding the esophagus in the azygoesophageal recess, although the esophagus itself is not identified unless filled with air. Similarly, the diaphragm itself is not seen unless it is silhouetted by ascites or air (Fig. 8-6).

Sagittal views of the thorax reveal anatomy in expected locations (Fig. 8-7). Laterally in the chest, the brachiocephalic and subclavian vessels may be noted in cross section, but they are at times difficult to see. More medially, the hilar vessels and bronchi come into view, distinguishable only by virtue of location. Posterior and anterior hilar masses may be well seen, but those more laterally situated may be difficult to detect. In the chest lateral to the hila, sagittal imaging is of limited usefulness, except in evaluating apical and basilar masses. Centrally in the mediastinum, however, sagittal imaging can provide important anatomic perspectives.

The anterior mediastinum is usually filled with high-intensity fat or low-intensity air. The sternum is well visualized and has a dark cortex and high-intensity marrow-filled center. Sternomanubrial and sternoxyphoid articulations may be recognized. Parasternal masses or adenopathy may be easily appreciated in this projection.

(Text continues on p. 191.)

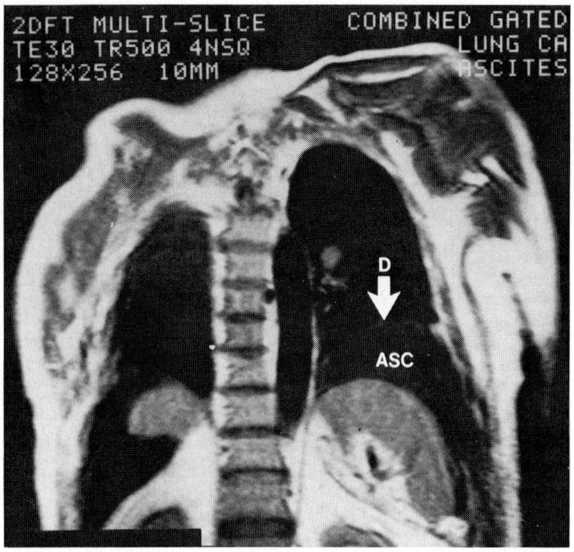

FIGURE 8-6

The diaphragm (D) is not usually seen unless silhouetted by ascites (ASC).

A	aortic arch
AA	ascending aorta
AJL	anterior junction line
APM	anterior papillary muscle
AR	aortic root
AXA	axillary artery
AZ	azygous vein
BCA	brachiocephalic artery
C	coronary sinus
CL	clavicle
CX	left circumflex coronary artery
D	diaphragm
DA	descending aorta
E	esophagus
ES	erector spinae muscle
H	humeral shaft
HH	humeral head
HI	hilum
IS	infraspinatus muscle
ITV	internal thoracic vein
IVC	inferior vena cava
IVS	interventricular septum
L	liver
LA	left atrium
LBV	left brachiocephalic vein
LCC	left common carotid artery
LD	latissimus dorsi muscle
LIJ	left internal jugular vein
LMB	left mainstem bronchus
LPA	left pulmonary artery
LPV	left pulmonary vein
LSCA	left subclavian artery
LSV	left superior pulmonary vein
LV	left ventricle
LVOT	left ventricular outflow tract
MHV	middle hepatic vein
MPA	main pulmonary artery
PC	pericardium
PF	pericardial fat
PMI	pectoralis minor muscle
PMJ	pectoralis major muscle
PV	portal vein
RA	right atrium
RCA	right coronary artery
RCC	right common carotid artery
RH	rhomboid muscles
RIJ	right internal jugular vein
RIJ	right internal jugular vein
RMB	right mainstem bronchus
RPA	right pulmonary artery
RPV	right superior pulmonary vein
RSCA	right subclavian artery
RV	right ventricle
SA	serratus anterior muscle
SAM	scalene anterior muscle
SCM	sternocleidomastoid muscle
SM	scalene medius muscle
SP	spinal cord
St	sternum
ST	stomach
SU	supraspinatus muscle
SVC	superior vena cava
T	trachea
TC	transverse colon
TH	thyroid
TR	trapezius muscle
TV	tricuspid valve

FIGURE 8-7

Sagittal cardiac-gated SE images of the chest and heart. (Courtesy of Fonar Corporation, 110 Marcus Drive, Melville, NY 11747)

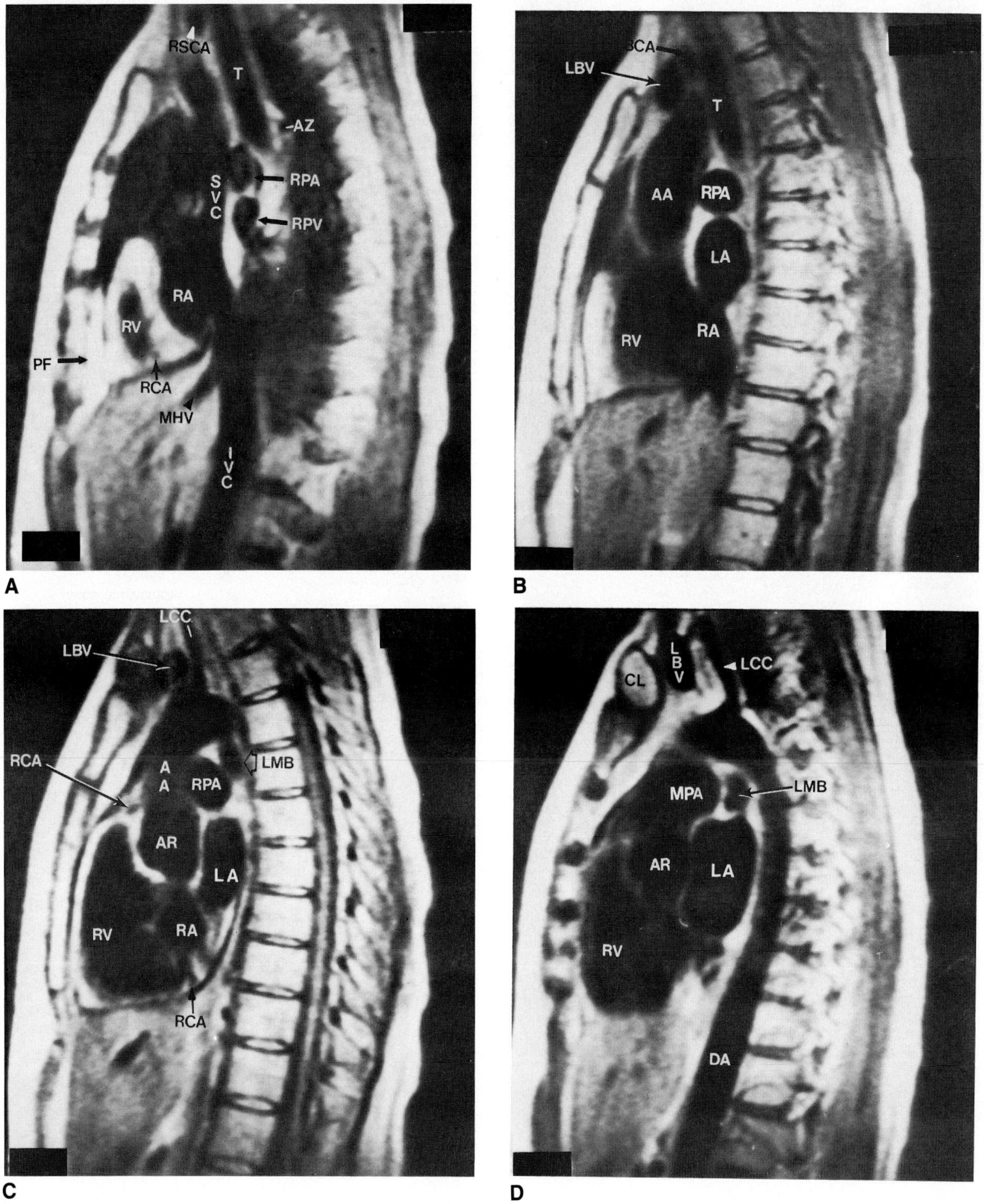

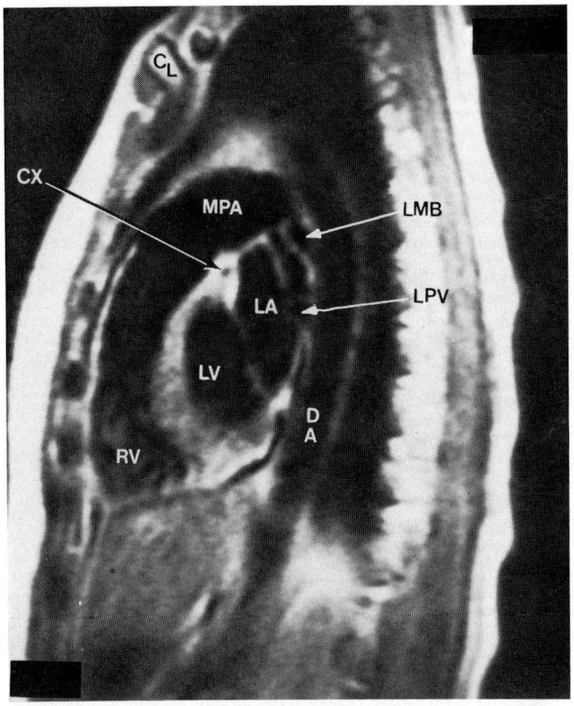

E

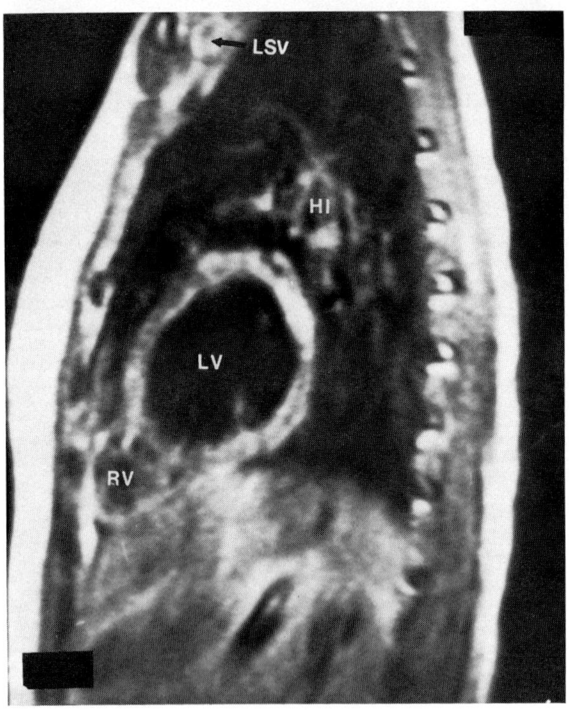

F

FIGURE 8-7 *(cont.)*

Sagittal cardiac-gated SE images of the chest and heart. (Courtesy of Fonar Corporation, 110 Marcus Drive, Melville, NY 11747)

A	aortic arch
AA	ascending aorta
AJL	anterior junction line
APM	anterior papillary muscle
AR	aortic root
AXA	axillary artery
AZ	azygous vein
BCA	brachiocephalic artery
C	coronary sinus
CL	clavicle
CX	left circumflex coronary artery
D	diaphragm
DA	descending aorta
E	esophagus
ES	erector spinae muscle
H	humeral shaft
HH	humeral head
HI	hilum
IS	infraspinatus muscle
ITV	internal thoracic vein
IVC	inferior vena cava
IVS	interventricular septum
L	liver
LA	left atrium
LBV	left brachiocephalic vein
LCC	left common carotid artery
LD	latissimus dorsi muscle
LIJ	left internal jugular vein
LMB	left mainstem bronchus
LPA	left pulmonary artery
LPV	left pulmonary vein
LSCA	left subclavian artery
LSV	left superior pulmonary vein
LV	left ventricle
LVOT	left ventricular outflow tract
MHV	middle hepatic vein
MPA	main pulmonary artery
PC	pericardium
PF	pericardial fat
PMI	pectoralis minor muscle
PMJ	pectoralis major muscle
PV	portal vein
RA	right atrium
RCA	right coronary artery
RCC	right common carotid artery
RH	rhomboid muscles
RIJ	right internal jugular vein
RIJ	right internal jugular vein
RMB	right mainstem bronchus
RPA	right pulmonary artery
RPV	right superior pulmonary vein
RSCA	right subclavian artery
RV	right ventricle
SA	serratus anterior muscle
SAM	scalene anterior muscle
SCM	sternocleidomastoid muscle
SM	scalene medius muscle
SP	spinal cord
St	sternum
ST	stomach
SU	supraspinatus muscle
SVC	superior vena cava
T	trachea
TC	transverse colon
TH	thyroid
TR	trapezius muscle
TV	tricuspid valve

The aortic arch is identified in two or three consecutive sagittal slices, arching over the pulmonary arteries and mainstem bronchi. Origins of the arch vessels can usually be seen. The carotid arteries may be followed up into the neck. The sagittal projection is useful in evaluating the spread of disease from the thorax into the neck, and vice versa.

The trachea is usually seen in one or two consecutive sagittal images as a long, low-intensity tubular structure. Mainstem bronchi are seen in cross section. The subcarinal space may be well evaluated and is usually filled with fat. Relationships of subcarinal masses to the left atrium are easy to appreciate in this projection.

Inferiorly, the contour of the diaphragm may be visualized, especially when respiratory gating is employed. The inferior vena cava is consistently imaged passing through the liver and diaphragm. The middle hepatic vein may be seen joining the inferior vena cava near the diaphragm.

Cardiac MRI

Two-dimensional echocardiography (2DE) is an excellent technique for imaging the heart. It allows real-time evaluation of wall motion, chamber size, and valve dynamics. It is doubtful that cardiac MRI will ever totally replace 2DE in the future of cardiac imaging, but MRI will probably come to play unique adjunctive and primary roles.

What MRI offers is a *global* perspective of the heart and great vessels, rather than piecemeal views through a narrow echocardiographic window. In complex congenital heart disease, MRI provides better assessment of anomalies of the great vessels, pulmonary veins, and postoperative shunts than is possible with 2DE. However, 2DE still remains superior to MRI in delineation of valvular abnormalities. In acquired heart disease, MRI may provide flow information, and recognition of ischemia and infarction. The latter diagnoses may be aided by future advances in spectroscopy and paramagnetic contrast agents.

It is possible to obtain acceptable diagnostic images of the heart in a nongated mode using spin-echo sequences, provided both TR and TE are very short (*e.g.,* SE 150/15). More detailed delineation of anatomy or detection of less obvious pathological processes, however, requires cardiac or combined gating. Surface coils may be needed to demonstrate coronary artery or valvular lesions.

When cardiac gating is used, it is not possible to specify the TR interval uniquely, since TR depends on the cardiac period. Estimations of tissue T1 and T2 values can be made in two ways: (1) by varying the TE parameter or (2) recording signals at TR and $2 \times$ TR by gating to every heartbeat or to alternate beats.

Some manufacturers (*e.g.,* Diasonics) permit a cycled acquisition of data from the heart. Using this technique, it is possible to view the same slice at staggered times through the cardiac cycle. Figure 8-8 demonstrates the same axial plane through the ventricles, obtained at successive 100-msec intervals through the cardiac cycle. This may be useful in evaluating wall motion, wall thickness, or blood flow dynamics.

A number of investigators believe that oblique planes should be used when quantitative cardiac information is needed. The reason for this is that the major cardiac axes do not lie parallel to the conventional axial, coronal, or sagittal planes used to image the rest of the thorax. Furthermore, it is not strictly possible to compare conventional orthogonal images of the heart between patients, because changes in body habitus will change the orientation of the heart.

Accordingly, those clinical problems requiring accurate cardiac measurements (*e.g.,* ventricular volume, wall thickness, ejection fraction) would be more ideally performed along oblique planes parallel and perpendicular to the cardiac axes. Conventional orthogonal planes (which pass at angles through the myocardium) may produce images with falsely increased ventricular wall thickness. Likewise, there is also a potential for error in evaluating tissue signal from myocardium in the epicardial and subendocardial areas. Oblique imaging may also be helpful in certain aortic lesions, like a long dissection. In this way it may be possible to display the entire arch in a single projection.

Oblique images of the heart and thorax may be obtained in one of two ways. The patient may be positioned in the scanner on foam pads in either 30° left posterior oblique or 30° right posterior oblique, like for conventional angiocardiography. The chest may then be imaged in the routine coronal and sagittal planes relative to the scanner axis, producing oblique views of the heart and major vessels (Table

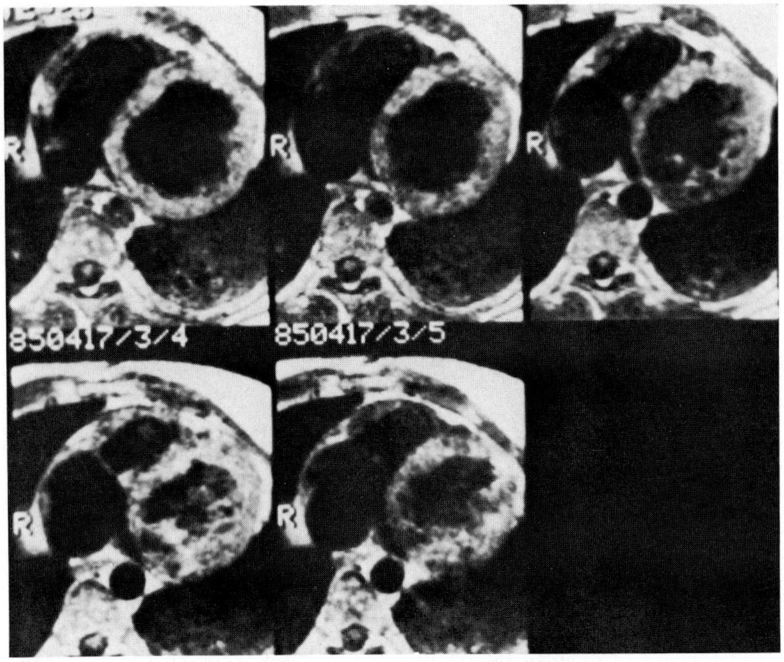

FIGURE 8-8

"Cycled" cardiac images. Same axial SE image through the heart recorded at successive 100-msec intervals after the R wave. The first image represents diastole; the fourth image is ventricular systole.

TABLE 8-3

Obtaining Oblique Projections of the Heart by Patient Positioning

Patient Position	Coronal MR Plane	Sagittal MR Plane
30° RPO	Profiled aortic arch Short axis of left ventricle (equivalent to conventional 30° RPO)	Long axis of left ventricle (equivalent to conventional 60° LAO)
30° LPO	Long axis of left ventricle (equivalent to conventional 60° LAO)	Profiled aortic arch Short axis of left ventricle (equivalent to conventional 30° RPO)

Note that the LPO sagittal image is the same as the RPO Coronal image and that the RPO sagittal image is the same as the LPO coronal image.

(Modified from Murphy WA, Gutierrez FR, Levitt RG, Glazer HS, Lee JKT: Oblique views of the heart by magnetic resonance imaging. Radiology 155:225–226, 1985)

8-3). A second method for obtaining oblique images of the thorax is currently available only in certain scanners but holds promise for future cardiac applications. Several manufacturers have developed methods to permit image acquisition in arbitrary planes by adjusting a set of gradient angles through the body. It is thus possible to image the heart along axes parallel and perpendicular to those of the left ventricle, producing views equivalent to the short-axis and long-axis views of echocardiography (Fig. 8-9 and 8-10).

Normal Cardiac Anatomy

Transverse, coronal, and sagittal images of the heart have already been presented in conjunction with the mediastinum (Figs. 8-3, 8-5, and 8-7). Several normal anatomic features, variants, and artifacts commonly encountered in cardiac MR imaging are presented in the paragraphs that follow.

The normal pericardium may not be perceived where it is adjacent to lung. With cardiac gating, it can be seen in nearly every case anterior to the

FIGURE 8-9

Oblique long-axis cardiac images. (Courtesy of Fonar Corporation, 110 Marcus Drive, Melville, NY 11747)

A	aortic arch
AA	ascending aorta
AJL	anterior junction line
APM	anterior papillary muscle
AR	aortic root
AXA	axillary artery
AZ	azygous vein
BCA	brachiocephalic artery
C	coronary sinus
CL	clavicle
CX	left circumflex coronary artery
D	diaphragm
DA	descending aorta
E	esophagus
ES	erector spinae muscle
H	humeral shaft
HH	humeral head
HI	hilum
IS	infraspinatus muscle
ITV	internal thoracic vein
IVC	inferior vena cava
IVS	interventricular septum
L	liver
LA	left atrium
LBV	left brachiocephalic vein
LCC	left common carotid artery
LD	latissimus dorsi muscle
LIJ	left internal jugular vein
LMB	left mainstem bronchus
LPA	left pulmonary artery
LPV	left pulmonary vein
LSCA	left subclavian artery
LSV	left superior pulmonary vein
LV	left ventricle
LVOT	left ventricular outflow tract
MHV	middle hepatic vein
MPA	main pulmonary artery
PC	pericardium
PF	pericardial fat
PMI	pectoralis minor muscle
PMJ	pectoralis major muscle
PV	portal vein
RA	right atrium
RCA	right coronary artery
RCC	right common carotid artery
RH	rhomboid muscles
RIJ	right internal jugular vein
RIJ	right internal jugular vein
RMB	right mainstem bronchus
RPA	right pulmonary artery
RPV	right superior pulmonary vein
RSCA	right subclavian artery
RV	right ventricle
SA	serratus anterior muscle
SAM	scalene anterior muscle
SCM	sternocleidomastoid muscle
SM	scalene medius muscle
SP	spinal cord
St	sternum
ST	stomach
SU	supraspinatus muscle
SVC	superior vena cava
T	trachea
TC	transverse colon
TH	thyroid
TR	trapezius muscle
TV	tricuspid valve

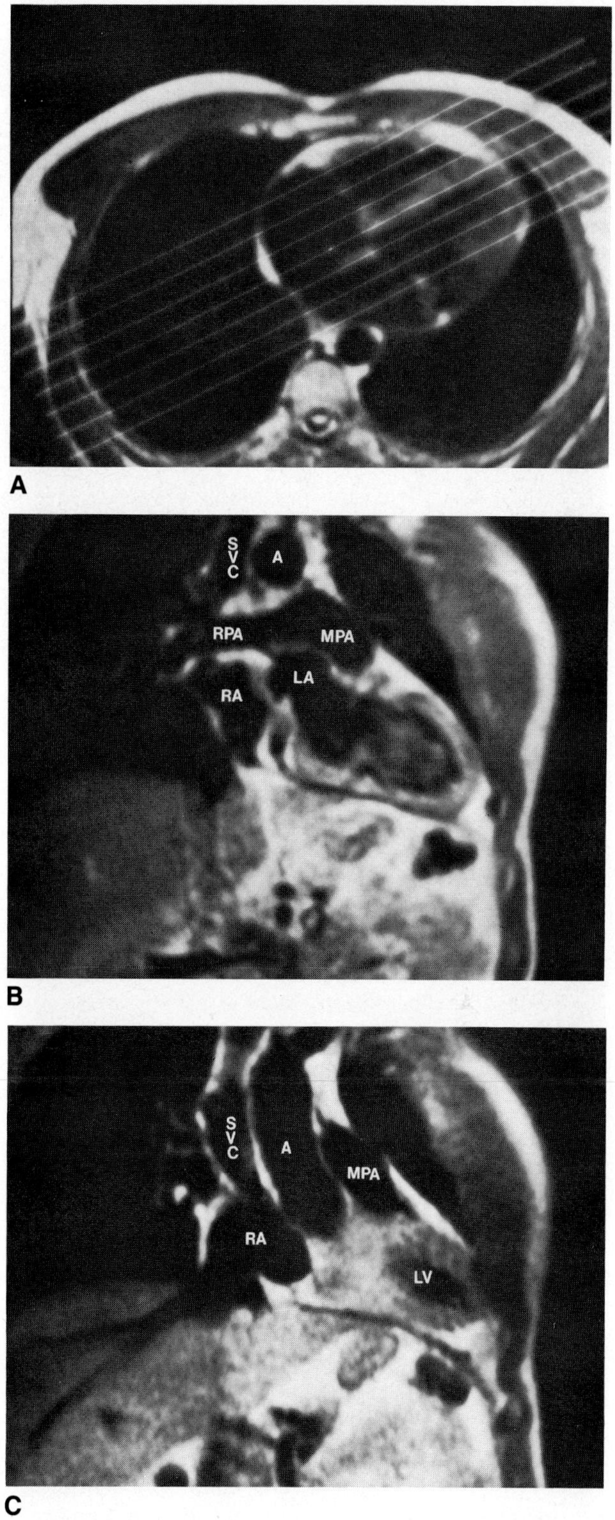

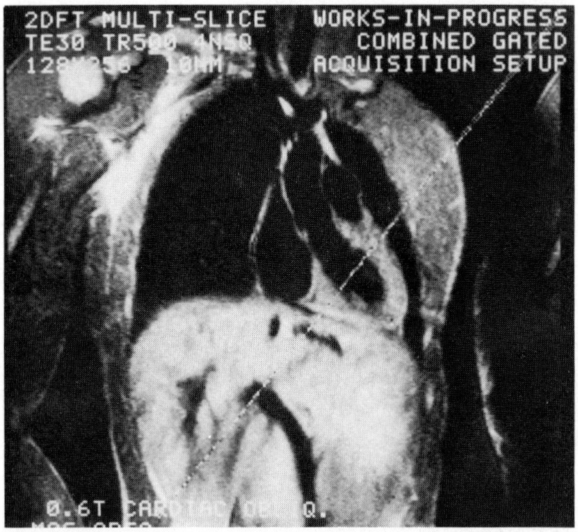

A

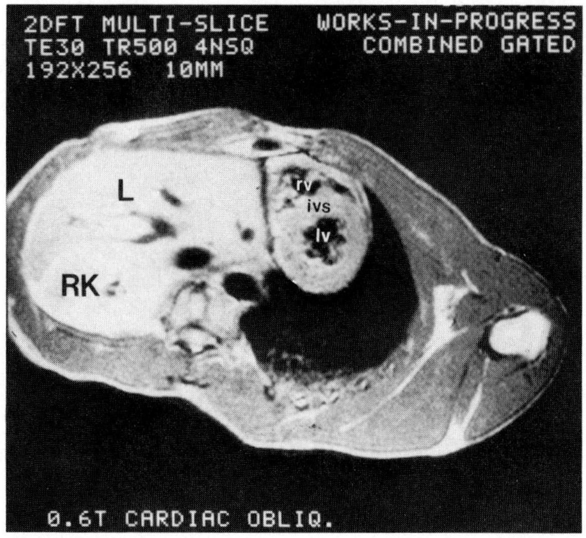

B

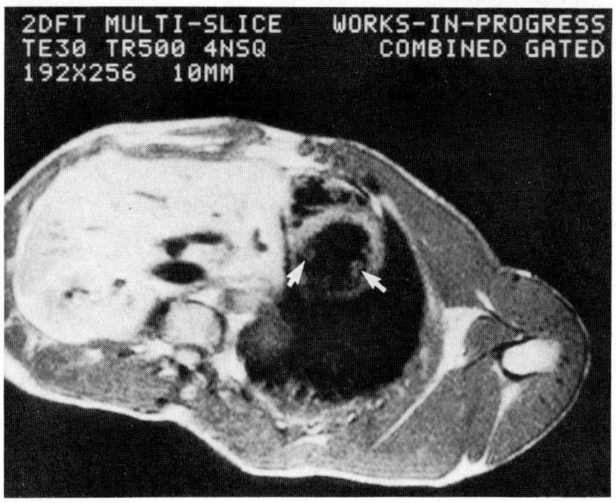

C

FIGURE 8-10

Oblique short-axis cardiac images. (*A*) Scout view to select oblique plane. (*B*) Oblique view shows the right ventricle (rv), left ventricle (lv), interventricular septum (ivs), liver (L), and right kidney (RK). (*C*) Oblique view demonstrates papillary muscles of the left ventricle (arrows). (Images provided courtesy of Technicare Corporation, Technicare Corp. © 1985)

ventricles. The normal pericardium can be identified as a 1-mm to 2-mm-thick curvilinear, low-intensity band between the high-intensity epicardial fat or myocardium and the pericardial fat (Fig. 8-3F). During systole, the low-intensity band representing pericardium may appear slightly thicker than on images obtained during diastole. This is a normal variation.

The myocardium is imaged with a medium signal intensity on most spin-echo sequences. The axial, coronal, and sagittal planes each demonstrate portions of the left ventricular walls to varying advantages (Table 8-4). The left ventricular walls should be relatively equal in thickness and in signal intensity. The ventricular septum is normally thinner than the other walls. Perhaps as a result of respiratory

TABLE 8-4

Left Ventricular Myocardial Segments Visualized on Each Projection

Plane of Imaging	Visualized Ventricular Segments
Axial	Lateral
	Septal
	Also portions of anterior and posterior walls
Coronal	Inferior (diaphragmatic)
	Also apical and lateral
Sagittal	Inferior
	Posterior
	Also portion of anteroseptal (apical) wall

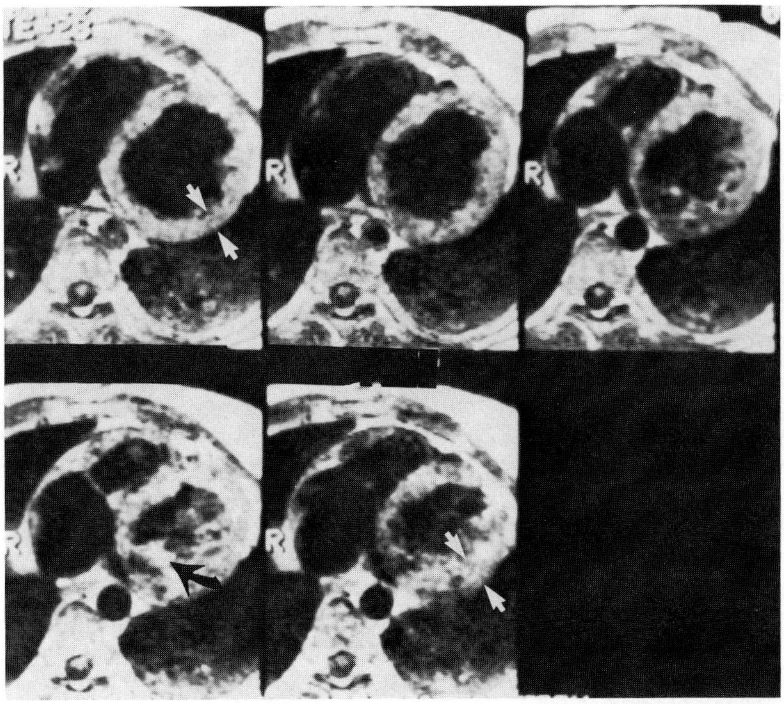

FIGURE 8-11

Increase in ventricular wall thickness between diastole and systole (white arrows). The actual wall thickness is overestimated on axial scans, because the scanning plane intersects the ventricular wall obliquely. Note also the "pseudoclot" (black arrow), a high-intensity signal recorded from the left ventricle during end-systole.

motion, the inferior (diaphragmatic) wall of the left ventricle frequently appears thinner and less intense than the other walls. This should not be misconstrued as representing a pathological condition.

The left ventricular wall thickness increases at least 35% between diastole and systole (Fig. 8-11). If only conventional axial images are obtained, estimated increase in thickness may be much higher (as great as 70%). This is a spurious thickening that results in the transverse imaging plane passing obliquely through the myocardium.

In general, blood flowing within the cardiac chambers and aorta is turbulent or rapidly moving. For reasons discussed in Chapter 2, very little MR signal is usually recorded. At various times during the cardiac cycle, however, blood may be nearly stationary in various chambers, particularly in patients with slow heart rates. It is not surprising that intraluminal signal may be recorded in normal patients when cardiac gated single- or double-echo sequences are used.

Signal is nearly always seen in the aorta during diastole; it is virtually never seen in normal patients in late systole (Fig. 8-12). Left ventricular signal is noted in more than half of normal patients at end-diastole or early systole; this most prominent in the anteroapical and posterior ventricular regions (Fig., 8-13). Most patients exhibit signal along the left side of the left atrium in late systole; no signal is usually seen in late diastole (Fig. 8-14). Ventricular luminal signal is less commonly seen in the right ventricle and occurs during end-diastole. Signal in the right atrium is only occasionally noted at end-systole (Fig. 8-15A). Intraluminal signal in the pulmonary arteries during systole is not normally seen and when present may be evidence of slow flow due to thrombus or pulmonary hypertension.

The coronary arteries may be identified in various planes, using standard gated as well as surface coil techniques (Fig. 8-15). Portions of the right coronary artery, left main coronary artery, left anterior descending artery, and left circumflex coronary artery may be routinely visualized. At present, however, limited spatial resolution does not permit detection of coronary artery narrowing or flow anomalies.

Surface coil techniques combined with cardiac gating seem promising for displayed detailed intracardiac anatomy. It is possible to distinguish leaflets of the cardiac valves as well as papillary muscles and chordae tendineae. Examples of experimental surface coil cardiac images are shown in Fig. 8-16.

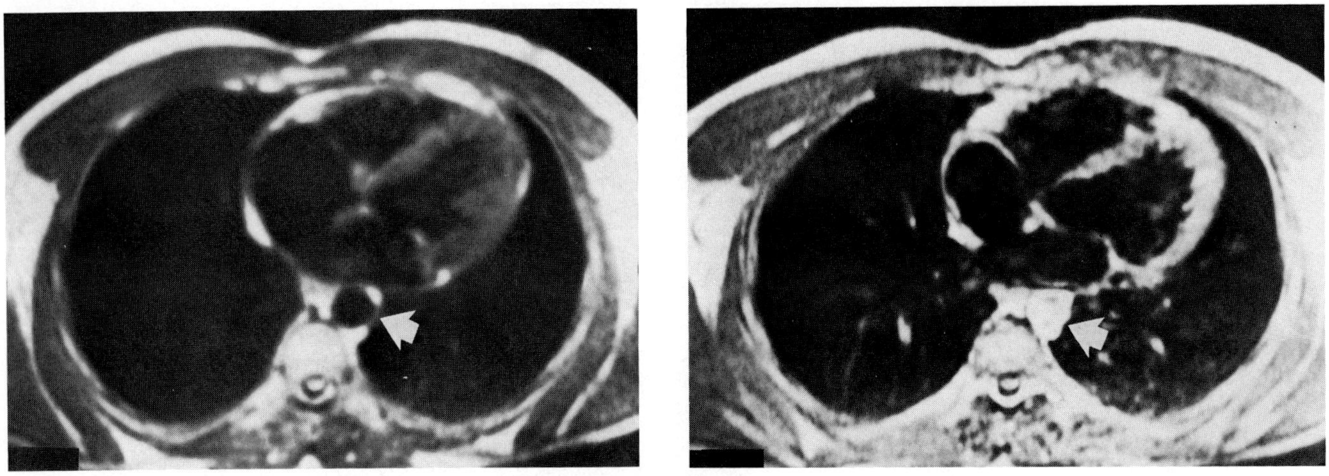

A B

FIGURE 8-12

(*A*) During systole, rapidly flowing aortic blood yields no signal (arrow). (*B*) During diastole, blood flow is stagnant and a signal is seen in aortas of nearly all patients (arrow). (Courtesy of Fonar Corporation, 110 Marcus Drive, Melville NY 11747)

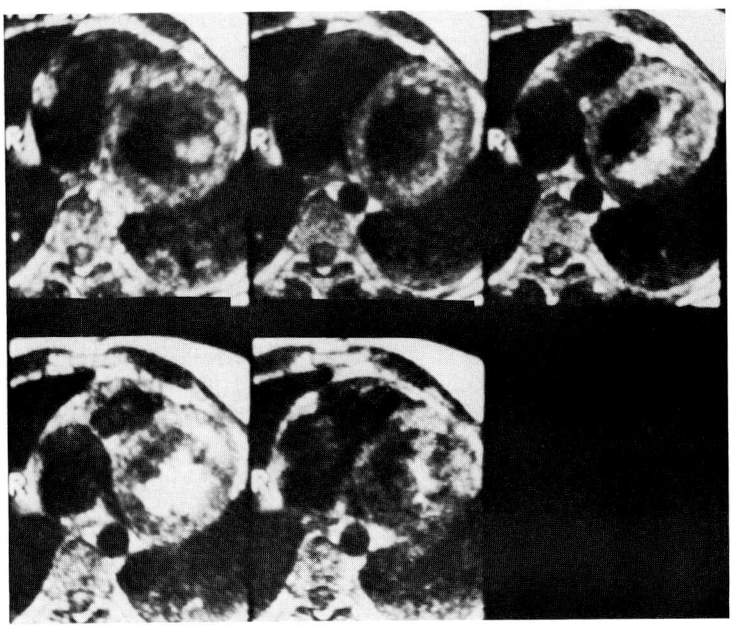

FIGURE 8-13

Some ventricular signal is seen in many normal patients because of relative stasis of blood during the cardiac cycle.

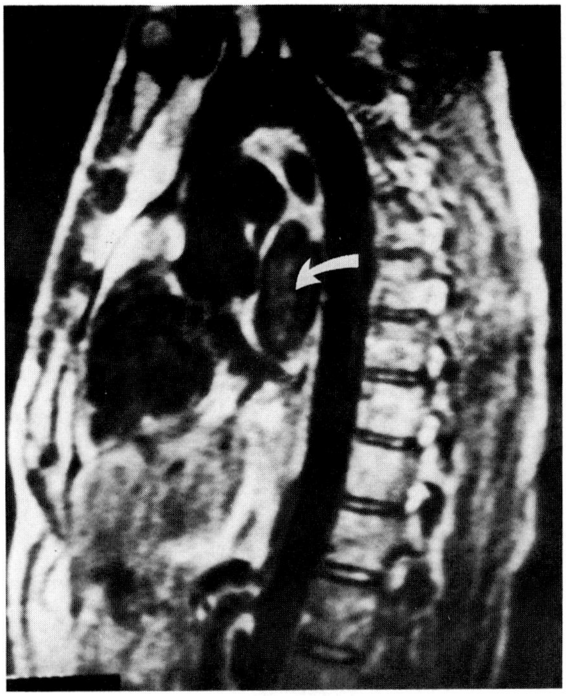

FIGURE 8-14

Signal may be seen in the normal left atrium during late systole (arrow). (Courtesy of Fonar Corporation, 110 Marcus Drive, Melville, NY 11747)

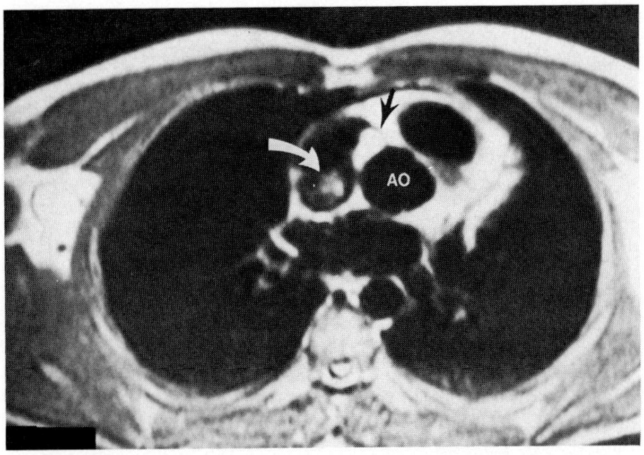

A

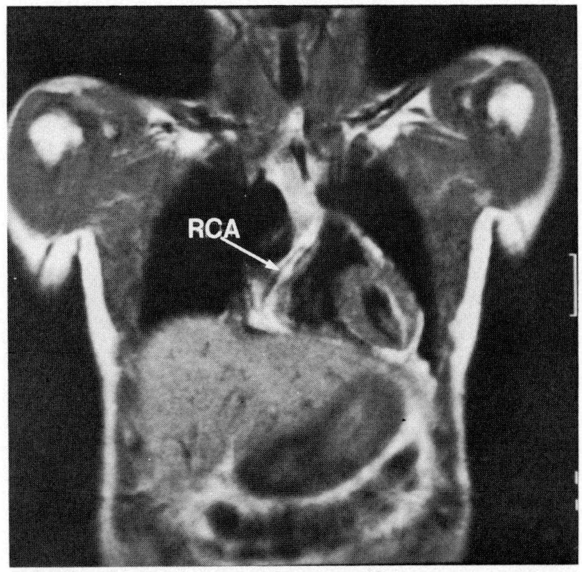

B

FIGURE 8-15

Coronary arteries by MR imaging. (*A*) Axial view shows origin of the right coronary artery (black arrow) from the aorta (AO). Note also signal in the right atrium (white arrow) due to stasis of flow in the cardiac cycle. (Courtesy of Fonar Corporation, 110 Marcus Drive, Melville, NY 11747) (*B*) Coronal image shows right coronary artery (RCA) along its length. (Courtesy of Siemens) (*C*) Axial views routinely demonstrate right coronary artery (arrowhead) and left circumflex coronary artery (arrow), which lie in the epicardial fat. (Courtesy of Fonar Corp.) (*D*) Left circumflex coronary artery (arrow) seen on coronal view. (Courtesy of Siemens) (E) Left circumflex coronary artery (arrow) seen on sagittal image of the heart. (Courtesy of Fonar Corporation, 110 Marcus Drive, Melville, NY 11747)

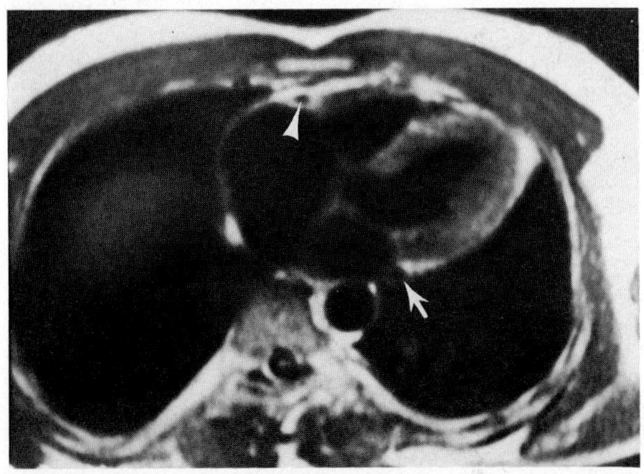

C

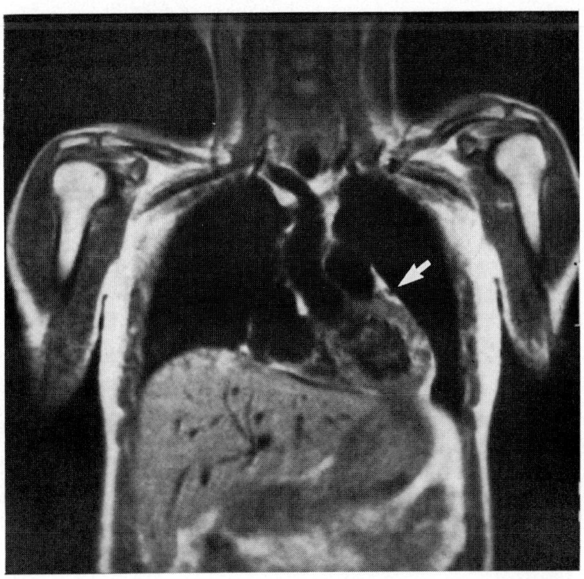

D

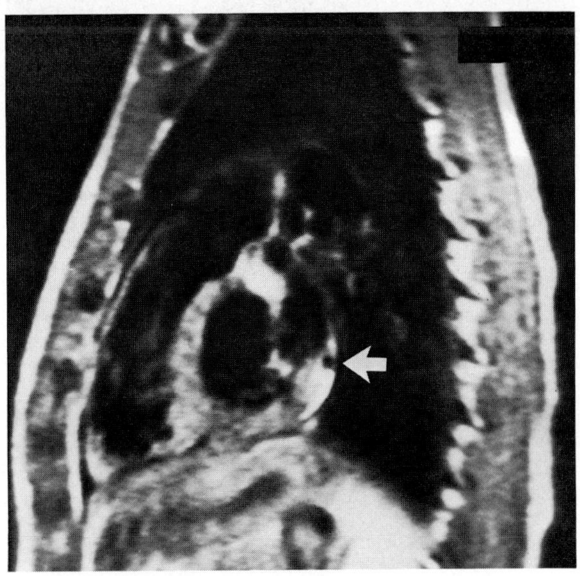

E

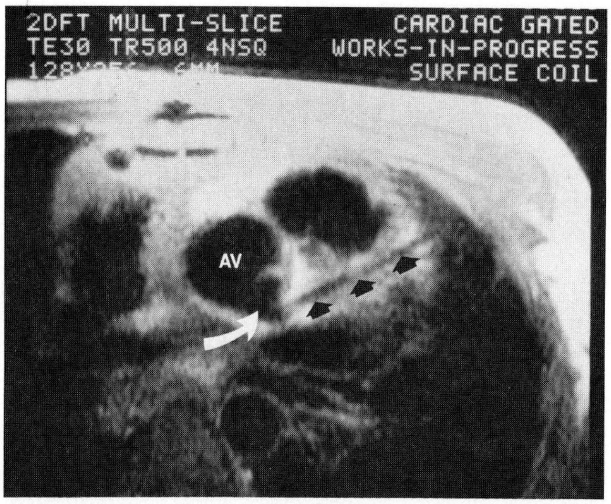

A

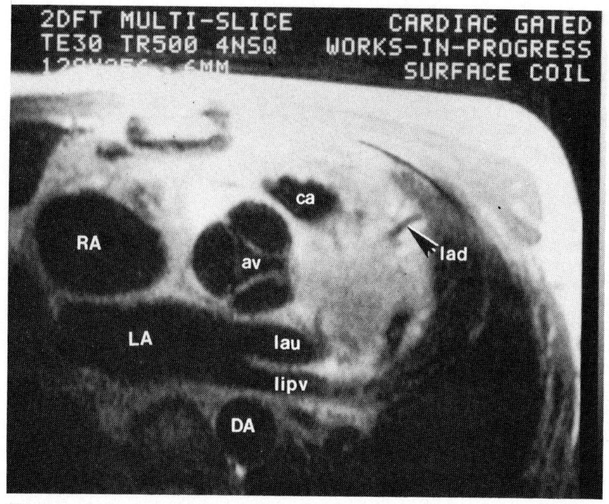

B

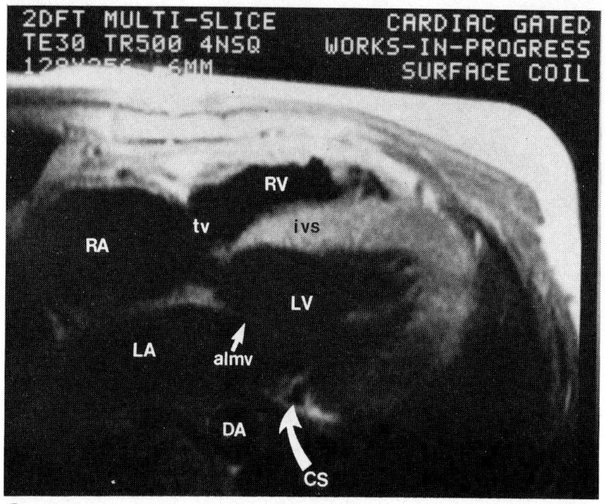

C

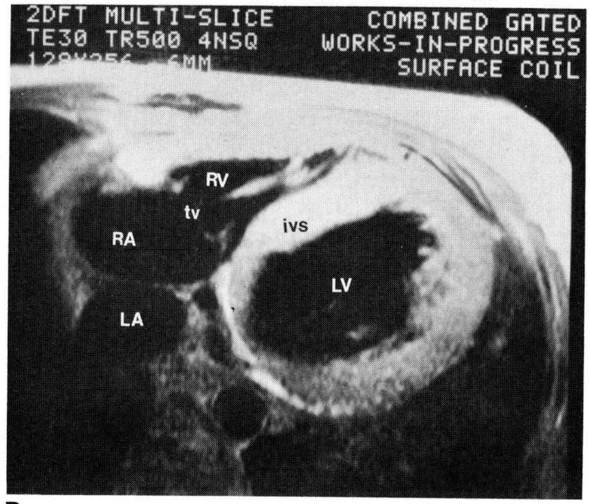

D

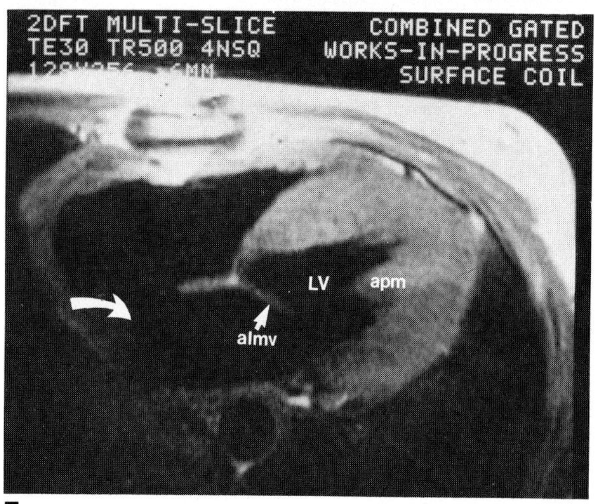

E

FIGURE 8-16

Surface coil images of the heart. (Courtesy of Technicare Corporation and Cleveland Clinic, Technicare Corp. © 1985) (*A*) Aortic valve (AV), sinus of Valsalva (white arrow), and left anterior descending coronary artery (black arrows). (*B*) Conus arteriosus (ca), left anterior descending coronary artery (lad), aortic valve (av), right atrium (RA), left atrium (LA), left auricular appendage (lau), left inferior pulmonary vein (lipv), and descending aorta (DA). (*C*) and (*D*) Right atrium (RA), tricuspid valve (tv), right ventricle (RV), interventricular septum (ivs), left ventricle (LV), anterior leaflet of mitral valve (almv), coronary sinus (CS), and descending aorta (DA). (E) Left ventricle (LV), anterior papillary muscle (apm), and anterior leaflet of mitral valve (almv). The interatrial septum is often not well seen (arrow) because it flutters and is not well imaged with conventional ECG gating.

CHAPTER 9

The Abdomen

MR has not been as successful in imaging the abdomen as it has other areas of the body. Respiratory motion is a problem in the upper abdomen, and respiratory gating brings with it an increase in imaging time to 30% to 100%. Peristaltic motion of the bowel also induces artifacts in scanning. No oral paramagnetic contrast agent has been found to opacify bowel satisfactorily. CT has a proven record of success in the abdomen, and its spatial resolution is superior to current MRI.

Despite these limitations, MRI may prove useful in certain capacities complementary to CT. It is hoped that masses and fluid collections will be more specifically identified using MR imaging characteristics. MR signal changes may be useful in diagnosing and monitoring the progress of certain medical diseases, such as hepatitis, hemochromatosis, and pyelonephritis.

The axial plane remains the single best direction for examining the abdomen by MRI. A routine screen for abdominal lesions should include both T1- and T2-weighted pulse sequences obtained in the axial plane. Glucagon and gas-forming crystals will distend the stomach and paralyze the bowel for better-quality images. If respiratory gating is not employed, sufficient detail may nevertheless be obtained for purposes of general diagnosis. However, the reliable delineation of small liver lesions and masses in the upper abdomen will probably require some sort of respiratory gating.

Although no high-concentration paramagnetic oral contrast agents to opacify bowel are currently on the market, a dilute iron-containing liquid may be given (*e.g.,* Geritol in water). This may sufficiently alter the MR imaging characteristics of bowel so that it may be distinguished from mass lesions in confusing situations. It is likely that in the next few years several safe and effective oral paramagnetic contrast agents will be on the market.

Routine coronal and sagittal images of the abdomen are not generally recommended except in specific situations. They may be useful in identifying the spread of intra-abdominal infections and tumors, particularly in the juxtadiaphragmatic regions. Special situations for each organ system in the abdomen where coronal or sagittal imaging may be useful will be detailed in the next few sections. For completeness, whole coronal and sagittal images of the abdomen are presented in Figures 9-1 and 9-2.

A	aorta
AC	ascending colon
AR	acetabular roof
B	bladder
BR	breast
CBD	common bile duct
CE	cecum
CIA,CIV	common iliac artery, vein
CL	caudate lobe
CRU	crus of the diaphragm
D	duodenum
DC	descending colon
DI	diaphragm
DS	dural sac
EIA, EIV	external iliac artery, vein
EM	erector spinae muscle
EO	external oblique muscle
FH	femoral head
G	gallbladder
GM	gluteus maximus muscle
GME	gluteus medius muscle
GMI	gluteus minimus muscle
HF	hepatic flexure
I	inferior vena cava
IL	ilium
IO	internal oblique muscle
IRF	ischiorectal fossa
ISC	ischium
K	kidney
L	liver
L1–L5	vertebral bodies (L1–L5)
LD	latissimus dorsi muscle
LHV	left hepatic vein
LM	longissimus muscle
LRA, LRV	left renal artery, vein
MHV	middle hepatic vein
NR	nerve root
OE	obturator externus muscle
OI	obturator internus muscle
P	prostate
PA	pancreas
PF	pericardial fat
PM	psoas major muscle
PV	portal vein
PY	pylorus
QL	quadratus lumborum muscle
R	rectum
RA	right adrenal
RHV	right hepatic vein
RK	right kidney
RM	rectus abdominus muscle
RPV	right portal vein
RRA, RRV	right renal artery, vein
S1, S2	sacral segments (S1, S2)
SA	serratus anterior muscle
SF	splenic flexure of colon
SIG	sigmoid colon
SMV	superior mesenteric vein
SP	spleen
SPA, SPV	splenic artery, vein
SPP	spinous process
ST	stomach
TA	transversus abdominus muscle
TSA	tuberosity of sacrum
TVS	transversospinalis muscle
U	ureter

FIGURE 9-1

Coronal MR images of the whole abdomen. (Courtesy of Picker International, Clinical Sciences Center)

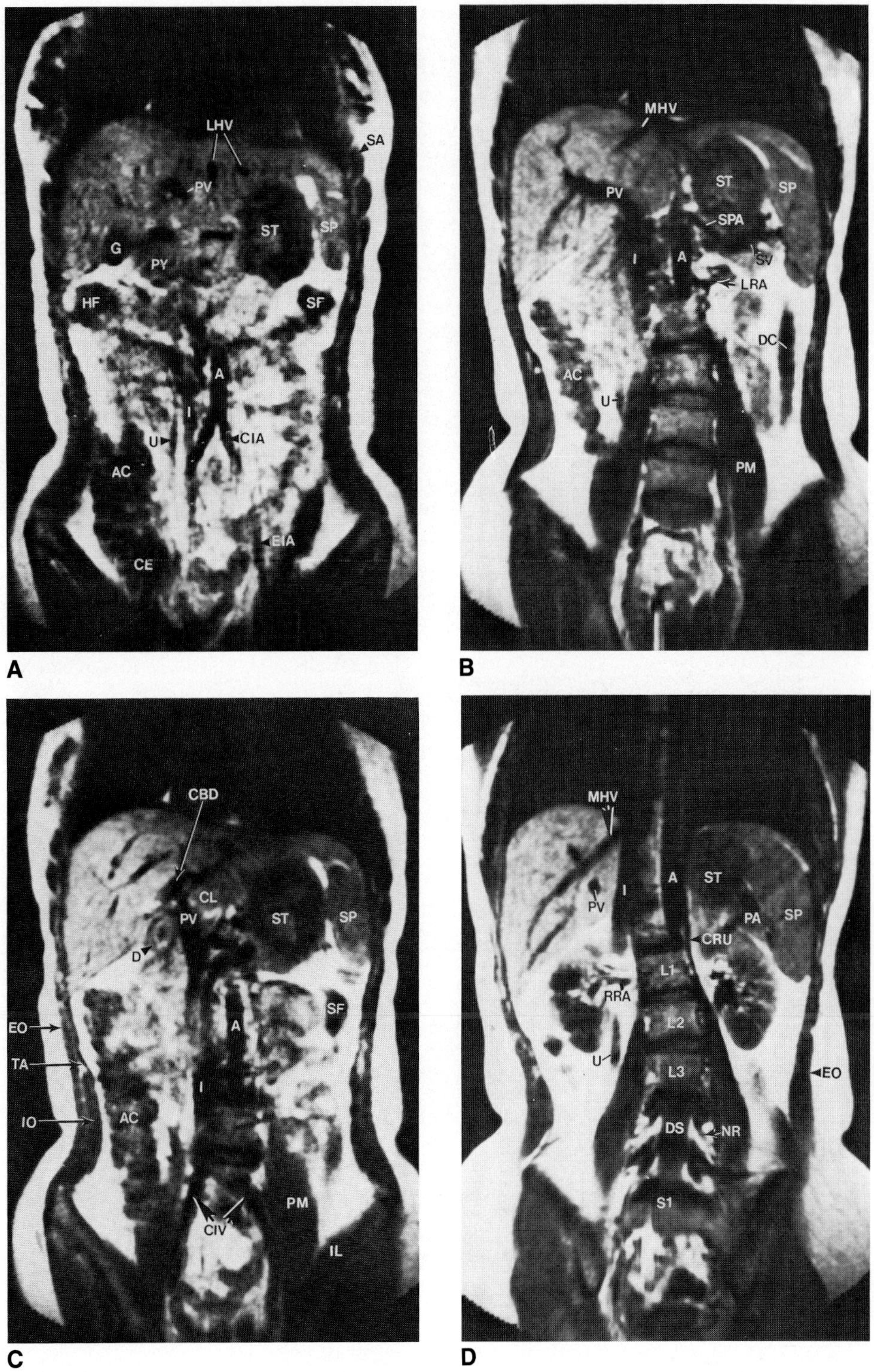

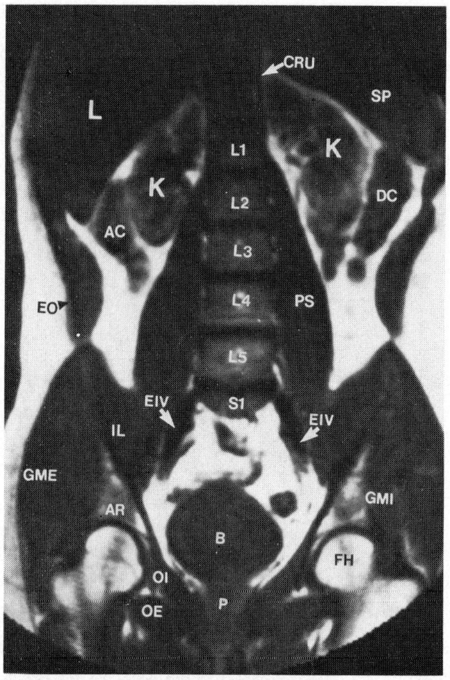

E

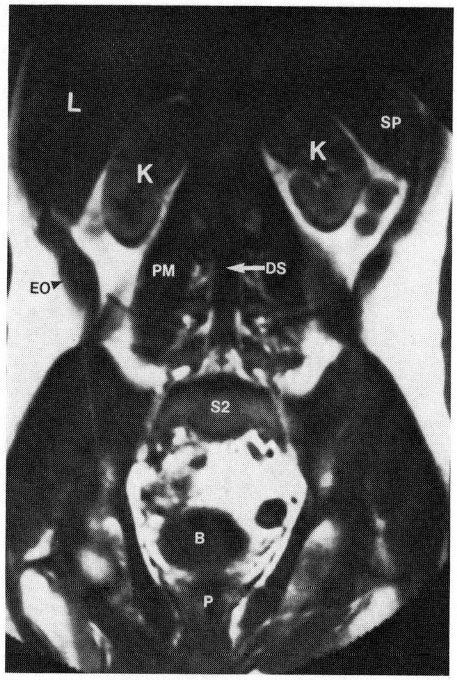

F

FIGURE 9-1 *(cont.)*

Coronal MR images of the w abdomen. (Courtesy of Pick ternational, Clinical Science ter)

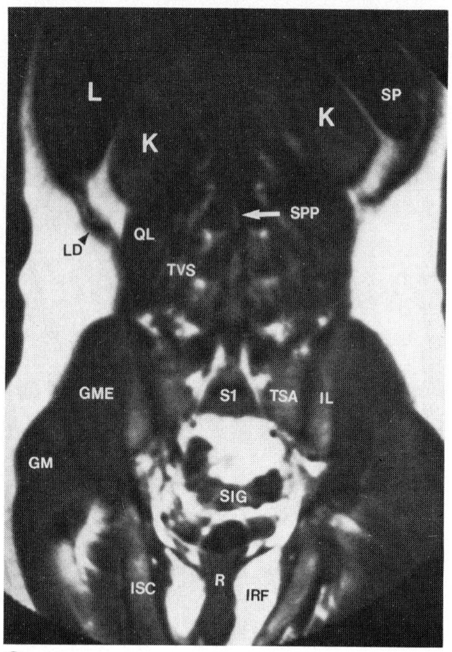

G

AC	ascending colon
AR	acetabular roof
B	bladder
BR	breast
CIA,CIV	common iliac artery, vein
CRU	crus of the diaphragm
DC	descending colon
DI	diaphragm
DS	dural sac
EIA, EIV	external iliac artery, vein
EM	erector spinae muscle
EO	external oblique muscle
GM	gluteus maximus muscle
GME	gluteus medius muscle
GMI	gluteus minimus muscle
IL	ilium
IRF	ischiorectal fossa
ISC	ischium
K	kidney
L	liver
L1–L5	vertebral bodies (L1–L5)
LD	latissimus dorsi muscle
LM	longissimus muscle
MHV	middle hepatic vein
OE	obturator externus muscle
OI	obturator internus muscle
P	prostate
PF	pericardial fat
PM	psoas major muscle
PV	portal vein
QL	quadratus lumborum muscle
R	rectum
RA	right adrenal
RHV	right hepatic vein
RK	right kidney
RM	rectus abdominus muscle
RPV	right portal vein
RRA, RRV	right renal artery, vein
S1, S2	sacral segments (S1, S2)
SIG	sigmoid colon
SMV	superior mesenteric vein
SP	spleen
SPP	spinous process
TA	transversus abdominus muscle
TSA	tuberosity of sacrum
TVS	transversospinalis muscle
U	ureter

FIGURE 9-2

Sagittal MR images of the abdomen, with emphasis on the liver and its relationships. (Courtesy of Picker International, Clinical Sciences Center)

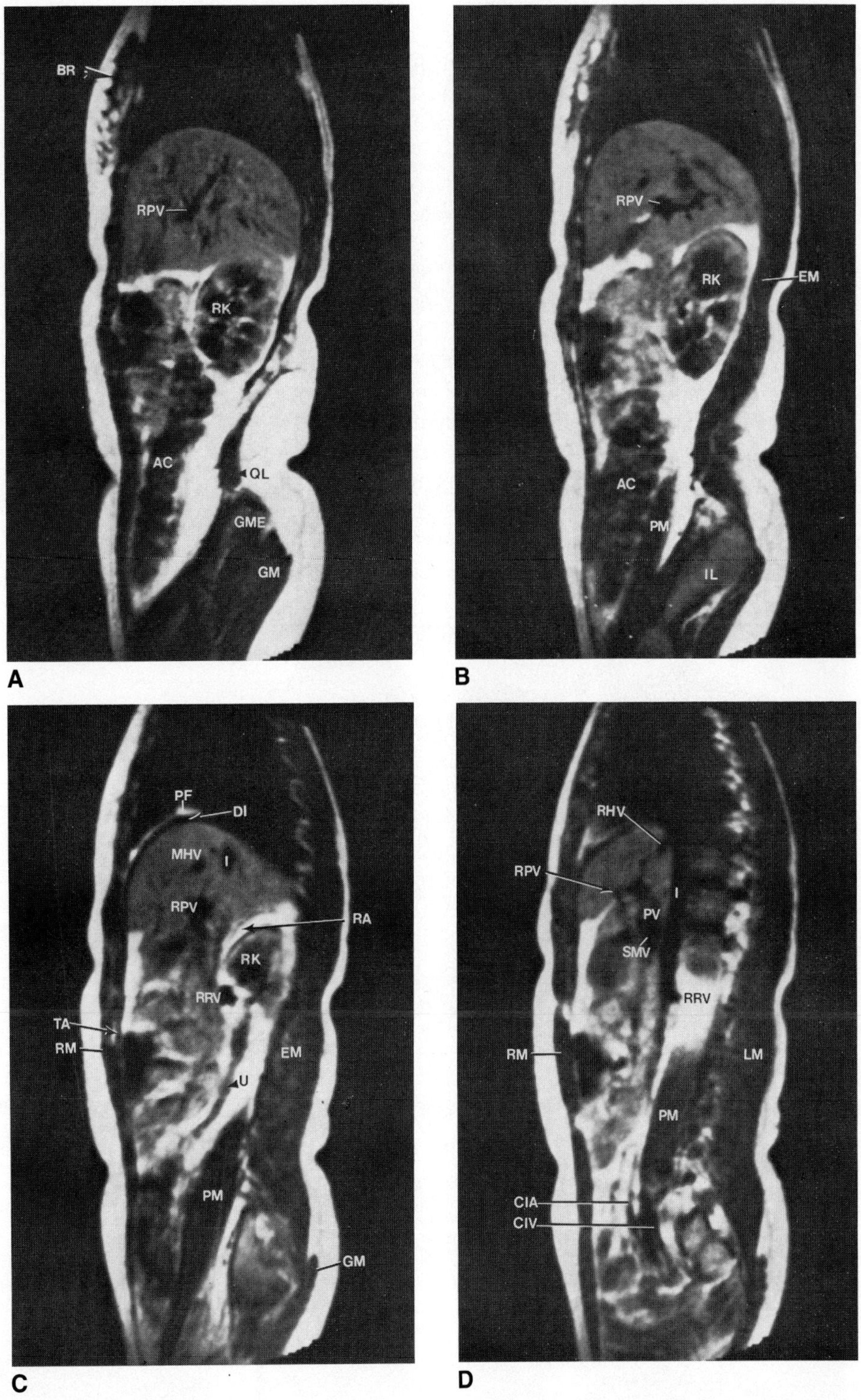

The Liver

The liver can be well imaged by MR, although optimal techniques and strategies are still open to debate. As in many other regions of the body, it has been found necessary to use both T1- and T2-weighted images to identify and characterize liver pathology sufficiently. The T1-weighted sequence may be a short spin-echo (*e.g.,* SE 250/20) or inversion recovery (*e.g.,* IR 1500/400). The T2-weighted sequence should be a long spin-echo such as SE 2000/120.

The identification of hepatic vascular anatomy is important for defining liver lobes and segments and for detecting subtle distortions by mass lesions. Intrahepatic arteries and the biliary radicles are normally not seen, but branches of the hepatic and portal veins are always identified. Hepatic vascular anatomy is probably best demonstrated on SE 2000/30 or similar sequences. Using this pulse sequence, maximal contrast is produced between high-intensity liver and venous structures, which remain dark because of flowing blood. On second echo images, such as SE 2000/56, the hepatic veins become isointense with liver parenchyma whereas the portal veins are seen to be of higher intensity (possibly a result of even echo rephasing of more slowly flowing blood in the portal system). Little or no signal should ever be present within the *main* portal veins, however. When seen, this should suggest portal hypertension or thrombosis.

The axial plane has proved to be the most consistent for demonstrating normal vascular structures as well as pathological lesions. Most hepatic vessels course perpendicularly to the axial plane, so they are more easily identified as rounded structures of signal void. The axial plane also possesses fewer problems with partial volume effects, except near the diaphragmatic surface. Routine axial images of the liver and upper abdomen are presented in Figure 9-3.

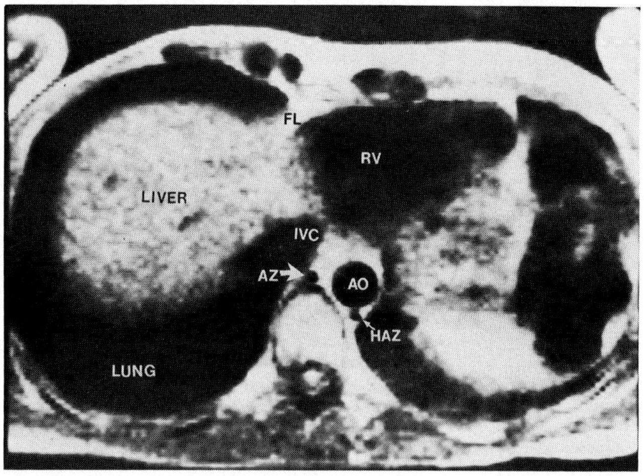

A

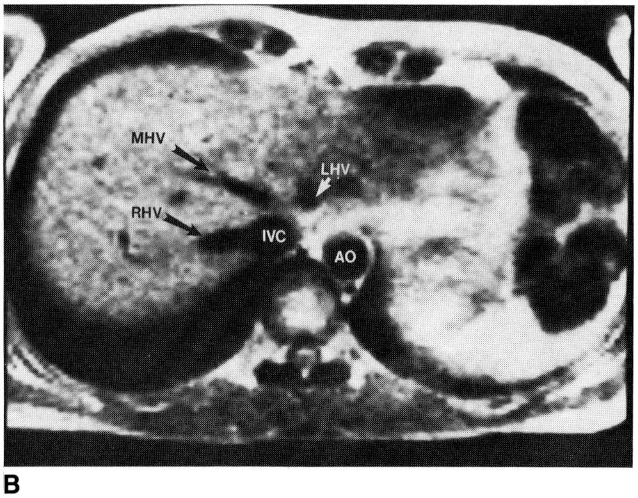

B

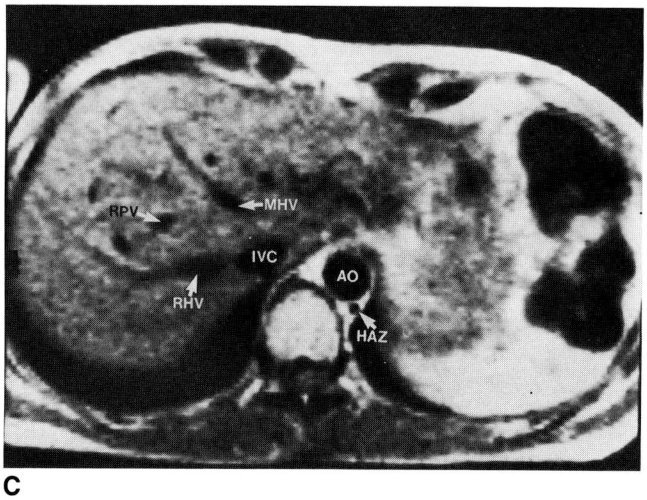

C

FIGURE 9-3

Axial spin-echo images of the upper abdomen. Arrows in F demonstrate a frequency shift artifact on the edge of the spleen. (F–I courtesy of Siemens)

AD	adrenal gland
AO	aorta
AZ	azygous vein
B	duodenal bulb
BP	body of pancreas
CBD	common bile duct
CE	celiac artery
FL	falciform ligament
GB	gallbladder
HAZ	hemiazygous vein
IVC	inferior vena cava
LK	left kidney
LHV	left hepatic vein
LLS	left hepatic lobe, lateral segment
LMS	left hepatic lobe, medial segment
LPV	left portal vein
LRV	left renal vein
LT	ligamentum teres
MHV	middle hepatic vein
PV	main portal vein
PY	pylorus
RA	right adrenal
RK	right kidney
RV	right ventricle
RHV	right hepatic vein
RPV	right portal vein
RRV	right renal vein
SA&V	splenic artery and vein
SMA, SMV	superior mesenteric artery, vein
SP	spleen
ST	stomach
SV	splenic vein
TP	tail of pancreas
UP	uncinate process of pancreas

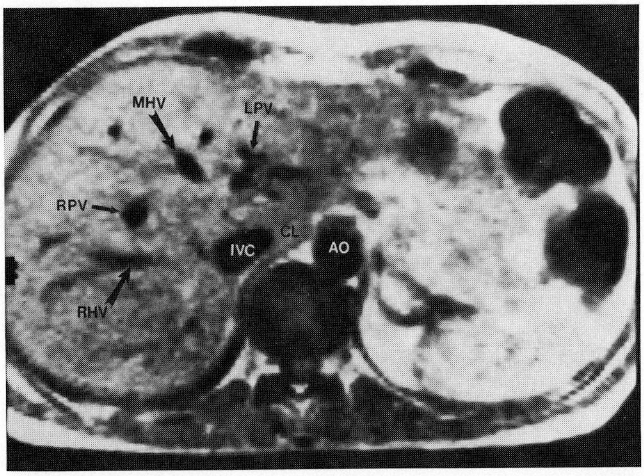

D

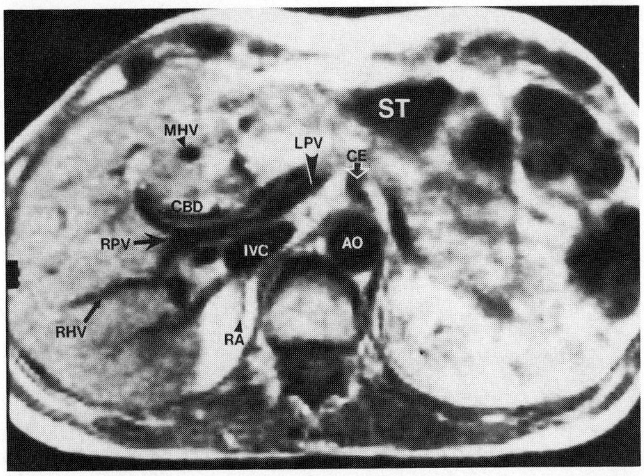

E

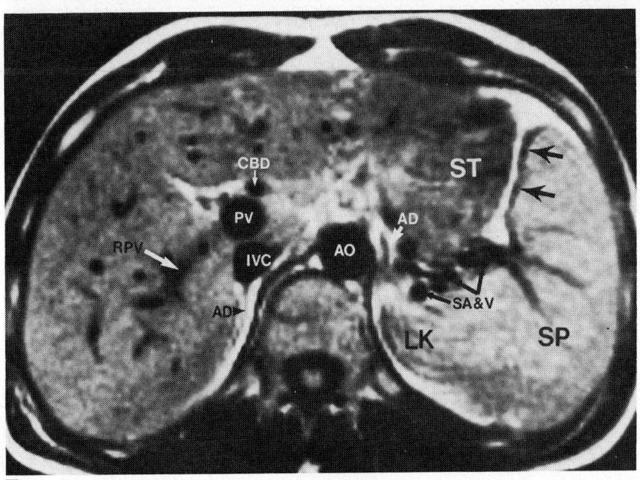

F

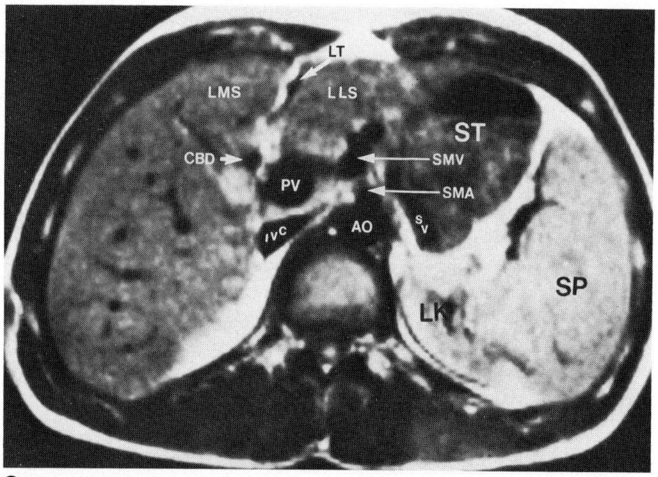

G

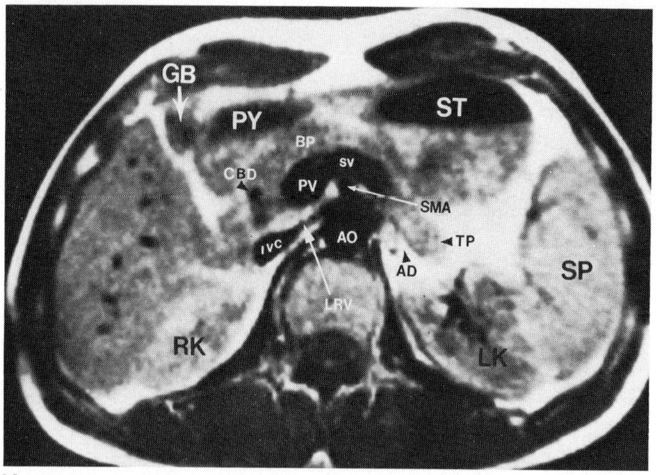

H

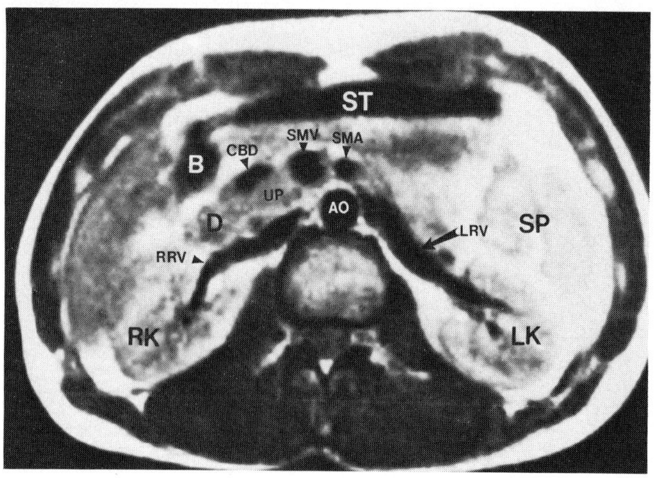

I

FIGURE 9-3 *(cont.)*

Axial spin-echo images of the upper abdomen. Arrows in F demonstrate a frequency shift artifact on the edge of the spleen. (F–I courtesy Siemens)

AD	adrenal gland
AO	aorta
AZ	azygous vein
B	duodenal bulb
BP	body of pancreas
CBD	common bile duct
CE	celiac artery
FL	falciform ligament
GB	gallbladder
HAZ	hemiazygous vein
IVC	inferior vena cava
LK	left kidney
LHV	left hepatic vein
LLS	left hepatic lobe, lateral segment
LMS	left hepatic lobe, medial segment
LPV	left portal vein
LRV	left renal vein
LT	ligamentum teres
MHV	middle hepatic vein
PV	main portal vein
PY	pylorus
RA	right adrenal
RK	right kidney
RV	right ventricle
RHV	right hepatic vein
RPV	right portal vein
RRV	right renal vein
SA&V	splenic artery and vein
SMA, SMV	superior mesenteric artery, vein
SP	spleen
ST	stomach
SV	splenic vein
TP	tail of pancreas
UP	uncinate process of pancreas

The sagittal plane is sometimes helpful in identification of lesions high in the dome of the liver. The sagittal plane also shows the relations of the liver to the lung bases, diaphragm, and subphrenic spaces. Additionally, if there is an abnormality of portal venous flow, it is best recognized in this plane, because the portal veins intersect the sagittal plane perpendicularly. The sagittal plane demonstrates the full course of the middle hepatic vein in at least 90% of patients; this allows accurate distinction between the left and right hepatic lobes.

The coronal plane is least helpful in liver imaging. It is useful at times to demonstrate the course of the inferior vena cava, main portal vein, and right portal vein. Occasionally, the coronal plane may aid in understanding the relations of masses or fluid collections to the liver. Table 9-1 lists the optimal planes for visualization of the hepatic vascular anatomy.

In addition to the hepatic and portal veins, several other normal structures may be seen in the liver. The low-intensity ligamentum teres is well seen on axial images surrounded by high-intensity fat (Fig. 9-4). The common bile duct is regularly identified in the porta and also in the head of the pancreas (Fig. 9-5 and 9-3E–I). The gallbladder is seen with about the same frequency as by CT (Fig. 9-6). On the SE 500/56 sequence, a normal gallbladder in a fasting adult should appear hyperintense compared with surrounding liver. Lower intensity (suggesting less concentrated bile) should raise suspicion of gallbladder disease. Stones are best seen as low intensity filling defects on T2-weighted sequences where bile is rendered white.

The Spleen

The spleen is easily recognized in the left upper quadrant of the abdomen in most planes and imaging sequences. The spleen contains about 5% more water than the liver, which probably accounts for its prolonged T1 and T2 values compared with the liver. On long spin-echo sequences (*e.g.,* SE 1500/30), the spleen will appear brighter than the liver, pancreas, or abdominal musculature (Fig. 9-3F–H).

TABLE 9-1

Visualization of Hepatic Vascular Anatomy by MRI*

	Axial	Coronal	Sagittal
Consistently visualized (more than 90% of scans)	IVC MPV RPV LPV MHV LHV RHV	IVC MPV RPV	IVC MPV RPV LPV MHV
Moderately well visualized (in 50% to 90% of scans)	HA	RHV MHV LPV	RHV LHV
Poorly visualized (fewer than 15% of scans)		HA LHV	HA

* Typical findings for scans of liver without respiratory gating using Diasonics MT/S 0.35T scanner with 7-mm slices and SE 2000/28.

Abbreviations: IVC = inferior vena cava; MPV = main portal vein; RPV = right portal vein; LPV = left portal vein; MHV = middle hepatic vein; RHV = right hepatic vein; LHV = left hepatic vein; HA = hepatic artery.

Note that the reliability for visualization of each vessel will increase with further technical developments as well as respiratory gating.

(Adapted from Fisher MR et al: Hepatic vascular anatomy on magnetic resonance imaging. AJR 144:739–746, 1985)

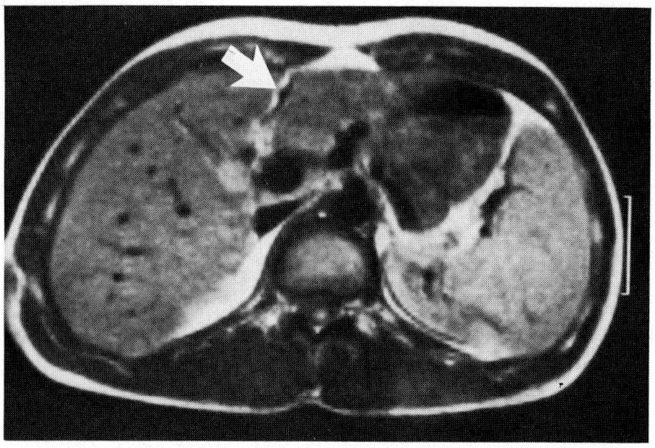

FIGURE 9-4

Ligamentum teres (arrow) is seen on axial MR images surrounded by high-intensity fat. (Courtesy of Siemens)

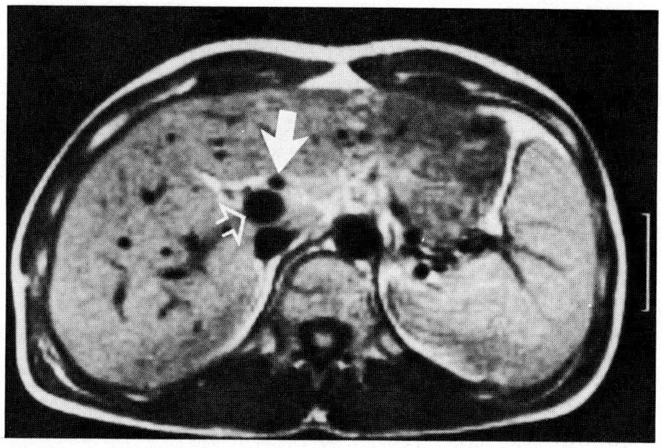

FIGURE 9-5

The porta hepatis on axial SE 500/30. Open arrow = main portal vein. Solid arrow = common bile duct. (Courtesy of Siemens)

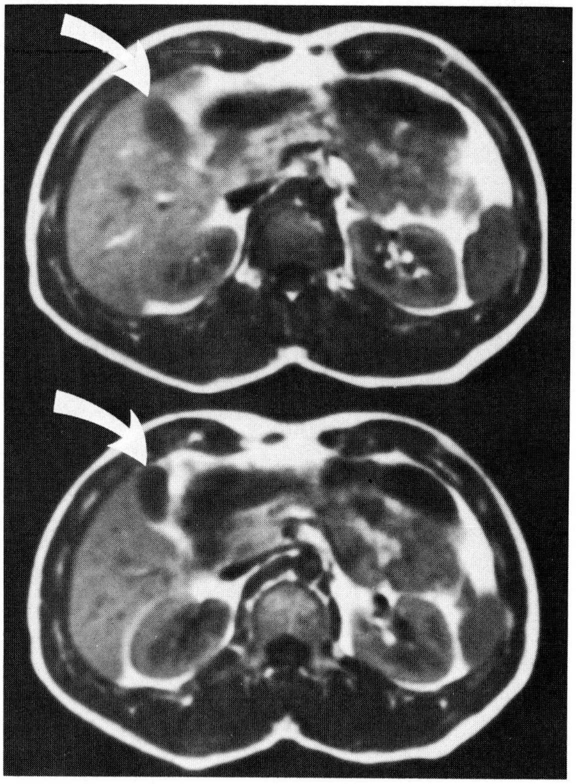

FIGURE 9-6

The gallbladder is seen on consecutive spin-echo axial images (arrows). (Courtesy of Siemens)

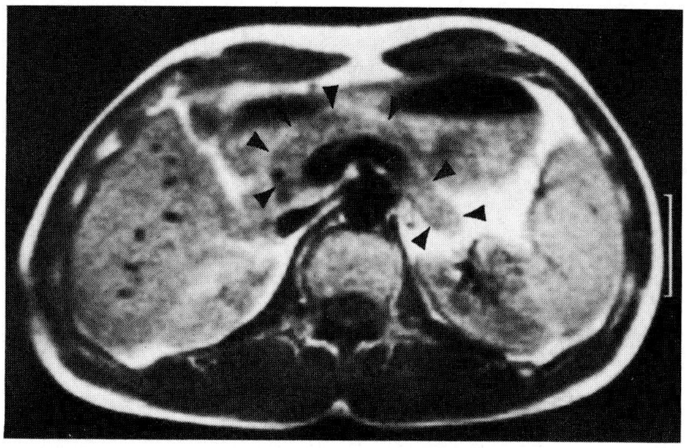

FIGURE 9-7

The pancreas (arrowheads) may be identified in the midabdomen on axial images if there is sufficient retroperitoneal fat. (Courtesy of Siemens)

Splenic vessels in the hilum may be routinely identified. A low-intensity band is often seen along one margin of the spleen where it abuts fat. This does not represent the splenic capsule, but rather is a frequency shift artifact as discussed in Chapter 5. The axial plane in T1- and T2-weighted sequences is best for evaluating splenic lesions.

The Pancreas

The pancreas is the most difficult organ to image reliably by MR. Its posterior border, composed of the splenic vein, aorta, and vena cava, is well outlined in nearly all patients. The anterior margin of the pancreas, however, is often difficult to define. If a large amount of retroperitoneal fat overlies it, the anterior border may be reasonably well seen. Unfortunately, in at least 40% of patients, this is not the case. Stomach or small bowel is intimately apposed to its anterior margin, obscuring it. Peristalsis of overlying bowel and respiratory motion artifacts further compromise its examination.

The T1 and T2 values of pancreas are similar to liver, and the pancreas is perhaps best visualized on intermediate spin-echo sequences (*e.g.,* SE 1000/30). Inversion recovery sequences may be constructed to intensify the pancreas (*e.g.,* IR 1200/400); other retroperitoneal organs and structures are less well visualized, and the overall signal is less intense. If possible, the stomach should be distended with glucagon and gas; respiratory gating may be employed. Only the axial plane has been of much value in defining anatomic relationships of the normal or diseased pancreas. It is conceivable that a sagittal image might occasionally prove helpful in defining the extent of tumor or the location of a pseudocyst or peripancreatic fluid collection.

Unfortunately, tissue relaxation times have not proved helpful in many pancreatic diseases. The T1 and T2 values of adenocarcinoma and lymphoma are similar to those of normal pancreas. However, pancreatic islet cell tumors have been shown to have prolonged T2 times, as have pseudocysts and pancreatic inflammatory processes. The inability to identify pancreatic calcifications by MR further limits its usefulness in this area. Whether MRI will in the future be useful for imaging the normal or diseased pancreas is unknown. A normal-appearing pancreas is shown in Figure 9-7.

The Kidneys and Adrenals

MRI has already proved useful in the diagnosis of both medical and surgical diseases of the kidneys. The ability to image in multiple planes directly makes possible clarification of the origin and extension of renal and retroperitoneal masses.

Changes in renal T1 and T2 values may be sensitive indicators of renal disease. A major disadvantage of MRI in the kidneys, however, lies in its poor demonstration of areas of calcification and small calculi. The extent to which the first two advantages of MRI will outweigh this one disadvantage remains to be seen.

What is the optimum plane for imaging the kidneys? The axial plane remains an excellent dimension for evaluating renal disease, especially tumors. The axial plane is probably superior for detecting renal hilar and periaortic lymphadenopathy. Likewise, it is useful for evaluation of renal vein invasion or thrombosis. The coronal plane is useful for correlating findings with those of excretory urography for demonstrating the relationship of masses to the renal pelvis, and for evaluating tumor extension in the inferior vena cava. Direct sagittal images are sometimes helpful to clarify whether a retroperitoneal tumor has arisen from the kidney or adrenal or from some other site. Presence or absence of liver invasion by tumor may at times be more reliably estimated with sagittal images.

What are the best imaging sequences for the kidneys? As in many other parts of the body, it has been found useful to image the kidneys with two techniques, one T1 weighted and the other T2 weighted. The T1-weighted sequence may be either an inversion recovery or short spin-echo. The T2-weighted sequence should be a long spin-echo type.

T1-weighted pulse sequences allow differentiation of the renal cortex and renal medulla. The renal medulla may be thought of as having more water (urine) than the renal cortex, and hence a longer T1 value. Thus on T1-weighted pulse sequences, the medulla will appear less intense than the cortex. In T2-weighted sequences, this corticomedullary differentiation will be lost. The sharpest corticomedullary differentiation by MRI has been obtained with inversion recovery sequences, such as IR 1500/400 or IR 1000/300 (Fig. 9-8). Reasonably good corticomedullary differentiation is also possible with short saturation recovery sequences (TR = 200 msec) or short

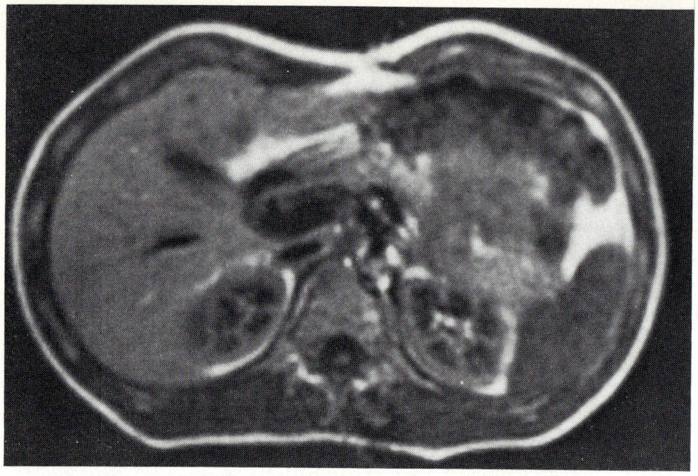

FIGURE 9-8

The best corticomedullary differentiation in the kidney is provided by inversion recovery sequences. (Image obtained on Magniscan 5000, Thomson-CGR MR system, IR 1500/400/28)

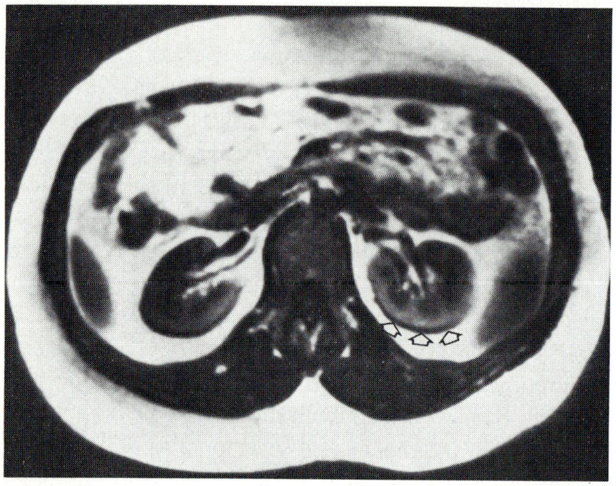

FIGURE 9-9

Reasonably good corticomedullary differentiation may be obtained using short spin-echo sequences (SE 500/30). Note the frequency shift artifact (arrows) that occurs where the kidney abuts retroperitoneal fat. (Courtesy of Picker International, Clinical Sciences Center)

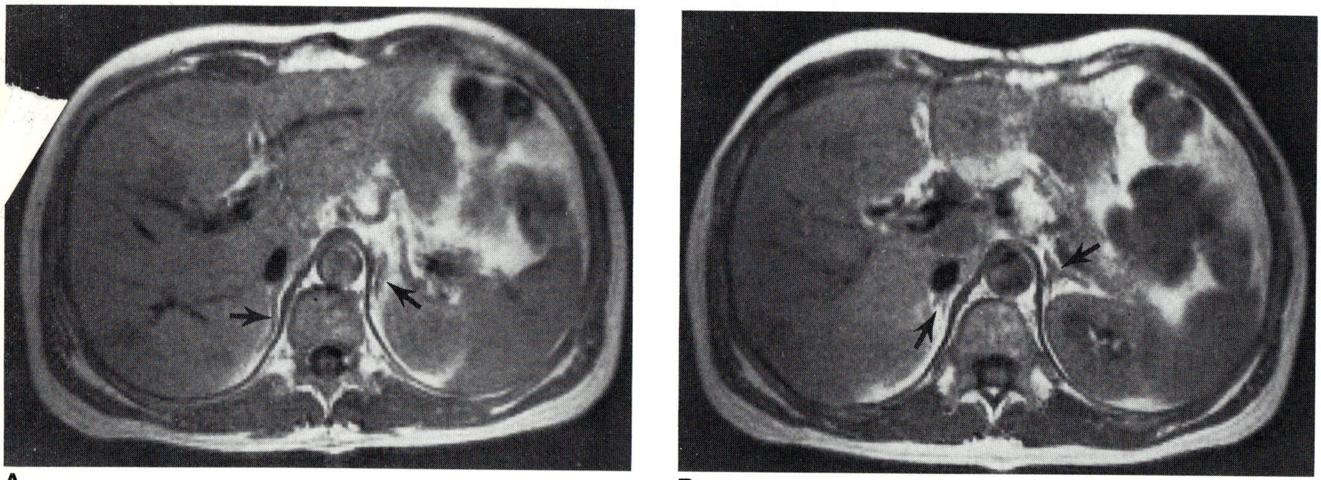

A B

FIGURE 9-10

In axial section, the adrenal glands (arrows) have characteristic V or Y shapes. (Images obtained on Magniscan 5000, Thomson-CGR MR system)

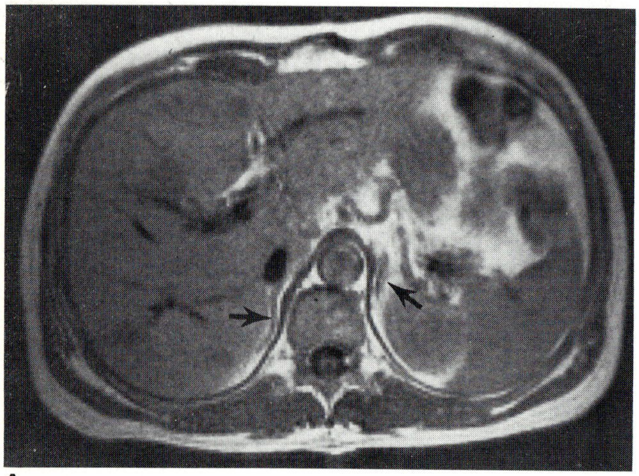

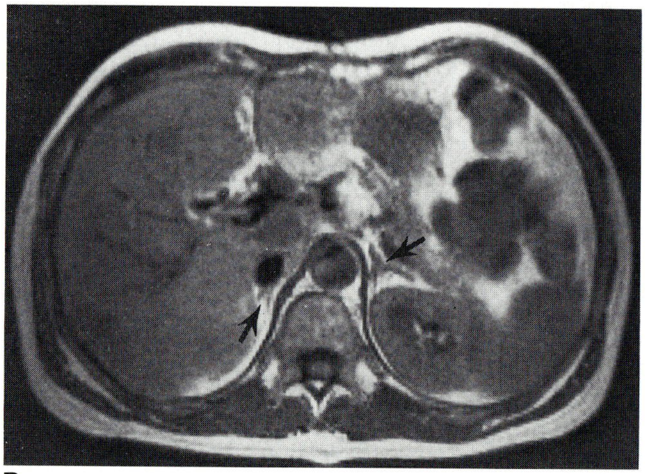

spin-echo sequences (SE 500/25) (Fig. 9-9). The short spin-echo sequence has the advantage of overall higher signal strength than the inversion recovery sequence and better definition of the renal collecting system, although its corticomedullary differentiation is not as great. Corticomedullary differentiation is important for the diagnosis of a number of renal diseases by MRI. Loss of distinction between the cortex and medulla is seen in several conditions, including glomerulonephritis, acute renal failure, chronic renal failure, renal artery stenosis, transplant rejection, and acute obstruction. Thus it is important always to include a T1-weighted sequence in the evaluation of renal disease by MR.

Addition of a T2-weighted pulse sequence allows evaluation of abnormalities noted on the T1-weighted sequence, based on T2 imaging characteristics. For example, a simple fluid-filled renal cyst will appear dark on the T1-weighted sequence but bright on a T2-weighted sequence. At times, calculated T2 images may be helpful. Examples have appeared in the literature in which a calculated T2 image was helpful in distinguishing tumor thrombus in the inferior vena cava from sluggish blood flow.

The renal hilum contains high-intensity fat and is bright on most imaging sequences. The renal artery and vein are of low intensity because of their content of rapidly flowing blood. The pelvicaliceal system contains urine of very high T1 and T2 values. It will appear dark on all but heavily T2-weighted images. The renal medulla will usually appear darker or isodense compared with the renal cortex, depending on whether the sequence is T1 or T2 weighted. Perirenal fat of high intensity is commonly seen surrounding the kidneys. Gerota's fascia is often identified as a low-intensity band within the bright perirenal fat.

The adrenal glands are best visualized on T1-weighted sequences (*e.g.,* SE 500/30), which optimize contrast between their lower intensity and the surrounding high-intensity retroperitoneal fat. The adrenal glands have characteristic inverted V or Y shapes as described in the CT literature. The right gland is best seen on axial images as appearing to hang off the back of the inferior vena cava. The left adrenal gland may perhaps better be seen on coronal images, between the left diaphragmatic crus and the left kidney (Figs. 9-10, 9-11). The normal adrenal is hypointense to liver on T1-weighted sequences and becomes isointense with progressive T2-weighting. By contrast, except for adenomas, most adrenal masses become hyperintense to liver on T2-weighted sequences.

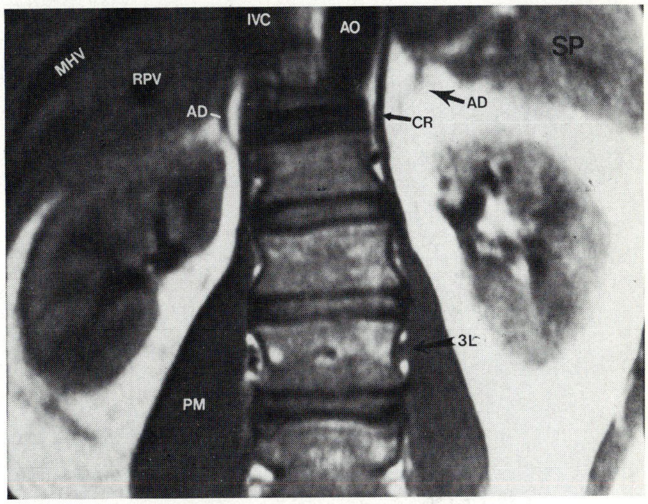

A

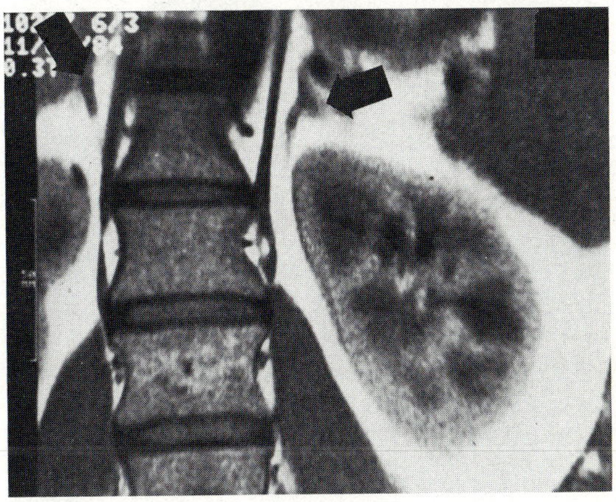

B

FIGURE 9-11

Adrenal glands in coronal section, SE 350/28. Also noted MHV = middle hepatic vein; RPV = right portal vein; IVC = inferior vena cava; AO = aorta; CR = crus of diaphragm; SP = spleen; AD = adrenal glands (also black arrows in 9-11B); PM = psoas major muscle; 3L = 3rd lumbar artery. (Courtesy of Fonar Corporation, 110 Marcus Drive, Melville, NY 11747)

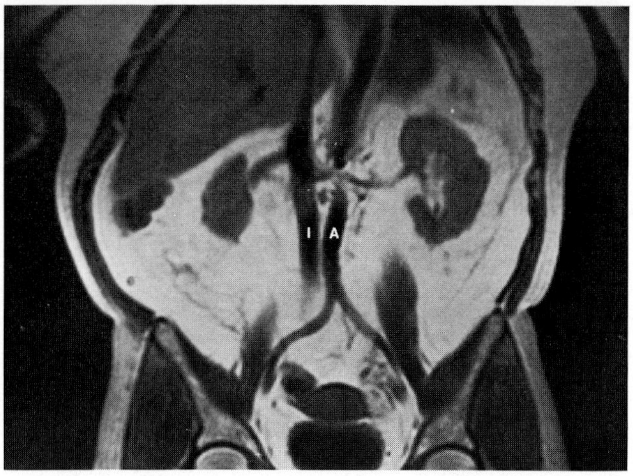

FIGURE 9-12

The aorta (A) and inferior vena cava (I) are only occasionally seen in their entire length on coronal scans because of lumbar lordosis. (Image obtained on Magniscan 5000, Thomson-CGR MR system)

FIGURE 9-13

Normal branching of the celiac axis. Small arrow = portal vein; arrowhead = hepatic artery; large arrow = splenic artery; open arrow = splenic vein.

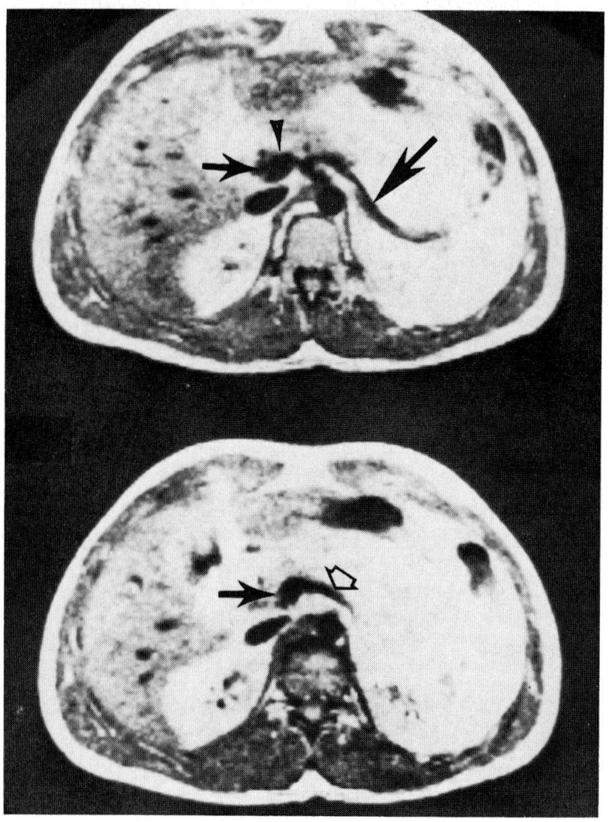

Abdominal Vasculature

The aorta, vena cava, and major vascular structures in the abdomen and retroperitoneum are well visualized by MRI as round or tubular structures with little or no signal produced by rapidly flowing blood. For simple anatomic visualization, axial sagittal images taken with short spin-echo (SE 500/25) or partial saturation sequences (PS 300/20) provide necessary contrast definition and speedy acquisition

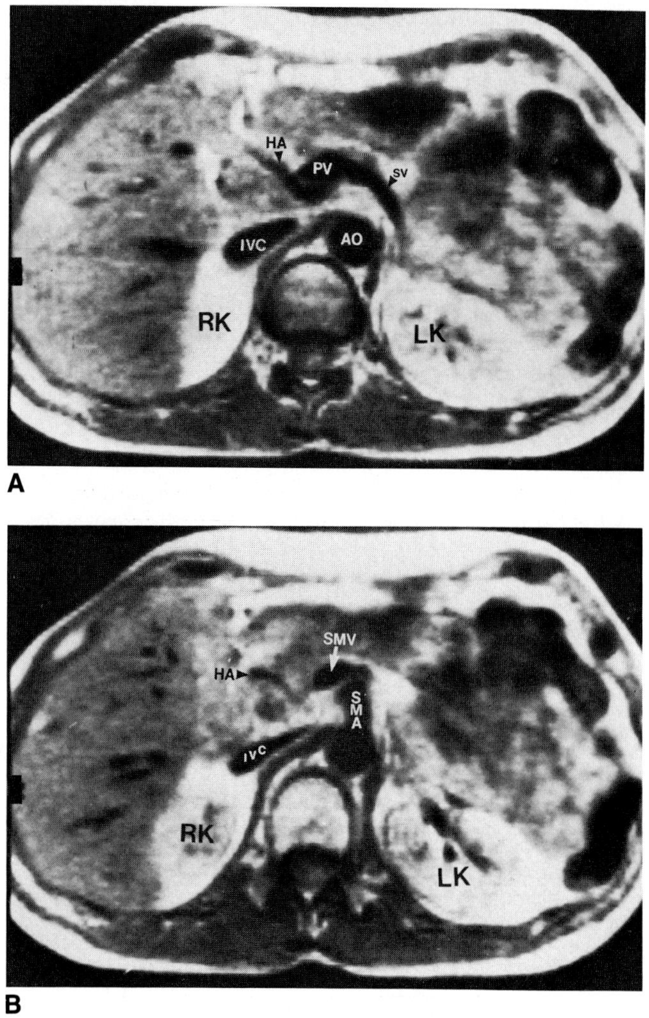

FIGURE 9-14

Replaced hepatic artery passes behind portal vein. HA = hepatic artery; PV = portal vein; SV = splenic vein; IVC = inferior vena cava; AO = aorta; RK = right kidney; LK = left kidney; SMA = superior mesenteric artery; SMV = superior mesenteric vein.

times. To distinguish the characteristics of clot, flow, tumor thrombus, and leakage areas from an aneurysm it is necessary to perform a second imaging sequence that is more T2-weighted.

Coronal and sagittal images are occasionally helpful in defining certain vascular relationships, such as the extension of an abdominal aortic aneurysm above the renal vessels or into the iliac vessels. Because of lumbar lordosis it may be difficult to image the entire aorta on a single coronal scan, and a sagittal plane may be more appropriate. With normal aging and increasing tortuosity of the aorta, neither the sagittal nor the coronal plane may be satisfactory for following its course. Figure 9-12 shows the entire abdominal aorta in coronal section.

Axial images through the upper abdomen routinely demonstrate the celiac axis dividing into the hepatic and splenic arteries (Fig. 9-13). The hepatic artery normally passes anterior to the portal vein. Occasionally a "replaced" hepatic artery may be identified where the artery passes posterior to the portal vein. (Fig. 9-14).

The superior mesenteric artery may be seen exiting anteriorly from the aorta at about the L1-2 level (Fig. 9-3G). The inferior mesenteric artery exits an interspace lower (Fig. 9-15). Mesenteric vasculature supplying the ileum and ileocolic regions may occasionally be identified on coronal images (Fig. 9-16).

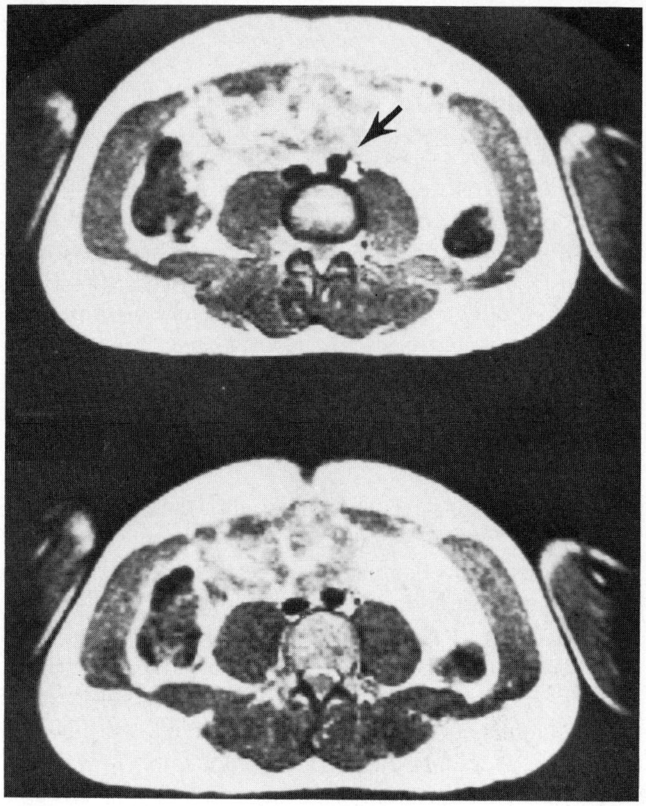

FIGURE 9-15

Inferior mesenteric artery seen exiting aorta at 1:30 position below kidneys (arrow).

FIGURE 9-16

Mesenteric vessel branches. (*A*) SB = small bowel; arrowheads = mesenteric branches; (*B*) arrowheads show branches of superior mesenteric artery to terminal ileum and cecum.

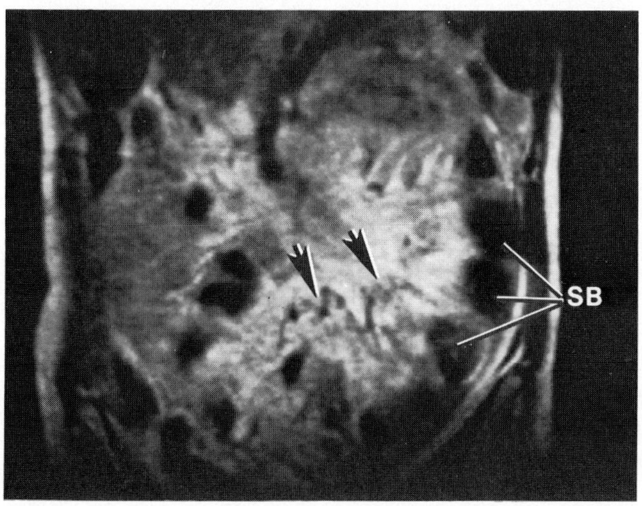

A

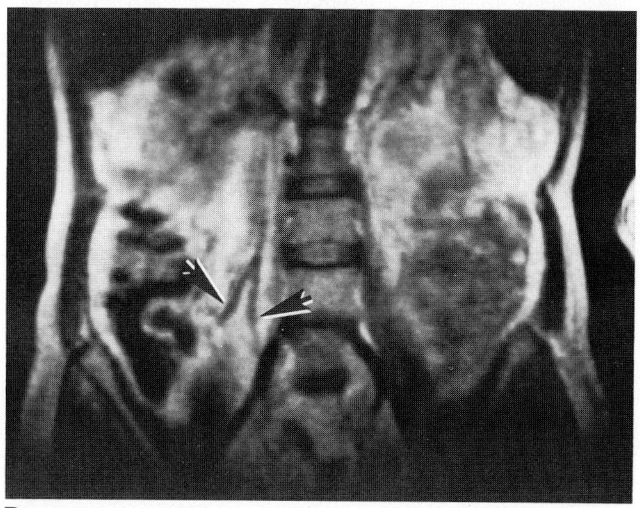

B

Abdominal and Pelvic Lymph Nodes

Analysis of the lymph node-bearing areas of the abdomen and pelvis is critical in many clinical situations, including the evaluation of lymphomas, metastatic disease, and inflammatory processes (Table 9-2). MRI has shown some promise in these regions. Again, axial imaging planes seem the most reliable for evaluation of abdominal and pelvic lymphadenopathy. Typical axial images through the abdomen below the kidneys reveal fat, blood vessels, and muscles only (Fig. 9-15).

The visualization of abdominal and pelvic lymph nodes depends on their contrast between three structures: (1) bowel, (2) retroperitoneal or mesenteric fat, and (3) muscles, especially the iliopsoas. Just as with CT, collapsed loops of bowel adjacent to the retroperitoneum, especially in thin patients, are a serious problem in MRI. The development of paramagnetic oral MR contrast agents will alleviate this problem somewhat, but not entirely. We now address the optimum pulse sequences for differentiating lymph nodes from fat and muscle.

In the evaluation of lymphadenopathy in the mediastinum, it is only necessary to use a pulse sequence that distinguishes nodes from fat, since there is no muscle and the other adjacent structures (lung and blood vessels) produce naturally high contrast regardless of the pulse sequence selected. In the abdomen and pelvis, a T1-weighted pulse sequence, such as SE with TR = 500, will adequately distinguish normal and pathologically involved lymph nodes from retroperitoneal fat. However, the distinction between lymph node and muscle will be poor with this technique. The best contrast between lymph nodes and muscle appears to be on heavily T2-weighted techniques; an intermediate spin-echo sequence of SE 900/30 has been suggested. This will allow visualization of lymph nodes with signal lower than fat but higher than paraspinous and psoas muscles. Unfortunately, the SE 900/30 technique is inadequate for evaluating focal hepatic lesions such as metastases or lymphoma. Therefore, unless only lymph node information is desired, a two-sequence technique using both T1- and T2-weighted formats as previously described is suggested.

TABLE 9-2

Possible Protocols for Imaging the Abdomen

"Routine" Screen for Abdominal Lesions

Protocol:
1. Glucagon and gas-forming crystals should be given to immobilize bowel and distend the stomach, NPO for 4 hours
2. May consider respiratory gating or abdominal cinch to diminish motion in upper abdomen if detailed anatomic information in this area is desired
3. Axial plane, SE 300/25
4. Axial plane, SE 2000/40,80,120

Liver

Protocol:
1. Axial plane, SE 250/20
2. Axial plane, SE 2000/60,120
3. If suspected near dome of liver, possible subphrenic or subhepatic fluid collection, use sagittal plane, SE 1000/30,60,90

Pancreas

Protocol:
1. Glucagon and gas essential
2. Axial SE 1000/30,60 or IR 1200/400

Kidneys and Adrenals

Protocol:
1. Axial plane, IR 1200/400 or SE 500/25 (These techniques best demonstrate corticomedullary differentiation)
2. Axial plane, SE 2000/40,80
3. Left adrenal gland and the relationship of certain renal masses is sometimes best appreciated in coronal plane

CHAPTER 10

Pelvis and Hips

MR has found more applications in the pelvis than in the abdomen proper. Organs in the pelvis are not appreciably affected by respiratory motion. Accordingly, gating is not required for obtaining good images. Furthermore, CT has been found to have more limitations in the pelvis than in the abdomen, particularly in imaging the female reproductive tract. MR may offer some advantages because of its multiplanar format, high sensitivity for detection of lesions, and ability to discriminate between lymph nodes and tortuous iliac vessels.

The ideal imaging planes and pulse sequences for the pelvis depend on the disease processes suspected. Table 10-1 gives some sample protocols for imaging pelvic lesions. Axial images of the pelvis from the level of the iliac crest to the dome of the bladder are shown in Figure 10-1. Note that the retroperitoneal blood vessels, muscles, and ureter are easily distinguished. Separate multiplanar images of the lower pelvis demonstrating male and female reproductive tracts appear in figures later in this chapter.

In terms of its MRI properties, urine is nearly pure water. As such, it has the longest T1 and T2 values of any substance in the body. The bladder wall, by contrast, is composed of smooth muscle, with relatively long T1 and short T2 values. On most T1-weighted pulse sequences, it is difficult to distinguish bladder wall from urine (Fig. 10-2). If more heavily T2-weighted sequences are used, the bladder wall may be seen as a dark rim surrounding whiter urine (contrast reversal phenomenon). The bladder wall may also be seen on short spin-echo sequences when markedly thickened or infiltrated by tumor (Fig. 10-3). In general, T1-weighted images are superior for evaluating the extension of bladder tumors into perivesical fat, whereas T2-weighted images best demonstarte bladder wall invasion or inflammation.

Sagittal or coronal images seem well-suited for imaging of the bladder, especially at its dome or neck. Axial images are useful for evaluating the lateral walls of the bladder but may be confusing near the dome because of partial volume sectioning with bowel (Fig. 10-4A). Such bowel resting on the bladder might simulate a mass unless followed on sequential axial images or recognized on sagittal or coronal scans.

TABLE 10-1

Sample Protocols For Pelvic MR Imaging

Routine Screen for Pelvic Lesions

Protocol:	1. Consider using water on air enema
	2. Tampon should be used in female patients
	3. Axial plane, SE 1000/30,60
	4. Coronal plane, SE 1500/30,60

Bladder

Protocol:	1. NPO for 8 hours before scan
	2. Glucagon, 1 mg IM at start
	3. Sagittal plane, SE 2000/40,80

Prostate

Protocol:	1. Axial plane, SE 1000/30
	2. Axial plane, SE 2000/30,60
	3. Sagittal plane, SE 1000/30
	4. Occasionally coronal images at SE 1500/30 are useful for base of prostate
	5. Occasionally sagittal IR 1500/100 images will help define plane between prostate and rectum

Seminal Vesicles

Protocol:	1. Axial plane, SE 500/30 or PS 400
	2. Sagittal plane, SE 500/30 or PS 400

Female Reproductive Tract (Vagina, Uterus, Ovaries)

Protocol:	1. Always use tampon in vagina
	2. Axial plane, SE 2000/30,60
	3. Axial plane, SE 500/30
	4. Sagittal plane, SE 2000/80

The Male Pelvis

The prostate, seminal vesicles, and male external genitalia are all well visualized by MR. Axial images of the male pelvis are shown in Figure 10-4. Coronal images appear in Figure 10-5. Sagittal images are shown in Figure 10-6. Sample protocols for imaging the male pelvis are found in Table 10-1.

The Prostate

Early reports concerning the utility of MR imaging in the examination of the prostate have been encouraging, although no specific imaging characteristic to distinguish benign from malignant conditions has yet been recognized. Axial, sagittal, and coronal planes all may at times be useful to show the spread of disease, especially carcinoma.

An SE 1000/30 technique is suitable for deline-

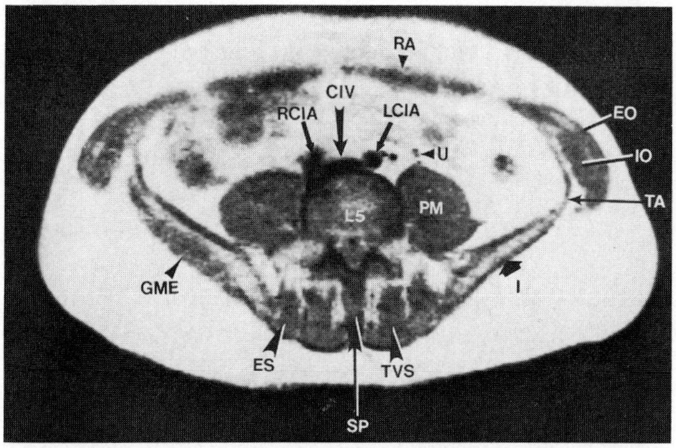

A

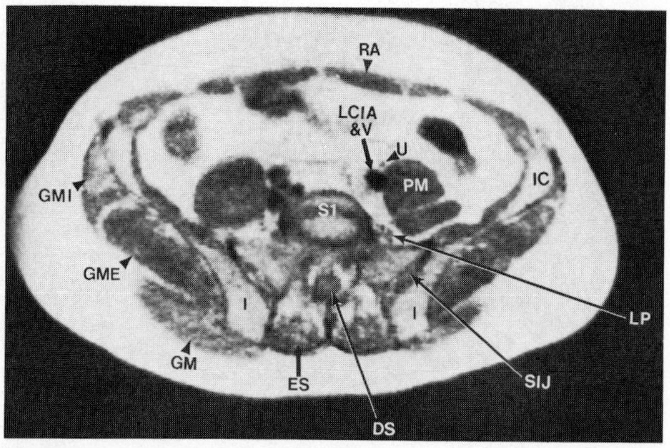

B

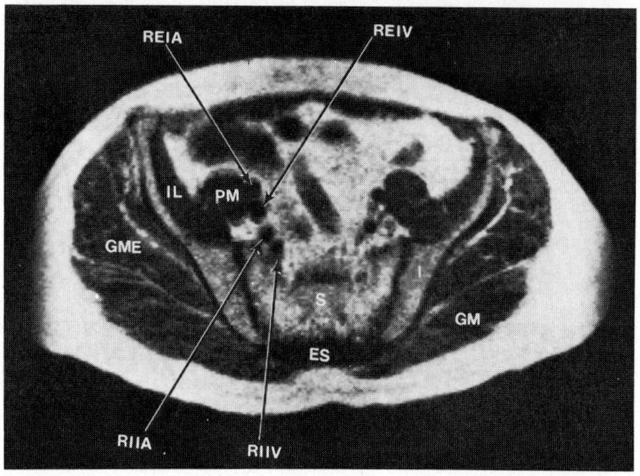

C

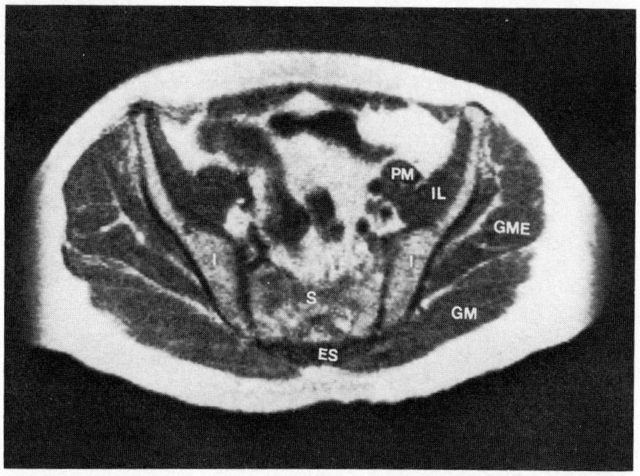

D

B	bladder	LP	lumbosacral plexus
CIV	common iliac veins	PI	piriformis muscle
DS	dural sac	PM	psoas major muscle
EO	external oblique muscle	RA	rectus abdominus muscle
ES	erector spinae muscle	RCIA	right common iliac artery
GM	gluteus maximus muscle	REIA, REIV	right external iliac artery, vein
GME	gluteus medius muscle	RIIA, RIIV	right internal iliac artery, vein
GMI	gluteus minimus muscle	S	sacrum
		S1	first sacral segment
I	ilium	SG	superior gluteal vessels
IC	iliac crest		
IL	iliacus muscle	SIJ	sacroliac joint
IO	internal oblique muscle	SP	spinous process
		TA	transversus abdominus muscle
IP	iliopsoas muscle		
L5	fifth lumbar vertebral body	TVS	transversospinalis muscle
LCIA, LCIV	left common iliac artery, vein	U	ureter

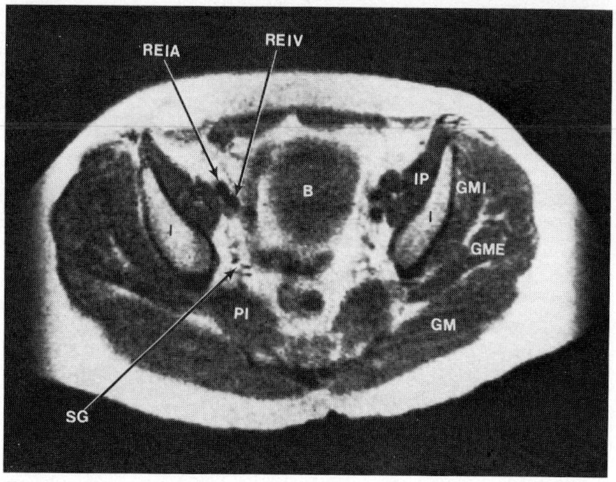

E

FIGURE 10-1

Axial images of the upper pelvis above the acetabular roofs (SE 2000/28).

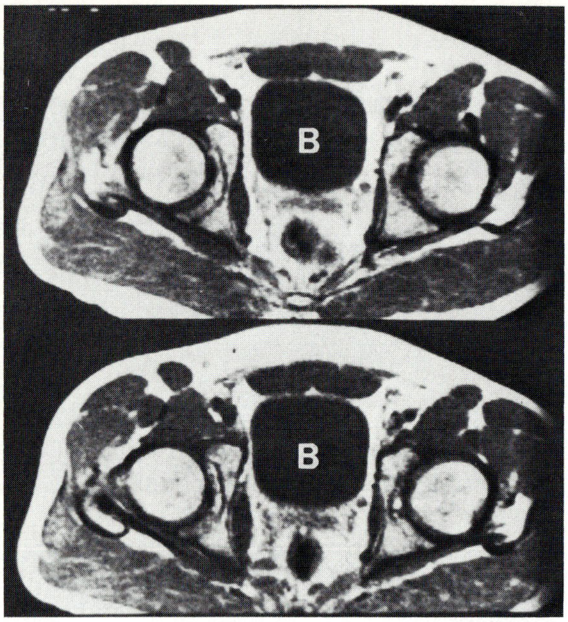

FIGURE 10-2

The bladder (*B*) on axial SE 1000/28 images. Note that the bladder wall cannot be distinguished from urine with this technique.

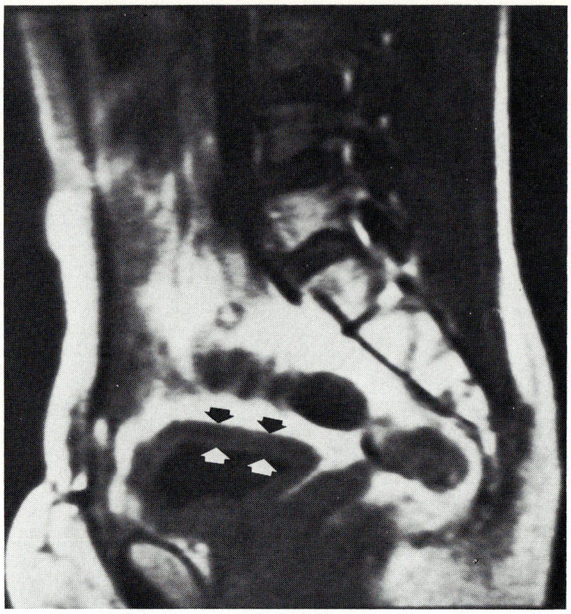

FIGURE 10-3

The bladder wall (arrows) is only seen at short spin-echo techniques (SE 500/28) when thickened or infiltrated by tumor. (Courtesy of Fonar Corporation, 110 Marcus Drive, Melville, NY 11747)

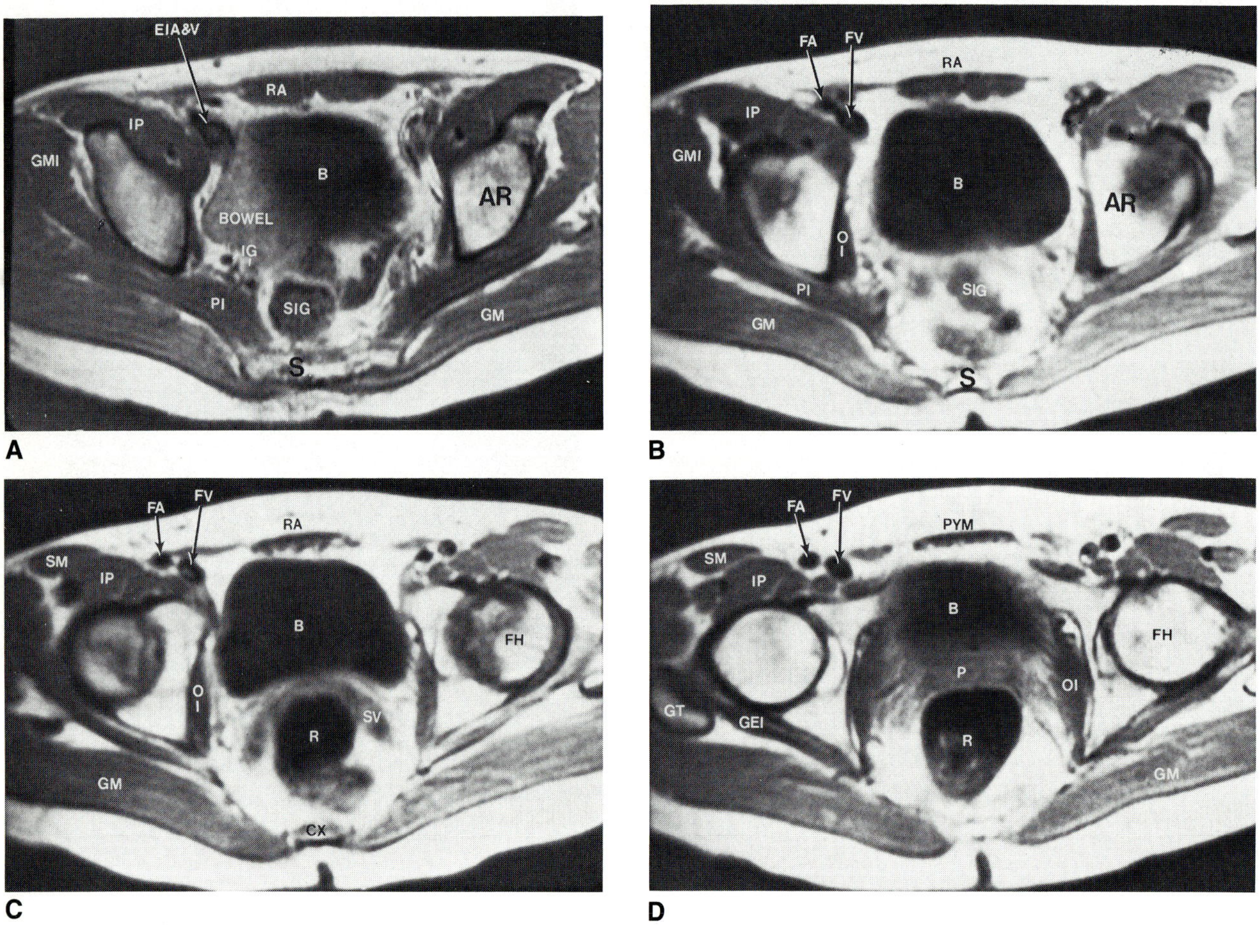

A	anus	FA, FV	femoral artery and vein
AB	adductor brevis muscle	FH	femoral head
AIIS	anterior inferior iliac spine	FN	femoral neck
AL	adductor longus muscle	GEI, GES	gemellus inferior, superior muscles
AR	acetabular roof	GF	gluteal fold
B	bladder	GM	gluteus maximus muscle
BF	biceps femoris muscle	GME	gluteus medius muscle
BP	bulb of penis	GMI	gluteus minimus muscle
CC	corpus cavernosum penis	GT	greater trochanter
CIA, CIV	common iliac artery, vein	I	ilium
CP	crus penis	IC	ischiocavernosus muscle
CS	corpus spongiosum penis	ICL	iliocostalis muscle
CX	coccyx	ICR	iliac crest
EIA, EIV	external iliac artery, vein	IE	inferior epigastic vessels
EO	external oblique muscle	IG	inferior gluteal vessels
EP	epididymis	IIA, IIV	internal iliac artery, vein
ES	erector spinae muscle	IL	ilium
IP	iliopsoas muscle	PR	pubic ramus
IR	ischial ramus	PYM	pyramidalis muscle
IRF	ischiorectal fossa	QF	quadratus femoris muscle
ISC	ischium	QL	quadratus lumborum muscle
IT	ischeal tuberosity	R	rectum
IVC	inferior vena cava	RA	rectus abdominus muscle
IVF	intervertebral foramen	RF	rectus femoris muscle
L3, 4, 5	lumbar vertebrae 3, 4, 5	S	sacrum
LA	levator ani muscle	SA	sphincter ani
LD	latissimus dorsi muscle	SAE	sphincter ani externus
LFC	lateral femoral circumflex artery	SAV	saphenous vein
LM	longissimus muscle	SC	spermatic cord
LNT	lumbar nerve trunk	SFA	superficial femoral artery
LS	lateral sacral vessels	SG	superior gluteal vessels
MFC	medial femoral circumflex artery	SH	short rotators of hip
OA	obturator artery	SIG	sigmoid colon
OI, OE	obturator internus, externus muscles	SM	sartorius muscle
P	pubis	SV	seminal vesicle
PD	pouch of Douglas	T	testicle
PE	pectineus muscle	TA	tunica albuginea
PF	profunda femoris artery	U	ureter
PI	piriformis muscle	VM	vastus medialis muscle
PM	psoas major muscle		

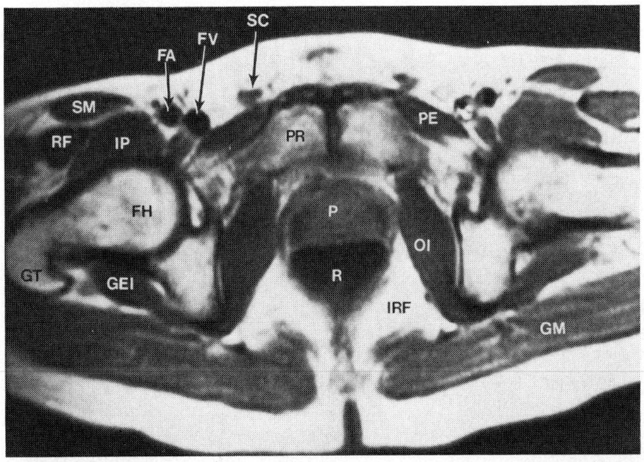

E

FIGURE 10-4

Axial MR images of the lower male pelvis using SE 500/28. The femoral heads exhibit aseptic necrosis, but the other anatomic structures are normal. (Courtesy of Fonar Corporation, 110 Marcus Drive, Melville, NY 11747)

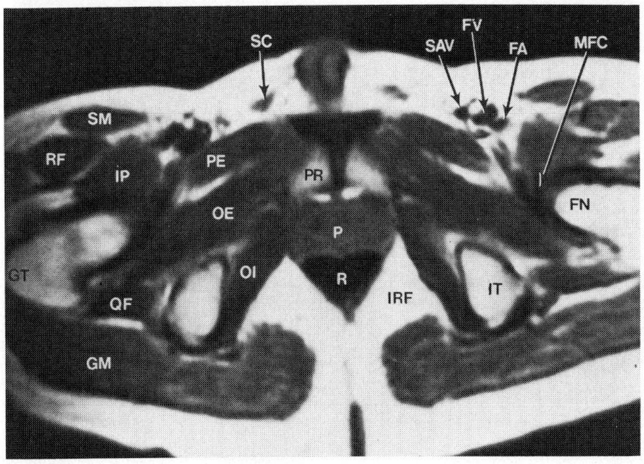

F

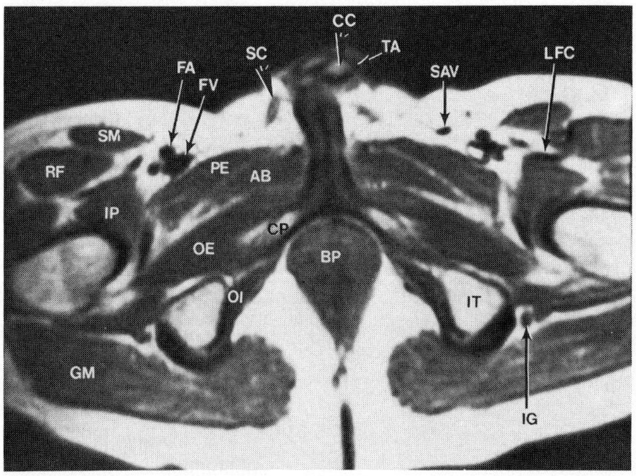

G

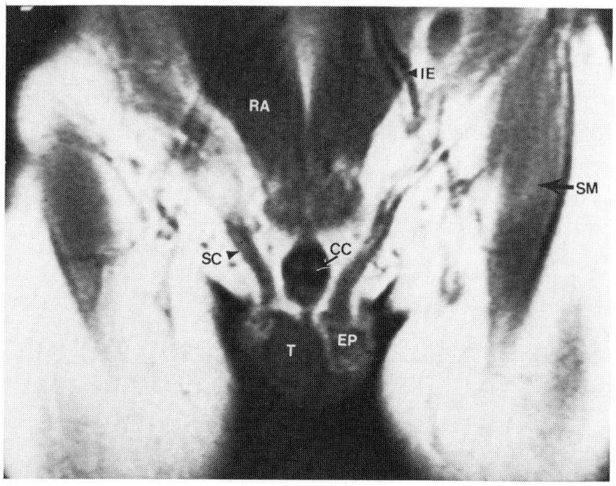
IE
RA
SM
SC
CC
T
EP
A

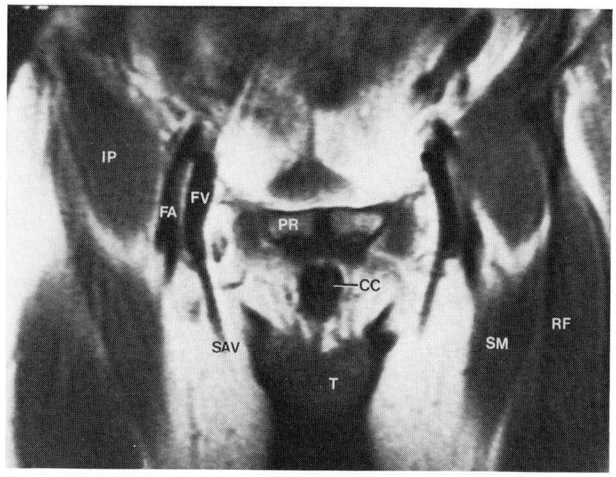
IP
FV
FA
PR
CC
SAV
SM
RF
T
B

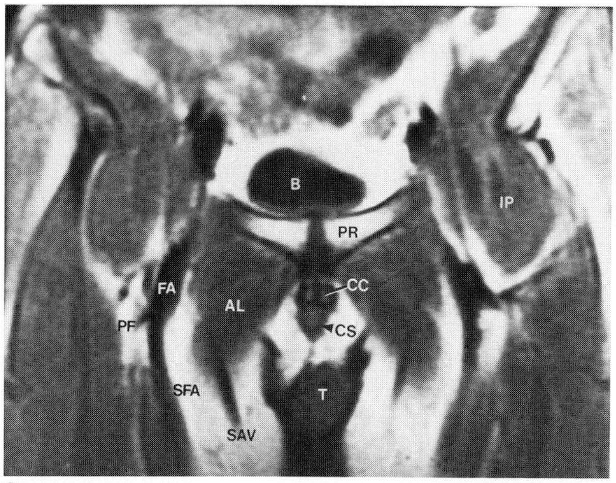
B
IP
PR
FA
AL
CC
CS
PF
SFA
SAV
T
C

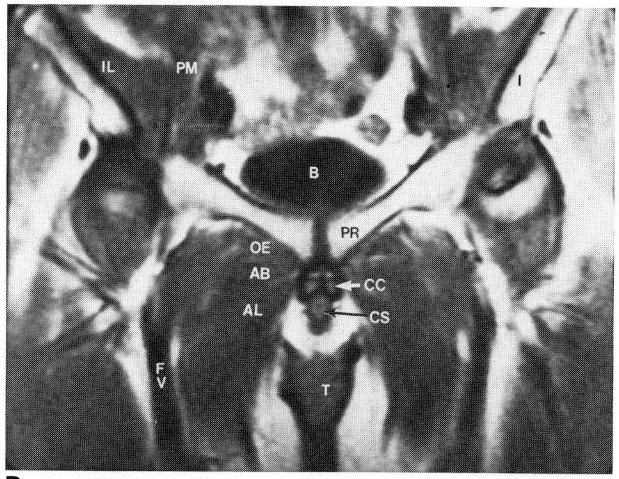
IL
PM
I
B
PR
OE
AB
CC
AL
CS
F
V
T
D

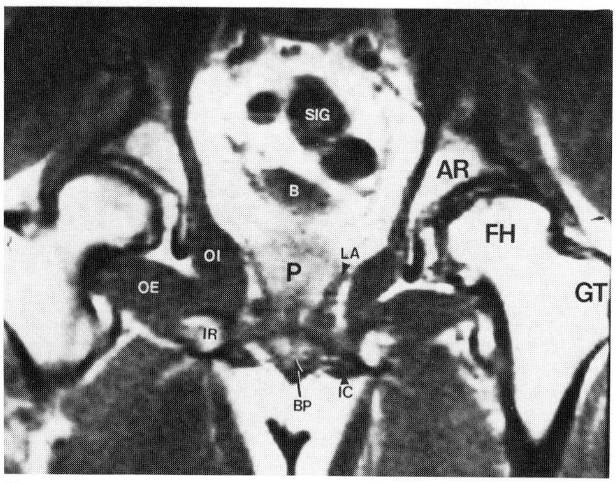
SIG
AR
B
FH
OI
P
LA
GT
OE
IR
BP
IC
E

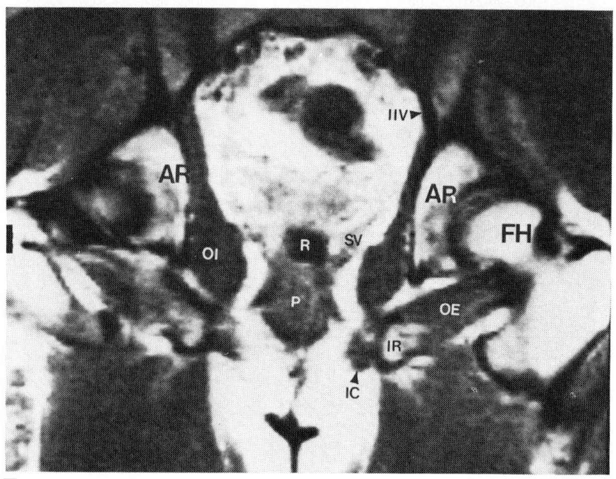
IIV
AR
AR
FH
OI
R
SV
P
OE
IR
IC
F

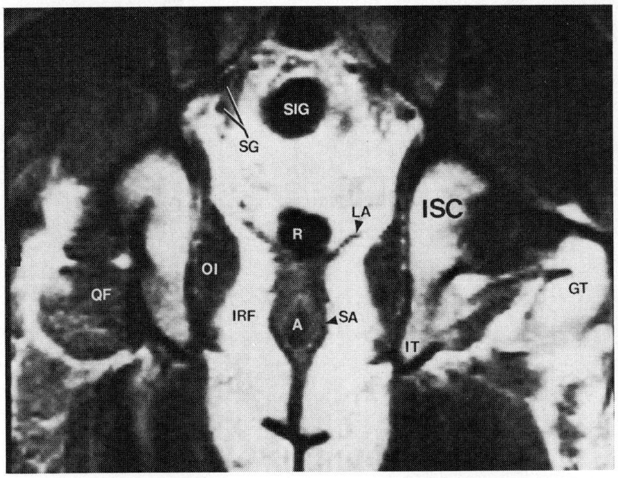

G

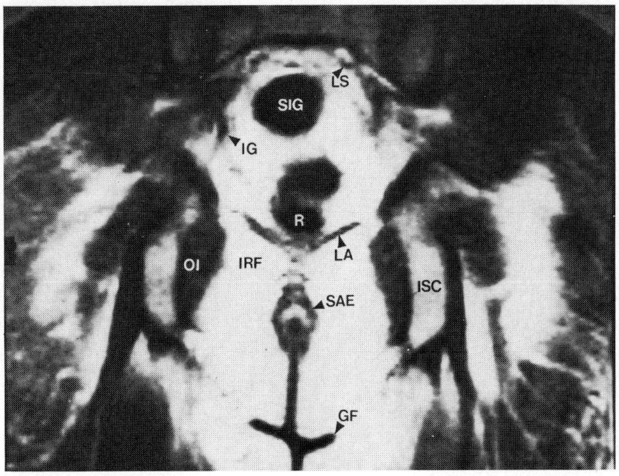

H

FIGURE 10-5

Coronal images of the normal male pelvis and hips. Images *A* through *D* performed at SE 500/28. (Courtesy of Fonar Corp.) Images *E* through *H* performed on Diasonics MT/S at 1500/28.

A	anus
AB	adductor brevis muscle
AIIS	anterior inferior iliac spine
AL	adductor longus muscle
AR	acetabular roof
B	bladder
BF	biceps femoris muscle
BP	bulb of penis
CC	corpus cavernosum penis
CIA, CIV	common iliac artery, vein
CP	crus penis
CS	corpus spongiosum penis
CX	coccyx
EIA, EIV	external iliac artery, vein
EO	external oblique muscle
EP	epididymis
ES	erector spinae muscle
FA, FV	femoral artery and vein
FH	femoral head
FN	femoral neck
GEI, GES	gemellus inferior, superior muscles
GF	gluteal fold
GM	gluteus maximus muscle
GME	gluteus medius muscle
GMI	gluteus minimus muscle
GT	greater trochanter
I	ilium
IC	ischiocavernosus muscle
ICL	iliocostalis muscle
ICR	iliac crest
IE	inferior epigastic vessels
IG	inferior gluteal vessels
IIA, IIV	internal iliac artery, vein
IL	ilium
IP	iliopsoas muscle
IR	ischial ramus
IRF	ischiorectal fossa
ISC	ischium
IT	ischeal tuberosity
IVC	inferior vena cava
IVF	intervertebral foramen
L3, 4, 5	lumbar vertebrae 3, 4, 5
LA	levator ani muscle
LD	latissimus dorsi muscle
LFC	lateral femoral circumflex artery
LM	longissimus muscle
LNT	lumbar nerve trunk
LS	lateral sacral vessels
MFC	medial femoral circumflex artery
OA	obturator artery
OI, OE	obturator internus, externus muscles
P	pubis
PD	pouch of Douglas
PE	pectineus muscle
PF	profunda femoris artery
PI	piriformis muscle
PM	psoas major muscle
PR	pubic ramus
PYM	pyramidalis muscle
QF	quadratus femoris muscle
QL	quadratus lumborum muscle
R	rectum
RA	rectus abdominus muscle
RF	rectus femoris muscle
S	sacrum
SA	sphincter ani
SAE	sphincter ani externus
SAV	saphenous vein
SC	spermatic cord
SFA	superficial femoral artery
SG	superior gluteal vessels
SH	short rotators of hip
SIG	sigmoid colon
SM	sartorius muscle
SV	seminal vesicle
T	testicle
TA	tunica albuginea
U	ureter
VM	vastus medialis muscle

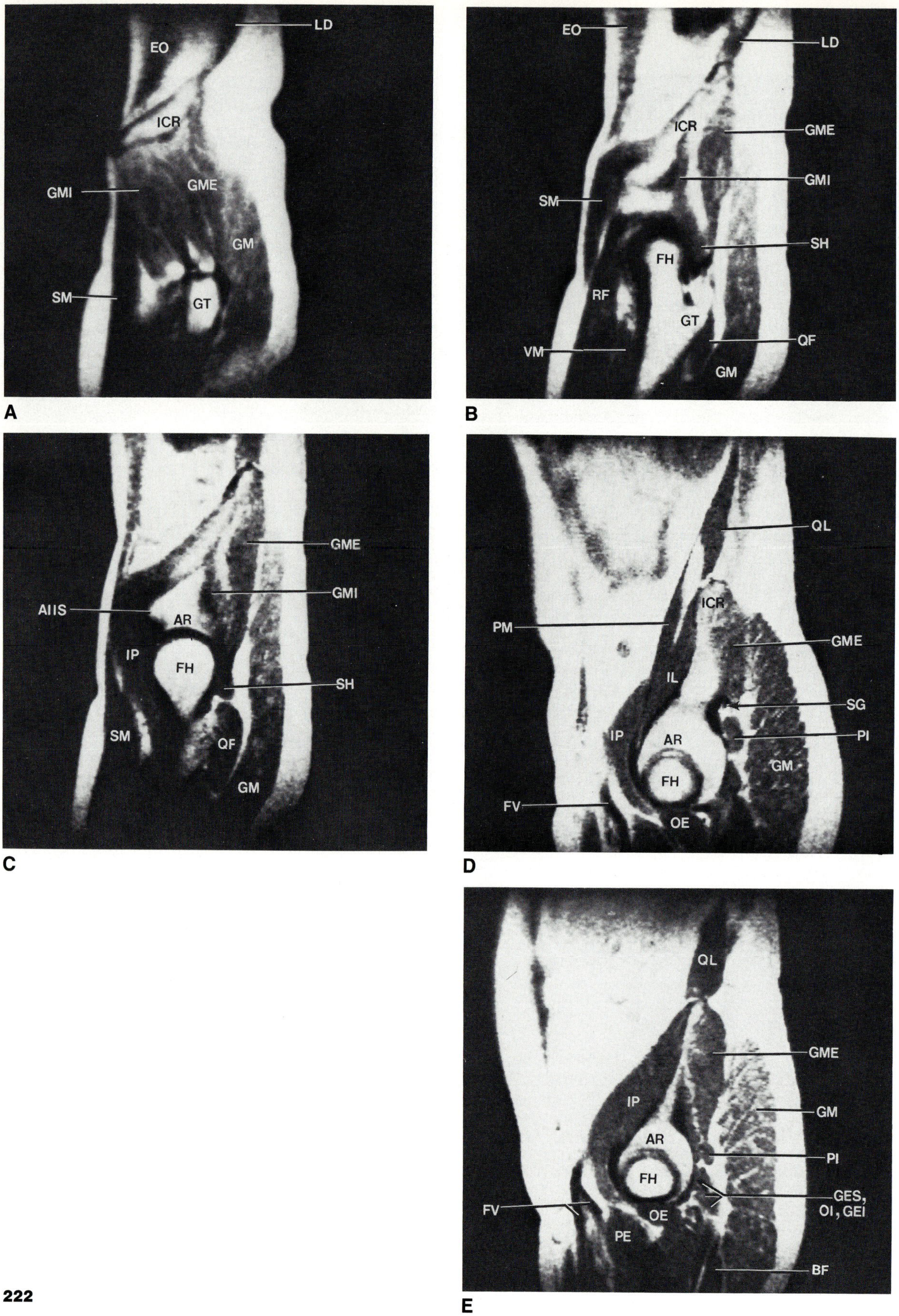
A
EO
LD
ICR
GMI
GME
GM
SM
GT
B
EO
LD
ICR
GME
GMI
SM
SH
FH
RF
GT
VM
QF
GM
C
GME
GMI
AIIS
AR
IP
FH
SH
SM
QF
GM
D
QL
ICR
PM
GME
IL
SG
IP
AR
PI
GM
FH
FV
OE
E
QL
GME
IP
GM
AR
PI
FH
GES,
OI, GEI
FV
OE
PE
BF

FIGURE 10-6

Sagittal images of the normal pelvis and hip, performed using SE 1000/28.

A	anus
AB	adductor brevis muscle
AIIS	anterior inferior iliac spine
AL	adductor longus muscle
AR	acetabular roof
B	bladder
BF	biceps femoris muscle
BP	bulb of penis
CC	corpus cavernosum penis
CIA, CIV	common iliac artery, vein
CP	crus penis
CS	corpus spongiosum penis
CX	coccyx
EIA, EIV	external iliac artery, vein
EO	external oblique muscle
EP	epididymis
ES	erector spinae muscle
FA, FV	femoral artery and vein
FH	femoral head
FN	femoral neck
GEI, GES	gemellus inferior, superior muscles
GF	gluteal fold
GM	gluteus maximus muscle
GME	gluteus medius muscle
GMI	gluteus minimus muscle
GT	greater trochanter
I	ilium
IC	ischiocavernosus muscle
ICL	iliocostalis muscle
ICR	iliac crest
IE	inferior epigastic vessels
IG	inferior gluteal vessels
IIA, IIV	internal iliac artery, vein
IL	ilium
IP	iliopsoas muscle
IR	ischial ramus
IRF	ischiorectal fossa
ISC	ischium
IT	ischeal tuberosity
IVC	inferior vena cava
IVF	intervertebral foramen
L3, 4, 5	lumbar vertebrae 3, 4, 5
LA	levator ani muscle
LD	latissimus dorsi muscle
LFC	lateral femoral circumflex artery
LM	longissimus muscle
LNT	lumbar nerve trunk
LS	lateral sacral vessels
MFC	medial femoral circumflex artery
OA	obturator artery
OI, OE	obturator internus, externus muscles
P	pubis
PD	pouch of Douglas
PE	pectineus muscle
PF	profunda femoris artery
PI	piriformis muscle
PM	psoas major muscle
PR	pubic ramus
PYM	pyramidalis muscle
QF	quadratus femoris muscle
QL	quadratus lumborum muscle
R	rectum
RA	rectus abdominus muscle
RF	rectus femoris muscle
S	sacrum
SA	sphincter ani
SAE	sphincter ani externus
SAV	saphenous vein
SC	spermatic cord
SFA	superficial femoral artery
SG	superior gluteal vessels
SH	short rotators of hip
SIG	sigmoid colon
SM	sartorius muscle
SV	seminal vesicle
T	testicle
TA	tunica albuginea
U	ureter
VM	vastus medialis muscle

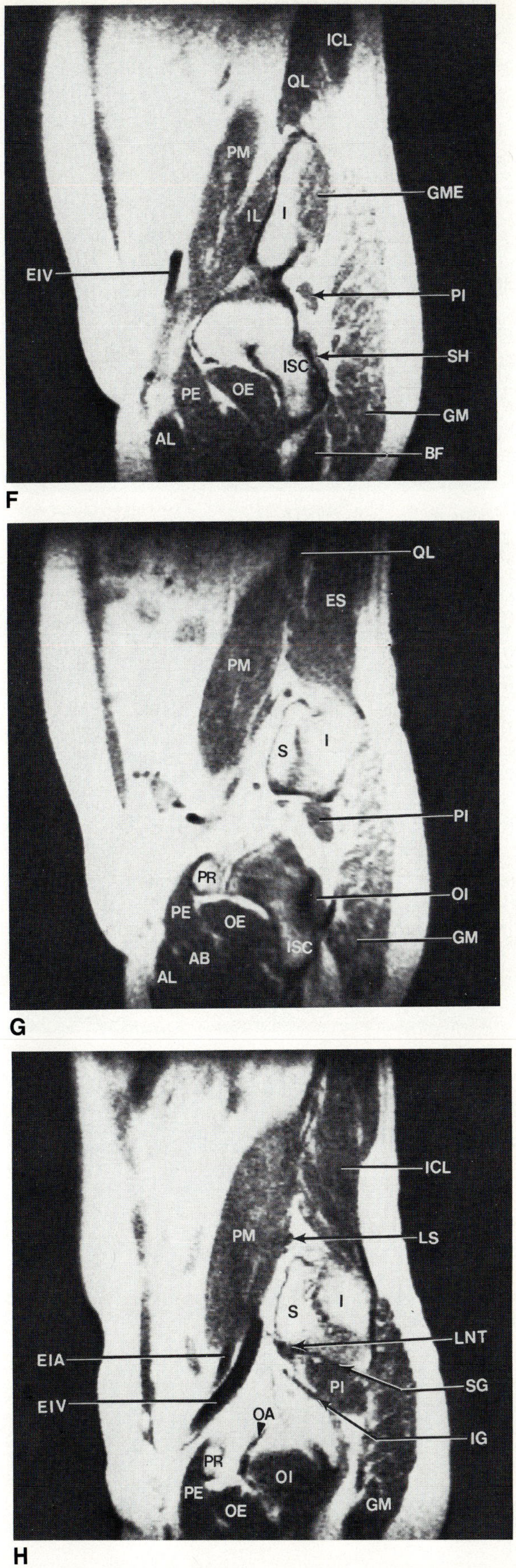

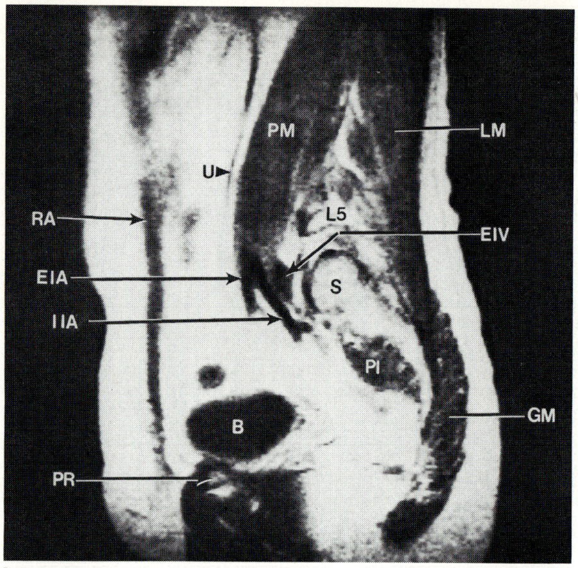

I

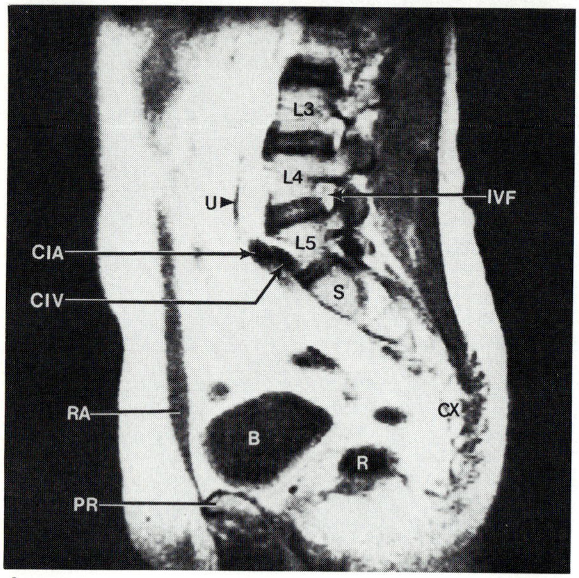

J

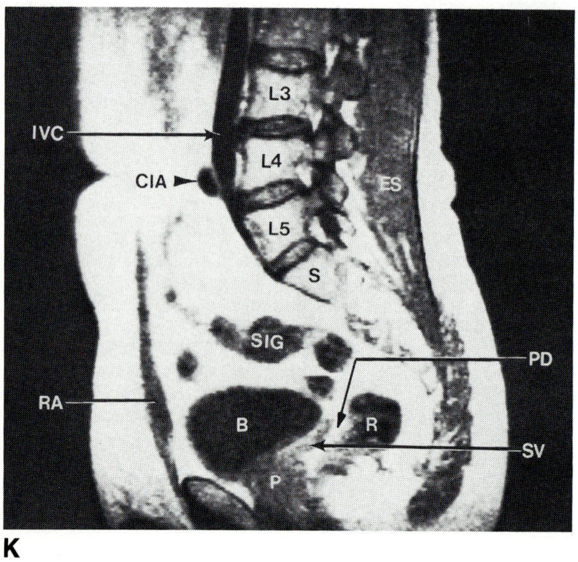

K

FIGURE 10-6 *(cont.)*

Sagittal images of the normal pelvis and hip, performed using SE 1000/28.

A	anus
AB	adductor brevis muscle
AIIS	anterior inferior iliac spine
AL	adductor longus muscle
AR	acetabular roof
B	bladder
BF	biceps femoris muscle
BP	bulb of penis
CC	corpus cavernosum penis
CIA, CIV	common iliac artery, vein
CP	crus penis
CS	corpus spongiosum penis
CX	coccyx
EIA, EIV	external iliac artery, vein
EO	external oblique muscle
EP	epididymis
ES	erector spinae muscle
FA, FV	femoral artery and vein
FH	femoral head
FN	femoral neck
GEI, GES	gemellus inferior, superior muscles
GF	gluteal fold
GM	gluteus maximus muscle
GME	gluteus medius muscle
GMI	gluteus minimus muscle
GT	greater trochanter
I	ilium
IC	ischiocavernosus muscle
ICL	iliocostalis muscle
ICR	iliac crest
IE	inferior epigastic vessels
IG	inferior gluteal vessels
IIA, IIV	internal iliac artery, vein
IL	ilium
IP	iliopsoas muscle
IR	ischial ramus
IRF	ischiorectal fossa
ISC	ischium
IT	ischeal tuberosity
IVC	inferior vena cava
IVF	intervertebral foramen
L3, 4, 5	lumbar vertebrae 3, 4, 5
LA	levator ani muscle
LD	latissimus dorsi muscle
LFC	lateral femoral circumflex artery
LM	longissimus muscle
LNT	lumbar nerve trunk
LS	lateral sacral vessels
MFC	medial femoral circumflex artery
OA	obturator artery
OI, OE	obturator internus, externus muscles
P	pubis
PD	pouch of Douglas
PE	pectineus muscle
PF	profunda femoric artery
PI	piriformis muscle
PM	psoas major muscle
PR	pubic ramus
PYM	pyramidalis muscle
QF	quadratus femoris muscle
QL	quadratus lumborum muscle
R	rectum
RA	rectus abdominus muscle
RF	rectus femoris muscle
S	sacrum
SA	sphincter ani
SAE	sphincter ani externus
SAV	saphenous vein
SC	spermatic cord
SFA	superficial femoral artery
SG	superior gluteal vessels
SH	short rotators of hip
SIG	sigmoid colon
SM	sartorius muscle
SV	seminal vesicle
T	testicle
TA	tunica albuginea
U	ureter
VM	vastus medialis muscle

FIGURE 10-7

The penis, axial SE1000/28. (*A*) Black arrow = bulb of penis; white arrow = crus of penis; white arrowhead = corpus cavernosum penis. (*B*) Short black arrow = muscle ischiocavernous; white arrow = bulbospongiosus muscle; black and white arrow = corpus spongiosum penis.

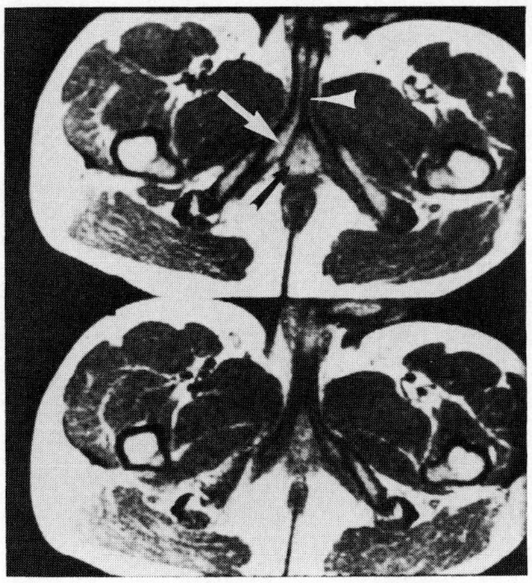
A

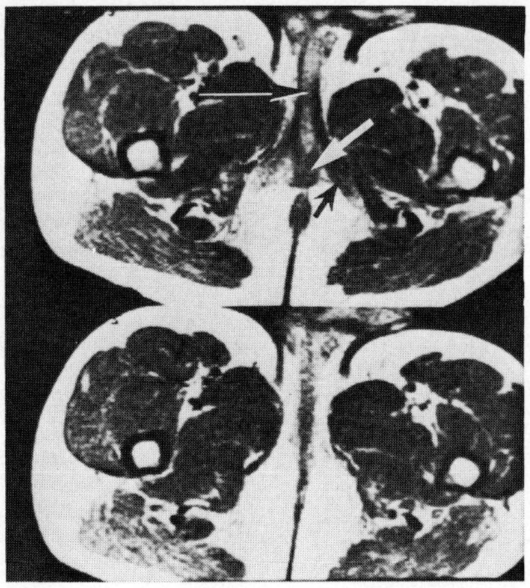
B

ating the prostate, bladder, and seminal vesicles; it is unsatisfactory for separating the prostate and the rectum, unless the rectum is filled with air. An inversion recovery sequence (IR 1500/100) will provide such a distinction between prostate and rectum; however, the overall image quality and signal-to-noise ratio is poor with this technique.

If a heavily T2-weighted sequence is used (*e.g.,* SE 2000/60), a bright rim of variable thickness may be seen around the prostate. It is possible that this represents the periprostatic venous plexus. Hricak has reported that on T2-weighted sequences the central and peripheral zones of the prostate may be distinguished. This may be an important anatomic finding, since most carcinomas arise from the peripheral zone. The distinction between zones is probably a result of the fact that the central zone contains striated muscle and hence has shorter T2 than the peripheral zone.

The relationship between the base of the prostate and the levator ani muscle is best appreciated on coronal planes (Fig. 10-5*E*). The border between the prostate and bladder is best appreciated on sagittal or coronal scans. The sagittal plane is also helpful in defining the preprostatic (Retzius) space, which is filled with fat, and, posteriorly, the pouch of Douglas and Denonvilliers' fascia. These features are shown in Fig. 10-6*K*.

The Seminal Vesicles

The seminal vesicles are best seen in the axial or sagittal planes on relatively short spin-echo sequences (*e.g.,* SE 500/30). The use of relatively T1-weighted sequences allows the vesicles to be distinguished from surrounding fat as lower-intensity structures. With more T2-weighted pulse sequences, the visualization of the seminal vesicles becomes difficult.

In the axial plane, the seminal vesicles are seen in their characteristic bow-tie appearance posterior to the bladder (Fig. 10-4*C*). These should normally be symmetrical, although distension of the rectum may produce a false asymmetry. In this situation, sagittal scans may be helpful in defining their size and position.

Penis and Scrotum

The corpora cavernosa and corpus spongiosum are well visualized with moderate intensity on most spin-echo sequences. Both the corpora cavernosa muscle and the bulbospongiosus muscle are imaged with low intensity and are easily distinguished from the corporal parenchyma (Fig. 10-7).

The spermatic cord includes the ductus deferens and the internal spermatic artery and vein. It may be imaged in both the axial and coronal planes. Occasionally it is possible to display the entire cord and testis in a single coronal slice (Fig. 10-5*A*). The testis and epididymis may be seen in the scrotum to have similar medium-intensity signals. They can be distinguished only by shape and location.

The Female Pelvis

The female reproductive tract is adequately imaged by MR. Multiplanar images of the normal female pelvis appear in Figures 10-8, 10-9, and 10-10. A suggested protocol for imaging the female pelvis is included in Table 10-1.

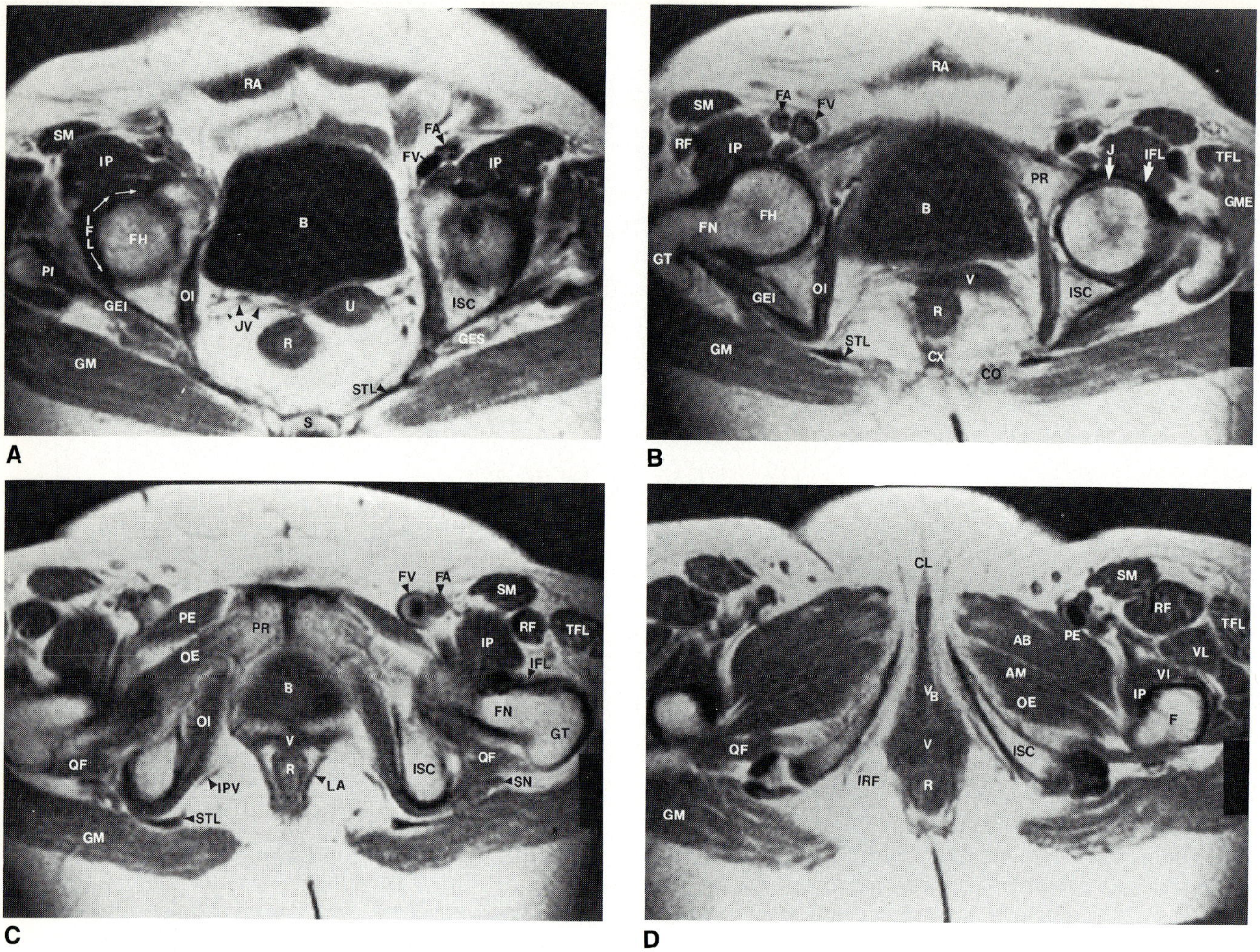

FIGURE 10-8

Axial SE 500/25 images of female pelvis and hips. (Images obtained on Magniscan 5000, Thompson-CGR MR system)

A	anus
AB	adductor brevis muscle
AC	ascending colon
AM	adductor magnus muscle
AO	aorta
AR	acetabular roof
B	bladder
BL	broad ligament
C	cervix
CE	cecum
CIA	common iliac arteries
CL	clitoris
CO	coccygeus muscle
CX	coccyx
ES	erector spinae muscle
FA, FV	femoral artery, vein
FH, FV	femoral head, neck
GEI, GES	gemelli inferior and superior muscles
GM	gluteus maximus muscle
GME	gluteus medius muscle
GMI	gluteus minimus muscle
GT	greater trochanter
I	ilium
IC	iliac crest
IFL	ischiofemoral ligament
IP	iliopsoas muscle
IPV	internal pudendal vessels
IRF	ischiorectal fossa
ISC	ischium
J	hip joint
L3, 4, 5	lumbar vertebrae 3, 4, 5
LA	levator ani muscle
LB	labia
LM	longissimus muscle
O	ovary
OE, OI	obturator externus and internus muscles
PE	pectineus muscle
PF	posterior fornix of vagina
PI	piriformis muscle
PM	psoas muscle
PR	pubic ramus
QF	quadratus femoris muscle
QL	quadratus lumborum muscle
R	rectum
RA	rectus abdominus muscle
RF	rectus femoris muscle
S	sacrum
S1	first sacral segment
SIG	sigmoid colon
SM	sartorius muscle
SN	sciatic nerve
SR	short rotators of the hip
STL	sacrotuberous ligament
TFL	tensor fascia lata muscle
U	uterus
UA, UV	uterine artery, vein
UM	umbilicus
V	vagina
VB	vaginal bulb
VI	vastus intermedius muscle
VL	vastus lateralis muscle

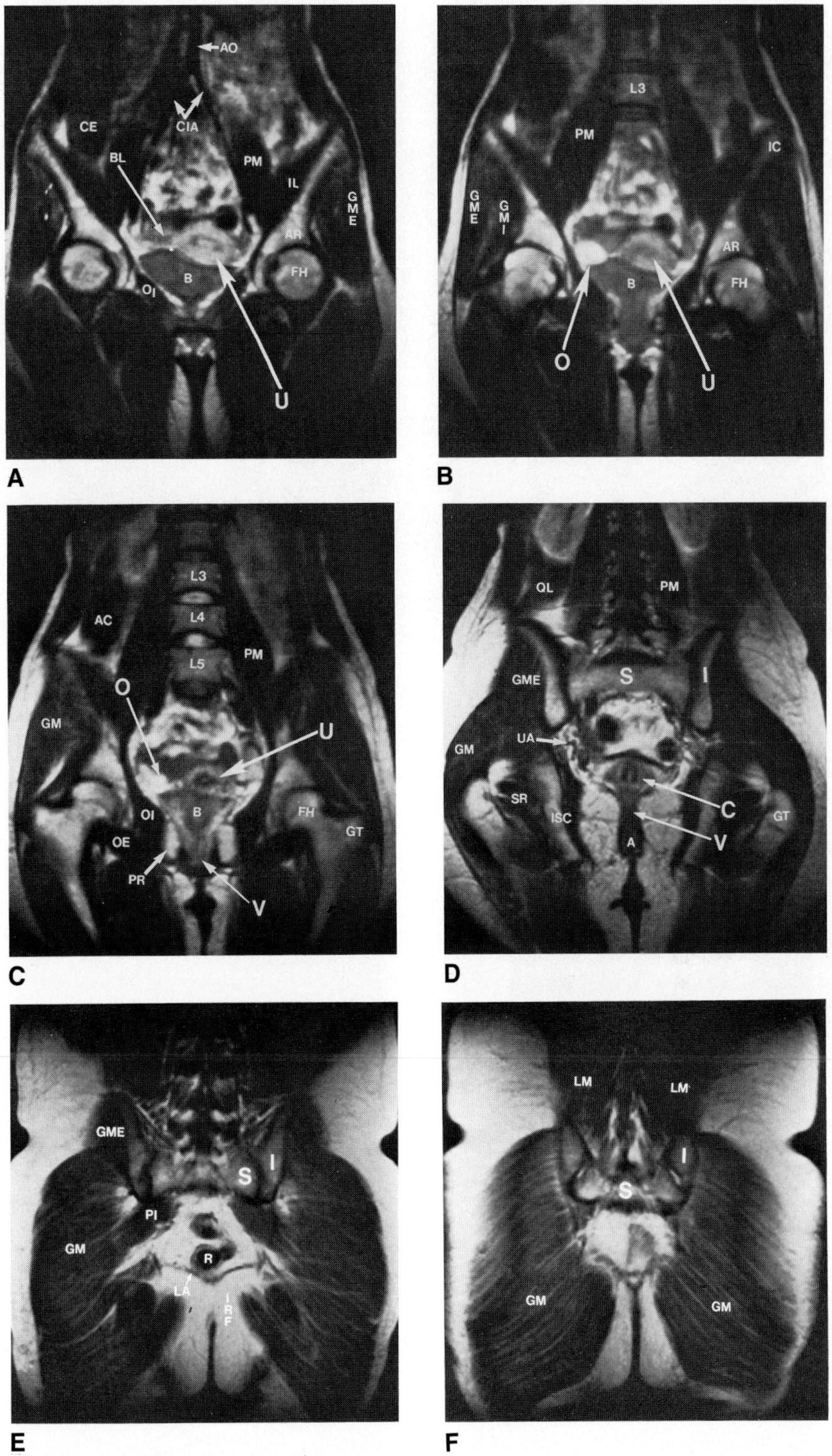

FIGURE 10-9

Coronal SE 1500/60 images of the female pelvis. (Courtesy of Picker International, Clinical Sciences Center)

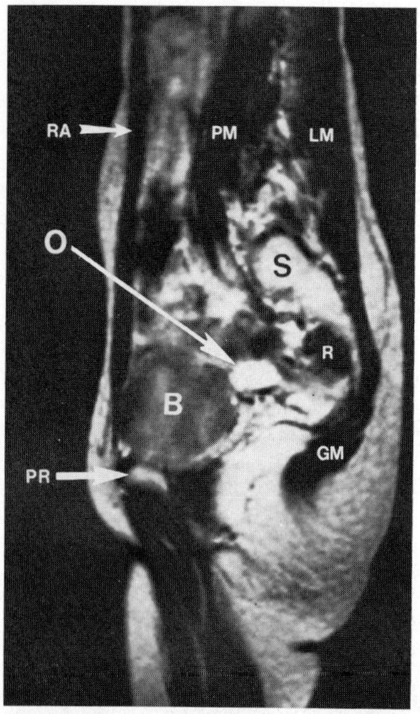

A

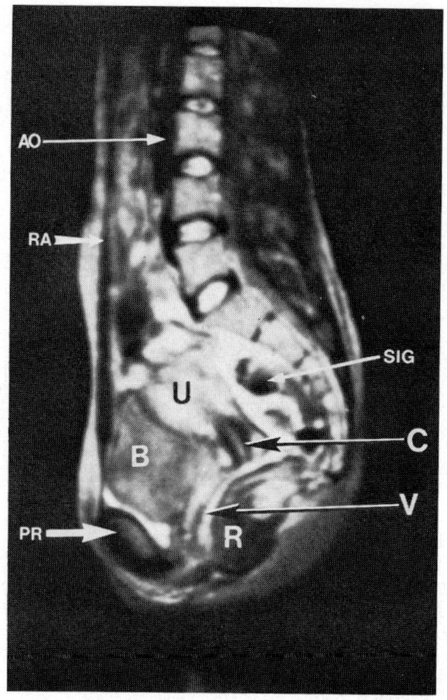

B

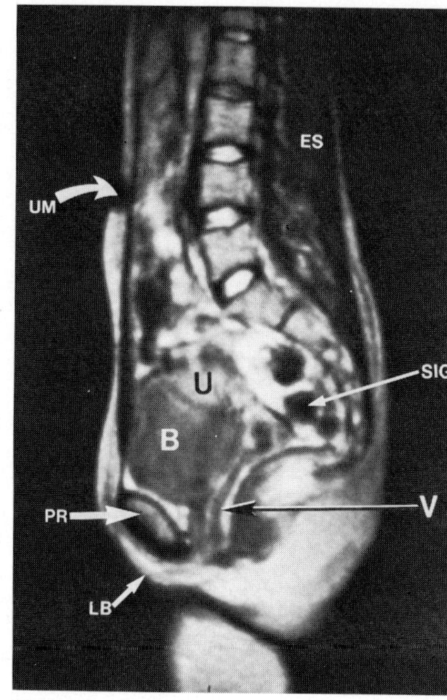

C

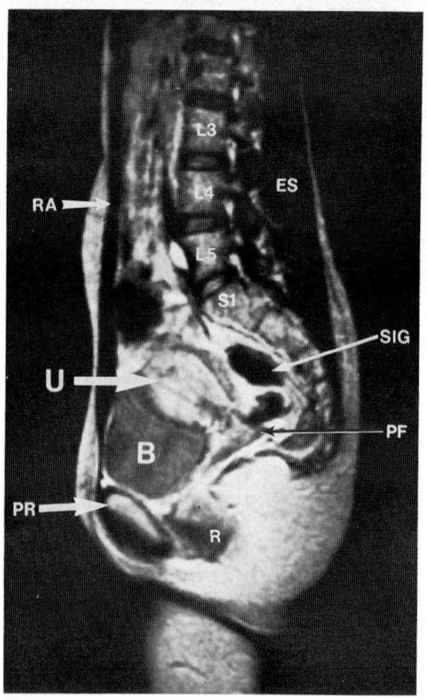

D

FIGURE 10-10

Sagittal SE 1500/60 images of the female pelvis. (Courtesy of Picker International, Clinical Sciences Center)

AO	aorta
B	bladder
C	cervix
ES	erector spinae muscle
GM	gluteus maximus muscle
L3, 4, 5	lumbar vertebrae 3, 4, 5
LB	labia
LM	longissimus muscle
O	ovary
PF	posterior fornix of vagina
PM	psoas muscle
PR	pubic ramus
R	rectum
RA	rectus abdominus muscle
S	sacrum
S1	first sacral segment
SIG	sigmoid colon
U	uterus
UM	umbilicus
V	vagina

FIGURE 10-11

(*A*) The uterus (U) is seen to have three signals. The highest intensity is seen centrally (E) and represents endometrium. A darker band separates the endometrium from the surrounding myometrium. (*B*) The dark band posterior to the uterus (open arrows) represents a frequency shift artifact and should not be misinterpreted as a normal structure. Note also B = bladder; O = ovary; U = uterus. (Courtesy of Picker International, Clinical Sciences Center) (*C*) The endometrial signal (arrow) becomes larger and more intense just before menses.

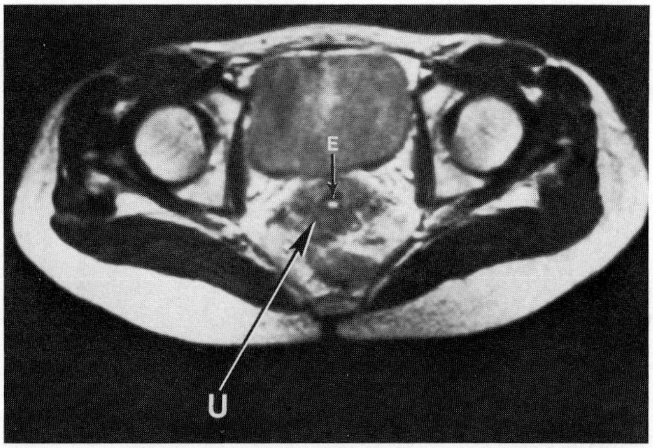

A

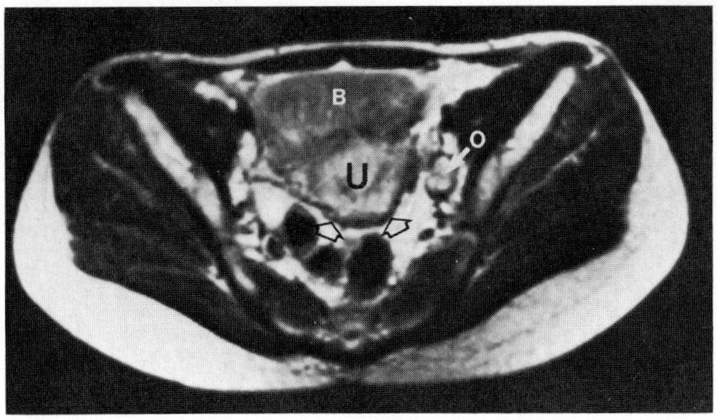

B

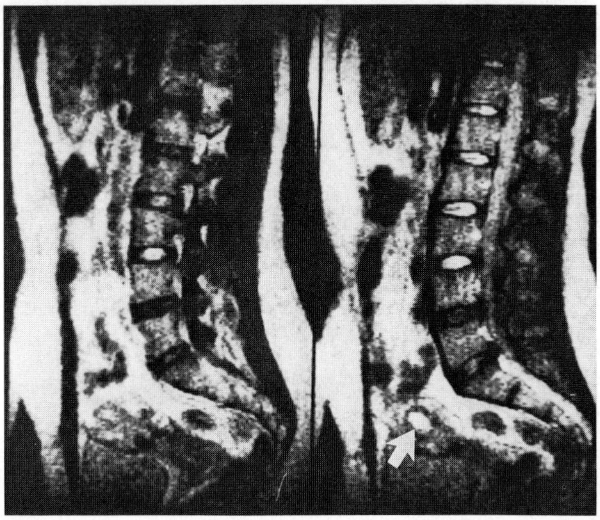

C

The Uterus

Depending on its degree of version, the uterus occupies a somewhat variable position in the pelvis. Accordingly, it may be imaged in all planes, although the sagittal and coronal planes are often preferable. Both T1- and T2-weighted sequences may be necessary to detect and characterize most types of lesions.

When a T2-weighted sequence is performed, it is possible to note three signals from within the uterus. The endometrium usually shows the highest signal intensity and is separated from the moderate-intensity myometrium by a low-intensity band (Fig. 10-11). Early investigators proposed that this band represented the stratum basale. No histologic proof, however, has been put forth to substantiate this claim. Indeed, since the stratum basale is only a few cells thick, it seems unlikely that it is being imaged *per se*. The precise anatomic correlate of this structure remains unknown.

Endonmetrial thickness and MR signal vary through the menstrual cycle, being minimal immediately after menses and maximal at midsecretory phase. The T2 of myometrium is also higher during the secretory phase. Women on birth control pills often show endometrial atrophy, lack of junctional zone, and poor separation of endometrial and myometrial signals. Postmenarchal uteri become atrophic, and the length of the corpus equals that of the cervix.

The Cervix

The normal cervix usually demonstates only two zones on T2-weighted images. The central high-intensity region represents cervical endothelium and mucus. A low-intensity zone representing fibrous

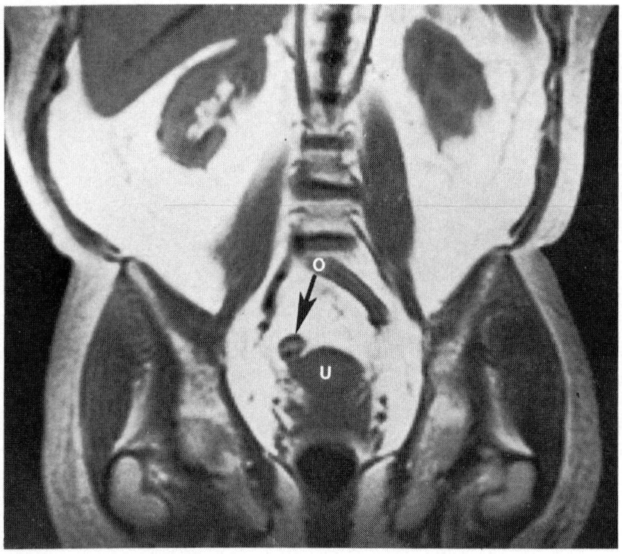

A

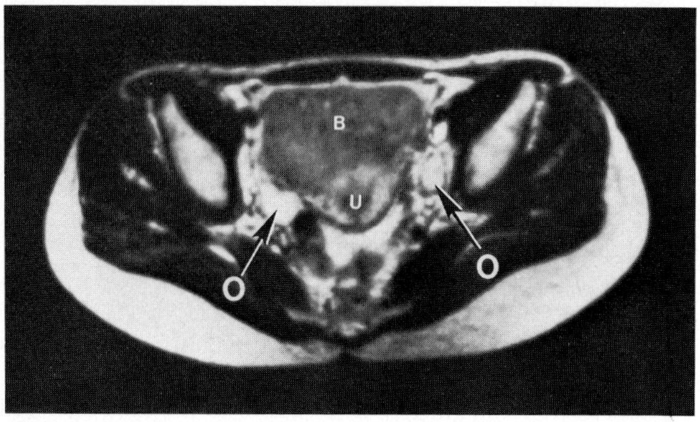

B

FIGURE 10-12

(*A*) The ovaries appear darker relative to retroperitoneal fat on T1-weighted sequences. O = ovary; U = uterus; (Images obtained on Magniscan 5000, Thompson-CGR MR system, SE 500/25) (*B*) The ovaries (O) show high intensity on T2-weighted pulse sequences, such as SE 1500/60. B = bladder; U = uterus. (Courtesy of Picker International, Clinical Sciences Center)

cervical stroma surrounds the first. Occasionally, a third intermediate band similar to that in the uterus is also noted. Cervical signal changes during the menstrual cycle. The cervix is best visualized on axial or sagittal T2-weighted images.

The Adnexae

The broad ligament of the uterus with its vessels maybe identified on axial or coronal images (Fig. 10-8*A*). The fallopian tubes are difficult to define reliably. The ovaries are surrounded by fat but possess relatively long T1 and T2 values. On T2-weighted sequences, they may become of quite bright intensity (Fig. 10-12*B*). At intermediate ranges near this contrast reversal point, they may be difficult to distinguish from surrounding fat. The axial plane seems adequate for imaging the normal ovary and for evaluating spread of ovarian malignancy.

The Vagina and Female Genitalia

Use of a tampon during scanning facilitates accurate evaluation of the vagina. Long spin-echo sequences define the vaginal wall and lower-intensity lumen. The sagittal or coronal planes seem best for vaginal imaging (Fig. 10-10*B,C*) The clitoris and vaginal bulb are seen in axial section (Fig. 10-8*D*).

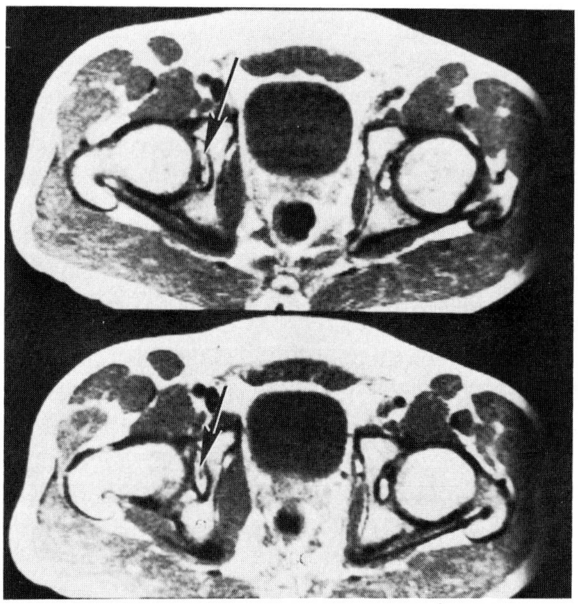

FIGURE 10-13

Acetabular cartilage of hip (arrows) seen on axial SE 1000/28 image.

The Hips

The bony acetabulum is composed of low-intensity cortical bone surrounding a high-intensity central medullary cavity. The articular cartilage may be identified as a thin layer of tissue of higher intensity than cortical bone but less than bone marrow (Fig. 10-13). The iliofemoral ligaments may be noted, especially on axial images, as thick low-intensity bands (Fig. 10-8*A*,*B* and 10-14). These ligaments merge with the capsule of the hip and cannot be distinguished from the capsule. The surrounding musculature is well visualized on all imaging sequences because of a naturally high contrast between muscle and fat.

The femoral head, like the acetabulum and other large bones, consists of a thin rim of low-intensity cortex and a high-intensity central medullary cavity containing fat and blood. Two low-intensity bands traverse the femoral head (Fig. 10-15). The first of these runs transversely and is quite narrow. This represents the physis. The second low-intensity band is much broader and more vertically oriented; this corresponds to a collection of central weight-bearing trabeculae.

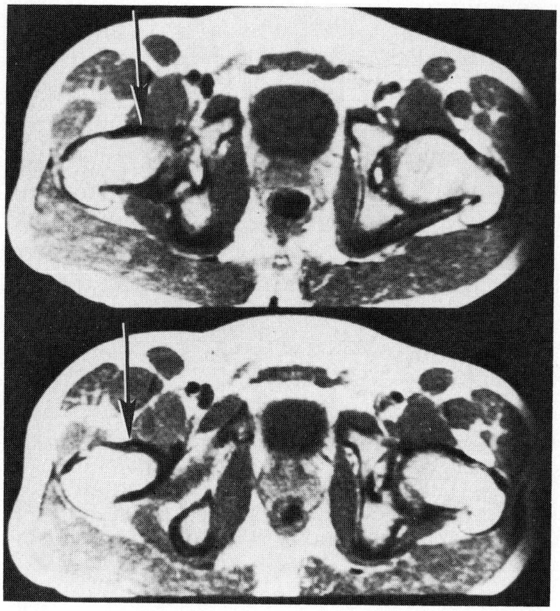

FIGURE 10-14

The hip capsule merges with the ischiofemoral ligaments, both being seen as dark bands anteriorly (arrows).

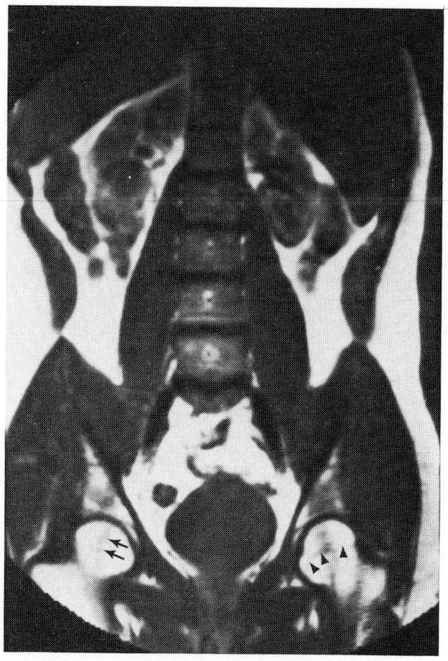

FIGURE 10-15

Two dark bands normally traverse the femoral head. Arrowheads show the horizontal band representing the physis. Arrows on opposite hip show a band representing weight-bearing trabeculae. (Courtesy of Picker International, Clinical Sciences Center)

To the present, most MR studies of the hip have centered on diseases of the femoral head, usually aseptic necrosis. Relatively little is known about other diseases affecting this area. The femoral head seems best imaged on short spin-echo sequences (*e.g.,* SE 500/30). Coronal images are most easily correlated with radiographs and are most readily accepted by referring physicians. Additionally, coronal images seem best suited for displaying the subcortical cancellous bone of the superior femoral head, which may be the earliest region involved by aseptic necrosis. Axial images may be useful for visualizing surrounding muscle and fascial planes. Joint effusions in the hip are most easily detected in this projection.

Axial, coronal, and sagittal views of the hip have been included with those of the male and female pelvis in Figures 10-4 through 10-10. A suggested protocol for imaging the hip is presented in Table 10-2.

TABLE 10-2

Possible Protocol for MRI of the Hips

Indications:

1. Early aseptic necrosis (best seen in coronal plane)
2. Joint effusion (best seen in axial plane)
3. Tumors, masses

Protocol:

1. Axial plane SE 1500/30,60
2. Coronal plane SE 1000/30,60

CHAPTER 11

Surface Coil Applications: Spine, Breast, and Knee

Surface coil technology may be used for MRI of other regions of the body, in addition to the orbit and temporal bone, discussed in Chapter 7. These regions include the cervical spine, thoracic spine, lumbar spine, breast, and knee. Other superficial structures in the body are potentially amenable to surface coil imaging, including all the extremities and their articulations. Because general clinical experience worldwide is limited in these other regions, they will not be discussed here. Instead, we will concentrate on the anatomy and MRI strategies of the spine, breast, and knee, visualized with and without surface coils.

The Cervical Spine

MR holds an advantage over CT in the evaluation of the cervical spine and spinal cord similar to that in the posterior fossa. Namely, dense bone beam-hardening artifacts in these regions, which plague CT, are not a problem for MRI. MRI also allows accurate delineation of the cord and lower brain stem. It is thus much more sensitive than CT for detecting intramedullary tumors and other lesions.

Inversion recovery techniques appear to offer no advantage in the cervical spine but are useful where subtle T1 differentiation may be needed. However, in the spinal canal, the T1 values of vertebrae, fat, cerebrospinal fluid (CSF), and cord are sufficiently different so that the longer image acquisition times and loss of T2 information make inversion recovery seem unwarranted. Short spin-echo techniques (*e.g.,* SE 500/30) have been found to be ideal for anatomic definition. Short spin-echo techniques have proved most useful in evaluation of Chiari malformations and syringomyelia, in which the short spin-echo technique has been called the sequence of choice.

Longer spin-echo sequences (*e.g.,* SE 3000/60 or 1500/90) provide T2-weighted information. These are useful in evaluating tumors and other mass lesions within or adjacent to the spinal cord (*e.g.,* abscess, hematoma). Intramedullary lesions of multiple sclerosis may also be appreciated. Intervertebral disk protrusions are also best evaluated using these longer spin-echo techniques. A change in signal of the degenerating disk may be better appreciated than on the short spin-echo sequence. Furthermore, the CSF is rendered relatively white compared with the vertebral body and disk. An "MR myelogram" may thus be obtained.

Sagittal imaging is recommended in nearly all cases for several reasons. It allows visualization of the entire cervical cord with a minimum number of slices. It allows accurate assessment of the lower brain stem and cerebellar tonsils in cases of suspected Chiari malformation. The extent of upward or downward migration of herniated disk may be assessed. Likewise, the extent of tumor may be estimated.

Axial imaging is recommended in addition to sagittal projection because it may better demonstrate the lateral extension of disk herniation or tumor. Occasionally, slit-like syrinxes may only be appreciated in the axial plane. Coronal projections are not generally as helpful. However, occasional asymmetries such as unilateral tonsilar herniation and internal architecture of hydromyelic cavities may be better appreciated coronally.

Routine axial, coronal, and sagittal views of the cervical spine and paraspinous musculature have been included with the images of the neck in Chapter 7 (Fig. 7–30 through 7–32). The use of specialty surface coils for the neck allows even greater detail to be obtained. Examples of coronal and sagittal surface coil images of the cervical spine are presented in Figures 11-1 and 11-2.

The precise boundaries of the craniocervical junction may be somewhat difficult to define by MRI. Note that the posterior rim of the foramen magnum is not as consistently localized as is the anterior rim (clivus) because it is composed of cortical bone, which casts little MR signal (Fig. 11-3). Similarly, the odontoid process of C2 contains primarily cortical bone and casts little MR signal compared with the C2 vertebral body. On the T1-weighted images, it is difficult to distinguish the posterior margins of the vertebral bodies and the CSF. The cortical posterior margins appear dark because they have few hydrogen protons. The CSF appears dark because of its long T1 value (recalling the inverse relationship between T1 and signal intensity on short spin-echo sequences.)

For completeness, note that it is possible to obtain direct oblique images of the cervical spine on certain commercial scanners, as shown in Figure 11-4. The clinical utility of such a technique in the cervical spine is yet to be determined, although the oblique anatomy is elegantly displayed.

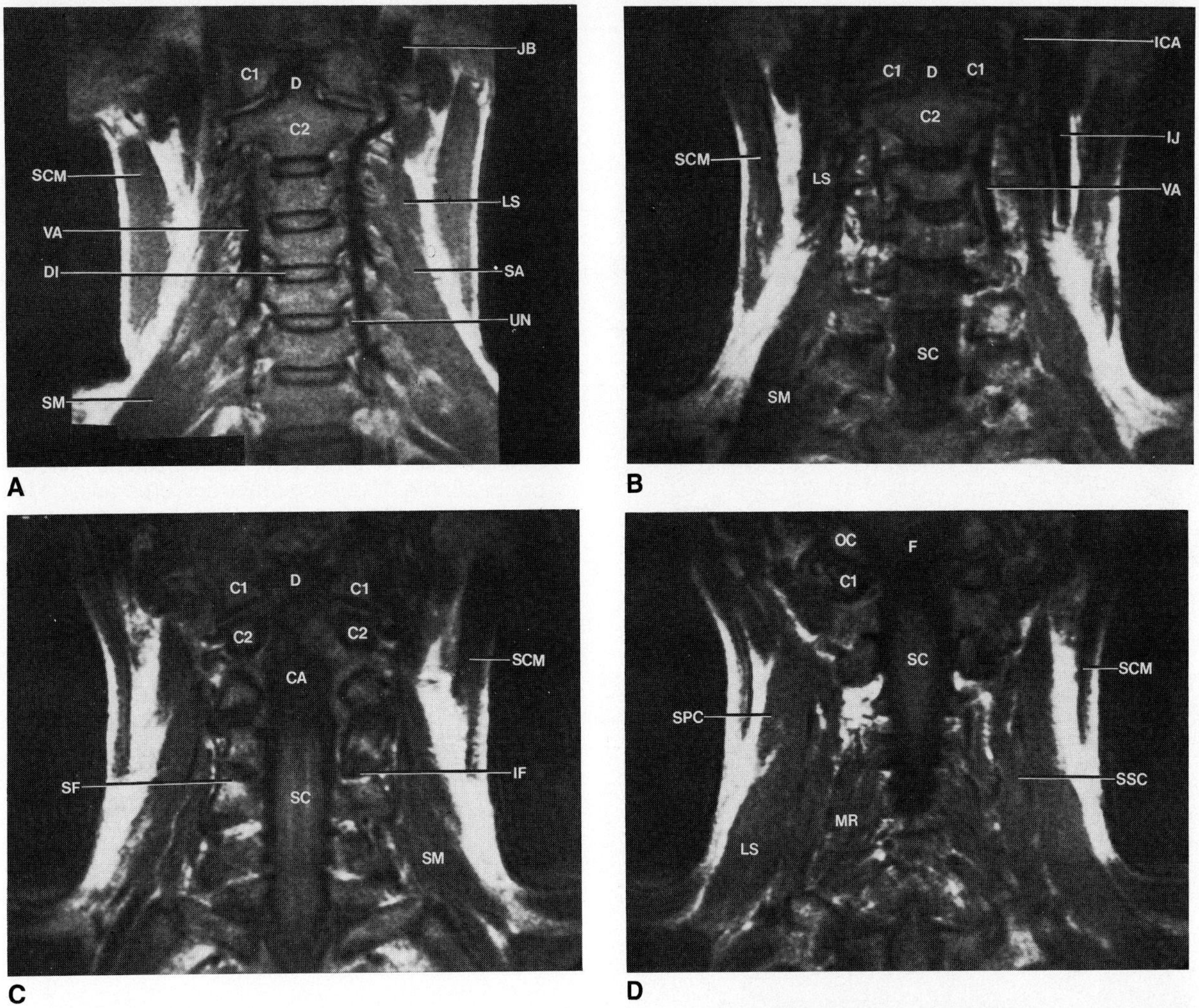

FIGURE 11-1

Coronal surface coil SE 388/28 images of the cervical spine. (Courtesy of Fonar Corporation, 110 Marcus Drive, Melville, NY 11747)

C1, C2	vertebral bodies (atlas, axis)
CA	spinal canal
D	dens
DI	intervertebral disk
F	foramen magnum
ICA	internal carotid artery
IF	inferior articular facet C4
IJ	internal jugular vein
JB	jugular bulb
LC	longus colli muscle
LS	levator scapulae muscle
MR	multifidus and rotatores cervicis muscles
OC	occipital condyle
SA	scalenus anterior muscle
SC	spinal cord
SCM	sternocleidomastoid muscle
SF	superior articular facet C5
SM	scalene middle muscle
SPC	splenius cervicis muscle
SSC	semispinalis capitis muscle
UN	uncinate process C6
VA	vertebral artery

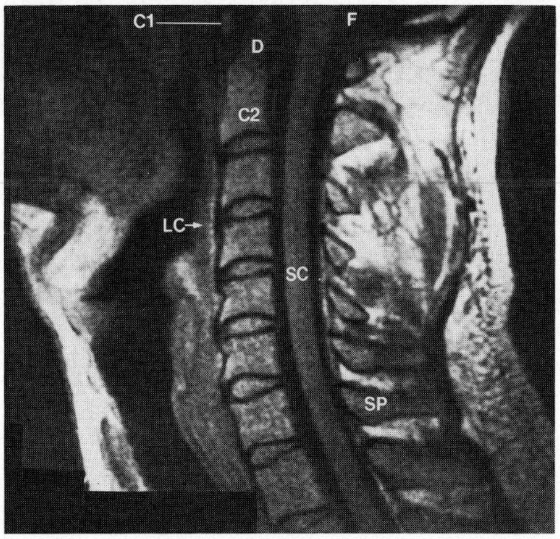

FIGURE 11-2

Sagittal surface coil SE 388/28 image of the cervical spine and cord. (Courtesy of Fonar Corporation, 110 Marcus Drive, Melville, NY 11747)

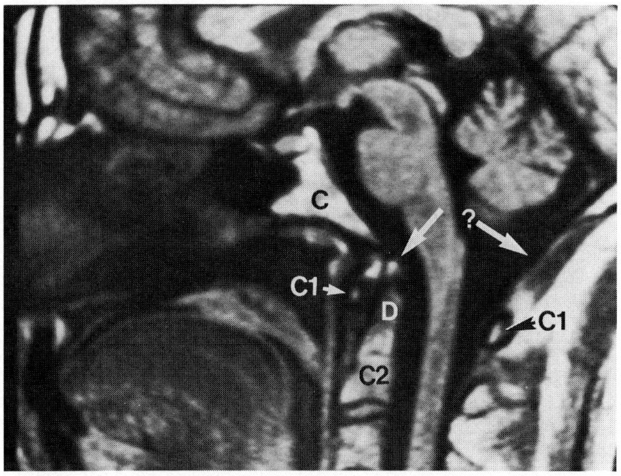

FIGURE 11-3

The cervicocranium is seen on this SE 400/28 sagittal image. The anterior and posterior arches of the atlas (C1) are seen, as well as the dens (D) and body of the axis (C2). Note that on such heavily T1-weighted images the posterior cortex of the vertebral body is difficult to distinguish from spinal fluid. The anterior rim of the foramen magnum (white arrow) is barely discernible here, aided by the large component of fatty marrow in the clivus (C). The posterior margin of the foramen magnum is difficult to define precisely (? arrow). Determination of tonsilar herniation can sometimes be unreliable. (Courtesy of Fonar Corporation, 110 Marcus Drive, Melville, NY 11747)

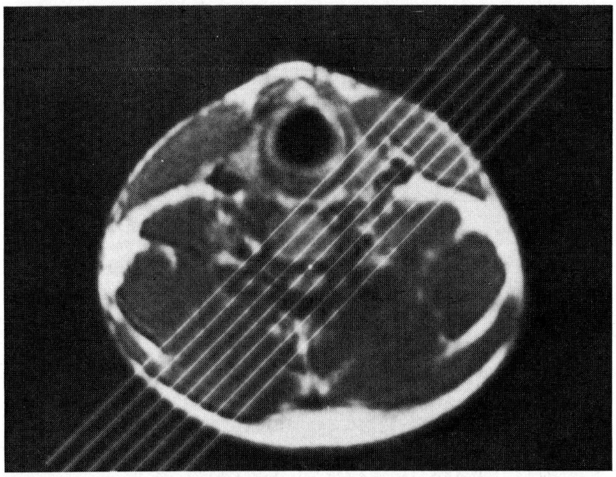

A

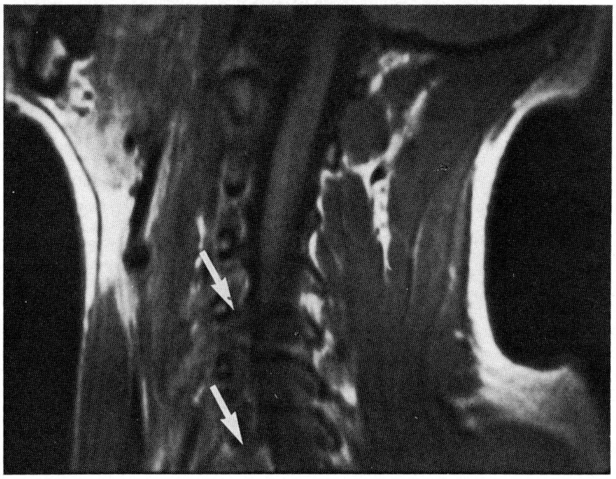

B

FIGURE 11-4

On some commercial scanners, oblique imaging is possible by selecting lines through a scout axial image (*A*). In the cervical spine, this allows visualization of nerve roots (arrows, 11-4*B*) as they exit beneath the pedicles. (Courtesy of Fonar Corporation, 110 Marcus Drive, Melville, NY 11747)

Thoracic Spine

Experience with MR imaging of the thoracic spine is limited. Except for posttraumatic problems and occasional tumors, pathological conditions confined to the thoracic spine are much less common than those of the cervical or lumbar regions. Since disk herniation is most unusual in the thoracic spine, it is probably more critical for MR techniques to be sensitive to tumors and vascular malformations.

In general, the same imaging principles discussed for the cervical and lumbar spine apply to the thoracic spine. Because of the large number of levels that must be scanned, direct sagittal imaging may be the only plane chosen. Because of normal thoracic kyphosis, coronal imaging displays only short, discontinuous segments of the thoracic spine and is of limited use. When an abnormality is suspected clinically or on sagittal images, direct axial scans through the region of interest should be performed.

Sagittal SE 1000/28 images through the upper thoracic spine are shown in Figure 11-5. The more lateral image demonstrates nerve roots in the intervertebral foramina. Figure 11-6 shows sagittal images from the lower thoracic spine. Here can be seen some Schmorl's nodes and the conus medullaris. Note that in sagittal images just off the midline, partial volume effects with the cord and pedicles may cast confusing signals, which should not be misinterpreted as pathological processes.

FIGURE 11-5

Sagittal SE 1000/28 image of the upper thoracic spine. In *A*, vertebral bodies T1 through T6 and their spinous processes (arrowheads) are noted. The variation in size and signal intensity in the cord is due to a slight degree of scoliosis, which takes it in and out of the plane of imaging. In *B*, about 1 cm laterally to *A*, the pedicles (P) may be seen, as well as nerve roots (arrowheads) in the intervertricular foramina.

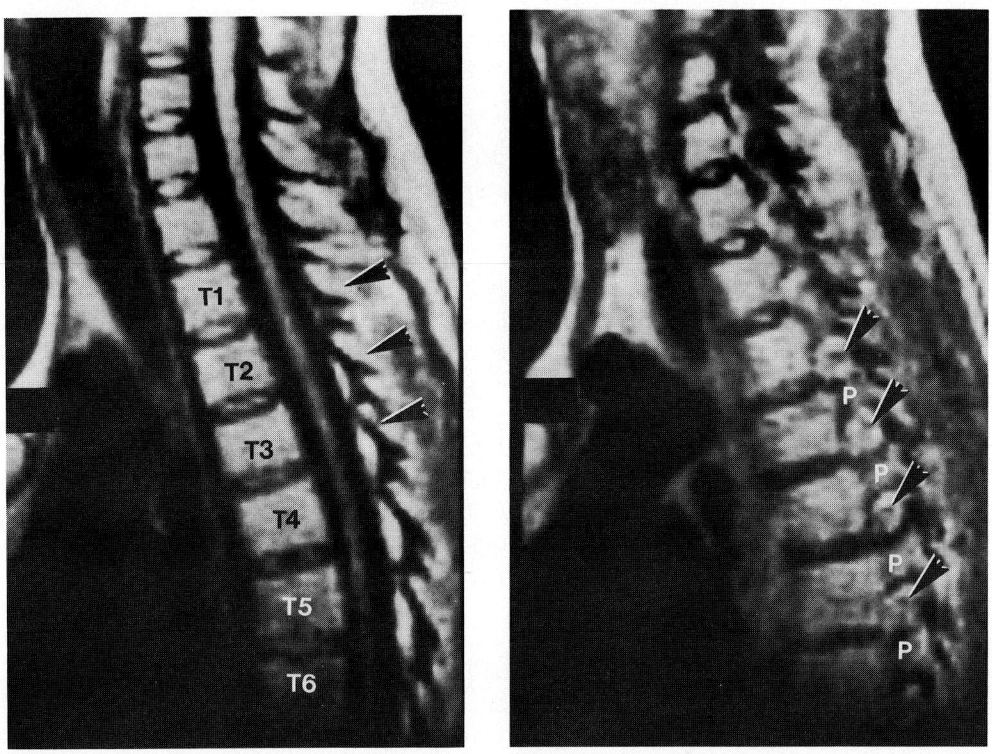

A **B**

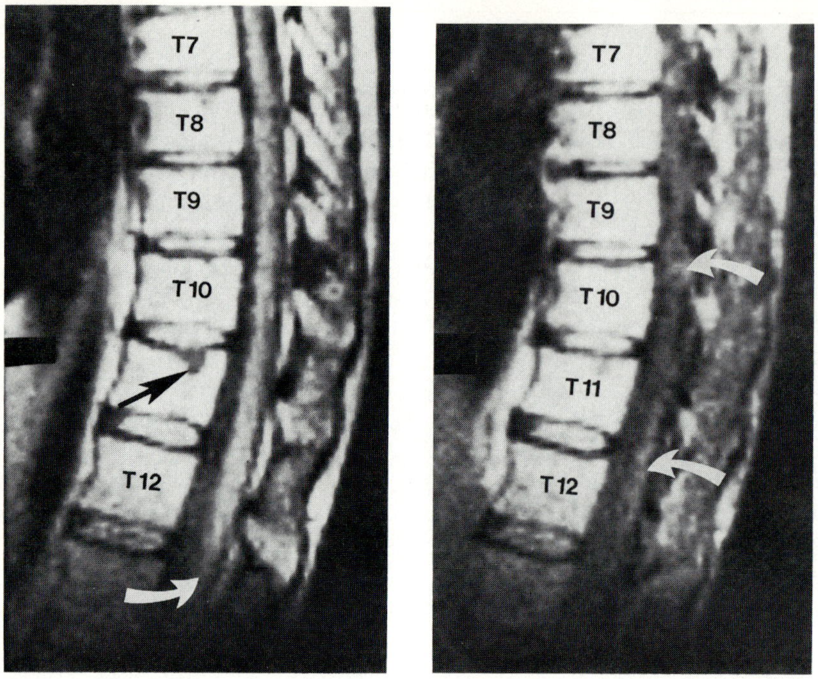

FIGURE 11-6
Sagittal SE 1000/28 images of the lower thoracic spine. In *A* can be noted a Schmorl's node (black arrow) and the conus medullaris (white arrow) at T12–L1. In *B*, partial voluming of the cord and conus produces confusing signals within the spinal canal (arrows), which should not be construed as representing a pathological process.

Lumbar Spine

During the past 5 years, CT has established a record of high sensitivity and accuracy in the evaluation of the lumbar spine. A great advantage of CT has been its ability to detect soft tissue lesions (such as disk herniation) as well as bony disease (such as spinal stenosis) in a single noninvasive examination. MR thus faces a formidable opponent if it seeks to replace CT as a primary imaging modality for the lumbar spine.

Despite the advances of CT, several limitations have become apparent. First of all, CT covers a relatively limited field of view (routine scanning is usually performed only from L3 to S1 at most centers). Second, high-resolution CT scans can be performed only in the axial plane, and the resolution of reformatted sagittal or coronal images is limited. Third, the lower thoracic cord and conus medullaris are not well evaluated by CT, even when the field of scanning is expanded to include these structures. Finally, certain clinical problems such as differentiating postoperative scar from recurrent disk herniation remain unsatisfactorily solved by CT.

MRI offers the potential to overcome some of these limitations of CT. Routine direct sagittal imaging allows visualization of the thoracic cord, conus medullaris, and the entire lumbar canal. In addition to providing anatomic information, MRI also offers the ability to detect subtle changes in signal intensity of degenerating disks and spinal tumors. The capacity to distinguish postoperative scar from disk has already been proved in many cases.

Nevertheless, certain features of MR spinal imaging still limit its full application. First of all, MRI is not yet accurate in defining spinal lesions that are primarily bony (stenosis and facet disease). Cortical bone and osteophytes have little MR signal because of their paucity of hydrogen protons. The effects of such bony abnormalities must be indirectly witnessed with MR imaging, by the distortion of the dural sac or obliteration of extradural fat planes. Similarly, calcified disk fragments may be "MR-invisible," their presence being detected only by indirect effects. Finally, the resolution of MRI in the axial plane is still inferior to that possible with the best CT scanners. Further refinements with surface coil technology should eliminate this final disadvantage.

Knowledge of several biophysical features will assist in understanding the imaging characteristics of the spine in health and disease. Table 11-1 lists approximate T1 and T2 values for normal and abnormal disk material. Note that normal nucleus pulposus has relatively long T1 and T2 values compared with either degenerating nucleus pulposus or normal annulus fibrosus. This might be expected, because the gelatinous normal nucleus pulposus has a higher water content.

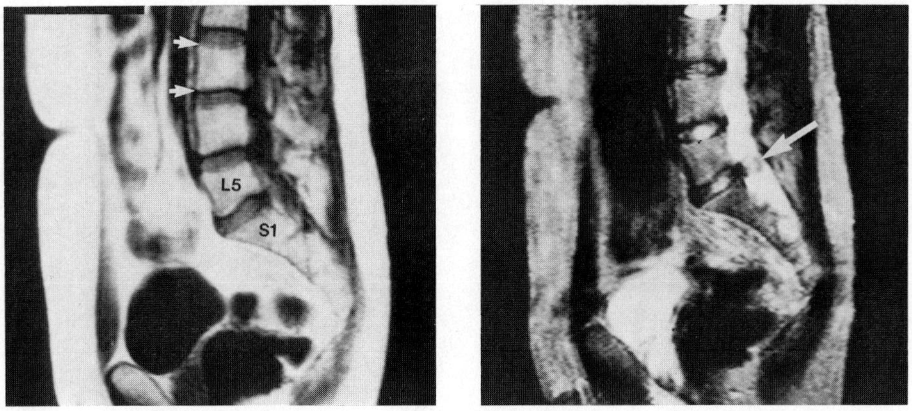

A B

FIGURE 11-7

Pulse sequences in spinal imaging. A T1-weighted sequence such as this SE 500/30 allows for rapid localization and visualization of anatomic relationships. The CSF appears black, disk material gray, and marrow in the vertebral bodies white. Note that the lower vertebral end-plate is dark whereas the upper one is white (arrows). This represents a frequency shift artifact, as discussed in Chapter 5. Note also that there is some separation of the CSF from the posterior margins of L5 and S1, suggesting disk herniation, although its margins are somewhat ill defined. (*B*) The sagittal image, performed with SE 3000/120 technique. The nucleus pulposus is now very bright, as is CSF. Herniated disk at L5–S1 is easily seen silhouetted in this MR myelogram. (Courtesy of Technicare Corporation and Cleveland Clinic, Technicare Corp © 1985)

With aging and degeneration, a number of biochemical changes occur in the intervertebral disk. In young patients, the water content of the nucleus pulposus is approximately 85% to 90%, but this value drops to 70% in old age and with degeneration. The annulus fibrosus water content in youth is about 78%; this decreases to 70% with aging and degeneration. Changes in water content alone only incompletely explain imaging characteristics of the disk. Complex biochemical changes such as mucopolysaccharide and chondroitin sulfate content must also be considered.

TABLE 11-1

Approximate T1 and T2 Values of Normal and Abnormal Intervertebral Disks*

	T1 (msec)	T2 (msec)
Normal anulus fibrosus	420	30
Normal nucleus pulposus	740	85
Degenerated nucleus pulposus	625	38

* Average of *in vivo* and *in vitro* measurements.

(Adapted from Modic MT, Pavlicek W, Weinstein MA et al: Magnetic resonance imaging of intervertebral disk disease. Radiology 152:103, 1984)

MR imaging strategies for the lumbar spine at present are open to debate. Investigators at several centers have shown equivalent diagnostic power between MR and CT for demonstrating intervertebral disk disease. The final and optimal strategies will not be determined until surface coils and thin-section capabilities are fully implemented.

As elsewhere in the body, it is generally recognized that both T1- and T2-weighted pulse sequences are needed for optimum anatomic delineation and detection of pathological conditions. What these sequences should be, however, is still controversial.

A short spin-echo technique (*e.g.,* SE 500/30) is useful initially for several reasons (Fig. 11-7*A*). First, it allows for rapid localization and patient positioning. Epidural fat is well delineated with high-intensity signal (short T1). The recognition of this fat is im-

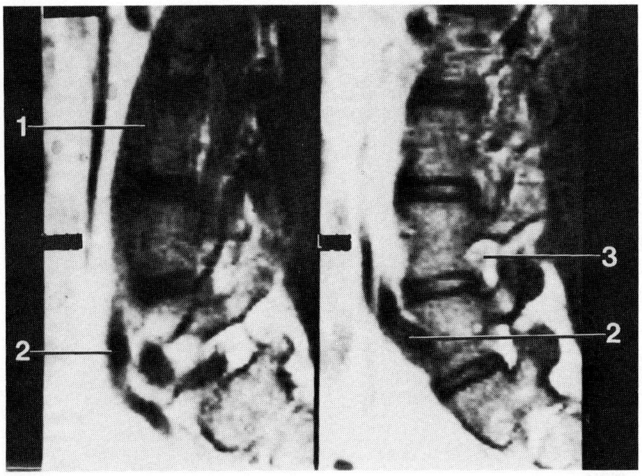

A

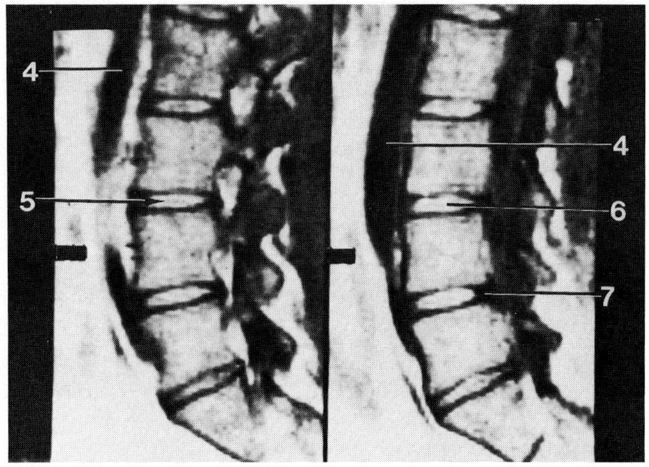

B

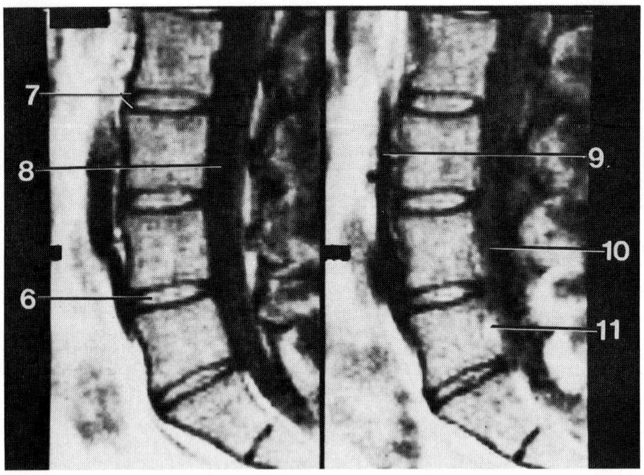

C

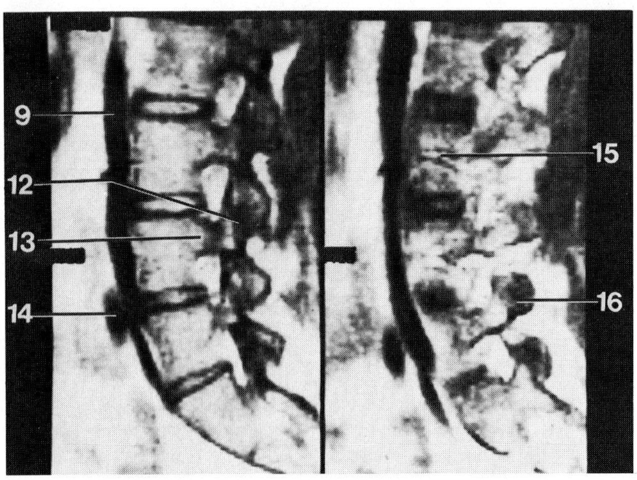

D

FIGURE 11-8

Sagittal SE 1000/28 images of the lumbar spine in a normal volunteer, from left to right in 5-mm increments. Note especially the components of the intervertebral disk. The anulus fibrosus (7) and vertebral end-plates are both low intensity and difficult to distinguish except anteriorly and posteriorly. The nucleus pulposus (6) is of rather high signal intensity. Centrally within the nucleus pulposus is a low-intensity intranuclear cleft (5), which corresponds to the central region seen on diskography.

1 psoas muscle
2 left iliac vein
3 nerve root in intervertebral foramen
4 aorta
5 intranuclear cleft
6 nucleus pulposus
7 anulus fibrosus
8 dural sac
9 inferior vena cava
10 lateral recess
11 epidural fat
12 facet joint
13 pedicle
14 right iliac artery
15 lumbar vein
16 spinous process
17 nerve root in spinal canal
18 lamina

portant in evaluating the size of neural foramina, which may become obscured by high-intensity CSF on longer spin-echo sequences. Finally, short spin-echo techniques allow good differentiation of low-intensity CSF from higher-intensity spinal cord, conus, and nerve roots.

A second pulse sequence that is more T2 weighted should also be used. How heavily T2-weighted this sequence needs to be is still open to debate. At a minimum, SE 1500/30 or equivalent is required. It may be that very heavily T2-weighted sequences such as SE 3000/120 are needed for optimum diagnostic accuracy. Such sequences produce a stark white CSF (Fig. 11-7*B*) and have been termed an *MR-myelogram.*

Routine sagittal imaging has been the most reliable plane for defining spinal lesions by MRI to date. Examples of a series of parasagittal lumbar spine images are shown in Figure 11-8. Sagittal imaging has the advantage of scanning a long segment of the spinal canal in a short time with relatively few slices. Continuity of extruded disk material and deformities with spondylolisthesis may be better appreciated in this projection. However, it is often difficult to distinguish central from posterolateral disk herniations. Surprisingly, it can also be difficult to distinguish between right-and left-sided herniation as well, particularly if there is a small degree of scoliosis.

If on sagittal view an abnormality is suspected, a series of transaxial sections is mandatory. (Some would argue for routine axial imaging anyway.) Thinner slices will improve the accuracy of axial MR scanning; the price, of course, will be increased scanning time. Axial views through the upper and lower lumbar spine appear in Fig. 11-9.

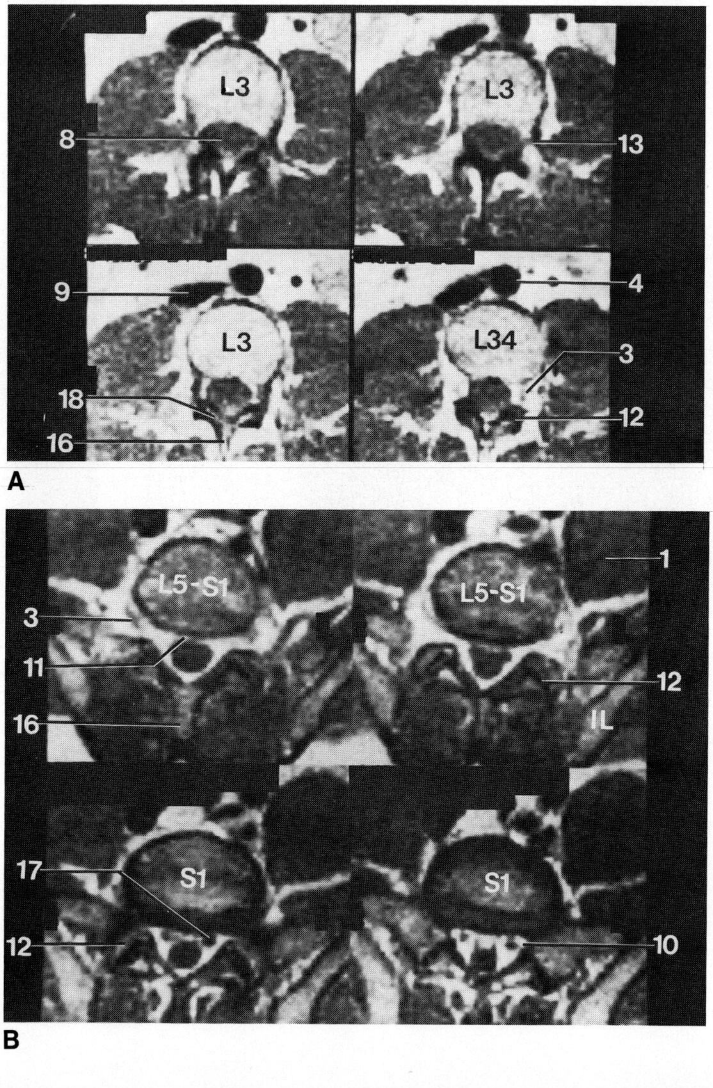

FIGURE 11-9

(*A*) Axial SE 1000/28 images at the L3–4 level. (*B*) Axial SE 1000/28 images at the L5–S1 level. Note similar anatomy to CT, although bony margins are not as well defined and spatial resolution is less.

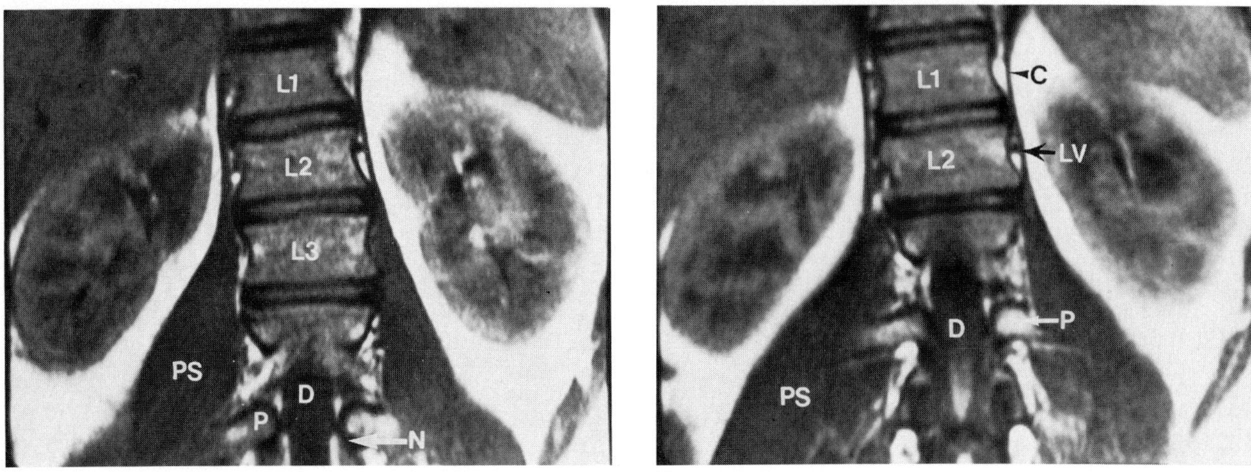

A B

FIGURE 11-10

Coronal SE 500/28 images of the midlumbar spine are of relatively limited usefulness (C = crus; D = dural sac; LV = lumbar vein; N = nerve root; P = pedicle; PS = psoas muscle). (Courtesy of Fonar Corporation, 110 Marcus Drive, Melville, NY 11747)

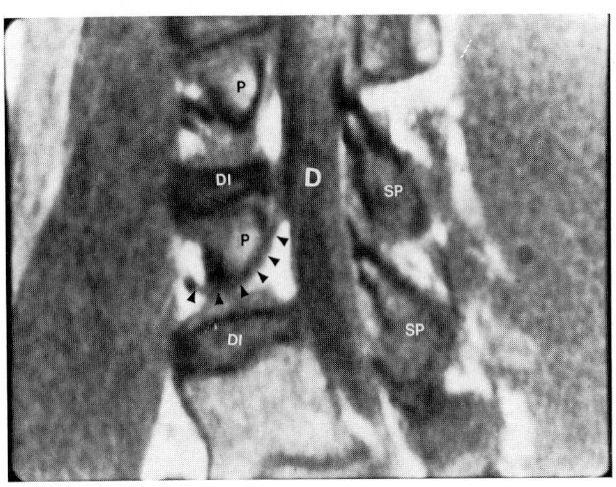

FIGURE 11-11

Oblique imaging of the lumbar spine may one day prove useful (D = dural sac; DI = disk; P = pedicle; SP = spinous process; arrowheads = spinal nerve exiting under pedicle). (Courtesy of Fonar Corporation, 110 Marcus Drive, Melville, NY 11747)

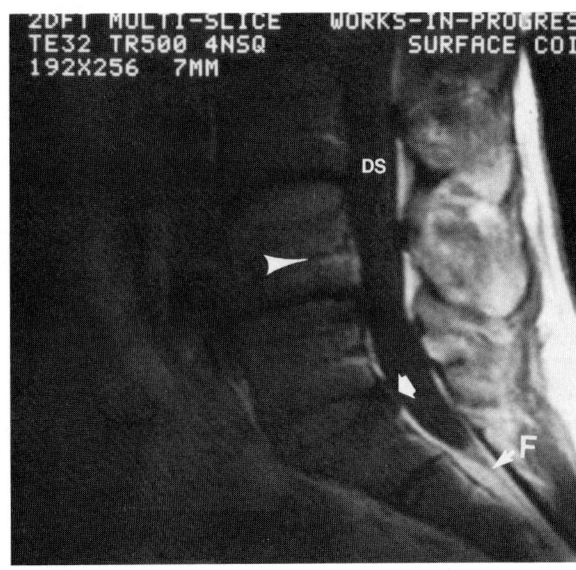

FIGURE 11-12

Experimental surface coils allow increased resolution and signal-to-noise ratios (DS = dural sac; F = filum terminale; arrowhead = basivertebral vein; short arrow = herniated disk obliterating epidural fat). (Courtesy of Technicare Corporation © 1985)

Coronal imaging (Fig. 11-10) may occasionally be useful but should probably not be part of a routine scanning protocol. As in the thoracic spine, normal spinal curvature (lordosis) allows one to view only short, discontinuous segments of the lumbar spine using conventional coronal imaging. On scanners that allow oblique imaging, 45° to 60° LPO and RPO projections may have diagnostic use (Fig. 11-11). In the future, surface coil technology will allow even greater delineation of normal anatomy and spinal lesions in a multiplanar format (Fig. 11-12).

The Breast

MRI will probably never surpass mammography for the detection and screening of breast cancer, although it may come to play an adjunctive role. MRI is incapable of detecting microcalcifications, and its resolution is limited. It is possible that MRI will be able to characterize larger lesions that are indeterminate by mammographic or ultrasonic criteria. MRI also allows evaluation of the prepectoral fascial plane. This advantage is at least equivalent to CT and ultrasonography and is superior to that of mammography. Finally, MRI uses no ionizing radiation and may be practical for certain patients who refuse mammography because of perceived x-irriadiation risks.

Table 11-2 lists some approximate T1 and T2 values recorded in the normal and abnormal breast. Unfortunately, there is sufficient overlap between malignant and nonmalignant tumor relaxation times to make certain distinction impossible. Cysts may be reliably diagnosed on the basis of prolonged T1 and T2 times. The distribution of fibroglandular and fatty tissues within the breast may be determined well enough to permit correlation with the mammographic patterns of Wolfe.

Table 11-3 presents a possible protocol for MRI of the breast. Although authorities may disagree about precise imaging strategies, several features seem clear. First, surface coils are needed to demonstrate optimum anatomic detail. Second, it is probably best to evaluate the patient in the prone position, since this will maximally stretch breast tissues away from the chest wall. Finally, at least two different pulse sequences are necessary to characterize various lesions.

(Text continues on p. 246.)

TABLE 11-2

Approximate T1 and T2 Measurements of Normal and Abnormal Breast Tissue

Tissue	T1 (msec)	T2 (msec)
Normal breast fat	174	57
Normal breast ductal tissue	286	53
Masses (including carcinoma and benign tumors)	258–532	47–66
Predominantly cystic disease	954	83

(Adapted from el-Yousef SJ, O'Connell DM, Duchesneau RH et al: Benign and malignant breast disease: Magnetic resonance and radiofrequency pulse sequences. AJR 145:1, 1985)

TABLE 11-3

Protocol for MRI of the Breast

1. Patient should be scanned in prone position using surface coil
2. Axial plane preferred
3. Sequence 1: SE 250/30 or PS 400 (distinguishes fat from ductal tissue and masses, which will be lower intensity)
4. Sequence 2: SE 1000/120 or similar heavily T2-weighted sequence (cysts become high-intensity, whereas solid masses either decrease, remain the same, or minimally increase)
5. Sequence 3: IR 1000/300/30 or IR 1500/450 (use only for fibrocystic breast disease to distinguish fibroadenomas and other masses from underlying fibrous tissue)

Examples of surface coil imaging of the normal breast are shown in Figures 11-13 through 11-16.

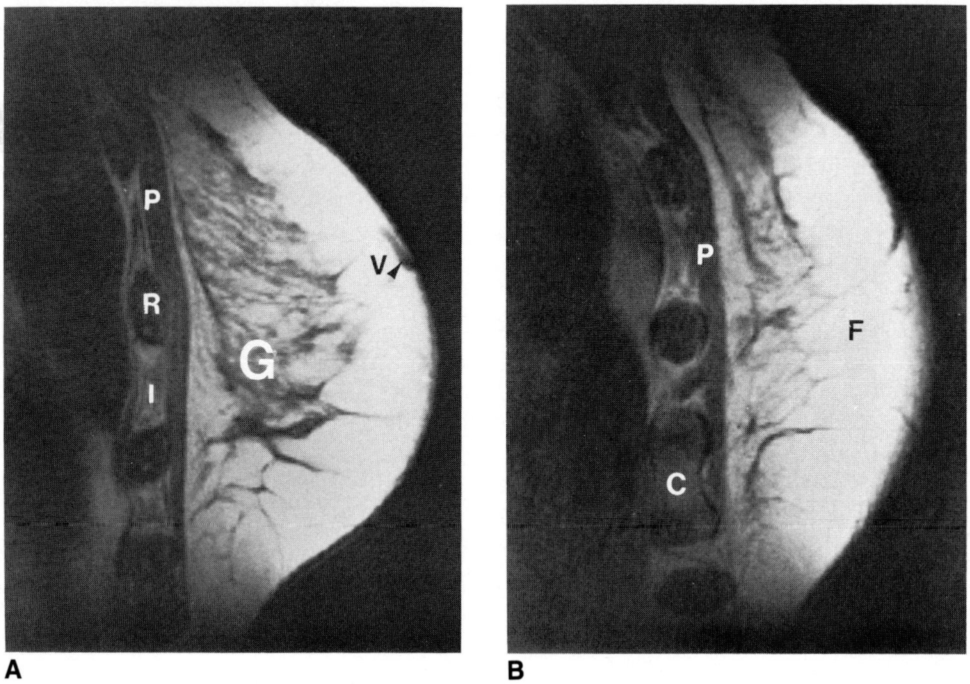

FIGURE 11-13

Sagittal surface coil SE 400/30 images of a normal breast shows fat (F), fibroglandular tissue (G), pectoral muscles (P), ribs (R), intercostal muscles (I), costal cartilages (C), and a surface vein (V). (Images obtained on Magniscan 5000, Thomson-CGR MR system)

FIGURE 11-14

Axial SE 400/30 surface coil images of the same patient in Figure 11-13. N = nipple; G = fibroglandular tissue; P = pectoral muscles. (Images obtained on Magniscan 5000, Thomson-CGR MR system)

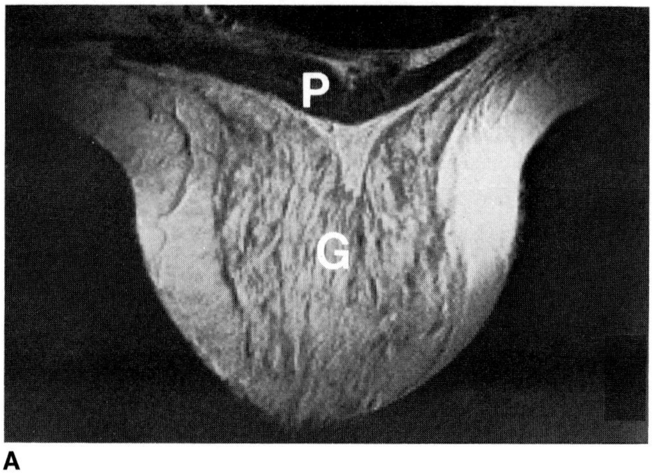

FIGURE 11-15

A very dense breast, Wolfe Classification DY, imaged by surface coils. (Courtesy of Philips Medical Systems)

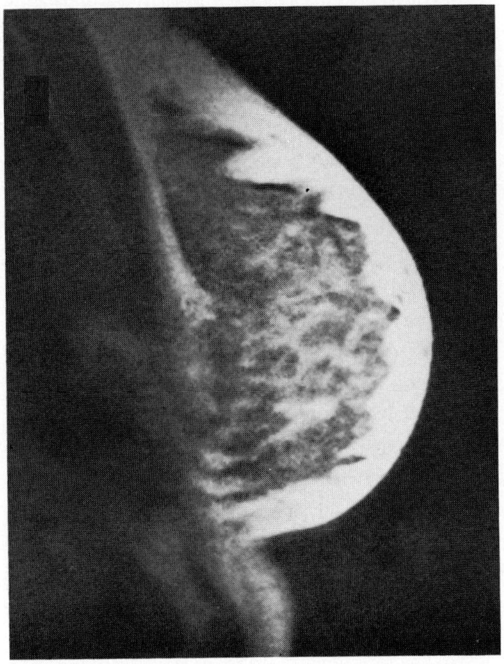

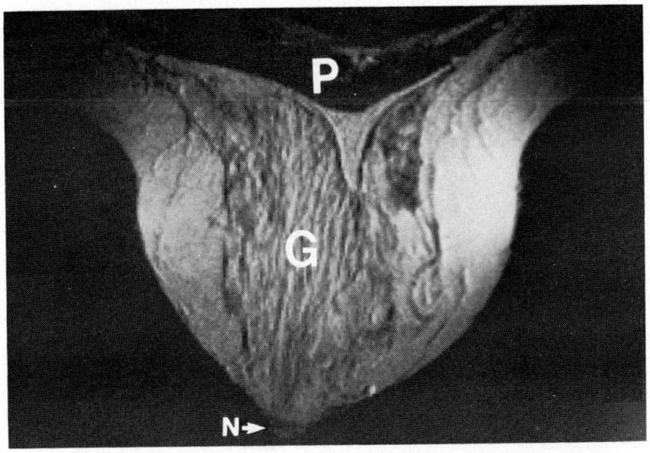

B

FIGURE 11-16

Larger surface coils that cover both breasts save imaging time and allow side-to-side comparisons to be made. (Courtesy of Technicare Corporation, Technicare Corp. © 1985)

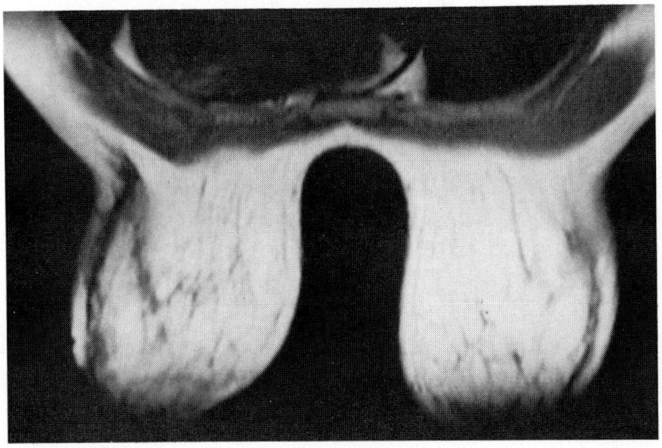

The Knee

MRI of the knee may be useful in a number of situations, ranging from the evaluation of acute ligamentous injury to the staging of tumors and chronic disease. Coronal and sagittal images are most appropriate for evaluation of ligamentous structures and the bony articulations. Axial images may be more appropriate for defining the extent of mass lesions around the knee.

As with other sites in the musculoskeletal system, T1-weighted sequences accentuate the contrast between high-intensity fat and lower-intensity muscles and ligaments. Thus, for optimal anatomic delineation of tissue planes, short spin-echo or partial saturation sequences have been recommended. Longer, more T2-weighted sequences provide less anatomic delineation but are helpful in identifying musculoskeletal abnormalities, such as edema, hemorrhage, and tumor. Inversion recovery sequences are more time-consuming, have a lower signal-to-noise ratio, and have been found to be of little advantage in imaging the knee or musculoskeletal system.

The knee may be examined with a standard head or neck coil. Several companies have developed surface coils especially for the knee. Many of the images in this chapter were produced with the Philips surface coil, using a short spin-echo sequence.

The medial and lateral collateral ligaments of the knee are silhouetted by fat and run in the coronal plane. As such, they are optimally imaged with a short spin-echo sequence in the coronal plane. These ligaments will appear as low-intensity linear structures against a background of intense fat (Fig. 11-17).

The cruciate ligaments, on the other hand, are surrounded by joint fluid with long values T1 and T2. A T2-weighted sequence will allow these ligaments to be imaged as low-intensity structures against a high-intensity background of joint fluid (Fig. 11-18). The sagittal plane is especially well suited to visualize them because of their course and location. Acute injuries of the collateral and cruciate ligaments have been diagnosed based on whether they appeared discontinuous or contained a focus of high-intensity hemorrhage.

Meniscal cartilages, like the cruciate ligaments, are best seen on T2-weighted sequences in which they appear dark compared with higher-intensity fat

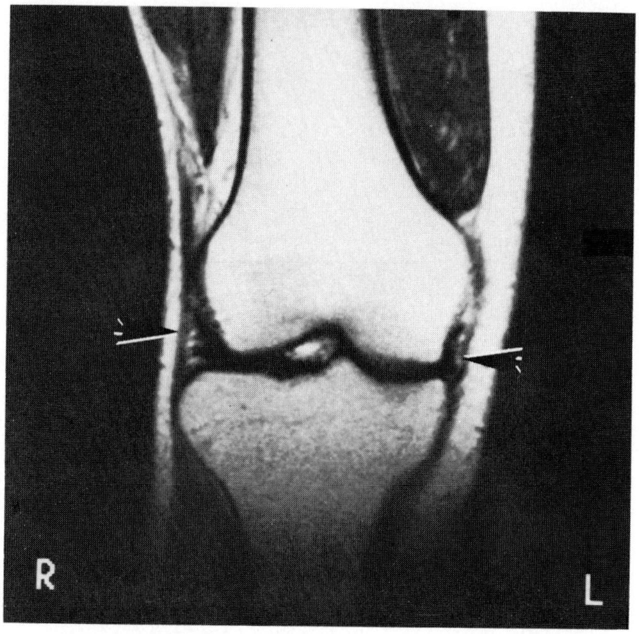

FIGURE 11-17

The medial and lateral collateral ligaments are well seen on this midline coronal SE 800/50 image. (Courtesy of Philips Medical Systems and W. Steinbrich, M.D.)

FIGURE 11-18

Posterior cruciate ligament is well seen in its characteristic location on this SE 388/28 surface coil image. Anterior cruciate ligament is seen in Figures 11-21 and 11-23G. (Courtesy of Fonar Corporation, 110 Marcus Drive, Melville, NY 11747)

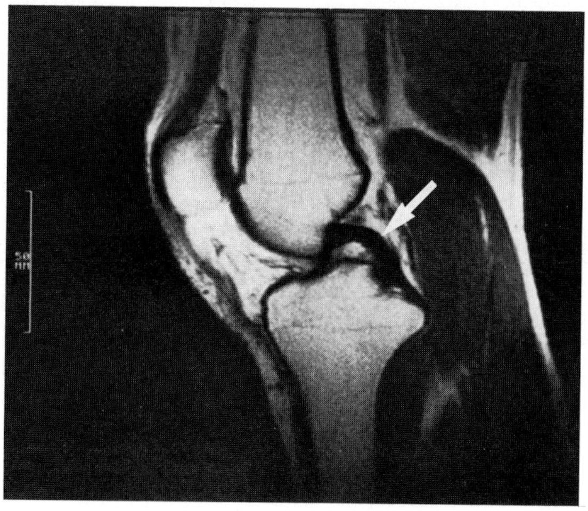

FIGURE 11-19

Anterior and posterior horns of medial meniscus (M) are well seen in this sagittal SE 388/28 surface coil image of the knee. Also note cortex of the femoral condyle (C) and a small amount of synovial fluid (SF). (Courtesy of Fonar Corporation, 110 Marcus Drive, Melville, NY 11747)

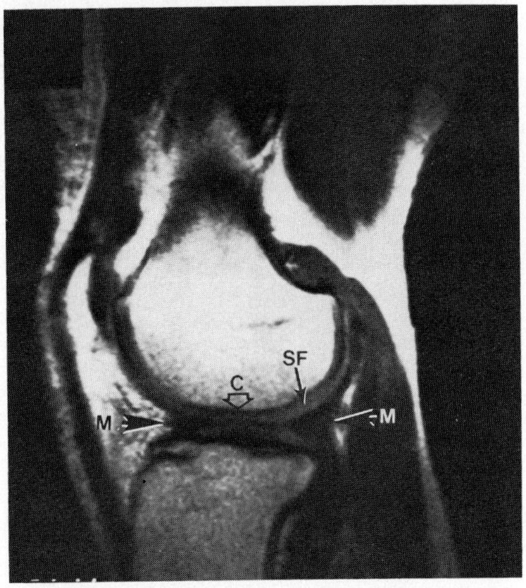

and joint fluid (Fig. 11-19). At present, spatial resolution does not reliably allow detection of meniscal tears by MR imaging. The coronal plane provides the most consistent views of the menisci in their characteristic triangular shape.

The distal femur at the knee is seen to have a low-intensity cortex and a higher-intensity marrow and fat-filled medulla. The intercondylar notch produces an infolding of cortical bone, which may be partially volumed, producing a lower-intensity signal in the distal femur. This should not be misinterpreted as a low-intensity lesion in the bone (Fig. 11-20).

Table 11-4 lists the optimal imaging planes and techniques for visualizing the ligaments and cartilages of the knee. Figures 11-21 through 11-23 illustrate the normal anatomy of the knee in axial, coronal, and sagittal planes, as seen by a spin-echo sequence using a knee coil.

TABLE 11-4

MRI of the Ligaments and Cartilages of the Knee

Structure	Optimal Plane	Optimal Technique
Collateral ligaments	Coronal	Short SE (300/30)
Cruciate ligaments	Sagittal	Long SE (2000/30)
Menisci	Coronal	Lone SE (2000/30)

FIGURE 11-20

Infolding of cortical bone at the intercondylar notch produces a low-intensity signal on certain sections through the distal femur; this should not be misinterpreted as a pathological process. (Courtesy of Philips Medical Systems and W. Steinbrich, M.D.)

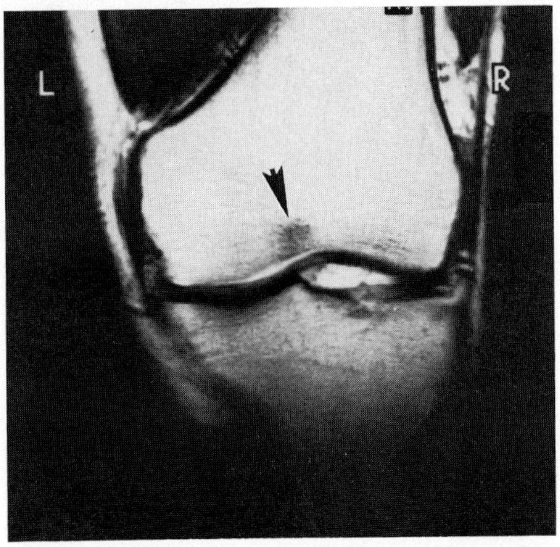

A

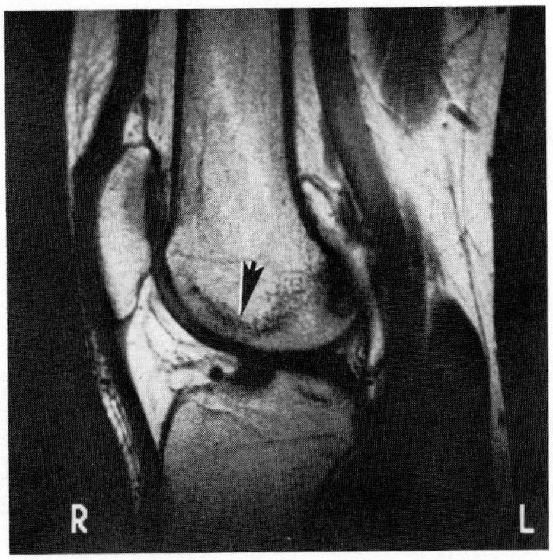

B

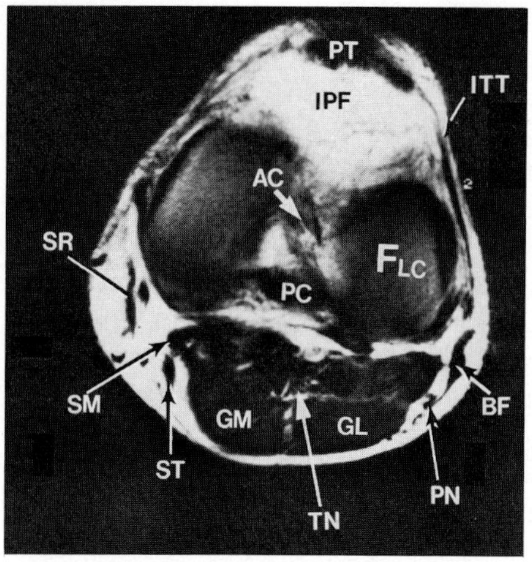

FIGURE 11-21

Axial SE 800/50 image using surface coil through the right knee. (Courtesy Philips Medical Systems and W. Steinbrich, M.D.)

AC	anterior cruciate ligament
BF	biceps femoris muscle
F	femur
FI	fibula
FLC	femur (lateral condyle)
GL, GM	lateral and medial heads gastrocnemius muscle
IPF	infrapatellar fat pad
ITT	iliotibial tract
LM	lateral meniscus
LCL	lateral collateral ligament
MCL	medial collateral ligament
P	patella
PA	popliteal artery
PC	posterior cruciate ligament
PL	plantaris muscle
PN	peroneal nerve
PO	popliteus tendon
PT	patellar tendon
PV	popliteal vein
QT	quadriceps tendon
RF	rectus femoris muscle
SGA	superior genicular artery
SM	semimembranosus muscle/tendon
SO	soleus muscle
SR	sartorius muscle
ST	semitendinosus muscle/tendon
T	tibia
TN	tibial nerve
VI	vastus intermedius muscle
VL	vastus lateralis muscle
VM	vastus medius muscle

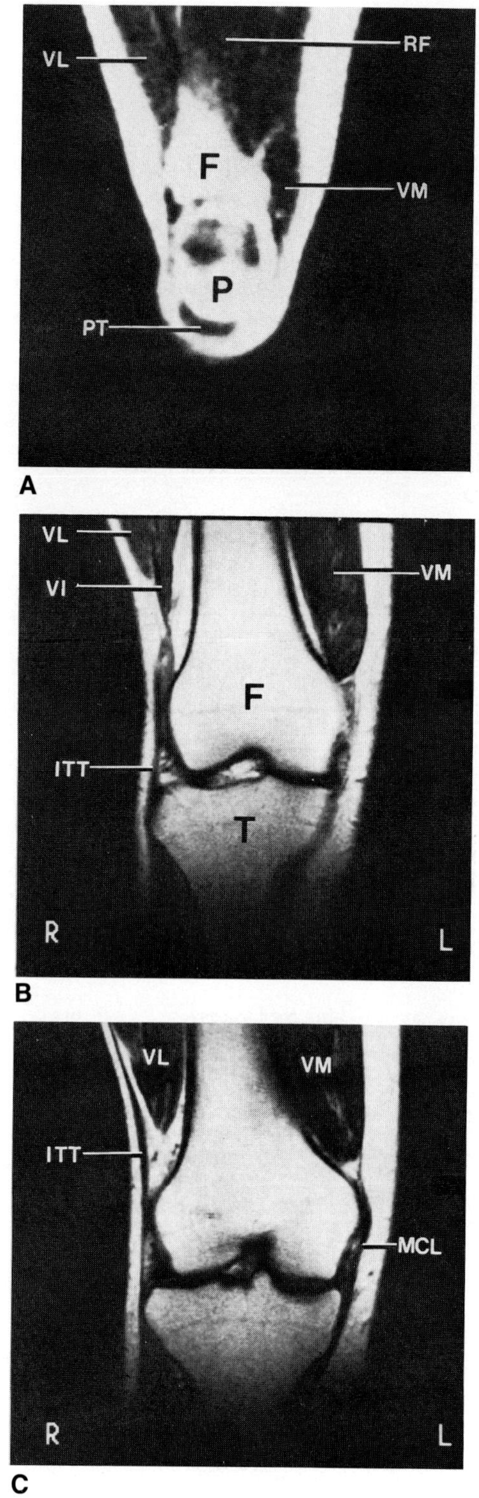

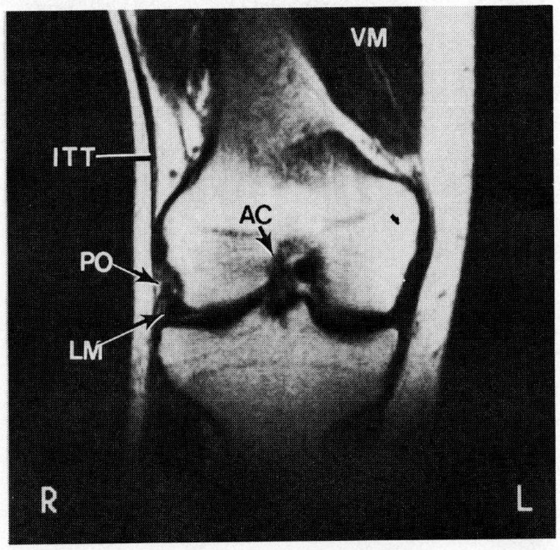

D

FIGURE 11-22

Coronal SE 800/50 images of the normal right knee from anterior to posterior. (Courtesy of Philips Medical Systems and W. Steinbrich, M.D.)

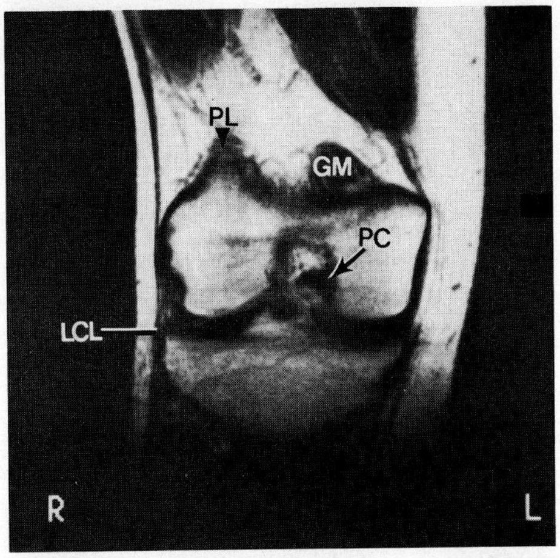

E

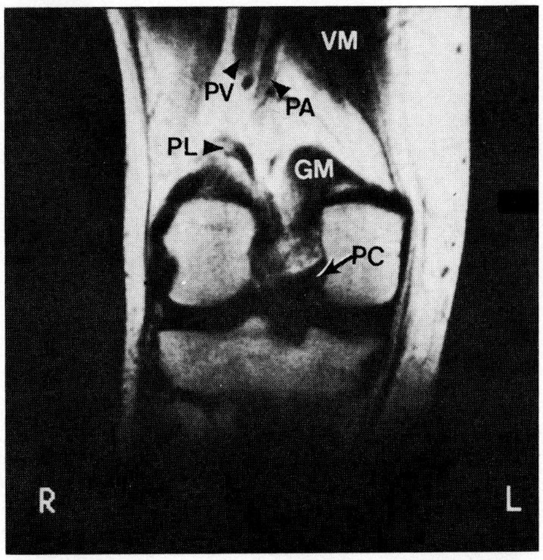

F

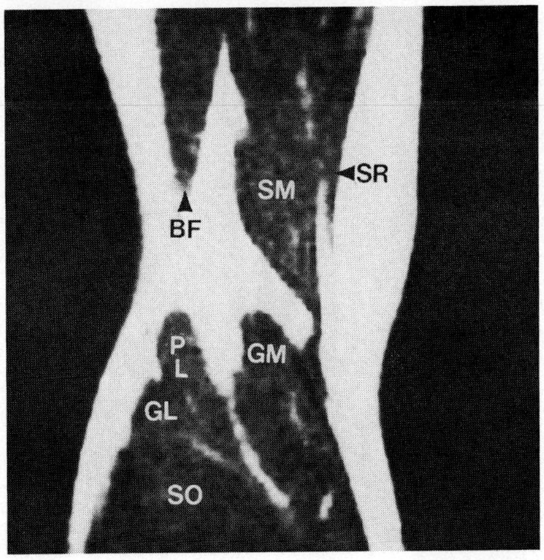

G

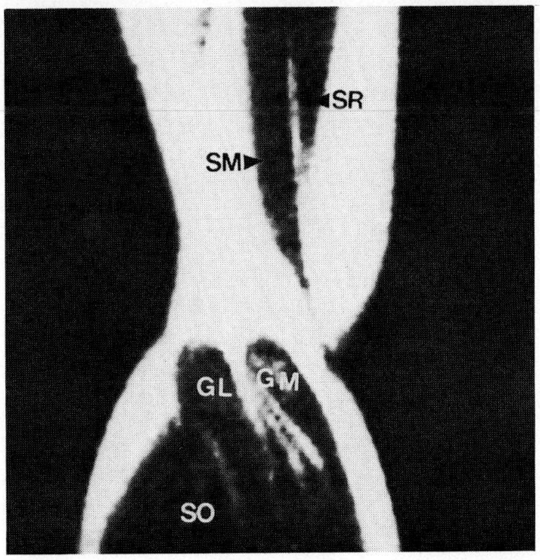

H

AC	anterior cruciate ligament	PN	peroneal nerve
BF	biceps femoris muscle	PO	popliteus tendon
F	femur	PT	patellar tendon
FI	fibula	PV	popliteal vein
F_{LC}	femur (lateral condyle)	QT	quadriceps tendon
GL, GM	lateral and medial heads gastrocnemius muscle	RF	rectus femoris muscle
IPF	infrapatellar fat pad	SGA	superior genicular artery
ITT	iliotibial tract	SM	semimembranosus muscle/tendon
LM	lateral meniscus	SO	soleus muscle
LCL	lateral collateral ligament	SR	sartorius muscle
MCL	medial collateral ligament	ST	semitendinosus muscle/tendon
P	patella	T	tibia
PA	popliteal artery	TN	tibial nerve
PC	posterior cruciate ligament	VI	vastus intermedius muscle
PL	plantaris muscle	VL	vastus lateralis muscle
		VM	vastus medius muscle

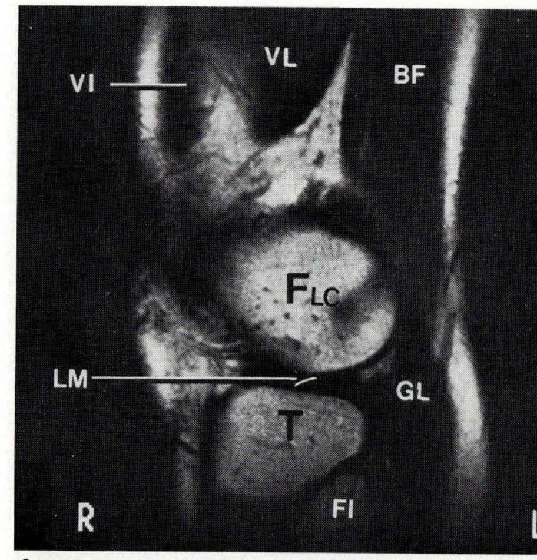

A

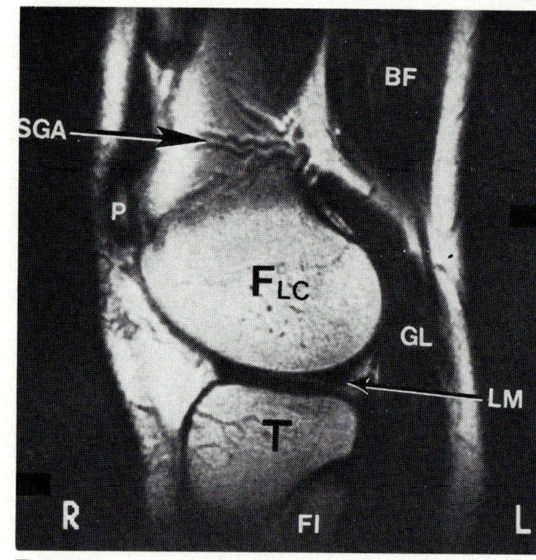

B

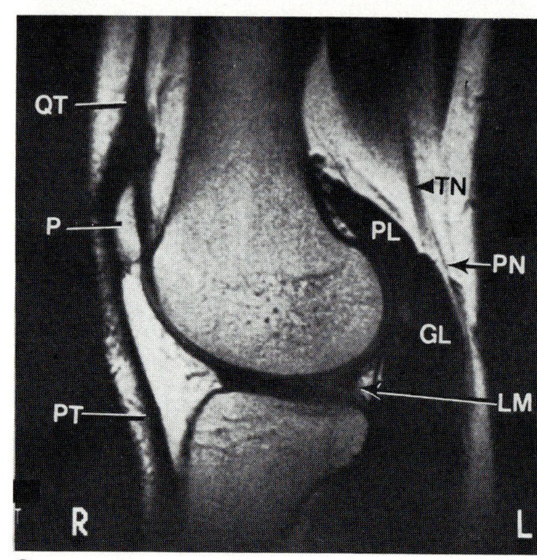

C

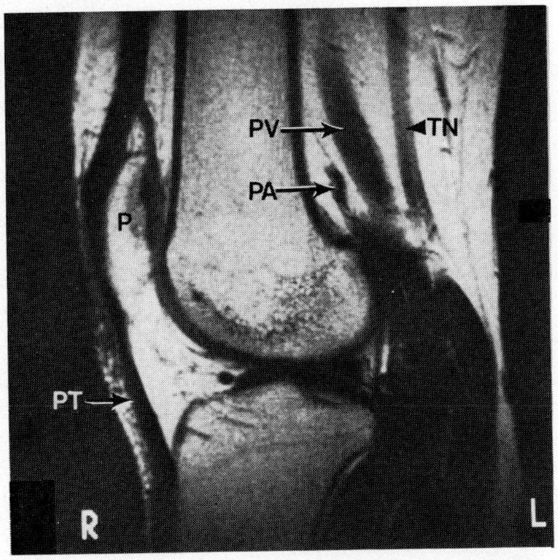

D

FIGURE 11-23

Sagittal SE 800/50 images of the right knee, laterally to medially. (Courtesy of Philips Medical Systems and W. Steinbrich, M.D.)

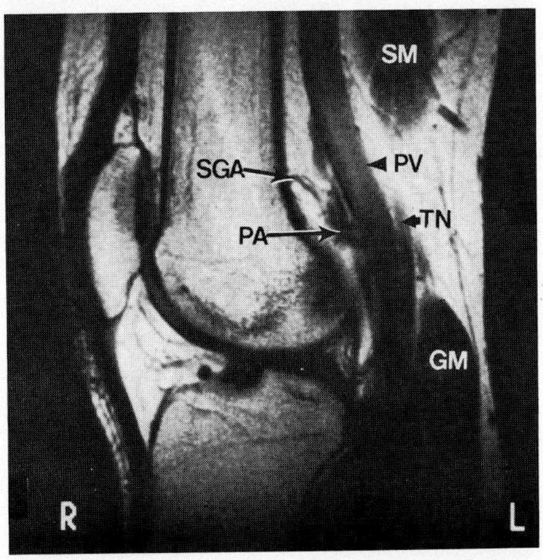

E

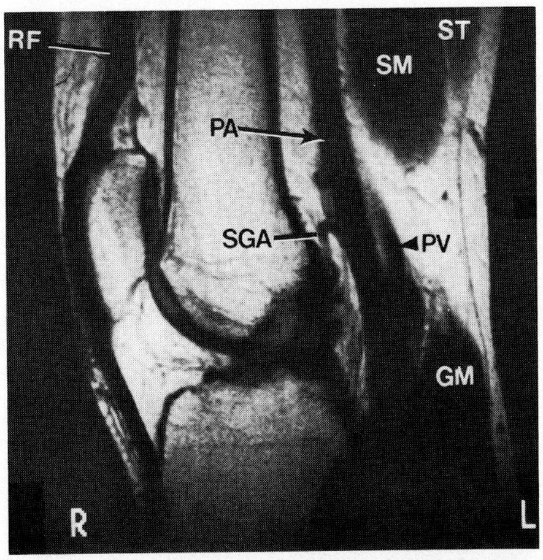

F

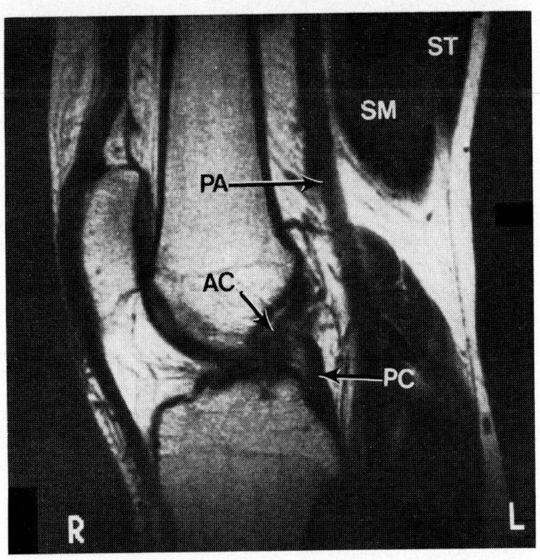

G

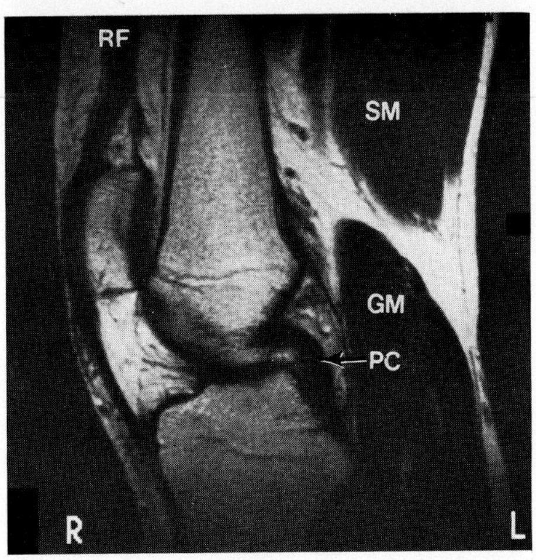

H

APPENDIX A

Specifications of Nine Major Commercial MR Scanners, 1985

All information contained in this appendix has been obtained from published surveys* and promotional literature supplied by each manufacturer. Every attempt has been made to ensure accuracy of this information, but because of potential typographical errors and changing specifications in rapidly advancing technology, neither the author nor the publisher can guarantee all facts presented. It is therefore recommended that interested readers contact each company directly for complete and current specifications and prices.

At least five companies that produce MR scanners have not been included in this appendix. Information was not available at the time this book went to press concerning the specifications and options available on each. The fact that these scanners were not included is in no way intended to reflect upon the quality of these machines or the companies that manufacture them. Complete information about these scanners may be obtained by writing to the following addresses:

1. Bruker Medical Instruments, Inc.
   D-7512 Rheinstetten 4
   Karlsruhe, Germany
2. Esacontrol
   Ansaldo Electric Biomedicale
   Via Pesce, 5, 16151
   Genova, Italy
3. M & D Technology Ltd.
   Unit 1, Whitemyres Avenue
   Aberdeen, Scotland, UK AB2 6HQ
4. NMR Imaging, Inc.
   2501 Central Parkway, Suite C-17
   Houston, TX 77092
5. Palmex Instrumentation Oy
   Elimaenkatu 22-24
   PO Box 357 SF-0010
   Helsinki, Finland

*Business Briefs, Diagnostic Imaging, November 1985, pp. 219–226

Industrial Corner, J Comput Assist Tomogr 9:1155–1165, 1985

Diasonics, Inc.
533 Cabot Road
South San Francisco, CA 94080

Model(s): MT/S

List price: $1,500,000

Number operational in North America: 35

Magnet type: Superconducting

Field strength (T): 0.5–2.0

Field uniformity (ppm over 30 cm dia. sphere): 50

Size of 5G fringe field (ft): 39 × 39 × 50

Magnet bore/minimum aperture (cm): 105

Maximum gradient field (G/cm): 1

RF coils: Head (30 × 20) cm); body (56 × 25 cm), (50 × 50 × 25 cm)

RF transmitter power (kW): 1

RF tuning method: Manual/automatic

Surface coils: General purpose circular (5 cm), (10 cm); breast (20 × 20 cm); extremities (15 × 25 cm)

Computer/Memory size: DEC PDP11 (256 kByte); DEC VAX-11 (1 MByte)

Array processor: CSPI Minimap

Imaging parameter range:
TR: 0.1–5.0 sec
TI: 100–600 msec
TE: 30–150 msec

Slice thickness (mm): 2.5, 5.0, 10.0
Maximum spatial resolution (mm): 0.95
Image acquisition matrix: 128 × 256, 256 × 256
Display matrix: 256 × 256, 512 × 512
Size magnet assembly, L × W × H (cm): 200 × 285 × 262
Installed weight (kg): 6350
Cooling method(s): Air only
Maximum cryogen usage (L/hr):
    Helium: 0.5
    Nitrogen: 1.0
Special features:
    Cryogen recirculation system available
    Color monitor available
    Off-center shift of image plane by frequency offset
    Cardiac-gated phase cycled multislice acquisition
    T1, T2 images

Elscint, Inc.
930 Commonwealth Avenue
Boston, MA 02215

Model(s): Gyrex
List price: $1,400,000–$2,000,000
Number operational in North America: 2
Magnet type: Superconducting
Field strength (T): 0.5–1.95
Field uniformity (ppm over 30 cm dia. sphere): 10–15
Size of 5G fringe field (ft): 32 × 32 × 40
Magnet bore/Minimum aperture (cm): 100
Maximum gradient field (G/cm): 1
RF coils: Head (30 × 30 cm); Body (56 × 56 cm)
RF transmitter power (kW): NA
RF tuning method: Automatic
Surface coils: Expandable neck
Computer/memory size: DEC PDP-11 (4 MByte)
Array processor: CSPI Minimap
Imaging parameter range:
TR: 0.15–999 sec
TI: 0.2–999 sec
TE: 18 msec–999 sec
Slice thickness (mm): 3–99
Maximum spatial resolution (mm): 0.5 (head); 1.2 (body)
Image acquisition matrix: 128 × 128, 128 × 256, 256 × 256
Display matrix: 512 × 512
Size magnet assembly, L × W × H (cm): 200 × 250 × 250
Installed weight (kg): 5500–9500
Cooling method(s): Air and water
Maximum cryogen usage (L/hr):
    Helium: 0.4
    Nitrogen: 1.5
Special features:
    Cryogen conservation system
    Local RF shielding possible
    Simultaneous image acquisition and manipulation
    Color monitor available
    Detachable patient couch optional
    Power and manual couch positioning
    Oblique and double oblique imaging
    Whole volume (3DFT) imaging
    Spectroscopic capability
    Sodium imaging capability

Fonar Corporation
110 Marcus Drive
Melville, NY 11747

Model(s): Beta 3000
List price: $1,648,000
Number operational in North America: 14
Magnet type: Permanent
Field strength (T): 0.3
Field uniformity (ppm over 30 cm dia. sphere): 6
Size of 5G fringe field (ft): 8 × 10 × 6
Magnet bore/Minimum aperture (cm): 42
Maximum gradient field (G/cm): 1
RF coils: Head (27 × 36 cm); Body (56 × 32 × 31 cm)
RF transmitter power (kW): 0.5
RF tuning method: Manual and automatic
Surface coils: General purpose circular (20 cm); expandable for neck, knee, body
Computer/memory size: Data General Eclipse S-140 (1MByte)
Array processor: Analogic AP 400
Imaging parameter range:
    TR: 0.1–5.0 sec
    TI: 0.1–1.0 sec
    TE: 28–112 msec
Slice thickness (mm): 3–20
Maximum spatial resolution (mm): 0.33
Image acquisition matrix: 1024 × 512, 1024 × 256
Display matrix: 256 × 256, 512 × 512
Size magnet assembly, L × W × H (cm): 461 × 205 × 277
Installed weight (kg): 18,000–90,000
Cooling method(s): Air only
Maximum cryogen usage (L/hr):
    Helium: Not needed
    Nitrogen: Not needed

Special features:
- Variable RF pulse profile
- Simultaneous image acquisition and manipulation
- Color monitor available
- Power and manual patient couch
- All scanning sequences performed in oblique format with continuous choice of slice angle, 0° to 90°
- No power consumption or cryogen cost (permanent magnet)
- Shielded room provided by Fonar as part of base price
- Off-center shift of image plane by frequency offset
- Cardiac-gated phase cycled multislice acquisition

General Electric Company
P.O. Box 414
Milwaukee, WI 53201

Model(s): Signa
List price: $1,999,000
Number operational in North America: 30

Magnet type: Superconducting
Field strength (T): 1.5
Field uniformity (ppm over 30 cm dia. sphere): 5
Size of 5G fringe field (ft): 31 × 31 × 39
Magnet bore/Minimum aperture (cm): 100
Maximum gradient field (G/cm): 1

RF coils: Head (28 × 33 cm); Body (55 × 92 cm)
RF transmitter power (kW): 10
RF tuning method: Manual and automatic
Surface coils: 5 General purpose circular coils

Computer/Memory size: Data General MV4000 (4 MByte)
Array processor: FPS 3000

Imaging parameter range:
- TR: 0.25–2.25 sec
- TI: NA
- TE: 25–250 msec

Slice thickness (mm): 3–20
Maximum spatial resolution (mm): 0.3
Image acquisition matrix: 128 × 256, 256 × 256
Display matrix: 512 × 512

Size magnet assembly, L × W × H (cm): 300 × 250 × 250 (approx)
Installed weight (kg): 8050
Cooling method(s): Air and water
Maximum cryogen usage (L/hr):
- Helium: 0.5
- Nitrogen: 2.0

Special features:
- Simultaneous image acquisition and manipulation
- Detachable patient couch
- Power couch positioning
- Mirrors on head coil to reduce claustrophobia
- Power conditioner included in base price
- Spectroscopic capability
- Sodium imaging capability

Philips Medical Systems, Inc.
710 Bridgeport Avenue
Shelton, CT 06484

Model(s) : Gyroscan S5, S15
List price: $1,800,000–$2,200,000
Number operational in North America: 6

Magnet type: Superconducting
Field strength (T): S5 = 0.5; S15 = 1.5
Field uniformity (ppm over 30 cm dia. sphere): 3
Size of 5G fringe field (ft): NA
Magnet bore/Minimum aperture (cm): 105
Maximum gradient field (G/cm): 0.3

RF coils: Head (26 × 31 × 36 cm); body (36 × 58 × 64)
RF transmitter power (kW): S5 = 1.5; S15 = 5.0
RF tuning method: Automatic
Surface coils: General purpose rectangular (10 × 40 cm), (10 × 20 cm):
General purpose circular (8 cm, 11 cm, 14 cm, 17 cm)

Computer/Memory size: DEC VAX 11-750 (2 MByte)
Array processor: AP 500

Imaging parameter range:
- TR: 0.45–10.0 sec
- TI: 100–800 msec
- TE: 30–200 msec

Slice thickness (mm): 5–100
Maximum spatial resolution (mm): Head (0.7); body (1.4)
Image acquisition matrix: 64 × 64, 128 × 128, 128 × 256, 256 × 256
Display matrix: 512 × 512

Size magnet assembly, L × W × H (cm): S5 × 1955 × 230 × 242; S15 = 2220 × 217 × 275
Installed weight (kg): S5 = 4800; S15 + 8215
Cooling method(s): Air only
Maximum cryogen usage (L/hr):
- Helium: 0.3
- Nitrogen: 1.0

Special features:
- Cryogen recirculation system available
- Internal RF shielding
- Simultaneous image acquisition and manipulation
- Power patient couch
- Oblique and double oblique imaging
- Echoplanar or hybrid image acquisition

Whole volume (3DFT) isotropic and anisotropic imaging
Off-center shift of image plane by frequency offset
Cardiac-gated phase cycled multislice
T1, T2 images
Spectroscopic capability
Sodium imaging capability

Picker International
5500 Avion Park Drive
Highland Heights, OH 44143

Model(s): Vista MR
List price: $975,000–$2,120,000
Number operational in North America: 29
Magnet type: Superconducting (resistive also available)
Field strength (T): 0.5–2.0 (resistive = 0.15)
Field uniformity (ppm over 30 cm dia. sphere): 10
Size of 5G fringe field (ft): 30 × 30 × 36–70 × 70 × 84
Magnet bore/minimum aperture (cm): 100
Maximum gradient field (G/cm): 1.2
RF coils: Head (30 × 60 cm); body (60 × 60 cm)
RF transmitter power (kW): 15
RF tuning method: Automatic
Surface coils: C-spine (22.3 cm); L-spine (14.5 cm); orbit (21.4 cm);
T-bone (9.5 cm); knee (13.3 cm); breast (9 cm)
Computer/memory size: Perkin-Elmer 3210 (1 MByte)
Array processor: 32-bit microprocessor
Imaging parameter range:
TR: <60 sec
TI: 100–900 msec
TE: 10–240 msec
Slice thickness (mm): 2–20
Maximum spatial resolution (mm): 0.39
Image acquisition matrix: 128 × 256, 256 × 256, 512 × 512
Display matrix: 512 × 512
Size magnet assembly, L × W × H (cm): 229 × 210 × 259
Installed weight (kg): 9090
Cooling method(s): Air only
Maximum cryogen usage (L/hr):
Helium: 0.4
Nitrogen: 1.0
Special features:
Cryogen recirculation system available
Internal RF shielding
Power patient couch
Oblique and double oblique imaging
Echoplanar or hybrid imaging
Whole volume (3DFT) anisotropic imaging possible
Off-center shift of image plane by frequency offset
Power conditioner included in base price
T1, T2 images

Siemens Medical Systems, Inc.
186 Wood Avenue South
Iselin, NJ 08830

Model(s): Magnetom
List price: NA
Number operational in North America: 33
Magnet type: Superconducting
Field strength (T): 0.5–2.0
Field uniformity (ppm over 30 cm dia. sphere): 5
Size of 5G fringe field (ft): 22 × 22 × 27–34 × 34 × 42
Magnet bore/Minimum aperture (cm): 100
Maximum gradient field (G/cm): 0.3–0.6
RF coils: Head (30 × 25 cm); body (57 × 55 cm)
RF transmitter power (kW): 10–15
RF tuning method: Automatic
Surface coils: General purpose circular (16 cm)
Computer/Memory size: DEC VAX 11-730 (2 MByte)
Array processor: Siemens BSP 11/MR
Imaging parameter range:
TR: 0.1–20 sec
TI: 30 msec–20 sec
TE: 25 msec–20 sec
Slice thickness (mm): 3–200
Maximum spatial resolution (mm): 0.6 (head; 0.95 (body)
Image acquisition matrix: 128 × 128, 128 × 256, 256 × 512
Display matrix: 256 × 256, 512 × 512
Size magnet assembly, L × W × H (cm): 255 × 210 × 254
Installed weight (kg): 6350–7600
Cooling method(s): Air and water
Maximum cryogen usage (L/hr):
Helium: 0.3–0.5
Nitrogen: 1.2–2.0
Special features:
Cryogen recirculation system available
Simultaneous image acquisition and manipulation
Independent display console is included in base price
Power patient couch
Oblique imaging possible
Whole volume (3DFT) anisotropic imaging possible
Cardiac-gated phase cycled multislice imaging
Off-center shift of image plane by frequency offset
T1, T2 images

P-31 spectroscopy possible
Sodium imaging capability

Technicare Corporation
P.O. Box 5130
Cleveland, OH 44101-0130

Model(s): Teslacon
List price: \$850,000–\$2,400,000
Number operational in North America: 64
Magnet type: Superconducting (resistive also available)
Field strength (T): 0.15–2.0
Field uniformity (ppm over 30 cm dia. sphere): 10
Size of 5G fringe field (ft): 12 × 12 × 15–35 × 35 × 44
Magnet bore/Minimum aperature (cm): 100
Maximum gradient field (G/cm): 0.25
RF coils: Head (23 × 30 cm); body (50 × 48 cm)
RF transmitter power (kW): 10
RF tuning method: Manual
Surface coils: 6 general purpose coils, also breast and orbit coils
Computer/Memory size: PDP 11-24 (512 kByte)
Array processor: FPS 100
Imaging parameter range:
TR: 0.23–4.0 sec
TI: 0.1–1.0 sec
TE: 32–256 msec
Slice thickness (mm): 4–15
Maximum spatial resolution (mm): 1.1 (head); 1.8 (body)
Image acquisition matrix: 256 × 128, 256 × 192, 256 × 256
Display matrix: 512 × 512
Size magnet assembly, L × W × H (cm): 261 × 226 × 223
Installed weight (kg): 9090
Cooling method(s): Air only
Maximum cryogen usage (L/hr):
Helium: 0.5
Nitrogen: 2.0
Special features:
Liquid helium recirculation system available
Gaussian or sinc RF pulse profiles
Simultaneous image acquisition and manipulation
Color monitor available
Oblique and double oblique imaging
Whole volume (3DFT) isotropic and anisotropic imaging possible
Cardiac-gated phase cycled multislice acquisition
T1 images
Spectroscopy possible
Sodium imaging possible

Thomson-CGR Medical Corporation
10150 Old Columbia Road
Columbia, MD 21046

Model(s): Magniscan 5000
List price: NA
Number operational in North America: 3
Magnet type: Superconducting
Field strength (T): 0.5
Field uniformity (ppm over 30 cm dia. sphere): <5
Size of 5G fringe field (ft): NA
Magnet bore/Minimum aperture (cm): 55
Maximum gradient field (G/cm): 0.8
RF coils: Head (30 × 28 cm); body (55 × 42 cm)
RF transmitter power (kW): NA
RF tuning method: Semiautomatic
Surface coils: Under development
Computer/Memory size: DEC VAX 11-730 (1 MByte)
Array processor: CDA MSP 3000
Imaging parameter range:
TR: 0.2–4.0 sec
TI: 0.05–2.0 sec
TE: 28–200 msec
Slice thickness (mm): 4–300
Maximum spatial resolution (mm): 0.8 (head); 1.0 (body)
Image acquisition matrix: 128 × 128, 256 × 256
Display matrix: 256 × 256
Size magnet assembly, L × W × H (cm): NA
Installed weight (kg): 5000
Cooling method(s): Air only
Maximum cryogen usage (L/hr):
Helium: 0.35
Nitrogen: 1.3
Special features:
Simultaneous image acquisition and manipulation
Color monitor available
Power patient couch
Image addition, subtraction, histogramming
T1, T2 images

APPENDIX B

Glossary of Magnetic Resonance Terminology*

B_0 A symbol for the constant magnetic field produced by the large magnet in an MR scanner. B_0 is measured in units of tesla.

B_1 A symbol for the much smaller rotating radio-frequency magnetic field, which in conjunction with B_0 excites hydrogen nuclei to resonance.

Chemical shift The change in resonance frequency a given proton experiences by virtue of its position within a molecule. A given hydrogen proton will experience more or less than the applied external magnetic field because of shielding effects from neighboring atoms. Measurement of chemical shifts makes possible the analysis of molecular structure.

Coherence Rotation or oscillation of protons harmoniously in phase with one another. The transverse component of magnetization (Mxy) is generated by coherent precession at resonance.

Coil Multiple loops of wire that may be used to produce a magnetic field (by passing current through it) or to detect a changing magnetic field (by measuring the voltage induced in the wire).

Contrast The relative difference in signal intensities between two adjacent regions of an image. If I_1 is the image intensity in one region and I_2 is the image intensity in an adjacent region, the contrast may be written as $C = (I_1 - I_2)/(I_1 + I_2)$.

Diamagnetic A substance whose molecular regions tend to realign themselves to oppose an externally applied magnetic field. Examples of diamagnetic substances include certain nuclei like ^{19}F and ^{23}Na and certain large molecules like paraffins and glycerol. Compare *Paramagnetic.*

Echo time (TE) A parameter used to specify a spin-echo pulse sequence. It represents the time in milliseconds between application of the 90° pulse and echo signal. Usual TEs are on the order of 30 msec to 100 msec. If more than one echo is recorded, the times between the 90° pulse and each echo are called TE1, TE2, TE3, and so on.

Fourier transform A mathematical procedure used in MR scanners to analyze and separate amplitude and frequency components of the complex detected signal. In conjunction with magnetic field encoding gradients applied to the patient during scanning, Fourier transform analysis allows spatial information to be reconstructed from the raw data. Most MR scanners in clinical use today use two-dimensional or three-dimensional Fourier transformation reconstruction techniques (2DFT or 3DFT). A particularly fast and efficient computer program to perform these calculations is called the *fast Fourier transform* (FFT).

Free induction decay (FID) The signal recorded in the transverse plane resulting after a radio-frequency pulse has excited a system to resonance. Detection of this FID signal forms the basis for the more complicated pulse imaging techniques such as spin-echo and inversion recovery.

Frequency (f) The number of cycles or repetitions of an event per unit time, usually expressed in *hertz* (Hz), where 1 Hz = 1 cycle per second. When a rotation system is studied, the term *angular frequency* is sometimes used. Angular frequency, ω, is related to plain frequency, f, by the equation $\omega = 2\pi f$.

Gauss (G) A unit of magnetic field strength that is the approximate strength of the earth's magnetic field

* Modified from Glossary of NMR Terms prepared under the auspices of The American College of Radiology, 1983

on its surface. The unit gauss has been largely replaced by the larger unit tesla (T), and 1 T = 10,000 G.

Gradient magnetic field A small magnetic field applied in addition to the large static field in an MR scanner. This gradient field varies in strength in a certain direction. The application of gradient fields in different directions allows each small volume element in a sample to experience a different magnetic field, and hence resonate at a different frequency. In this way, spatial encoding may be performed.

Gyromagnetic ratio (γ) A constant relating the nuclear MR frequency and the strength of the external magnetic field (see Larmor frequency).

Hertz (Hz) A unit of frequency equal to 1 cycle per second. The larger unit megahertz (MHz) = 1,000,000 Hz.

Image (data) acquisition time The time required to pulse and collect MR signals for processing. Total time for performing a scan includes image acquisition time + image reconstruction time.

Inversion recovery (IR) An imaging sequence that involves successive 180° and 90° pulses, after which a heavily T1-weighted signal is obtained. The inversion recovery sequence is specified in terms of two parameters, the inversion time (TI) and the repetition time (TR). These are discussed in Chapter 3.

Inversion time (TI) The time between the 180° and subsequent 90° pulse in an inversion recovery sequence. This usually chosen to be 100 msec to 1000 msec.

Larmor frequency (ω_0) The frequency at which nuclear magnetic resonance occurs. The Larmor frequency is related to magnetic field strength (B_0) and a constant called the gyromagnetic ratio (γ) by an equation known as the Larmor equation.

Magnetic moment A measure of the torque exerted on a magnet or spinning proton that tends to align it with an externally applied magnetic field.

Magnetization The net effect that an externally applied magnetic field has on a material placed within it and that tends to polarize and turn that material into a magnet. Most body tissues are weakly susceptible to this process, and their protons tend to align with the field, producing a net magnetization vector. Some substances called *paramagnetics* have a more marked tendency to align with the field. Other substances have a tendency to align opposite to the field and are called *diamagnetics.*

Nuclear magnetic resonance (NMR) A phenomenon exhibited by hydrogen and certain atoms with odd numbers of protons and neutrons, such as ^{13}C, ^{19}F, ^{23}Na, and ^{31}P. When these atoms are placed in a strong external magnetic field, B_0, and excited by a suitable induction field, B_1, rotating at the Larmor frequency, energy absorption and emission occur, constituting NMR. NMR is often referred to simply as magnetic resonance (MR).

Nucleon A term for either a neutron or a proton.

Paramagnetic Materials with a small but positive magnetizability. These substances usually possess an unpaired electron and include certain transition elements, rare earths, and free radicals. They may one day be used as contrast agents for MRI.

Partial saturation (PS) An NMR pulse sequence consisting of repetitive 90° pulses after which a free induction decay is recorded. This produces a strongly T1-weighted image.

Phantom A usually oil-filled plastic cylinder of known dimensions and properties used to test and calibrate an MR scanner.

Phase The position relative to a particular part of the cycle of a periodic function, such as a sine wave.

Pixel A "picture element," the smallest discrete part of a digital image display.

Precession The wobbling of spinning protons when placed in an external magnetic field, analogous to the wobbling of a spinning top in the earth's gravitational field.

Precessional frequency Same as the Larmor frequency. The frequency of a radio-frequency pulse that induces MR as well as the frequency of the emitted NMR signal.

Pulse sequence A set of radio-frequency and gradient magnetic field pulses used to induce nuclear resonance and produce an image. Examples of commonly used pulse sequences include inversion recovery and spin-echo techniques.

Quenching A potential disaster that may occur when a superconductive magnet suddenly loses its superconductivity. The magnet suddenly becomes resistive and a large amount of heat is released, causing liquid helium to evaporate rapidly. Superconductive magnets have special gas-release safely valves to prevent an explosion due to quenching.

Radio-frequency (RF) High-frequency electromagnetic waves used in MRI similar to those used in commercial radio transmission, usually in the range of megahertz (MHz).

Receiver coil A coil of wire that is placed around the patient and that detects the MR signal.

Reconstruction The computer manipulation of the many complex MR signals to decode spatially and produce an image.

Relaxation times After excitation with the applied radio-frequency pulse, spinning protons tend to realign with the static magnetic field. The time it takes for this to occur is known as relaxation time. Two relaxation time constants may be defined parallel and perpendicular to the static magnetic field. These are known as the T1 and T2 relaxation times, respectively.

Repetition time (TR) The time interval between the beginning of a pulse sequence and the succeeding pulse sequence, usually chosen in the range 300 msec to 3.0 seconds.

Resistive magnet A magnet that uses electric current in coils to generate a magnetic field and that operates at temperatures higher than superconductive range (*i.e.,* > −360° C). Resistive magnets are cheaper to build than superconductive magnets, but their fields are not as uniform or as strong.

Resonance The rapid oscillation between high- and low-energy states of a system that occurs when the system is stimulated or excited at a specific frequency known as the *resonance frequency.*

RF pulse A brief burst of electromagnetic radiation at radio frequencies that excite the net magnetization vector to rotate a certain amount. Commonly used RF pulses include the 90° and 180° pulses.

Saturation A nonequilibrium state in MR in which equal numbers of spinning protons are aligned with and opposite to the static magnetic field, resulting in no net magnetization.

Saturation recovery (SR) An MR imaging pulse sequence similar to partial saturation but in which recovery from total saturation occurs before the next repetition. Like PS, SR produces a heavily T1-weighted image.

Shimming Placing electromagnets or metal bars on the outer surface of the large main magnet to correct in homogeneities (irregularities) in its field.

Signal-to-noise ratio (S/N or SNR) The ratio between the amplitude of the recorded signal and background noise, which distorts that signal. Signal-to-noise ratio (and hence image quality) may be improved by taking more averages of the signal, by using longer sampling times, and by sampling larger volumes.

Spin A property of nuclei with an odd number of protons or neutrons accounts for their magnetic moments and allows for MR to occur.

Spin-echo An MR pulse sequence technique in which alternating 90° and 180° pulses are applied to the sample and an echo signal recorded. The spin-echo sequence is sensitive to both T1 and T2 values.

Spin-lattice relaxation time See T1.

Spin–spin relaxation time See T2.

Superconductive magnet A magnet whose field is produced by current flowing through a substance near absolute zero. Although its is more expensive to build than a resistive magnet, its field strength and field homogeneity are higher.

Surface coil MR A new technique in MR imaging in which a specially constructed flat receiver coil is placed directly on or near the skin surface. This allows excellent high resolution of organs and tissues that are within a few centimeters of the coil.

T1 Also called the spin-lattice or longitudinal relaxation time. This represents the time constant for spins to realign themselves after perturbation with the externally applied field. When starting from zero magnetization in a direction parallel to the field, T1 represents the time for this magnetization to grow to 63% of its final value.

T2 Also called the spin–spin or transverse relaxation time. This represents the time constant for loss of phase coherence between spins along a plane perpendicular to the static field. Starting from a magnetization in this transverse plane, T2 represents the time it takes for this magnetization to decay to 63% of its initial value.

Tesla (T) A unit of magnetic field flux density, equal to 10,000 gauss.

Torque A force that produces rotation.

Transverse relaxation time See T2.

Vector A physical quantity with both magnitude and direction.

Voxel A volume element, which corresponds in three-dimensional space to the *pixel.*

APPENDIX C

Abbreviations Commonly Used in MR Imaging

B	Magnetic induction or flux density
B_0	Magnetic induction field
B_1	Radio-frequency magnetic field
f	Frequency
FT	Fourier transform
FFT	Fast Fourier transform
FID	Free induction decay
G	Gauss
H	Magnetic field
Hz	Hertz
IR	Inversion recovery
M	Macroscopic magnetization vector
MHz	Megahertz
MR	Magnetic resonance
MRI	Magnetic resonance imaging
NMR	Nuclear magnetic resonance
PS	Partial saturation
RF	Radio-frequency
SR	Saturation recovery
SE	Spin-echo
S/N	Signal-to-noise ratio
SSFP	Steady-state free precession
T	Tesla
T1	Spin-lattice or longitudinal relaxation time
T2	Spin–spin or transverse relaxation time
TE	Echo time
TI	Inversion time
TR	Repetition time
2DFT	Two-dimensional Fourier transform
3DFT	Three-dimensional Fourier transform
γ	Gyromagnetic ratio
δ	Chemical shift
ω	Angular frequency
ω_0	Larmor frequency

BIBLIOGRAPHY

The following bibliography lists all major English language references in clinical and basic science aspects of Nuclear Magnetic Resonance between January 1980 and July 1985. For a complete bibliography for the period 1962 to 1982 see:

Jaklovsky J: NMR imaging: A comprehensive bibliography. Reading Mass, Addison–Wesley Publishing Co., 1983.

Selected Textbooks

Abragam A: The Principles of Nuclear Magnetic Resonance. Oxford, Oxford University Press, 1961

Andrew ER: Nuclear Magnetic Resonance. London, Cambridge University Press, 1969

Becker ED: High Resolution NMR: Theory and Clinical Application. New York, Academic Press, 1969

Bradley WG, Adey WR, Hasso AN: Magnetic Resonance Imaging of the Brain, Head, and Neck. Rockville, Maryland, Aspen Systems Corporation, 1985

Carrington A, McLachlan AD: Introduction to Magnetic Resonance: With Applications to Chemistry and Chemical Physics. New York, Harper & Row, 1967

Dwek RA: *Nuclear Magnetic Resonance (NMR) in Biochemistry.* Oxford, Clarendon Press, 1975

Farrar TC, Becker ED: Pulse and Fourier Transform NMR: Introduction to Theory and Methods. New York, Academic Press, 1971

Fukushima E, Roeder SBW: Experimental Pulse NMR. A Nuts and Bolts Approach. Reading, MA, Addison–Wesley Publishing Company, 1981

Gonzales CF, Grossman CB, Masdeu JC (eds): Head and Spine Imaging. New York, John Wiley & Sons, 1985

James TL, Margulis AR (eds): Biomedical Magnetic Resonance. San Francisco, Radiology Research and Education Foundation, 1985

Knowles PF, March D, Rattle HWE: Magnetic Resonance of Biomolecules: An Introduction to the Theory and Practice of NMR and ESR in Biological Systems. New York, John Wiley & Sons, 1976

Kressel HY (ed): Magnetic Resonance Annual 1985. New York, Raven Press, 1985

Margulis AR, Higgins CB, Kaufman L, Crooks LE: Clinical Magnetic Resonance Imaging. San Francisco, Radiology Research and Education Foundation, 1983

Newton TH, Potts DG (eds): Advanced Imaging Techniques. San Anselmo, CA, Clavadel Press, 1983

Slichter CP: Principles of Magnetic Resonance. New York, Springer-Verlag, 1978

Witcofski RL, Karstaedt N, Partain CL (eds): NMR Imaging. (proceedings of international symposium on nuclear magnetic resonance imaging). Winston-Salem, NC, Bowman Gray School of Medicine, 1982

Biological Effects of MRI

Adey WR: Tissue interactions with nonionizing electromagnetic fields. Physiol Rev 61:435, 1981

Bawin SM, Adey WR: Sensitivities of calcium binding in cerebral tissue to weak environmental electric fields oscillating at low frequency. Proc Natl Acad Sci USA 73:1999, 1976

Bawin SM, Kaczmarek LK, Adey WR: Effects of modulated VHF fields on the central nervous system. Ann NY Acad Sci 247:74, 1975

Bergstrom K, Jung B, Hemmingsson A et al: Nuclear magnetic resonance—a new diagnostic imaging method with wide possibilities. Lakartidningen 79:4665, 1982

Boijsen E, Persson BR: Nuclear magnetic resonance and relations to diagnostic radiology. Skeletal artefacts and genetic effects are avoided in nuclear resonance technic. Lakartidningen 81:91, 1984

Bradley WG Jr: Magnetic resonance imaging of the central nervous system. Neurol Res 6:91, 1984

Byus CV, Lundak RL, Fletcher RM et al: Altered protein kinase activity following exposure of cultured human lymphocytes to modulated microwave fields. Bioelectromagnetics 5:2, 1984

Davydov AS: Solitons in molecular systems. Physica Scripta 20:387, 1979

Delgado JMR, Leal J, Monteagudo JL et al: Embryological changes induced by weak, extremely low frequency electromagnetic fields. J Anat (London) 134:533, 1982

Dixey R, Rein G: ^{3}H-nonadrenaline release potentiated in a clonal nerve cell line by low-intensity pulsed magnetic fields. Nature 296:253, 1982

Genzel L, Kremer F, Poglitsch A et al: Relaxation processes on a picosecond time scale in hemoglobin and poly-l-alanine observed by mm-wave-spectroscopy. Biopolymers 22:1715, 1983

Ghandi OP, Hagman MJ: Some recent results on the deposition of electromagnetic energy in animals and models of man. In Taylor LS, Cheung AY (eds): The Physical Basis of Electromagnetic Interactions with Biological Systems, p 243. College Park, University of Maryland, 1977.

Grundler W, Keilmann F, Putterlik V et al: Nonthermal resonant action of millimeter microwaves on yeast growth. In Frohlich H, Kremer F (eds): Coherent Excitations in Biological Systems, p 25. New York, Springer-Verlag, 1983

Illinger KH: Electromagnetic field interaction with biological systems in the microwave and far-infrared region. In Illinger KH (ed): Biological Effects of Nonionizing Radiation, p 1. Washington, DC, American Chemical Society, 1981

Johnston DL, Liu P, Wismer GL et al: Magnetic resonance imaging: Present and future applications. Can Med Assoc J 132:765, 1985

Jolley WB, Hinshaw DB, Knierim K et al: Magnetic field effects on calcium efflux and insulin secretion in isolated rabbit islets of Langerhans. Bioelectromagnetics 4:103, 1983

Kritikos HN, Schwan HP: Potential temperature rise induced by electromagnetic field in brain tissue. IEEE Trans Biomed Eng 26:29, 1979

Luben RA, Cain CD, Chen MC-Y et al: Effects of electromagnetic stimuli on bone and bone cells in vitro: Inhibition of responses to parathyroid hormone by low-energy low-frequency fields. Proc Natl Acad Sci USA 79:4180, 1982

Lyle DB, Schechter P, Adley WR et al: Suppression of T-lymphocyte cytotoxicity following exposure to sinusoidally amplitude-modulated fields. Bioelectromagnetics 4:281, 1983

Mei WN, Kohli M, Van Zandt LL et al: Long-range forces in DNA. In Illinger KH (ed): Biological Effects of Nonunizing Radiation, p 95. Washington, DC, American Chemical Society, 1981

Palmer J: Nuclear magnetic resonance imaging. Med J Aust 1:252, 1983

Polk C: Time varying magnetic fields and DNA synthesis: Magnitude of forces due to magnetic fields on surface-bound counter-ions (abstr). Proc 6th Ann Meet. Bioelectromagnetics Soc 77, 1984

Prohofsky LL: Calculated microwave absorption by double-helical DNA. In Illinger KH (ed): Biological Effects of Nonionizing Radiation, p 101. Washington DC, American Chemical Society, 1981

Rinck PA: Risk and dangers in nuclear magnetic resonance tomography. Suggestions for protection and surveillance. Dtsch Med Wochenschr 108:992, 1983

Scott AC: The lasar-Raman spectrum of a Davydov soliton. Physics Letters 86A:60, 1981

Semm P: Neurobiological investigations on the magnetic sensitivity of the pineal gland in rodents and pigeons. Comp Biochem Physiol 76A: 683, 1983

Sheppard AR, Pickard WF, Bawin SM: Measurements in Aplysia neurons detect no transmembrane demodulation of extremely low frequency amplitude modulated 450 MHz fields (abstr). Proc 6th Ann Meet Bioelectromagnetics Soc 50, 1984

Shulman GI, Alger JR, Prichard JW et al: Nuclear magnetic resonance spectroscopy in diagnostic and investigative medicine. J Clin Invest 74:1127, 1984

Soulen RL, Budinger TF, Higgins CB: Magnetic resonance imaging of prosthetic heart valves. Radiology 154:705, 1985

Tenforde TS, Gaffey CT, Moyer BR et al: Cardiovascular alteration in Macaca monkeys exposed to stationary magnetic fields: Experimental observations and theoretical analysis. Bioelectromagnetics 4:1, 1983

Vbeda A, Leal J, Trilla MA et al: Pulse shape of magnetic fields influences chick embryogenesis. J Anat 137:513, 1983

Wolff S, James TL, Young GB et al: Magnetic resonance imaging: Absence of in vitro cytogenetic damage. Radiology 155:163, 1985

Cardiovascular

Amparo EG, Higgins, CB, Farmer D et al: Gated MRI of cardiac and paracardiac masses: Initial experience. AJR 143:1151, 1984

Amparo EG, Higgins CB, Hoddick W et al: Magnetic resonance imaging of aortic disease: Preliminary results. AJR 143:1203, 1984

Amparo EG, Higgins CB, Hricak H: Primary diagnosis of abdominal arteriovenous fistula by MR imaging. J Comput Assist Tomogr 8:1140, 1984

Amparo EG, Higgins CB, Hricak H et al: Aortic dissection: Magnetic resonance imaging. Radiology 155:399, 1985

Amparo EG, Hoddick WK, Hricak H et al: Comparison of magnetic resonance imaging and ultrasonography in the evaluation of abdominal aortic aneurysms. Radiology 154:451, 1985

Amparo EG, Higgins CB, Shafton EP: Demonstration of coarctation of the aorta by magnetic resonance imaging. AJR 143:1192, 1984

van As H, Schaafsma TJ, de Jager PA et al: Flow imaging by nuclear magnetic resonance. Ann Radiol (Paris) 27:405, 1984

Barth K, Deimling M, Fritschy P et al: Visualization and measurement of flow with magnetic resonance imaging. Biomed Tech (Berlin) 30:12, 1985

Battocletti JH: NMR proton imaging. Crit Rev Biomed Eng 11:313, 1984

Becker RC, Hobbs RE, Ratliff NB: Cardiac rhabdomyosarcoma: Case report with review of clinical and pathologic features. Cleve Clin Q 51:83, 1984

Berger HJ, Pettigrew RI: The future of cardiovascular imaging: A shift from anatomy to in vivo biochemistry. J Am Coll Cardiol 5:750, 1985

Bryant DJ, Payne JA, Firmin DN et al: Measurement of flow with NMR imaging using a gradient pulse and phase difference technique. J Comput Assist Tomogr 8:588, 1984

Budinger TF: Dynamic transmission computed tomography, emission tomography, and nuclear magnetic resonance methods of measuring physiologic parameters. Mayo Clin Proc (Suppl):57 67, 1982

Byrd BF 3rd, Schiller NB, Botvinick EH et al: Normal cardiac dimensions by magnetic resonance imaging. Am J Cardiol 55:1440, 1985

Choyke PL, Kresel HY, Reichek N et al: Nongated cardiac magnetic resonance imaging: preliminary experience at 0.12 T. AJR 143:1143, 1984

Crooks LE, Barker B, Chang H et al: T1 magnetic resonance imaging strategies for heart studies. Radiology 153:459, 1984

Crooks LE, Kaufman L: NMR imaging of blood flow. Br Med Bull 40:167, 1984

Crooks LE, Mills CM, Davis PL et al: Visualization of cerebral and vascular abnormalities by NMR imaging. The effects of imaging parameters on contrast. Radiology 144:843, 1982

Cushley RJ, Forrest BJ, Grover AK et al: ^{13}C and ^{31}P nuclear magnetic resonance of lipid dispersions from human aorta. Can J Biochem 58:206, 1980

van Dijk P: Direct cardiac NMR imaging of heart wall and blood flow velocity. J Comput Assist Tomogr 8:429, 1984

van Dijk P: EGC-triggered NMR imaging of the heart. Diagn Imag Clin Med 53:29, 1984

Dinsmore RE, Wismer GL, Levine RA et al: Magnetic resonance imaging of the heart: Positioning and gradient angle selection for optimal imaging planes. AJR 143:1135, 1984

Farmer D, Higgins CB, Yee E et al: Tissue characterization by magnetic resonance imaging in hypertrophic cardiomyopathy. Am J Cardiol 55:230, 1985

Farmer DW, Moore E, Amparo E et al: Calcific fibrosing mediastinitis: Demonstration of pulmonary vascular obstruction by magnetic resonance imaging. AJR 143:1189, 1984

Feiglin DH, George CR, MacIntyre WJ et al: Gated cardiac magnetic resonance structural imaging: Optimization by electronic axial rotation. Radiology 154:129, 1985

Feinberg DA, Crooks L, Hoenninger J 3d et al: Pulsatile blood velocity in human arteries displayed by magnetic resonance imaging. Radiology 153:177, 1984

Flak B, Li DK, Ho BY et al: Magnetic resonance imaging of aneurysms of the abdominal aorta. AJR 144:991, 1985

Gadian DG: Metabolic studies of whole animals and humans using phosphorus nuclear magnetic resonance. Biosci Rep 1:449, 1981

Geisinger MA, Risius B, ODonnell JA et al: Thoracic aortic dissections: Magnetic resonance imaging. Radiology 155:407, 1985

George CR, Jacobs G, MacIntyre WJ et al: Magnetic resonance signal intensity patterns obtained from continuous and pulsatile flow models. Radiology 151:421, 1984

Goldman MR, Pohost GM, Ingwall JS et al: Nuclear magnetic resonance imaging: Potential cardiac applications. Am J Cardiol 46:1278, 1980

Gould KL, Goldstein RA: Cardiovascular imaging metabolic and functional. Physiologist 27:27, 1984

Gutierrez FR, Glazer HS, Levitt RG et al: NMR imaging of pulmonary arteriovenous fistulae. J Comput Assist Tomogr 8:750, 1984

Gutierrez FR, Shackelford GD, McKnight RC et al: Diagnosis of congenital absence of left pericardium by MR imaging. J Comput Assist Tomogr 9:551, 1985

Heidelberger E, Peterson SB, Lauterbur PC: Aspects of cardiac diagnosis using synchronized NMR imaging. Eur J Radiol 3 (Suppl)1:281, 1983

Hawkes RC, Holland GN, Moore WS et al: Nuclear magnetic resonance (NMR) tomography of the normal heart. J Comput Assist Tomogr 5:605, 1981

Higgins CB, Goldberg H, Hricak H et al: Nuclear magnetic resonance imaging of vasculature of abdominal viscera: Normal and pathologic features. AJR 140:1217, 1983

Herfkens RJ, Higgins CB, Hricak H et al: Nuclear magnetic resonance imaging of the cardiovascular system: Normal and pathologic findings. Radiology 147:749, 1983

Herfkens RJ, Higgins CB, Hricak H et al: Nuclear magnetic resonance imaging of atherosclerotic disease. Radiology 148:161, 1983

Higgins CB, Byrd BF 3rd, Farmer DW et al: Magnetic resonance imaging in patients with congenital heart disease. Circulation 70:851, 1984

Higgins CB, Byrd BF 3rd, Stark D et al: Magnetic resonance imaging in hypertrophic cardiomyopathy. Am J Cardiol 55:1121, 1985

Higgins CB, Kaufman L, Crooks LE: Magnetic resonance imaging of the cardiovascular system. Am Heart J 109:136, 1985

Higgins CB, Lanzer P, Stark D et al: Imaging by nuclear magnetic resonance in patients with chronic ischemic heart disease. Circulation 69:523, 1984

Higgins CB, Lanzer P, Stark D et al: Assessment of cardiac anatomy using nuclear magnetic resonance imaging. J Am Coll Cardiol 5:77S, 1985

Higgins CB, Stark D, McNamara M et al: Multiplane magnetic resonance imaging of the heart and major vessels: Studies in normal volunteers. AJR 142:661, 1984

Jacobstein MD, Fletcher BD, Goldstein S et al: Evaluation of atrioventricular septal defect by magnetic resonance imaging. Am J Cardiol 55:1158, 1985

Jacobstein MD, Fletcher BD, Nelson AD et al: Magnetic resonance imaging: evaluation of palliative systemic-pulmonary artery shunts. Circulation 70:650, 1984

Jacobstein MD, Fletcher BD, Nelson AD et al: ECG-gated nuclear magnetic resonance imaging: Appearance of the congenitally malformed heart. Am Heart J 107:1014, 1984

Justich E, Amparo EG, Hricak H et al: Infected aorto-iliofemoral grafts: Magnetic resonance imaging. Radiology 154:133, 1985

Kaufman L, Crooks L, Sheldon P et al: The potential impact of nuclear magnetic resonance imaging on cardiovascular diagnosis. Circulation 67:251, 1983

Kaufman L, Crooks LE, Sheldon PE et al: Evaluation of NMR imaging for detection and quantification of obstructions in vessels. Invest Radiol 17:554, 1982

Lanzer P, Botvinick EH, Schiller NB et al: Cardiac imaging using gated magnetic resonance. Radiology 150:121, 1984

Lee JK, Ling D, Heiken JP et al: Magnetic resonance imaging of abdominal aortic aneurysms. AJR 143:1197, 1984

Lees RS, Kistler JP: Noninvasive diagnosis of extracranial cerebrovascular disease Clin Neurol 2:667, 1984

Lieberman JM Alfidi RJ, Nelson AD et al: Gated magnetic resonance imaging of the normal and diseased heart. Radiology 152:465, 1984

Lieberman JM, Botti RE, Nelson AD: Magnetic resonance imaging of the heart. Radiol Clin North Am 22:847, 1984

Martin KW, Morian JP Jr, Lee JK et al: Demonstration of a splenic artery pseudoaneurysm by MR imaging. J Comput Assist Tomogr 9:190, 1985

McCarthy S, Stark DD, Higgins CB: Demonstration of the fetal cardiovascular system by MR imaging. J Comput Assist Tomogr 8:1168, 1984

McNamara MT, Higgins CB: Cardiovascular applications of magnetic resonance imaging. Magn Reson Imaging 2:167, 1984

McNamara MT, Higgins CB, Schechtmann N et al: Detection and characterization of acute myocardial infarction in man with use of gated magnetic resonance. Circulation 71:717, 1985

Menasche P, Fauchet M, Fossel ET et al: Nuclear magnetic resonance: A new method for non-invasive assessment of cardiac metabolism. Med Prog Technol 8:183, 1982

Merritt CR, Bluth EI: Techniques for diagnostic imaging. Computed tomography, ultrasound, and magnetic resonance imaging. Postgrad Med 77:56, 1985

Mills CM, Brant-Zawadzki M, Crooks LE et al: Nuclear magnetic resonance: Principles of blood flow imagins. AJR 142:165, 1984

Moore EH, Webb WR, Verrier ED et al: MRI of chronic posttraumatic false aneurysms of the thoracic aorta. AJR 143:1195, 1984

Murphy WA, Gutierrez FR, Levitt RG et al: T1 oblique views of the heart by magnetic resonance imaging. Radiology 154:225, 1985

Nishikawa J, Machida K, Iio M et al: ECG-gated NMR-CT for cadiovascular disease. Radiat Med 1:274, 1983

O'Donnell M: NMR blood flow imaging using multiecho, phase contrast sequences. Med Phys 12:59, 1985

Osbakken M, Briggs RW: Nuclear magnetic resonance: Theory and review of cardiac application. Am Heart J 108:574, 1984

Pflugfelder PW, Wisenberg G, Boughner DR: Detection of atrial myxoma by magnetic resonance imaging. Am J Cardiol 55:242, 1985

Pizzarello RA, Goldberg SM, Goldman MA et al: Tumor of the heart diagnosed by magnetic resonance imaging. J Am Coll Cardiol 5:989, 1985

Pohost GM, Ratner AV: Nuclear magnetic resonance. New methods for the assessment of cardiac structure and function. Cardiology 71:162, 1984

Pohost GM, Ratner AV: Nuclear magnetic resonance. Potential applications in clinical cardiology. JAMA 251:1304, 1984

Pohost GM, Ratner AV, Okada RD: Proton NMR imaging: A new approach for the evaluation of cardiac structure and function. Int J Cardiol 4:87, 1983

Radda GK: Potential and limitations of nuclear magnetic resonance for the cardiologist. Br Heart J 50:197, 1983

Rehr RB, Filipchuk NG, Malloy CR, et al: Magnetic resonance imaging in aortic valve, ascending aortic and isthmic aortic disease. Am J Cardiol 55:1243, 1985

Reynolds JR, Mikulin T, Hopkinson BR et al: A comparison of nuclear magnetic resonance and intravenous xeroangiography with conventional arteriography in popliteal artery imaging. Clin Radiol 35:409, 1984

Rhodes RS, Cohen AM: Magnetic resonance imaging and spectroscopy in the study of cardiovascular disease. J Vasc Surg 2:354, 1985

Ringertz HG, Brasch RC, Brody A et al: Magnetic resonance imaging of vascular lesions in children. Assessment of flow patterns. Acta Radiol [Diagn] (Stockh) 25:449, 1984

Rollo FD: Future vistas in cardiovascular nuclear medicine. Clin Nucl Med 6:P6, 1981

Ross RS, Barnes RW, Budinger TF et al: Summary of NHLBI-sponsored workshop on noninvasive techniques for assessment of atherosclerosis. IEEE Trans Biomed Eng 27:677, 1980

Rowlands DJ: Imaging the heart. J R Coll Physicians Lond 18:253, 1984

Rzedzian R, Chapman B, Mansfield P et al: Real-time nuclear magnetic resonance clinical imaging in paediatrics. Lancet 2(8362):1281, 1983

Rzedzian R, Doyle M, Mansfield P et al: Echo planar imaging in paediatrics: Real-time-nuclear magnetic resonance. Ann Radiol (Paris) 27:182, 1984

Salles-Cunha SX, Halbach RE, Battocletti JH et al: The NMR blood flowmeter–applications. Med Phys 8:452, 1981

Schelbert HR, Phelps ME, Shine KL: Imaging metabolism and biochemistry—a new look at the heart. Am Heart J 105:522, 1983

Schiavone WA, ODonnell JK: Congenital absence of the left portion of parietal pericardium demonstrated by nuclear magnetic resonance imaging. Am J Cardiol 55:1439, 1985

Schultz CL, Morison S, Bryan PJ: Azygos continuation of the inferior vena cava: Demonstration by NMR imaging. J Comput Assist Tomogr 8:774, 1984

Seeger JF, Carmody RF: Radiologic evaluation of the carotid arteries. CRC Crit Rev Diagn Imaging 22:127, 1984

Singer JR, Crooks LE: Nuclear magnetic resonance blood flow measurements in the human brain. Science 221:654, 1983

Skorton DJ, Collins SM: New directions in cardiac imaging. Ann Intern Med 102:795, 1985

Solen RL, Stark DD, Higgins CB: Magnetic resonance imaging of constrictive pericardial disease. Am J Cardiol 55:480, 1985

Stark DD, Higgins CB, Lanzer P et al: Magnetic resonance imaging of the pericardium: Normal and pathologic findings. Radiology 150:469, 1984

Steiner RE: Nuclear magnetic resonance imaging of the heart and mediastinum. Br Med Bull 40:191, 1984

Steiner RE, Bydder GM, Selwyn A et al: Nuclear magnetic resonance imaging of the heart. Current status and future prospects. Br Heart J 50:202, 1983

Thickman D, Kressel HY, Axel L: Demonstration of pulmonary embolism by magnetic resonance imaging. AJR 142:921, 1984

Tripathi A, Bydder GM, Hughes JM et al: Effect of oxygen tension on NMR spin-lattice relaxation rate of blood in vivo. Invest Radiol 19:174, 1984

Urry DW, Trapane TL, Andrews SK et al: NMR observation of altered sodium interaction with human erythrocyte membranes of essential hypertensives. Biochem Biophys Res Commun 96:514, 1980

Waluch V, Bradley WG: NMR even echo rephasing in slow laminar flow. J Comput Assist Tomogr 8:594, 1984

Wehrli FW, Shimakawa A, MacFall JR et al: MR imaging of venous and arterial flow by a selective saturation-recovery spin echo (SSRSE) method. J Comput Assist Tomogr 9:537, 1985

Whitman GJ, Chance B, Bode H et al: Diagnosis and therapeutic evaluation of a pediatric case of cardiomyopathy using phosphorus-31 nuclear magnetic resonance spectroscopy. J Am Coll Cardiol 5:745, 1985

Zeitler E, Schuierer G: Diagnosis of cardiovascular diseases with NMR imaging. Prog Nucl Med 8:100, 1984

Urinary Tract

Altwein JE: New imaging techniques in the staging of urological tumors (kidney, retroperitoneal lymph nodes and tumors). Prog Clin Biol Res 153:23, 1984

Bales JR, Higham DP, Howe I et al: Use of high-resolution proton nuclear magnetic resonance spectroscopy for rapid multicomponent analysis of urine. Clin Chem 30:426, 1984

Brown CE, Battocletti JH, Johnson LF: Nuclear magnetic resonance (NMR) in clinical pathology: Current trends. Clin Chem 30:606, 1984

Bryan PJ, Butler HE, LiPuma JP: Magnetic resonance imaging of the pelvis. Radiol Clin North Am 22:897, 1984

Bryan PJ, Butler HE, LiPuma JP et al: NMR scanning of the pelvis: Initial experience with a 0.3 T system. AJR 141:1111, 1983

Bydder GM: Clinical NMR imaging of the abdomen. Prog Nucl Med 8:124, 1984

Carr DH: The use of proton relaxation enhancers in magnetic resonance imaging. Magn Reson Imaging 3:17, 1985

Carr DH, Brown J, Bydder GM et al: Gadolinium-DTPA as a contrast agent in MRI: Initial clinical experience in 20 patients. AJR 143:215, 1984

Choyke PL, Kressel HY, Pollack HM et al: Focal renal masses: Magnetic resonance imaging. Radiology 152:471, 1984

Choyke PL, Meranze S, Pahira JJ et al: Imaging of urinary tract disease. Current approaches. Med Clin North Am 68:1565, 1984

Demas BE, Hricak H, Williams RD: Magnetic resonance imaging in the evaluation of urologic malignancies. Semin Urol 3:27, 1985

Dwyer AJ, Knop RH, Hoult DI: Frequency shift artifacts in MR imaging. J Comput Assist Tomogr 9:16, 1985

Ehman RL, Wesbey GE, Moon KL et al: Enhanced MRI of tumors utilizing a new nitroxyl spin label contrast agent. Magn Reson Imaging 3:89, 1985

Gadian DG, Payne JA, Bryant DJ et al: Gadolinium-DTPA as a contrast agent in MR imaging—theoretical projections and practical observations. J Comput Assist Tomogr 9:242, 1985

Gatenby RA: Diagnostic evaluation of a renal mass. Semin Oncol 10:401, 1983

Geisinger MA, Risius B, Jordan ML et al: Magnetic resonance imaging of renal transplants. AJR 143:1229, 1984

Gupta RK, Gupta P, Moore RD: NMR studies of intracellular metal ions in intact cells and tissues. Annu Rev Biophys Bioeng 13:221, 1984

Hadley MD, Nichols DM, Smith FW: Nuclear magnetic resonance tomographic imaging in xanthogranulomatous pyelonephritis. J Urol 127:301, 1982

Hricak H: MR imaging of the retroperitoneum and pelvis. Br Med Bull 40:197, 1984

Hricak H, Crooks L, Sheldon P et al: Nuclear magnetic resonance imaging of the kidney. Radiology 146:425, 1983

Hricak H, Demas BE, Williams RD et al: Magnetic resonance imaging in the diagnosis and staging of renal and perirenal neoplasms. Radiology 154:709, 1985

Hricak H, Newhouse JH: MR imaging of the kidney. Radiol Clin North Am 22:287, 1984

Hricak H, Williams RD: Magnetic resonance imaging and its application in urology. Urology 23:442, 1984

Hricak H, Williams RD, Moon KL Jr et al: Nuclear magnetic resonance imaging of the kidney: Renal masses. Radiology 147:765, 1983

Kokko J: Applications of nuclear magnetic resonance (NMR) in nephrology. Adv Exp Med Biol 178:465, 1984

Kulkarni MV, Shaff MI, Sandler MP et al: Evaluation of renal masses by MR imaging. J Comput Assist Tomogr 8:861, 1984

Lang EK: Neoplasms of the bladder, prostate, and urethra. Semin Roentgenol 18:288, 1983

Laniado M, Weinmann HJ, Schorner W et al: First use of GdDTPA/dimeglumine in man. Physiol Chem Phys 16:157, 1984

Lantz EJ, Hattery RR: Diagnostic imaging of urothelial cancer. Urol Clin North Am 11:567, 1984

Leung AW, Bydder GM, Steiner RE et al: Magnetic resonance imaging of the kidneys. AJR 143:1215, 1984

LiPuma JP: Magnetic resonance imaging of the kidney. Radiol Clin North Am 22:925, 1984

Malet-Martino MC, Martino R, Lopez A et al: New approach to metabolism of 5′-deoxy-5-flourouridine in humans with flourine-19 NMR. Cancer Chemother Pharmacol 13:31, 1984

Marshall V, Ross B, Smith M et al: Organ and tissue preservation for transplantation: Monitoring by ^{31}P nuclear magnetic resonance. Transplant Proc 17:1693, 1985

Narayanan S, Appleton HD: Creatinine: A review. Clin Chem 26:1119, 1980

Newhouse JH: Urinary tract imaging by nuclear magnetic resonance. Urol Radiol 4:171, 1982

Pettersson H, Springfield D, Hamlin D et al: Magnetic resonance imaging and tissue characterization of a renal cell carcinoma and its osseous metastasis. Report of a case. Acta Radiol [Diagn] (Stockh) 26:193, 1985

Radda GK, Gadian DG, Ross BD: Energy metabolism and cellular pH in normal and pathological conditions. A new look through 31-phosphorus nuclear magnetic resonance. Ciba Found Symp 87:36, 1982

Resnick MI, Kursh ED, Bryan PD: Nuclear magnetic resonance imaging and bladder cancer. Prog Clin Biol Res 162A:255, 1984

Ross B, Marshall V, Smith M et al: Monitoring response to chemotherapy of intact human tumours by ^{31}P nuclear magnetic resonance. Lancet 1(8378):641, 1984

Smith FW: NMR proton imaging at 3.4 MHz—genitourinary tract and pelvis. Prog Nucl Med 8:135, 1984

Smith FW, Hutchinson JM, Mallard JR et al: Renal cyst or tumour? Differentiation by whole-body nuclear magnetic resonance imaging. Diagn Imaging 50:61, 1981

Smith FW, Reid A, Mallard JR et al: Nuclear magnetic resonance tomographic imaging in renal disease. Diagn Imaging 51:209, 1982

Soila KP, Viamonte M Jr, Starewicz PM: Chemical shift misregistration effect in magnetic resonance imaging. Radiology 153:819, 1984

Streem SB, Novick AC: Pelvic imaging techniques in renal transplantation. Urol Clin North Am 10:301, 1983

Sugisaki H, Onohara M, Kunitomo T: Phosphate in dialysis patients. Trans Am Soc Artif Intern Organs 29:38, 1983

te Strake L, van der Hem GK, Hooijkaas JA, et al: Nuclear magnetic resonance imaging of the kidney. Diagn Imag Clin Med 53:198, 1984

Thornbury JR, Wicks JD, Eckel CG: Imaging methods for evaluating the adult bladder and urethra: An overview. Semin Roentgenol 18:250, 1983

Todd LE, Perez JL, Elizondo G et al: In vivo T1 relaxation times in transplanted kidneys of human subjects. Physiol Chem Phys 15:27, 1983

van Ypersele de Strihou C: Non-invasive assessment of the kidney. What do nuclear medicine, ultrasonography, digital vascular imaging, computed tomography, and magnetic resonance contribute to diagnosis in nephrology? Proc Eur Dial Transplant Assoc 21:771, 1985

Weiner MW, Adam WR: Magnetic resonance spectroscopy for evaluation of renal function. Semin Urol 3:34, 1985

Weinmann HJ, Laniado M, Mutzel W: Parmacokinetics of GdDTPA/ dimeglumine after intravenous injection into healthy volunteers. Physiol Chem Phys 16:167, 1984

Wesbey GE, Engelstad BL, Brasch RC: Paramagnetic pharmaceuticals for magnetic resonance imaging. Physiol Chem Phys 16:145, 1984

Williams RD, Hricak H: Magnetic resonance imaging in urology. J Urol 132:641, 1984

Yoshikawa K, Matsushita K, Ohsaka A: ^{1}H-NMR spectroscopy in aqueous mediums. Examination of experimental conditions with human urine as a model sample. Physiol Chem Phys 14:385, 1982

Brain

Aaron J, New PF, Strand R et al: NMR imaging in temporal lobe epilepsy due to gliomas. J Comput Assist Tomogr 8:608, 1984

Andrews BT, Halks-Miller M, Berger MS et al: Neuroepithelial cysts of the posterior fossa: Pathogenesis and report of two cases. Neurosurgery 15:91, 1984

Bailes DR, Young IR, Thomas DJ et al: NMR imaging of the brain using spin-echo sequences. Clin Radiol 33:395, 1982

Battocletti JH: NMR proton imaging. Crit Rev Biomed Eng 11:313, 1984

Behnke EE, Schindler RA: Dermoid of the petrous apex. Laryngoscope 94:779, 1984

Bewermeyer H, Dreesbach HA, Hunermann B et al: MR imaging of familiar basilar impression. J Comput Assist Tomogr 8:953, 1984

Besson JA, Corrigan FM, Foreman EI et al: Nuclear magnetic resonance (NMR). II. Imaging in dementia. Br J Psychiatry 146:31, 1985

Besson JA, Foreman EI, Eastwood LM et al: Cognitive evaluation following NMR imaging of the brain. J Neurol Neurosurg Psychiatry 47:314, 1984

Besson JA, Glen AI, Foreman EI et al: Nuclear magnetic resonance observations in alcoholic cerebral disorder and the role of vasopressin. Lancet 2(8252):923, 1981

Bilaniuk LT: Magnetic resonance imaging of the brain—the present and the future. Psychopharmacol Bull 20:371, 1984

Bosley TM, Cohen DA, Schatz NJ et al: Comparison of metrizamide computed tomography and magnetic resonance imaging in the evaluation of lesions at the cervicomedullary junction. Neurology 35:485, 1985

Bottomley PA, Edelstein WA, Foster TH et al: In vivo solvent-suppressed localized hydrogen nuclear magnetic resonance spectroscopy: A window to metabolism? Proc Natl Acad Sci USA 82:2148, 1985

Bottomley PA, Foster TH, Leue WM: Chemical imaging of the brain by NMR (letter). Lancet 1(8386):1120, 1984

Bottomley PA, Hart HR Jr, Edelstein WA et al: Anatomy and metabolism of the normal human brain studied by magnetic resonance at 1.5 tesla. Radiology 150:441, 1984

Bottomley PA, Hart HR, Edelstein WA et al: NMR imaging/ spectroscopy system to study both anatomy and metabolism (letter). Lancet 2(8344):273, 1983

Brant-Zadawzki M, Davis PL, Crooks LE et al: NMR demonstration of cerebral abnormalities: Comparison with CT. AJR 140:847, 1983

Brant-Zawadzki M, Kelly W, Kjos B et al: Magnetic resonance imaging and characterization of normal and abnormal intracranial cerebrospinal fluid (CSF) spaces. Neuroradiology 27:3, 1985

Brenton DP, Garrod PJ, Krywawych S et al: Phosphoethanolamine is major constituent of phosphomonester peak detected by ^{31}P NMR in newborn brain (letter). Lancet 1(8420):115, 1985

Buonanno FS, Pykett IL, Brady TJ et al: Clinical relevance of two different nuclear magnetic resonance (NMR) approaches to imaging of a low grade astrocytoma. J Comput Assist Tomogr 6:529, 1982

Burton K, Farrell K, Li D et al: Lesions of the putamen and dystonia: CT and magnetic resonance imaging. Neurology 34:962, 1984

Bydder GM: Magnetic resonance imaging of the brain. Radiol Clin North Am 22:779, 1984

Bydder GM, Butsen PC, Harman RR et al: Use of spherical receiver coils in MR imaging of the brain. J Comput Assist Tomogr 9:413, 1985

Bydder GM, Steiner RE: NMR imaging of the brain. Neuroradiology 23:231, 1982

Bydder GM, Steiner RE, Spencer DH et al: NMR imaging of the brain: current status and perspectives. Ann Radiol (Paris) 26:39, 1983

Bydder GM, Steiner RE, Thoman DJ et al: Nuclear magnetic resonance imaging of the posterior fossa: 50 cases. Clin Radiol 34:173, 1983

Bydder GM, Steiner RE, Young IR et al: Clinical NMR imaging of the brain: 140 cases. AJR 139:215, 1982

Bydder GM, Whitelaw A: Nuclear magnetic resonance imaging of the brain. Arch Dis Child 58:401, 1983

Cady EB, Costello AM, Dawson MJ et al: Non-invasive investigation of cerebral metabolism in newborn infants by phosphorus nuclear magnetic resonance spectroscopy. Lancet 1(8333):1059, 1983

Carr WA, Baumann RJ, Baker RS: Nuclear magnetic resonance imaging in neuro-ophthalmology. Demonstration of a pontine glioma. Surv Ophthalmol 29:79, 1984

Carr DH, Brown J, Bydder GM et al: Gadolinium-DTPA as a contrast agent in MRI: Initial clinical experience in 20 patients. AJR 143:215, 1984

Daniels DL, Pech P, Mark L et al: Magnetic resonance imaging of the cavernous sinus. AJR 144:1009, 1985

Davidson HD, Abraham R, Steiner RE: Agenesis of the corpus callosum: Magnetic resonance imaging. Radiology 155:371, 1985

DeWitt LD, Buonanno FS, Kistler JP et al: Central pontine myelinolysis: demonstration by nuclear magnetic resonance. Neurology 34:570, 1984

Doyle FH, Gore JC, Pennock JM et al: Imaging of the brain by nuclear magnetic resonance. Lancet 2(8237):53, 1981

Drayer BP, Barrett L: Magnetic resonance imaging and CT scanning in multiple sclerosis. Ann NY Acad Sci 436:294, 1984

Dubowitz LM, Bydder GM: Nuclear magnetic resonance imaging in the diagnosis and follow-up of neonatal cerebral injury. Clin Perinatol 12:243, 1985

Eastwood LM, Hutchinson JM, Besson JA: Nuclear magnetic resonance (NMR): I. Imaging biochemical change. Br J Psychiatry 146:26, 1985

Flannigan BD, Bradley WG Jr, Mazziotta JC et al: Magnetic resonance imaging of the brainstem: Normal structure and basic functional anatomy. Radiology 154:375, 1985

Furman JM, Brownstone PK, Baloh RW: Atypical brainstem encephalitis: Magnetic resonance imaging and oculographic features. Neurology 35:438, 1985

Gadian DG: Metabolic studies of whole animals and humans using phosphorus nuclear magnetic resonance. Biosci Rep 1:449, 1981

Gandy SE, Snow RB, Zimmerman RD et al: Cranial nuclear magnetic resonance imaging in head trauma. Ann Neurol 16:254, 1984

Ganz E: Positron emission tomography and nuclear magnetic resonance. Clin Neurosurg 31:441, 1983

Gerard G, Rossi DR: Nuclear magnetic resonance imaging of the brain. Hosp Pract 19:143, 1984

Grossman RI, Lynch RM: Neuroimaging in neuro-ophthalmology. Neurol Clin 1(4):831, 1983

Gyulai L, Bolinger L, Leigh JS Jr et al: Phosphorylethanolamine—the major constituent of the phosphomonoester peak observed by ^{31}P-NMR on developing dog brain. FEBS Lett 178:137, 1984

Han JS, Benson JE, Kaufman B et al: MR imaging of pediatric cerebral abnormalities. J Comput Assist Tomogr 9:103, 1985

Han JS, Bonstelle CT, Kaufman B et al: Magnetic resonance imaging in the evaluation of the brainstem. Radiology 150:705, 1984

Han JS, Huss RG, Benson JE et al: MR imaging of the skull base. J Comput Assist Tomogr 8:944, 1984

Hawkes RC, Holland GN, Moore WS et al: Craniovertebral junction pathology: Assessment by NMR. AJNR 4:232, 1983

Hawkes RC, Holland GN, Moore WS et al: Nuclear magnetic resonance (NMR) tomography of the brain: A preliminary clinical assessment with demonstration of pathology. J Comput Assist Tomogr 4:577, 1980

Heinzerling J: New developments in nuclear magnetic resonance (NMR) imaging. Neurosurg Rev 7:281, 1984

Holland BA, Brant-Zawadzki M, Norman D et al: Magnetic resonance imaging of primary intracranial tumors: A review. Int J Radiat Oncol Biol Phys 11:315, 1985

Holland GN, Moore WS, Hawkes RC: NMR neuroradiology. Br J Radiol 53:253, 1980

Holland GN, Moore WS, Hawkes RC: Nuclear magnetic resonance tomography of the brain. J Comput Assist Tomogr 4:1, 1980

Hope PL, Costello AM, Cady EB et al: Cerebral energy metabolism studied with phosphorus NMR spectroscopy in normal and birth-asphyxiated infants. Lancet 2(8399):366, 1984

Hope PL, Reynolds EO: Investigation of cerebral energy metabolism in newborn infants by phosphorus nuclear magnetic resonance spectroscopy. Clin Perinatol 12:261, 1985

Hueftle MG, Han JS, Kaufman B et al: MR imaging of brain stem gliomas. J Comput Assist Tomogr 9:263, 1985

Hughes DW, Stollery JG, Moscarello MA et al: Binding of myelin basic protein to phospholipid micelles. J Biol Chem 257:4698, 1982

Huk W, Heindel W, Deimling M et al: Nuclear magnetic resonance (NMR) tomography of the central nervous system: Comparison of two imaging sequences. J Comput Assist Tomogr 7:468, 1983

Iivanainen M, Hakola P, Erkinjuntti T et al: Cerebral MR and CT imaging in polycystic lipomembraneous osteodysplasia with sclerosing leukoencephalopathy. J Comput Assist Tomogr 8:940, 1984

Inouye T, Satoh K, Kose K et al: Experimental results with a whole body NMR-CT scanner using a resistive magnet. Radiol Med 1:8, 1983

Jackson JA, Derman HS, Harper RL et al: Nuclear magnetic resonance diagnosis of an anaplastic astrocytoma. Magn Reson Imaging 2:227, 1984

Johnson MA, Bydder GM: NMR imaging of the brain in children. Br Med Bull 40:175, 1984

Johnson MA, Pennock JM, Bydder GM et al: Clinical NMR imaging of the brain in chidren: Normal and neurologic disease. AJR 141:1005, 1983

Jolesz FA: Functional imaging of the brain. Med Instrum 17:59, 1983

Joseph R, Pullicino P, Goldberg CD et al: Bilateral pontine gaze palsy. Nuclear magnetic resonance findings in presumed multiple sclerosis. Arch Neurol 42:93, 1985

Kamman RL, Go KG, Muskiet FA et al: Proton spin relaxation studies of fatty tissue and cerebral white matter. Magn Reson Imaging 2:211, 1984

Kaufman BA, Kaufman B, Rekate HL: Cervicomedullary junction tumor diagnosed by nuclear magnetic resonance scanning: Case report. Neurosurgery 15:878, 1984

Kean DM, Smith MA, Douglas RH et al: Two examples of CNS lipomas demonstrated by computed tomography and low field (0.08 T) MR imaging. J Comput Assist Tomogr 9:494, 1985

Kramer DM, Schneider JS, Rudin AM et al: True three-dimensional nuclear magnetic resonance zeumatographic images of a human brain. Neuroradiology 21:239, 1981

Kressel HY: The principles of NMR imaging and a review of early clinical results. Radiat Med 1:197, 1983

Laster DW, Penry JK, Moody DM et al: Chronic seizure disorders: Contribution of MR imaging when CT is normal. AJNR 6:177, 1985

Lawler GA, Pennock JM, Steiner RE et al: Nuclear magnetic resonance (NMR) imaging in Wilson disease. J Comput Assist Tomogr 7:1, 1983

Lee BC, Deck MD, Kneeland JB et al: MR imaging of the craniocervical junction. AJNR 6:209, 1985

Lee BC, Kneeland JB, Deck MD et al: Posterior fossa lesions: Magnetic resonance imaging. Radiology 153:137, 1984

Lee BC, Kneeland JB, Walker RW et al: MR imaging of brainstem tumors. AJNR 6:159, 1985

Leksell L, Herner T, Leksell D et al: Visualisation of stereotactic radiolesions by nuclear magnetic resonance. J Neurol Neurosurg Psychiatry 48:19, 1985

Levene MI, Whitelaw A, Dubowitz V et al: Nuclear magnetic resonance imaging of the brain in children. Br Med J [Clin Res] 285:774, 1982

Littrup PJ, Gebarski SS: MR imaging of Hallervorden-Spatz disease. J Comput Assist Tomogr 9:491, 1985

Lukes SA, Aminoff MJ, Crooks L et al: Nuclear magnetic resonance imaging in movement disorders (letters). Ann Neurol 13:690, 1983

Lukes SA, Crooks LE, Aminoff MJ et al: Nuclear magnetic resonance imaging in multiple sclerosis. Ann Neurol 13:592, 1983

Maravilla KR, Weinreb JC, Suss R et al: Magnetic resonance demonstration of multiple sclerosis plaques in the cervical cord. AJR 144:381, 1985

Mark L, Pech P, Daniels D et al: The pituitary fossa: A correlative anatomic and MR study. Radiology 153:453, 1984

McGinnis BD, Brady TJ, New PF et al: Nuclear magnetic resonance (NMR) imaging of tumors in the posterior fossa. J Comput Assist Tomogr 7:575, 1983

Mills CM, Brant-Zawadzki M, Crooks LE et al: Nuclear magnetic resonance imaging: Applications for neurological abnormalities. Radiat Med 1:1, 1983

Morrison AW, King TT: Space-occupying lesions of the internal auditory meatus and cerebellopontine angle. Adv Otorhinolaryngol 34:121, 1984

Nagashima C, Kubota S: Craniocervical abnormalities. Modern diagnosis and a comprehensive surgical approach. Neurosurg Rev 6:187, 1983

Noseworthy JH, Paty DW, Eders GC: Neuroimaging in multiple sclerosis. Neurol Clin 2:759, 1984

Novetsky GJ, Berlin L: Aqueductal stenosis: Demonstration by MR imaging. J Comput Assist Tomogr 8:1170, 1984

Oldendorf WH: The use and promise of nuclear magnetic resonance imaging in epilepsy. Epilepsia 25(Suppl)2:S105, 1984

Packer RJ, Zimmerman RA, Luerssen TG et al: Brainstem gliomas of childhood: Magnetic resonance imaging. Neurology 35:397, 1985

Petroff OA, Prichard JW: Cerebral pH by NMR (letter). Lancet 2(8341):105, 1983

Pettegrew JW, Minshew NJ, Diehl J et al: Anatomical considerations for interpreting topical P-31 NMR (letter). Lancet 2(8355):913, 1983

Poole CJ: Argyll Robertson pupils due to neurosarcoidosis: Evidence for site of lesion. Br Med J [Clin Res] 289:356, 1984

Pykett IL, Buonanno FS, Brady TJ et al: Techniques and approaches to proton NMR imaging of the head. Comput Radiol 7:1, 1983

Radda GK, Bore PJ, Rajagopalan B: Clinical aspects on ^{31}P NMR spectroscopy. Br Med Bull 40:155, 1984

Randell CP, Collins AG, Young IR et al: Nuclear magnetic

resonance imaging of posterior fossa tumors. AJR 141:489, 1983
Rangel-Guerra RA, Perez-Payan H, Minkoff L et al: Nuclear magnetic resonance in bipolar affective disorders. AJNR 4:229, 1983
Runge VM, Price AC, Kirshner HS et al: Magnetic resonance imaging of multiple sclerosis: A study of pulse-technique efficacy. AJR 143:1015, 1984
Scott JA, Augustyn GT, Gilmor RL et al: Magnetic resonance imaging of a venous angioma. AJNR 6:284, 1985
Simmonds D, Banks LM, Steiner RE et al: NMR anatomy of the brain using inversion-recovery sequences. Neuroradiology 25:113, 1983
Singer JR, Crooks LE: Nuclear magnetic resonance blood flow measurements in the human brain. Science 221:654, 1983
Sostman HD, Spencer DD, Gore JC et al: Preliminary observations on magnetic resonance imaging in refractory epilepsy. Magn Reson Imaging 2:301, 1984
Steiner RE, Bydder GM: Clinical NMR imaging of the brain and cord. Diagn Imag Clin Med 53:13, 1984
Stewart WA, Hall LD, Berry K et al: Correlation between NMR scan and brain slice data in multiple sclerosis (letter). Lancet 2(8399):412, 1984
Takeda KK, Sukuta M, Saeki F: Central pontine myelinolysis diagnosed by magnetic resonance imaging. Ann Neurol 17:310, 1985
Thickman D, Mintz M, Mennuti M et al: MR imaging of cerebral abnormalities in utero. J Comput Assist Tomogr 8:1058, 1984
Tofts PS, Cady EB, Delpy DT et al: Surface coil NMR spectroscopy of brain (letter). Lancet 1(8374):459, 1984
Tsementzis SA: Surgical management of intracerebral hematomas. Neurosurgery 16:562, 1985
Tychsen L, Hoyt WF: Occipital lobe dysplasia. Magnetic resonance findings in two cases of isolated congenital hemianopia. Arch Ophthalmol 103:680, 1985
Valvassori GE: New imaging tests for otology. Am J Otol 5:434, 1984
Vermess M, Bernstein RM, Bydder Gm et al: Nuclear magnetic resonance (NMR) imaging of the brain in systemic lupus erythematosus. J Comput Assist Tomogr 7:461, 1983
Weinstein MA, Modic MT, Pavlicek W et al: Nuclear magnetic resonance for the examination of brain tumors. Semin Roentgenol 19:139, 1984
Wiet RJ, Kazan R, Sacy G: Skull base mapping. Laryngoscope 92:515, 1982
Young IR, Burl M, Clarke GJ et al: Magnetic resonance properties of hydrogen: Imaging the posterior fossa. AJR 137, 895, 1981
Young IR, Bydder GM, Hall AS et al: The role of NMR imaging in the diagnosis and management of acoustic neuroma. AJNR 4:223, 1983
Young IR, Hall AS, Pallis CA et al: Nuclear magnetic resonance imaging of the brain in multiple sclerosis. Lancet 2((8255):1063, 1981
Young IR, Randell CP, Kaplan PW et al: Nuclear magnetic resonance (NMR) imaging in white matter disease of the brain using spin-echo sequences. J Comput Assist Tomogr 7:290, 1983
Younkin DP, Delivoria-Papadopoulos M, Leonard JC et al: Unique aspects of human newborn cerebral metabolism evaluated with phosphorus nuclear magnetic resonance spectroscopy. Ann Neurol 16:581, 1984
Zimmerman RA, Bilaniuk LT, Goldberg HI et al: Cerebral NMR imaging: Early results with a 0.12 T resistive system. AJR 141:1187, 1983
Zimmerman RA, Bilaniuk LT, Packer R et al: Resistive NMR of brain stem gliomas. Neuroradiology 27:21, 1985

Temporomandibular Joint

Helms CA, Richardson ML, Moon KL et al: Nuclear magnetic resonance imaging of the temporomandibular joint: Preliminary observations. J Craniomandibular Pract 2:219, 1984
Katzberg RW, Schenck J, Roberts D et al: Magnetic resonance imaging of the temporomandibular joint meniscus. Oral Surg 59:332, 1985
Roberts D, Schenck J, Joseph P et al: Temporomandibular joint: Magnetic resonance imaging. Radiology 154:829, 1985

Technical Considerations/Physics

Ackerman JJ, Grove TH, Wong GG et al: Mapping of metabolites in whole animals by ^{31}P NMR using surface coils. Nature 283:167, 1980
Alger JR, Shulman RG: NMR studies of enzymatic rates in vitro and in vivo by magnetization transfer. Q Rev Biophys 17:83, 1984
Arakawa M, Crooks LE, McCarten B et al: A comparison of saddle-shaped and solenoidal coils for magnetic resonance imaging. Radiology 154:227, 1985
Baker D: A systematic approach to the design and installation of NMR suites with particular reference to the briefing and feasibility stage. Prog Nucl Med 8:157, 1984
Baker HL Jr, Berquist TH, Kispert DB et al: Magnetic resonance imaging in a routine clinical setting. Mayo Clin Proc 60:75, 1985
Balaban RS: The application of nuclear magnetic resonance to the study of epithelial tissues. Prog Clin Biol Res 126:73, 1983

Balaban RS: The application of nuclear magnetic resonance to the study of cellular physiology. Am J Physiol 246:C10, 1984

Balban RS, Gadian DG, Radda GK: Phosphorus nuclear magnetic resonance study of the rat kidney in vivo. Kidney Int 20:575, 1981

Balban RS, Gadian DG, Radda GK et al: An NMR probe for the study of aerobic suspensions of cells and organelles. Anal Biochem 116:450, 1981

Battocletti JH: NMR proton imaging. Crit Rev Biomed Eng 11:313, 1984

Battocletti JH: Medical applications of NMR spectroscopy. I. Clinical applications of phosphorus-31 NMR. Crit Rev Biomed Eng 10:1, 1984

Bergstrom M, Martin W, Pate B: A look at anatomical and physiological brain images. Dimens Health Serv 60:36, 1983

Bernhardt JH, Kossel F: Recommendations for the safe use of NMR equipment. Clin Phys Physiol Meas 6:65, 1985

Bradley WG, Opel W, Kassabian JP: Magnetic resonance installation: Siting and economic considerations. Radiology 151:719, 1984

Burt CT, Koutcher JA: Multinuclear NMR studies of naturally occurring nuclei. J Nucl Med 25:237, 1984

Bydder GM, Butsen PC, Harman RR et al: Use of spherical receiver coils in MR imaging of the brain. J Comput Assist Tomogr 9:413, 1985

Chance B, Eleff S, Leigh JS Jr: Noninvasive nondestructive approaches to cell bioenergetics. Proc Natl Acad Sci USA 77:7430, 1980

Chilton HM, Jackels SC, Hinson WH et al: Use of a paramagnetic substance, colloidal manganese sulfide, as an NMR contrast material in rats. J Nucl Med 25:604, 1984

Cowen AR: Practical considerations in the assessment of noise-limited medical images: With special reference to nuclear magnetic resonance imaging. Ann 1st Super Sanita 19:175, 1983

Damadian R: Field focusing n.m.r. (FONAR) and the formation of chemical images in man. Philos Trans R Soc Lond [Biol] 289:489, 1980

Derbyshire W: Standard phantoms for NMR imaging equipment. Ann 1st Super Sanita 19:163, 1983

Edelstein WA, Schenck JF, Hart HR et al: Surface coil magnetic resonance imaging. JAMA 253:828, 1985

Field J, Irving MG, Brooks WM et al: In vivo ^{13}C nuclear magnetic resonance spectroscopy using a solenoid transmit/receiver coil. Biochem Biophys Res Commun 123:882, 19984

Gadian D, Radda G, Ross B et al: Examination of a myopathy by phosphorus nuclear magnetic resonance. Lancet 2(8250):774, 1981

Gadian DG: Metabolic studies of whole animals and humans using phosphorus nuclear magnetic resonance. Biosci Rep 1:449, 1981

Gordon RE: Topical magnetic resonance. Biosci Rep 2:701, 1982

Gordon RE, Timms WE: Magnet systems used in medical NMR. Comput Radiol 8:245, 1984

Halbach RE, Battocletti JH, Sances A Jr et al: Blood flow detection using the flat crossed-coil nuclear magnetic resonance flowmeter. IEEE Trans Biomed Eng 28:40, 1981

Hanley P: Magnets for medical applications of NMR. Br Med Bull 40:125, 1984

Hargest TS: Nuclear magnetic resonance: The state of the art from the clinical engineer's viewpoint. Med Instrum 18:187, 1984

Hendee WR, Morgan CJ: Magnetic resonance imaging. Part I—physical principles. West J Med 141:491, 1984

Hilberman M, Subramanian VH, Haselgrove J et al: In vivo time-resolved brain phosphorus nuclear magnetic resonance. J Cereb Blood Flow Metab 4:334, 1984

Hoult DI: Rotating frame zeugmatography. Philos Trans R Soc Lond [Biol] 289:543, 1980

Joseph PM, Axel L, O'Donnell M: Potential problems with selective pulses in NMR imaging systems. Med Phys 11:772, 1984

Kearfott KJ, Rottenberg DA, Knowles RJ: A new headholder for PET, CT, and NMR imaging. J Comput Assist Tomogr 8:1217, 1984

Keeler EK, Coyle PK: Contrast enhancement in NMR imaging by selection of radiofrequency pulse sequence and time: Examples in demyelinating disease. Physiol Chem Phys 15:235, 1983

Koretsky AP, Wang S, Murphy-Boesch J et al: ^{31}P NMR spectroscopy of rat organs, in situ, using chronically implanted radio-frequency coils. Proc Natl Acad Sci USA 80:7491, 1983

Lai CM, Lauterbur PC: True three-dimensional image reconstruction by nuclear magnetic resonance zeugmatography. Phys Med Biol 26:851, 1981

Leksell L, Leksell D, Schwebel J: Stereotaxis and nuclear magnetic resonance. J Neurol Neurosurg Psychiatry 48:14, 1985

Lerski RA: Physical principles of nuclear magnetic resonance imaging. Radiography 49:85, 1983

Levy GC, Craik DJ: Recent developments in nuclear magnetic resonance spectroscopy. Science 214:291, 1981

McRobbie D, Foster MA: Thresholds for biological effects of time-varying magnetic fields. Clin Phys Physiol Meas 5:67, 1984

Murphy WA, Totty WG, Gado M et al: Utilization characteristics of a superconductive MR system undergoing initial clinical trial. J Comput Assist Tomogr 9:258, 1985

Orr JS, Lerski RA, Straughan K: Preliminary results from phantoms for spatial and contrast resolution, standardisation and calibration, within NMR images. Ann 1st Super Sanita 19:191, 1983

Persson RB, Bolmsjo M, Helgesen H et al: Design and application of a proton NMR imaging system based on a window-frame type of magnet. Prog Nucl Med 8:28, 1984

Pykett IL: Instrumentation for nuclear magnetic resonance imaging. Semin Nucl Med 13:319, 1983

Redpath TW, Hutchinson JM: Estimating patient dielectric losses in NMR imagers. Magn Reson Imaging 2:295, 1984

Redpath TW, Selbie RD: A crossed ellipse RF coil for NMR imaging of the head and neck. Phys Med Biol 29:739, 1984

Salles-Cunha SX, Halbach RE, Battocletti JH et al: In vivo evaluation of nuclear magnetic resonance flowmetry: Blood flow through the normal forearm. Med Instrum 16:295, 1982

Schenck JF, Foster TH, Henkes JL et al: High-field surface-coil MR imaging of localized anatomy. AJNR 6:181, 1985

Scott AI, Baxter RL: Applications of ^{13}C NMR to metabolic studies. Annu Rev Biophys Bioeng 10:151, 1981

Segre AL: Synthetic polymers: A possible source of phantoms for NMR imaging. Ann 1st Super Sanita 19:169, 1983

Seiler T, Muller-Stolzenburg N, Wollensak J: Phase transitions in ocular tissue—NMR and temperature measurements. Graefes Arch Clin Exp Ophthalmol 221:122, 1983

Smith MA, Best JJ, Douglas RH et al: The installation of a commercial resistive NMR imager. Br J Radiol 57:1145, 1984

Stelling CB, Wang PC, Lieber A et al: Prototype coil for magnetic resonance imaging of the female breast. Work in progress. Radiology 154:457, 1985

Thomas SR, Ackerman JL, Kereiakes JG: Practical aspects involved in the design and set up of a 0.15 T 6-coil resistive magnet, whole body NMR imaging facility. Magn Reson Imaging 2:341, 1984

Tofts PS, Cady EB, Delpy DT et al: Surface coil NMR spectroscopy of brain (letter). Lancet 1(8374):459, 1984

Vollmann W: Influence of radiofrequency amplifier nonlinearities on nuclear magnetic resonance image quality. Magn Reson Imaging 2:221, 1984

Wolff S, Crooks LE, Brown P et al: Tests for DNA and chromosomal damage induced by nuclear magnetic resonance imaging. Radiology 136:707, 1980

Yamada K, Tanokura M: Post-contractile phosphocreatine splitting in muscle as revealed by time-resolved ^{31}P nuclear magnetic resonance. Jpn J Physiol 33:909, 1983

Abdomen (Including Liver, Pancreas, Spleen, GI Tract)

Aisen AM, Martel W, Glazer GM et al: Hepatic imaging: Positron emission tomography, digital angiography, and nuclear magnetic resonance imaging. Hepatology 3:1024, 1983

Amparo EG, Higgins CB, Hricak H: Primary diagnosis of abdominal arteriovenous fistula by MR imaging. J Comput Assist Tomogr 8:1140, 1984

Anacker H, Rupp N, Reiser M: Magnetic resonance (MR) in the diagnosis of pancreatic disease. Eur J Radiol 4:265, 1984

Arias IM: Nuclear magnetic resonance and the future of hepatology (editorial). Hepatology 3:763, 1983

Beall PT, Hazlewood CF, Rutzky LP: NMR relaxation times of water protons in human colon cancer cell lines and clones. Cancer Biochem Biophys 6:7, 1982

Bernardino ME, Small W, Goldstein J et al: Multiple NMR T_2 relaxation values in human liver tissue. AJR 141:1203, 1983

Borkowski GP, Buonocore E, George CR et al: Nuclear magnetic resonance (NMR) imaging in the evaluation of the liver: A preliminary experience. J Comput Assist Tomogr 7:768, 1983

Brasch RC, Wesbey GE, Gooding CA et al: Magnetic resonance imaging of transfusional hemosiderosis complicating thalassemia major. Radiology 150:767, 1984

Buonocore E, Borkowski GP, Pavlicek W et al: NMR imaging of the abdomen: Technical considerations. AJR 141:1171, 1983

Bury RW, Breen KJ, Desmond PV et al: Disposition of intravenous glycofurol: Effect of hepatic cirrhosis. Clin Pharmacol Ther 36:82, 1984

Bydder GM: Clinical NMR imaging of the abdomen. Prog Nucl Med 8:124, 1984

Carr DH: The use of iron and gadolinium chelates as NMR contrast agents: Animal and human studies. Physiol Chem Phys 16:137, 1984

Carr DH Brown J, Bydder GM et al: Gadolinium-DTPA as a contrast agent in MRI: Initial clinical experience in 20 patients. AJR 143:215, 1984

Church J, Bodie B, Jagelman DG et al: Primary rectal lymphoma staged by magnetic resonance imaging: Case report of an unusual cause of rectal bleeding. Cleve Clin Q 51:477, 1984

Cohen SM: Application of nuclear magnetic resonance to the study of liver physiology and disease. Hepatology 3:738, 1983

Dooms GC, Hricak H, Crooks LE et al: Magnetic resonance imaging of the lymph nodes: Comparison with CT. Radiology 153:719, 1984

Doyle FH, Pennock JM, Banks LM et al: Nuclear magnetic

resonance imaging of the liver: Initial experience. AJR 138:193, 1982

Edelstein WA, Hutchinson JM, Smith FW et al: Human whole-body NMR tomographic imaging: Normal sections. Br J Radiol 54:149, 1981

Ehman RL, Kjos BO, Hricak H et al: Relative intensity of abdominal organs in MR images. J Comput Assist Tomogr 9:315, 1985

Fisher MR, Wall SD, Hricak H et al: Hepatic vascular anatomy on magnetic resonance imaging. AJR 144:739, 1985

Glazer GM, Aisen AM, Francis IR et al: Hepatic cavernous hemangioma: Magnetic resonance imaging. Work in progress. Radiology 155:417, 1985

Goldstein EJ, Burnett KR, Hansell JR et al: Gadolinium DTPA (an NMR proton imaging contrast agent): Chemical structure, paramagnetic properties and pharmacokinetics. Physiol Chem Phys 16:97, 1984

Haaga JR: Magnetic resonance imaging of the pancreas. Radiol Clin North Am 22:869, 1984

Haaga JR: Magnetic resonance imaging of the liver. Radiol Clin North Am 22:879, 1984

Hawkes RC, Holland GN, Moore WS et al: Nuclear magnetic resonance (NMR) tomography of the normal abdomen. J Comput Assist Tomogr 5:613, 1981

Higgins CB, Goldberg H, Hricak H et al: Nuclear magnetic resonance imaging of vasculature of abdominal viscera: Normal and pathologic features. AJR 140:1217, 1983

Hricak H, Filly RA, Margulis AR et al: Work in progress: Nuclear magnetic resonance imaging of the gallbladder. Radiology 147:481, 1983

Itai Y, Ohtomo K, Furui S et al: Magnetic resonance of liver tumors: A preliminary report. Radiat Med 2:131, 1984

Jaffe MH, Goldstein HA, Zeman RK et al: Noninvasive imaging of the gastrointestinal tract. Med Clin North Am 68:1515, 1984

Kessing PH, Falke TH, Steiner RM et al: Magnetic resonance imaging in hemosiderosis. Diagn Imag Clin Med 54:7, 1985

Kerlan RK Jr, Hricak H, Gross BH et al: Nuclear magnetic resonance and computed tomographic angiography in the detection of hepatic metastases. J Clin Gastroenterol 5:461, 1983

Kressel HY, Axel L, Glover G et al: Coronal nuclear magnetic resonance (NMR) imaging of the abdomen at 0.5 tesla. J Comput Assist Tomogr 8:29, 1984

Kressel HY, Axel L, Thickman D et al: NMR imaging of the abdomen at 0.12 T: Clinical experience with a resistive magnet. AJR 141:1179, 1983

Lawler GA, Pennock JM, Steiner RE et al: Nuclear magnetic resonance (NMR) imaging in Wilson disease. J Comput Assist Tomogr 7:1, 1983

Lee JK, Dixon WT, Ling D et al: Fatty infiltration of the liver: Demonstration by proton spectroscopic imaging. Preliminary observations. Radiology 153:195, 1984

Lee JK, Heiken JP, Ling D et al: Magnetic resonance imaging of abdominal and pelvic lymphadenopathy. Radiology 153:181, 1984

Leung AW, Steiner RE, Young IR: NMR imaging of the liver in two cases of iron overload. J Comput Assist Tomogr 8:446, 1984

Margulis AR, Moss AA, Crooks LE et al: Nuclear magnetic resonance in the diagnosis of tumors of the liver. Semin Roentgenol 18:123, 1983

Martin KW, Morian JP Jr, Lee JK et al: Demonstration of a splenic artery pseudoaneurysm by MR imaging. J Comput Assist Tomogr 9:190, 1985

Mathur De Vre R, Grimee R, Rosa MP: Experimental protocol for tissue discrimination in vitro by NMR Biosci Rep 3:599, 1983

Moon KL Jr, Hricak H, Margulis AR et al: Nuclear magnetic resonance imaging characteristics of gallstones in vitro. Radiology 148:753, 1983

Moss AA, Goldberg HI, Stark DD et al: Hepatic tumors: Magnetic resonance and CT appearance. Radiology 150:141, 1984

Muhiudeen IA, Koerner TA, Samuelsson B et al: Characterization of human liver 3-0-beta-D-glucopyranuronosyl-cholesterol by mass spectrometry and nuclear magnetic resonance spectroscopy. J Lipid Res 25:1117, 1984

Myers MJ: Spleen imaging. Clin Haematol 12:395, 1983

Ohtomo K, Itai Y, Furui S et al: MR imaging of portal vein thrombus in hepatocellular carcinoma. J Comput Assist Tomogr 9:328, 1985

Ohtomo K, Itai Y, Furui S et al: Hepatic tumors: Differentiation by transverse relaxation time (T2) of magnetic resonance imaging. Radiology 155:421, 1985

Partain CL, James AE, Watson JT et al: Nuclear magnetic resonance and computed tomography: Comparison of normal human body images. Radiology 136:767, 1980

Runge VM, Clanton JA, Partain CL et al: Respiratory gating in magnetic resonance imaging at 0.5 tesla. Radiology 151:521, 1984

Runge VM, Clanton JA, Smith FW et al: Nuclear magnetic resonance of iron and copper disease states. AJR 141:943, 1983

Stark DD, Bass NM, Moss AA et al: Nuclear magnetic resonance imaging of experimentally induced liver disease. Radiology 148:743, 1983

Stark DD, Goldberg HI, Moss AA et al: Chronic liver disease: Evaluation by magnetic resonance. Radiology 150:149, 1984

Stark DD, Moseley ME, Bacon BR et al: Magnetic resonance imaging and spectroscopy of hepatic iron overload. Radiology 154:137, 1985

Stark DD, Moss AA, Goldberg HI et al: Computed tomography and nuclear magnetic resonance imaging of pancreatic islet cell tumors. Surgery 94:1024, 1983

Stark DD, Moss AA, Goldberg HI et al: Magnetic resonance and CT of the normal and diseased pancreas: A comparative study. Radiology 150:153, 1984

Smith FW: Diagnostic procedures in the evaluation of hepatic diseases. Nuclear magnetic resonance tomographic imaging. Lab Res Methods Biol Med 7:355, 1983

Smith FW: Proton imaging at 3.4 MHz. Thorax and abdomen. Prog Nucl Med 8:112, 1984

Smith FW, Hutchinson JM, Mallard JR et al: Oesophageal carcinoma demonstrated by whole-body nuclear magnetic resonance imaging. Br Med J [Clin Res] 282:510, 1981

Smith FW, Mallard JR: NMR imaging in liver disease. Br Med Bull 40:194, 1984

Smith FW, Mallard JR, Reid A et al: Nuclear magnetic resonance tomographic imaging in liver disease. Lancet 1(8227):963, 1981

Smith FW, Reid A, Hutchinson JM et al: Nuclear magnetic resonance imaging of the pancreas. Radiology 142:677, 1982

Steiner RE, Bydder GM: Nuclear magnetic resonance in gastroenterology. Clin Gastroenterol 13:265, 1984

Steiner RE, Bydder GM: Nuclear magnetic resonance imaging of the abdomen. Diagn Imag Clin Med 53:38, 1984

Tishler JM, Partain CL, Kulkarni M: Magnetic resonance imaging of the abdomen. Ala JA Med Sci 22:76, 1985

Volkholz HJ, Sailer D, Rodl W: New diagnostic and therapeutic possibilities in manifest idiopathic hemochromatosis. Hepatogastroenterology 31:289, 1984

Weinreb JC, Brateman L, Maravilla KR: Magnetic resonance imaging of hepatic lymphoma. AJR 143:1211, 1984

Weinreb JC, Maravilla KR, Redman HC et al: Improved MR imaging of the upper abdomen with glucagon and gas. J Comput Assist Tomogr 8:835, 1984

Wenker JC, Baker MK, Ellis JH et al: Focal fatty infiltration of the liver: Demonstration by magnetic resonance imaging. AJR 143:573, 1984

Wesbey GE, Brasch RC, Engelstad BL et al: Nuclear magnetic resonance contrast enhancement study of the gastrointestinal tract of rats and a human volunteer using nontoxic oral iron solutions. Radiology 149:175, 1983

Wesbey GE, Engelstad BL, Brasch RC: Paramagnetic pharmaceuticals for magnetic resonance imaging. Physiol Chem Phys 16:145, 1984

Wilcox DM, Weinreb JC, Lesh P: MR imaging of a hemorrhagic hepatic cyst in a patient with polycystic liver disease. J Comput Assist Tomogr 9:183, 1985

Woolfenden WR, Grant DM, Straight RC et al: Chemical characterization of pigment gallstones using ^{13}C nuclear magnetic resonance analysis. Biochem Biophys Res Commun 107:684, 1982

Zilm K, Grant DM, Englert E Jr et al: The use of solid ^{13}C nuclear magnetic resonance for the characterization of cholesterol and bilirubin pigment composition of human gallstones. Biochem Biophys Res Commun 93:857, 1980

Adrenal Glands

Cohen MD, Weetman R, Provisor A et al: Magnetic resonance imaging of neuroblastoma with a 0.15 T magnet. AJR 143:1241, 1984

Davis PL, Hricak H, Bradley WG Jr: Magnetic resonance imaging of the adrenal glands. Radiol Clin North Am 22:891, 1984

Fink IJ, Reinig JW, Dwyer AJ et al: MR imaging of pheochromocytomas. J Comput Assist Tomogr 9:454, 1985

Maris JM, Evans AE, McLaughlin AC et al: ^{31}P nuclear magnetic resonance spectroscopic investigation of human neuroblastoma in situ. N Engl J Med 312:1500, 1985

Moon KL Jr, Hricak H, Crooks LE et al: Nuclear magnetic resonance imaging of the adrenal gland: A preliminary report. Radiology 147:155, 1983

Schultz CL, Haaga JR, Fletcher BD et al: Magnetic resonance imaging of the adrenal glands: A comparison with computed tomography. AJR 143:1235, 1984

Musculoskeletal

Aue SP, Roufosse AH, Glimcher MJ et al: Solid-state phosphorus-31 nuclear magnetic resonance studies of synthetic solid phases of calcium phosphate: Potential models of bone mineral. Biochemistry 23:6110, 1984

Berquist TH: Magnetic resonance imaging: Preliminary experience in orthopedic radiology. Magn Reson Imaging 2:41, 1984

Bloem HL, Falke TH, Doornbos J: Re: Osteomyelitis in children: Detection by magnetic resonance (letter). Radiology 153:263, 1984

Brady TJ, Rosen BR, Pykett IL et al: NMR imaging of leg tumors. Radiology 149:181, 1983

Cherryman GR, Smith FW: NMR scanning for skeletal tumours (letter). Lancet 1(8391):1403, 1984

Cohen MD, Klatte EC, Baehner R et al: Magnetic resonance imaging of bone marrow disease in children. Radiology 151:715, 1984

Dooms GC, Fisher MR, Hricak H et al: Bone marrow imaging: Magnetic resonance studies related to age and sex. Radiology 155:429, 1985

Fletcher BD, Scoles PV, Nelson AD: Osteomyelitis in children: Detection by magnetic resonance. Work in progress. Radiology 150:57, 1984

Hudson TM, Hamlin DJ, Enneking WF et al: Magnetic resonance imaging of bone and soft tissue tumors: Early experience in 31 patients compared with computed tomography. Skeletal Radiol 13:134, 1985

Hudson TM, Hamlin DJ, Fitzsimmons JR: Magnetic resonance imaging of fluid levels in an aneurysmal bone cyst and in anticoagulated human blood. Skeletal Radiol 13:267, 1985

Hull RG, Rennie JA, Eastmond CJ et al: Nuclear magnetic resonance (NMR) tomographic imaging for popliteal cysts in rheumatoid arthritis. Ann Rheum Dis 43:56, 1984

Kean DM, Worthington BS, Preston BJ et al: Nuclear magnetic resonance imaging of the knee: Examples of normal anatomy and pathology. Br J Radiol 56:355, 1983

Li KC, Hendelman RM, Poon PY et al: MR imaging of the normal knee. J Comput Assist Tomogr 8:1147, 1984

Matthaei D, Frahm J, Haase A et al: Chemical-shift-selective magnetic-resonance imaging of avascular necrosis of the femoral head. Lancet 1(8425):370, 1985

Mechlin M, Thickman D, Kressel HY et al: Magnetic resonance imaging of postoperative patients with metallic implants. AJR 143:1281, 1984

Mizuta H, Yamasaki M: Nuclear magnetic resonance studies on experimental malignant bone tumors. Nippon Seikeigeka Gakkai Zasshi 58:83, 1984

Mizuta H, Yamasaki M: Nuclear magnetic resonance studies on human bone and soft tissue tumors. Nippon Seikeigeka Gakkai Zasshi 58:97, 1984

Moon KL Jr, Genant HK, David PL et al: Nuclear magnetic resonance imaging in orthopaedics: Principles and applications. J Orthop Res 1:101, 1983

Moon KL Jr, Genant HK, Helms CA et al: Musculoskeletal applications of nuclear magnetic resonance. Radiology 147:161, 1983

Muller RN, Marsh MJ, Bernardo ML et al: True 3-D imaging of limbs by NMR zeugmatography with off-resonance irradiation. Eur J Radio (Suppl) 1:286, 1983

Osterman AL, Heppenstall RB, Sapega AA et al: Muscle ischemia and hypothermia: A bioenergetic study using 31 phosphorus nuclear magnetic resonance spectroscopy. J Trauma 24:811, 1984

Pettersson H, Hudson T, Hamlin D et al: Magnetic resonance imaging of sacrococcygeal tumors. Acta Radiol [Diagn] (Stockh) 26:161, 1985

Pettersson H, Springfield D, Hamlin D et al: Magnetic resonance imaging and tissue characterization of a renal cell carcinoma and its osseous metastasis. Report of a case. Acta Radiol [Diagn] (Stockh) 26:193, 1985

Roufosse AH, Aue WP, Roberts JE et al: Investigation of the mineral phases of bone by solid-state phosphorus-31 magic angle sample spinning nuclear magnetic resonance. Biochemistry 23:6115, 1984

Sakar SK, Sullivan CE, Torchia DA: Solid state ^{13}C NMR study of collagen molecular dynamics in hard and soft tissues. J Biol Chem 258:9762, 1983

Scoles PV, Yoon YS, Makley JT et al: Nuclear magnetic resonance imaging in Legg-Calve-Perthes disease. J Bone Joint Surg [Am] 66:1357, 1984

Scott JA, Rosenthal DI, Brady TJ: The evaluation of musculoskeletal disease with magnetic resonance imaging. Radiol Clin North Am 22:914, 1984

Sepponen RE, Sipponen JT, Tanttu JI: A method for chemical shift imaging: Demonstration of bone marrow involvement with proton chemical shift imaging. J Comput Assist Tomogr 8:585, 1984

Smith R, Newman RJ, Radda GK et al: Hypophosphataemic osteomalacia and myopathy: Studies with nuclear magnetic resonance spectroscopy. Clin Sci 67:505, 1984

Stark DD, McCarthy SM, Filly RA et al: Pelvimetry by magnetic resonance imaging. AJR 144:947, 1985

Totty WG, Murphy WA, Ganz WI et al: Magnetic resonance imaging of the normal and ischemic femoral head. AJR 143: 1273, 1984

Turner DA, Prodromos CC, Petasnick JP et al: Acute injury of the ligaments of the knee: Magnetic resonance evaluation. Radiology 154:717, 1985

Zimmer WD, Berquist TH, McLeod RA et al: Bone tumors: Magnetic resonance imaging versus computed tomography. Radiology 155:709, 1985

Zimmer WD, Berquist TH, Sim FH et al: Magnetic resonance imaging of aneurysmal bone cyst. Mayo Clin Proc 59:633, 1984

Spine

Aguila LA, Priaino DW, Modic MT et al: The intranuclear cleft of the intervertebral disk: Magnetic resonance imaging. Radiology 155:155, 1985

Aubin ML, Vignaud J, Iba-Zizen MT et al: NMR imaging of the cranio-cervical junction and cervical spine. Normal and pathological features. J Neuroradiol 11:229, 1984

Battocletti JH: NMR proton imaging. Crit Rev Biomed Eng 11:313, 1984

Berquist TH: Magnetic resonance imaging: Preliminary experience in orthopedic radiology. Magn Reson Imaging 2:41, 1984

Bewermeyer H, Dreesbach HA, Hunermann B et al: MR

imaging of familial basilar impression. J Comput Assist Tomogr 8:953, 1984

Bluemm RG, Baleriaux D, Lausberg B et al: Initial experience with MR-imaging of intracranial midline-lesions and lesions of the cervical spine at half tesla. Neurosurg Rev 7:287, 1984

Bolton CF: The value of diagnostic imaging techniques in the management of diseases of the nervous system. Can Med Assoc J 130:1425, 1984

Bosley TM, Cohen DA, Schatz NJ et al: Comparison of metrizamide computed tomography and magnetic resonance imaging in the evaluation of lesions at the cervicomedullary junction. Neurology 35:485, 1985

Bradley WC Jr: Magnetic resonance imaging of the central nervous system. Neurol Res 6:91, 1984

Bradley WG Jr, Waluch V, Yadley RA et al: Comparison of CT and MR in 400 patients with suspected disease of the brain and cervical spinal cord. Radiology 152:695, 1984

Brown CE, Battocletti JH, Johnson LF: Nuclear magnetic resonance (NMR) in clinical pathology: Current trends. Clin Chem 30:606, 1984

Chafetz NI, Genant HK, Moon KL et al: Recognition of lumbar disk herniation with NMR. AJR 141:1153, 1983

Crawshaw C, Kean DM, Mulholland RC et al: The use of nuclear magnetic resonance in the diagnosis of lateral canal entrapment. J Bone Joint Surg 66:711, 1984

DeLaPaz RL, Brady TJ, Buonanno FS et al: Nuclear magnetic resonance (NMR) imaging of Arnold-Chiari type I malformation with hydromyelia. J Comput Assist Tomogr 7:126, 1983

Dooms GC, Fisher MR, Hricak H et al: Bone marrow imaging: Magnetic resonance studies related to age and sex. Radiology 155:429, 1985

Drayer BP, Barrett L: Magnetic resonance imaging and CT scanning in multiple sclerosis. Ann NY Acad Sci 436:294, 1984

Dwyer AJ, Knop RH, Hoult DI: Frequency shift artifacts in MR imaging. J Comput Assist Tomogr 9:16, 1985

Edelman RR, Shoukimas GM, Stark DD et al: High-resolution surface-coil imaging of lumbar disk disease. AJR 144:1123, 1985

Grafin von Einsiedel H, Stepan R: Magnetic resonance imaging of spinal cord syndromes. Eur J Radiol 5:127, 1985

Han JS, Benson JE, Yoon YS: Magnetic resonance imaging in the spinal column and craniovertebral junction. Radiol Clin North Am 22:805, 1984

Han JS, Kaufman B, El Yousef SJ et al: NMR imaging of the spine. AJR 141:1137, 1983

Hawkes RC, Holland GN, Moore WS et al: Craniovertebral junction pathology: Assessment by NMR. AJNR 4:232, 1983

Huk W, Heindel W, Diemling M et al: Nuclear magnetic resonance (NMR) tomography of the central nervous system: Comparison of two imaging sequences. J Comput Assist Tomogr 7:468, 1983

Huk WJ, Gademann G: Magnetic resonance imaging (MRI): Method and early clinical experiences in diseases of the central nervous system. Neurosurg Rev 7:259, 1984

Hyman RA, Edwards JH, Vacirca SJ et al: .6 T MR of the cervical spine: Multislice and multiecho techniques. AJNR 6:229, 1985

Jewel KL: Imaging: Magnetic resonance imaging of the spinal cord. J Med Soc NJ 82:399, 1985

Kaufman BA, Kaufman B, Rekate HL: Cervicomedullary junction tumor diagnosed by nuclear magnetic resonance scanning: Case report. Neurosurgery 15:878, 1984

Kean DM, Smith MA, Douglas RH et al: Two examples of CNS lipomas demonstrated by computed tomography and low field (0.08 T) MR imaging. J Comput Assist Tomogr 9:494, 1985

Kucharczyk W, Brant-Zawadzki M, Sobel D et al: Central nervous system tumors in children: Detection by magnetic resonance imaging. Radiology 155:131, 1985

Kulkarni MV, Burks DD, Price AC et al: Diagnosis of spinal arteriovenous malformation in a pregnant patient by MR imaging. J Comput Assist Tomogr 9:171, 1985

Lee BC, Zimmerman RD, Manning JJ et al: MR imaging of syringomyelia and hydromyelia. AJR 144:1149, 1985

Lee BC, Deck MD, Kneeland JB et al: MR imaging of the craniocervical junction. AJNR 6:209, 1985

Maravilla KR, Lesh P, Weinreb JC et al: Magnetic resonance of the lumbar spine with CT correlation. AJNR 6:237, 1985

Maravilla KR, Weinreb JC, Suss R et al: Magnetic resonance demonstration of multiple sclerosis plaques in the cervical cord. AJR 144:381, 1985

Meyer FB, Ebersold MJ, Reese DF: Benign tumors of the foramen magnum. J Neurosurg 61:136, 1984

Mikhael MA, Ciric IS, Tarkington JA: MR imaging in spinal echinococcosis. J Comput Assist Tomogr 9:398, 1985

Modic MT, Hardy RW Jr, Weinstein MA et al: Nuclear magnetic resonance of the spine: Clinical potential and limitation. Neurosurgery 15:583, 1984

Modic MT, Pavlicek W, Weinstein MA et al: Magnetic resonance imaging of intervertebral disk disease. Clinical and pulse sequence considerations. Radiology 152:103, 1984

Modic MT, Weinstein MA: Nuclear magnetic resonance of the spine. Br Med Bull 40:183, 1984

Modic MT, Weinstein MA, Pavlicek W et al: Magnetic reso-

nance imaging of the cervical spine: Technical and clinical observations. AJR 141:1129, 1983
Modic MT, Weinstein MA, Pavlicek W et al: Nuclear magnetic resonance imaging of the spine. Radiology 148:757, 1983
Moon KL Jr, Genant HK, Helms CA et al: Musculoskeletal applications of nuclear magnetic resonance. Radiology 147:161, 1983
Moon KL Jr, Genant HK, Davis PL et al: Nuclear magnetic resonance imaging in orthopaedics: Principles and applications. J Orthop Res 1:101, 1983
Nagashima C, Kubota S: Craniocervical abnormalities. Modern diagnosis and a comprehensive surgical approach. Neurosurg Rev 6:187, 1983
Norman D, Mills CM, Brant-Zawadzki M et al: Magnetic resonance imaging of the spinal cord and canal: Potentials and limitations. AJR 141:1147, 1983
Pettersson H, Hudson T, Hamlin D et al: Magnetic resonance imaging of sacrococcygeal tumors. Acta Radiol 26:161, 1985
Pojunas K, Williams AL, Daniels DL et al: Syringomyelia and hydromyelia: Magnetic resonance evaluation. Radiology 153:679, 1984
Ramsey RG, Zacharias CE: MR imaging of the spine after radiation therapy: Easily recognizable effects. AJR 144:1131, 1985
Rebner M, Gebarski SS: Magnetic resonance imaging of spinal-cord hemangioblastoma. AJNR 6:287, 1985
Rodziewicz GS, Kaufman B, Spetzler RF: Diagnosis of sacral perineural cysts by nuclear magnetic resonance. Surg Neurol 22:50, 1984
Schenck JF, Foster TH, Henkes JL et al: High-field surface-coil MR imaging of localized anatomy. AJNR 6:181, 1985
Scotti G, Scialfa G, Landoni L et al: Nuclear magnetic resonance in the diagnosis of syringomyelia. J Neuroradial 11:239, 1984
Smith FW, Runge V, Permezel M et al: Nuclear magnetic resonance (NMR) imaging in the diagnosis of spinal osteomyelitis. Magn Reson Imaging 2:53, 1984
Smith SJ, Greenberg M, Vogelzang RL et al: Diagnosis of syringomyelia. IMJ 167:128, 1985
Spetzler RF, Zabramski JM, Kaufman B: Clinical role of magnetic resonance imaging in the neurosurgical patient. Neurosurgery 16:511, 1985
Spinos E, Laster DW, Moody DM et al: MR evaluation of Chiari I malformations at 0.15 T. AJR 144:1143, 1985
Steiner RE, Bydder GM: Clinical NMR imaging of the brain and cord. Diagn Imag Clin Med 53:13, 1984
Tress BM, Stimac GK, Brant-Zawadzki M: Nuclear magnetic resonance imaging. Applications in the diagnosis of cerebrospinal diseases. Med J Aust 142:25, 1985
Yeates A, Brant-Zawadzki M, Norman D et al: Nuclear magnetic resonance imaging of syringomyelia. AJNR 4:234, 1983

Female Reproductive Tract

Bies JR, Ellis JH, Kopecky KK et al: Assessment of primary gynecologic malignancies: Comparison of 0.15 T resistive MRI with CT. AJR 143:1249, 1984
Butler H, Bryan PJ, LiPuma JP et al: Magnetic resonance imaging of the abnormal female pelvis. AJR 143:1259, 1984
Fisher M, Hricak H, Reinhold C et al: Female urethral carcinoma: MRI staging. AJR 144:603, 1985
Hricak H, Alpers C, Crooks LE et al: Magnetic resonance imaging of the female pelvis: Initial experience. AJR 141:1119, 1983
Johnson IR, Symonds EM, Worthington BS et al: Imaging ovarian tumours by nuclear magnetic resonance. Br J Obstet Gynaecol 91:260, 1984
Johnson IR, Symonds EM, Kean DM et al: Imaging the pregnant human uterus with nuclear magnetic resonance. Am J Obstet Gynecol 148:1136, 1984
Mann WJ, Mendonca-Dias MH, Lauterbur PC et al: Preliminary in vitro studies of nuclear magnetic resonance spin-lattice relaxation times and three-dimensional nuclear magnetic resonance imaging in gynecological oncology. Am J Obstet Gynecol 148:91, 1984
McCarthy SM, Filly RA, Stark DD et al: Obstetrical magnetic resonance imaging: Fetal anatomy. Radiology 154:427, 1985
McCarthy SM, Stark DD, Filly RA et al: Obstetrical magnetic resonance imaging: Maternal anatomy. Radiology 154:421, 1985
Mendonca-Dias MH, Mann WJ, Chumas J et al: Three-dimensional nuclear magnetic resonance zeugmatographic imaging of surgical specimens. Biosci Rep 2:713, 1982
Moore FA, Todd LE, DeJimenez RL: T_1 relaxation times in vivo of human normal pelvic tissues and gynecologic malignancies. Physiol Chem Phys 15:23, 1983
Rome RM: Is it possible to determine the extent of gynaecological malignancy by noninvasive methods? Aust NZ J Obstet Gynaecol 24:150, 1984
Snoep G, van Engelshoven JM, Falke TH: Magnetic resonance imaging of the normal female pelvis. Diagn Imag Clin Med 54:57, 1985
Thickman D, Kressel H, Gussman D et al: Nuclear magnetic resonance imaging in gynecology. Am J Obstet Gynecol 149:835, 1984

Male Reproductive Tract

Altwein JE: New imaging techniques in the staging of urological tumors (kidney, retroperitoneal lymph nodes and tumors). Prog Clin Biol Res 152:23, 1984

Buonocore E, Hesemann C, Pavlicek W et al: Clinical and in vitro magnetic resonance imaging of prostatic carcinoma. AJR 143:1267, 1984

Ellis JH, Bies JR, Kopecky KK et al: Comparison of NMR and CT imaging in the evaluation of metastatic retroperitoneal lymphadenopathy from testicular carcinoma. J Comput Assist Tomogr 8:709, 1984

Hricak H, Williams RD, Spring DD et al: Anatomy and pathology of the male pelvis by magnetic resonance imaging. AJR 141:1101, 1983

Lang EK: Neoplasms of the bladder, prostate, and urethra. Semin Roentgenol 18:288, 1983

Poon PY, McCallum RW, Henkelman MM et al: Magnetic resonance imaging of the prostate. Radiology 154:143, 1985

Steyn JH, Smith FW: Nuclear magnetic resonance imaging of the prostate. Br J Urol 54:726, 1982

Steyn JH, Smith FW: Nuclear magnetic resonance (NMR) imaging of the prostate. Br J Urol 56:679, 1984

Economics

Bradley WG Jr: Practical economic considerations of clinical nuclear magnetic resonance (editorial). JAMA 251:1302, 1984

Bradley WG, Opel W, Kassabial JP: Magnetic resonance installation: Siting and economic considerations. Radiology 151:719, 1984

Cinti DC, Hawkins HB: Two locomotives (letter). JAMA 253:775, 1985

Corday E, Berman DS, Corday SR: Development of diagnostic noninvasive imaging. Compr Ther 8:3, 1982

Christensen B: Competition thrives among NMR manufacturers. Hospitals 57:73, 1983

diMonda R: Is NMR right for your hospital? Hospitals 59:55, 1985

Evens RG: Economic costs of nuclear magnetic resonance imaging. J Comput Assist Tomogr 8:200, 1984

Fisher DW: NMR: Right approach, wrong target (editorial). Hosp Pract 19:17, 1984

Gift DA: Changes and challenges in diagnostic imaging. Mich Med 84:204, 1985

Goldsmith MF: NMR v CT: Questions of cost, complexity, and efficacy (news). JAMA 251:869, 1984

Here's what the American Hospital Association foresees for NMR. Mich Med 84:205, 1985

Hillman BJ, Winkler JD, Phelps CE et al: Adoption and diffusion of a new imaging technology: A magnetic resonance imaging prospective. AJR 143:913, 1984

James AE Jr, Partain CL, Patton JA et al: Current status of magnetic resonance imaging. South Med J 78:580, 1985

Magnetic resonance imaging (MRI) in Australia. Med J Aust 142:60, 1985

Marr J: Cost-effectiveness and proper use of NMR debated in Michigan. Mich Med 84:202, 1985

Murphy WA: How does magnetic resonance compare with computed tomography? Radiology 152:235, 1984

Palmer J: Nuclear magnetic resonance imaging. Med J Aust 1:252, 1983

Schroeder SA: Magnetic resonance imaging: Present costs and potential gains (editorial). Ann Intern Med 102:551, 1985

Schwartz S: Installing NMR scanners: Is your building ready? Dimens Health Serv 61:10, 1984

Skorton DJ, Collins SM: New directions in cardiac imaging. Ann Intern Med 102:795, 1985

Smith T: German science in six days. Br Med J [Clin Res] 285:961, 1982

Whitman GJ, Harken AH: Applications of nuclear magnetic resonance to surgical disease: A collective review. J Surg Res 38:187, 1985

Wortzman G: Management of neuroradiological investigations in relation to the clinical signs. J Neuroradiol 10:195, 1983

Temporal Bone

Behnke EE, Schindler RA: Dermoid of the petrous apex. Laryngoscope 94:779, 1984

Daniels DL, Herfkins R, Koehler PR: Magnetic resonance imaging of the internal auditory canal. Radiology 151:105, 1984

Longridge NS, Mallinson AI: Arnold-Chiari malformation and the otolaryngologist: Place of magnetic resonance imaging and electronystagmography. Laryngoscope 95:335, 1985

New PF, Bachow TB, Wismer GL et al: MR imaging of the acoustic nerves and small acoustic neuromas at 0.6 T: Prospective study. AJR 144:1021, 1985

Schenck JF, Foster TH, Henkes JL et al: High-field surface-coil MR imaging of localized anatomy. AJNR 6:181, 1985

Valvassori GE: New imaging tests for otology. Am J Otol 5:434, 1984

Head and Neck (Excluding Brain, Orbit, and Temporal Bone)

Baker HL Jr, Berquist TH, Kispert DB et al: Magnetic resonance imaging in a routine clinical setting. Mayo Clin Proc 60:75, 1985

de-Certaines J, Herry JY, Lancien G et al: Evaluation of human thyroid tumors by proton nuclear magnetic resonance. J Nucl Med 23:48, 1982

Dillon WP, Mills CM, Kjos B et al: Magnetic resonance imaging of the nasopharynx. Radiology 152:731, 1984

Han JS, Huss RG, Benson JE et al: MR imaging of the skull base. J Comput Assist Tomogr 8:944, 1984

Kreipke DL, Lingeman RE: Cross-sectional imaging (CT, NMR) of branchial cysts: Report of three cases. J Comput Assist Tomogr 8:114, 1984

Lufkin RB, Larsson SG, Hanafee WN: Work in progress: NMR anatomy of the larynx and tongue base. Radiology 148:173, 1983

Paushter DM, Modic MT, Borkowski GP et al: Magnetic resonance. Principles and applications. Med Clin North Am 68:1393, 1984

Redpath TW, Selbie RD: A crossed ellipse RF coil for NMR imaging of the head and neck. Phys Med Biol 29:739, 1984

Sandler MP, Patton JA, Sacks GA et al: Evaluation of intrathoracic goiter with I-123 scintigraphy and nuclear magnetic resonance imaging. J Nucl Med 25:874, 1984

Schenck JF, Foster TH, Henkes JL et al: High-field surface-coil MR imaging of localized anatomy. AJNR 6:181, 1985

Stark DD, Clark OH, Moss AA: Magnetic resonance imaging of the thyroid, thymus, and parathyroid glands. Surgery 96:1083, 1984

Stark DD, Moss AA, Gamsu G et al: Magnetic resonance imaging of the neck. Part I: Normal anatomy. Radiology 150:447, 1984

Stark DD, Moss AA, Gamsu G et al: Magnetic resonance imaging of the neck. Part II: Pathologic findings. Radiology 150:455, 1984

Tennvall J, Biorklund A, Moller T et al: Studies of NMR-relaxation times in malignant tumours and normal tissues of the human thyroid gland. Prog Nucl Med 8:142, 1984

Unger JM: The oral cavity and tongue: Magnetic resonance imaging. Radiology 155:151, 1985

Wiet RJ, Kazan R, Sacy G: Skull base mapping. Laryngoscope 92:515, 1982

Yamamoto K, Tsuji T, Tarutani O et al: Structural changes of carbohydrate chains of human thyroglobulin accompanying malignant transformations of thyroid glands. Eur J Biochem 143:133, 1984

Chest

Axel L, Kressel HY, Thickman D et al: NMR imaging of the chest at 0.12 T: Initial clinical experience with a resistive magnet. AJR 141:1157, 1983

Beall PT, Narayana PA, Amtey SR et al: The systemic effect of cancers on human sera proton NMR relaxation times. Magn Reson Imaging 2:83, 1984

Berquist TH, Brown LR, May GR et al: Magnetic resonance imaging of the chest: a diagnostic comparison with computed tomography and hilar tomography. Magn Reson Imaging 2:315, 1984

Bhattacharyya SN, Lynn WS, Dabrowski J et al: Structure elucidation by one- and two-dimensional 360- and 500-MHz ^{1}H NMR of the oligosaccharide units of two glycoproteins isolated from alveoli of patients with alveolar proteinosis. Arch Biochem Biophys 231:72, 1984

Bottomley PA, Foster TH, Argersinger RE et al: A review of normal tissue hydrogen NMR relaxation times and relaxation mechanisms from 1–100 MHz: Dependence on tissue type, NMR frequency, temperature, species, excision, and age. Med Phys 11:425, 1984

Brasch RC, Gooding CA, Lallemand DP et al: Magnetic resonance imaging of the thorax in childhood. Work in progress. Radiology 150:463, 1984

Chapman JD: The detection and measurement of hypoxic cells in solid tumors. Cancer 54:2441, 1984

Cohen AM: Magnetic resonance imaging of the thorax. Radiol Clin North Am 22:829, 1984

Cohen AM, Creviston S, LiPuma JP et al: Nuclear magnetic resonance imaging of the mediastinum and hili: Early impressions of its efficacy. AJR 141:1163, 1983

Cohen AM, Creviston S, LiPuma JP et al: NMR evaluation of hilar and mediastinal lymphadenopathy. Radiol 148:739, 1983

Dunlop D, Harvey J: Symptomless abnormalities. The solitary pulmonary nodule. Br J Hosp Med 28:138, 1982

Epstein DM, Kressel H, Gefter W et al: MR imaging of the mediastinum: A retrospective comparison with computed tomography. J Comput Assist Tomogr 8:670, 1984

Gamsu G, Webb WR, Sheldon P et al: Nuclear magnetic resonance imaging of the thorax. Radiology 147:473, 1983

Glazer HS, Levitt RG, Lee JK et al: Differentiation of radiation fibrosis from recurrent pulmonary neoplasm by magnetic resonance imaging. AJR 143:729, 1984

Gooding CA, Lallemand DP, Brasch RC et al: Magnetic resonance imaging in cystic fibrosis. J Pediatr 105:384, 1984

Greene R: Biochemical and physiologic phenomena: Relevance to new forms of radiologic imaging and functional mapping. AJR 138:1218, 1982

Inouye T, Satoh K, Kose K et al: Experimental results with a whole body NMR-CT scanner using a resistive magnet. Radiat Med 1:8, 1983

Kressel HY: The principles of NMR imaging and a review of early clinical results. Radiat Med 1:197, 1983

Krzanowski JJ, Szentivanyi A: Reflections on some aspects

of current research in asthma. J Allergy Clin Immunol 72:433, 1983
Kundel HL, Kressel HY, Epstein D: The potential role of NMR imaging in thoracic disease. Radiol Clin North Am 21:801, 1983
Lamblin G, Boersma A, Klein A et al: Primary structure determination of five sialylated oligosaccharides derived from bronchial mucus glycoproteins of patients suffering from cystic fibrosis. The occurrence of the NeuAc alpha (1—3)Gal beta (1—4)[Fuc alpha(1—3)] GlcNAc beta(1—.) structural element revealed by 500-MHz ^{1}H NMR spectroscopy. J Biol Chem 259:9051, 1984
Lamblin G, Boersma A, Lhermitte M et al: Further characterization, by a combined high-performance liquid chromatography/^{1}H-NMR approach, of the heterogeneity displayed by the neutral carbohydrate chains of human bronchial mucins. Eur J Biochem 143:227, 1984
Malet-Martino MC, Martino R, Lopez A et al: New approach to metabolism of 5′-deoxy-5-flourouridine in humans with flourine-19 NMR. Cancer Chemother Pharmacol 13:31, 1984
Munakata H, Nimberg RB, Snider GL et al: The structure of the carbohydrate units of the 36k glycoprotein derived from the lung lavage of a patient with alveolar proteinosis by high resolution ^{1}H-NMR spectroscopy. Biochem Biophys Res Commun 108:1401, 1982
Newell JD: Evaluation of pulmonary and mediastinal masses. Med Clin North Am 68:1463, 1984
Newhouse JH: Nuclear magnetic resonance studies of the chest. Clin Chest Med 5:307, 1984
O'Donovan PB, Ross JS, Sivak ED et al: Magnetic resonance imaging of the thorax: The advantages of coronal and sagittal planes. AJR 143:1183, 1984
Partain CL, James AE, Watson JT et al: Nuclear magnetic resonance and computed tomography: Comparison of normal human body images. Radiology 136:767, 1980
Ross JS, O'Donovan PB, Novoa R et al: Magnetic resonance of the chest: Initial experience with imaging and in vivo T1 and T1 calculations. Radiology 152:95, 1984
Runge VM, Clanton JA, Partain CL et al: Respiratory gating in magnetic resonance imaging at 0.5 tesla. Radiology 151:521, 1984
Rupp N, Reiser M, Stetter E: The diagnostic value of morphology and relaxation times in NMR-imaging of the body. Eur J Radiol 3:68, 1983
Rzedzian R, Chapman B, Mansfield P et al: Real-time nuclear magnetic resonance clinical imaging in paediatrics. Lancet 2:1281, 1983
Schultz CL, Alfidi RJ, Nelson AD et al: The effect of motion on two-dimensional Fourier transformation magnetic resonance images. Radiology 152:117, 1984
Smith FW: Proton imaging at 3.4 MHz. Thorax and abdomen. Prog Nucl Med 8:112, 1984
Staub NC: The measurement of lung water content. J Microwave Power 18:259, 1983
Stewart RG, Runge VM, Brenner DE et al: Nuclear magnetic resonance relaxation rates of serum from lung cancer patients: Work in progress. J Tenn Med Assoc 77:131, 1984
Van-Halbeek H, Dorland L, Vliegenthart JF et al: Primary-structure determination of fourteen neutral oligosaccharides derived from bronchial-mucus glycoproteins of patients suffering from cystic fibrosis, employing 500-MHz ^{1}H-NMR spectroscopy. Eur J Biochem 127:7, 1982
Vannier MW: Nuclear magnetic resonance imaging. The case for prudent use in clinical diagnosis. Postgrad Med 76:159, 1984
Webb WR, Gamsu G: Clinical NMR imaging of the chest and mediastinum. Diagn Imag clin Med 53:22, 1984
Webb WR, Gamsu G, Crooks LE: Multisection sagittal and coronal magnetic resonance imaging of the mediastinum and hila. Work in progress. Radiology 150:475, 1984
Webb WR, Gamsu G, Golden JA et al: Nuclear magnetic resonance of pulmonary arteriovenous fistula: Effects of flow. J Comput Assist Tomogr 8:155, 1984
Webb WR, Gamsu G, Stark DD et al: Evaluation of magnetic resonance sequences in imaging mediastinal tumors. AJR 143:723, 1984
Webb WR, Gamsu G, Stark DD et al: Magnetic resonance imaging of the normal and abnormal pulmonary hila. Radiology 152:89, 1984
Webb WR, Jensen BG, Gamsu G et al: Coronal magnetic resonance imaging of the chest: Normal and abnormal. Radiology 153:729, 1984
Webb WR, Jensen BG, Gamsu G et al: Sagittal MR imaging of the chest: Normal and abnormal. J Comput Assist Tomogr 9:471, 1985
Webb WR, Moore EH: Differentiation of volume averaging and mass on magnetic resonance images of the mediastinum. Radiology 155:413, 1985

Orbit

Axel L: Surface coil magnetic resonance imaging. J Comput Assist Tomogr 8:381, 1984
Daniels DL, Herfkins R, Gager WE et al: Magnetic resonance imaging of the optic nerves and chiasm. Radiology 152:79, 1984
Edelstein WA, Schenck JF, Hart HR et al: Surface coil magnetic resonance imaging. JAMA 253:828, 1985
Edwards JH, Hyman RA, Vacirca SJ et al: 0.6 T magnetic resonance imaging of the orbit. AJR 144:1015, 1985
Garner WH: Non-invasive techniques in the study of cata-

ract development at the metabolic and protein molecular level. Ciba Found Symp 106:248, 1984

Greiner JV, Kopp SJ, Mercola JM et al: Organophosphate metabolites of the human and rabbit crystalline lens: A phosphorus-31 nuclear magnetic resonance spectroscopic analysis. Exp Eye Res 34:545, 1982

Greiner JV, Lass JH, Glonek T: Ex vivo metabolic analysis of eye bank corneas using phosphorus nuclear magnetic resonance. Arch Ophthalmol 102:1171, 1984

Grossman RI, Lynch RM: Neuroimaging in neuro-ophthalmology. Neurol Clin 1:831, 1983

Han JS, Benson JE, Bonstelle CT et al: Magnetic resonance imaging of the orbit: A preliminary experience. Radiology 150:755, 1984

Hawkes RC, Holland GN, Moore WS et al: NMR imaging in the evaluation of orbital tumors. AJNR 4:254, 1983

Joseph R, Pullicino P, Goldberg CD et al: Bilateral pontine gaze palsy. Nuclear magnetic resonance findings in presumed multiple sclerosis. Arch Neurol 42:93, 1985

Kincaid MC, Green WR: Diagnostic methods in orbital diseases. Ophthalmology 91:719, 1984

Kopp SJ, Glonek T, Greiner JV: Interspecies variations in mammalian lens metabolites as detected by phosphorus-31 nuclear magnetic resonance. Science 215:1622, 1982

Kopp SJ, Greiner JV, Glonek T: Analysis of intact rat lens metabolites by P-31 NMR spectroscopy. Curr Eye Res 1:375, 1981

Lerman S: An experimental and clinical evaluation of lens transparency and aging. J Gerontol 38:293, 1983

Lerman S, Megaw JM, Gardner K et al: NMR analysis of the cold cataract. II. Studies on protein solutions. Invest Ophthalmol Vis Sci 24:99, 1983

Li KC, Poon PY, Hinton P et al: MR imaging of orbital tumors with CT and ultrasound correlations. J Comput Assist Tomogr 8:1039, 1984

Morrice GD, Smith FW: Early experience with nuclear magnetic resonance (NMR) imaging in the investigation of ocular proptosis. Trans Ophthalmol Soc UK 103:143, 1983

Moseley I, Brant-Zawadski M, Mills C: Nuclear magnetic resonance imaging of the orbit. Br J Ophthalmol 67:333, 1983

Poole CJ: Argyll Robertston pupils due to neurosarcoidosis: Evidence for site of lesion. Br Med J [Clin Res] 289:356, 1984

Pope JM, Chardra S, Balfa JD: Changes in the state of water in senile cataractous lenses as studied by nuclear magnetic resonance. Exp Eye Res 34:57, 1982

Racz P, Tompa K, Pocsik I et al: Water fractions in normal and senile cataractous eye lenses studied by NMR. Exp Eye Res 36:663, 1983

Safran AB: Neuro-ophthalmology in the recent European literature. Part III. Heredodegenerations, stroke, pain, and diagnostic techniques. J Clin Neuro Ophthalmol 4:275, 1984

Sassani JW, Osbakken MD: Anatomic features of the eye disclosed with nuclear magnetic resonance imaging. Arch Ophthalmol 102:541, 1984

Schenck JF, Hart HR Jr, Foster TH etal: Improved MR imaging of the orbit at 1.5 T with surface coils. AJR 144:1033, 1985

Schwartz AC, Weaver RG Jr, Bloomfield R et al: Cavernous hemangioma of the retina, cutaneous angiomas, and intracranial vascular lesion by computed tomography and nuclear magnetic resonance imaging. Am J Ophthalmol 98:483, 1984

Seiler T, Muller-Stolzenburg N, Wollensak J: Phase transitions in ocular tissue—NMR and temperature measurements. Graefes Arch Clin Exp Ophthalmol 221:122, 1983

Seiler T, Trahms L, Wollensak J: The distinction of corneal water in free and bound fractions. Graefes Arch Clin Exp Ophthalmol 219:287, 1982

Sobel DF, Kelly W, Kjos BO et al: MR imaging of orbital and ocular disease. AJNR 6:259, 1985

Sobel DF, Mills C, Char D et al: NMR of the normal and pathologic eye and orbit. AJNR 5:345, 1984

Tychsen L, Hoyt WF: Occipital lobe dysplasia. Magnetic resonance findings in two cases of isolated congenital hemianopia. Arch Ophthalmol 103:680, 1985

Worthington BS: NMR imaging of intracranial and orbital tumours. Br Med Bull 40:179, 1984

Worthington BS: Clinical prospects for nuclear magnetic resonance. Clin Radiol 34:3, 1983

Yeagle PL, Selinsky BS, Albert AD: Perturbations of phospholipid head groups by membrane proteins in biological membranes and recombinants. Biophys J 45:1085, 1984

Breast

Beall PT, Brinkley BR, Chang DC et al: Microtubule complexes correlated with growth rate and water proton relaxation times in human breast cancer cells. Cancer Res 42:4124, 1982

Bovee WM, Creyghton JH, Getreuer KW et al: NMR relaxation and images of human breast tumours in vitro. Philos Trans R Soc Lond [Biol] 289:535, 1980

Budinger TF, Lauterbur PC: Nuclear magnetic resonance technology for medical studies. Science 226:288, 1984

Chapman JD: The detection and measurement of hypoxic cells in solid tumors. Cancer 54:2441, 1984

Cohen AM: Magnetic resonance imaging of the thorax. Radiol Clin North Am 22:829, 1984

El Yousef SJ, Alfidi RJ, Duchesneau RH et al: Initial experience with nuclear magnetic resonance (NMR) imaging of the human breast. J Comput Assist Tomogr 7:215, 1983

El Yousef SJ, Duchesneau RH: Magnetic resonance imaging of the human breast: A phase I trial. Radiol Clin North Am 22:859, 1984

El Yousef SJ, Duchesneau RH, Alfidi RJ et al: Magnetic resonance imaging of the breast. Work in progress. Radiology 150:761, 1984

El Yousef SJ, O'Connell DM, Duchesneau RH et al: Benign and malignant breast disease: Magnetic resonance and radio-frequency pulse sequences. AJR 145:1, 1985

Evanochko WT, Ng TC, Glickson JD et al: Human tumors as examined by in vivo ^{31}P NMR in athymic mice. Biochem Biophys Res Commun 109:1346, 1982

Fossel ET, Brodsky G, deLayre JL et al: Nuclear magnetic resonance for the differentiation of benign and malignant breast tissues and axillary lymph nodes. Ann Surg 198:541, 1983

Glatstein E, Lichter AS, Fraass BA et al: The imaging revolution and radiation oncology: Use of CT, ultrasound, and NMR for localization, treatment planning and treatment delivery. Int J Radiat Oncol Biol Phys 11:299, 1985

Kopans DB: "Early" breast cancer detection using techniques other than mammography. AJR 143:465, 1984

Kopans DB, Meyer JE, Sadowsky N: Breast imaging. N Engl J med 310:960, 1984

Koutcher JA: Nuclear magnetic resonance: Preclinical and clinical studies in tumor detection. CRC Crit Rev Oncol Hematol 1:93, 1983

Mallard J, Hutchison JM, Edelstein WA et al: In vivo n.m.r. imaging in medicine: The Aberdeen approach, both physical and biological. Philos Trans R Soc Lond [Biol] 289:519, 1980

Mansfield P, Morris PG, Ordidge RJ et al: Human whole body imaging and detection of breast tumours by n.m.r. Philos Trans R Soc Lond [Biol] 289:503, 1980

McCormack SA, Bearden D, Dennison DK et al: Methodological aspects of analysing human breast cancer cell lines by NMR spectroscopy. Physiol Chem Phys Med NMR 16:359, 1984

McSweeney MB, Small WC, Cerny V et al: Magnetic resonance imaging in the diagnosis of breast disease: Use of transverse relaxation times. Radiology 153:741, 1984

Moskowitz M, Feig SA, Cole-Beuglet C et al: Evaluation of new imaging procedures for breast cancer. Recent Results Cancer Res 90:55, 1984

Paushter DM, Modic MT, Borkowski GP et al: Magnetic resonance. Principles and applications. Med Clin North Am 68:1393, 1984

Richardson JD, Cigtay OS, Grant EG et al: Imaging of the breast. Med Clin North Am 68:1481, 1984

Ross RJ, Thompson JS, Kim K et al: Nuclear magnetic resonance imaging and evaluation of human breast tissue: Preliminary clinical trials. Radiology 143:195, 1982

Small WC, McSweeney MB, Goldstein JG et al: Handling of in vitro human breast tissue samples: Protocol requirements for accurate NMR relaxation measurements. Biochem Biophys Res Commun 112:991, 1983

Stelling CB, Wang PC, Lieber A et al: Prototype coil for magnetic resonance imaging of the female breast. Work in progress. Radiology 154:457, 1985

Strax P: Imaging of the breast. A perspective. Surg Clin North Am 64:1061, 1984

Turner DA: Nuclear magnetic resonance in oncology. Semin Nucl Med 15:210, 1985

Wolfman NT, Moran R, Moran PR et al: Simultaneous MR imaging of both breasts using a dedicated receiver coil. Radiology 155:241, 1985

INDEX

Page numbers in italics indicate illustrations; page numbers followed by t indicate tabular material.

Abdomen, 200, *201–203, 206,* 212–213, *212–213*. *See also* Hips; Pelvis
Abdominal vasculature, *206,* 212–213, *212–213*
Adenocarcinoma, 209
Adenoidal tissue, 144, *145*
Adnexae, of female pelvis, 230, *230*
Adrenal glands, *210,* 211, *211*
Aerodigestive pathway, 162, *170–172*
Air-containing spaces, appearance of, 24
Aorta, 187, 195, *196–197*
  abdominal, *212,* 213
  blood flowing within, 195
  branches of, 187
Aortic arch, 191
Aorticopulmonary window region, 187
Areolar tissue, fatty, 158
Array processing errors, 60, *62*
Arteries. *See specific arteries*
Artifact(s)
  caused by ferromagnetic objects, 60, *61*
  frequency shift, *67,* 67–68
  lacking, with MR, 5
  motion, 58, *59–60,* 60. *See also* Gating
    cardiac, 58, 60, *60*
    of globe, 129, *130*
    peristaltic, 200
    respiratory, 58
  system, 60, *61–65,* 64
  wraparound, 66, *66*
Aspect ratio setup, improper, 66, *66*
Attenuation, lack of application to MR scanning, 14
Auditory canal, interior, neurovascular bundle of, 136, *137*
Axial images. *See* Plane(s)
Azygous vein, 187

B_0, defined, 259
B_1, defined, 259
Basilar artery, 80, *81*
Basiocciput, 76, *78*
Bile duct, common, 207, *208*
Bladder, 216, *218–219*
Bloch equation, 38–39, 41
Blood
  effect of hemoglobin on image and, 56
  flowing
    appearance of, 24–25, *25*
    in brain, 80
    within cardiac chambers and aorta, 195
    in jugular bulb, 136, *137*
    in jugular vein, 76, *78*
Blood vessels. *See specific blood vessels;* Vasculature
Body coils. *See* Surface coils
Bone(s). *See also specific bones*
  cortical, 234, *236*
    appearance of, 24
  of skull, 76, *76–79,* 79
Bowel, opacification of, 200
Brachial plexus, 162, *170–172*
Brachiocephalic veins, right and left, 187
Brain, 72–74, 76, *76–81,* 79–80, 82, *88–126*
  bones and soft tissues of the skull and, 76, *76–79,* 79
  cerebral vasculature and, 80, *81,* 82
  contrast with CSF, 73, *74,* 80, *95*
  CSF-containing spaces in, 79–80, *80*
  flowing blood in, 80
  imaging strategies for, 72–73
  protocols for, 73–74, 75t
  T1 and T2 values of, 72, 73t
Brain stem, 86, 87t, *99, 126*
  dorsal, *110*
Breast, 243, *244–245*
  protocol for, 243t
  T1 and T2 measurements of, 243t
Brightness scale, 39, 41t
Bronchi, 187, 191
Bruker Medical Instruments, Inc. scanner, 253
Bulbospongiosus muscle, 225, *225*

Calcification, effect on image, 53, 55, *55*
Camera, out of focus, 60, *63*
Cardiac chambers, blood flowing within, 195
Cardiac gating, 175–176, *177,* 191
  respiratory gating with, 176, *177,* 178
Cardiac motion artifacts, 58, 60, *60*
Cardiac pacemakers, as contraindication to MR, 4
Carotid arteries, 144, *147,* 191
  internal, 82, *82*
Carotid sheath, 144, *147*
Cavernous sinus, 85, *86*
Celiac axis, *212,* 213
Cerebellar arteries, 80
Cerebellum, *114, 116, 119, 126*
  tonsil tips of, *101*
Cerebral vasculature, 80, *81,* 82
Cerebral veins, great and internal, 82, *82*
Cerebrospinal fluid (CSF), 234, *239,* 241
  in brain, 79–80, *80*
  contrast between brain and, 73, *74, 95*
  in sella, 85, *85*
  in sulci and lateral ventricles, *92*
Cerebrum, *119*
Cervical cord, *101*
Cervicocranium, 234, *236*
Cervix, *228,* 229–230
Chemical shift, defined, 259
Chemical shift artifacts, *67,* 67–68
Chest
  gating and, 174, 176, *177,* 178, 180–181, 200
    techniques for, 175–176
  normal anatomy of mediastinum and, 178, *179–190,* 187, 191
  planes for imaging of, 174–175, 175t
  protocols for, 178, 178t

Cholesterol, T1 relaxation and, 23
Choroid, 129
Ciliary body, 129
Claustrophobia, as contraindication to MR, 5
Clinoid processes, anterior, fat in, 134, *134*
Clitoris, *226,* 230
Clivus, 76, *79*
Cochlea, 138, *138*
Coherence, defined, 259
Coils. *See also* RF coil; Surface coils
  defined, 259
  gradient, 8
    changes in frequency and phase produced by, 20
  receiver, defined, 260
  shim, 8
  surface, defined, 261
  tuning, 13
Collateral ligaments, medial and lateral, of knee, 246, *246*
Computed tomography (CT) compared with MR, 4t, 4–5
  for abdomen, 200
  for brain, 72
  for cervical spine, 234
  for lumbar spine, 238
  for nasopharynx, 144
  plane and, 30
Contrast, defined, 259
Contrast reversal phenomenon, 39, *39,* 41
Conus medullaris, 237, *238*
Coronal images. *See* Plane(s)
Coronary arteries, 195, *197*
Corpora cavernosa muscle, 225, *225*
Corporal parenchyma, 225, *225*
Cost(s)
  of brain MR scan, 14
  of MR equipment, 5, 253–257
Cranial nerve(s), 87t
Cranial nerve V, 85, *86*
Craniocervical junction, 234, *236*
Crisscross patterns, 60, *62*
Cruciate ligaments, 246, *246*
CSF. *See* Cerebrospinal fluid
CT. *See* Computed tomography
Cycled data acquisition, 191, *192*
Cyst(s), fluid-filled, effect on image, 53

Data acquisition
  cycled, 191, *192*
  interleaved, 47
    motion artifacts and, 58
Data acquistition time, 45, 47t, 47–48
  defined, 260
  slice interleaving and, 47
2DE. *See* Two-dimensional echocardiography
Diamagnetic, defined, 259
Diaphragm, 187, 191
Diasonics, Inc. scanners, 6
  cycled acquisition of data with, 191, *192*
  specifications of, 253–254
Diploic space, 76, *76–77*
Disks, intervertebral, T1 and T2 values of, 238–239, 239t
Douglas and Denonvilliers' fascia, pouch of, *224,* 225

Echo, *36,* 37. *See also* Spin-echo
  multiecho nonuniformities and, 64, *64*
Echocardiography, two-dimensional, 191
Echo-planar methods, 176
Echo time (TE), 37
  defined, 259
Edema
  differentiation from tumor, 53
  effect on image, 52
Electronic equipment, peripheral, *11,* 11–12
Elscint, Inc. scanners, specifications of, 254
Endometrium, 229, *229*
Entry phenomenon, 25
Epididymis, 225
Epidural fat, 239, 241
Esacontrol scanners, specification of, 253
Esophagus, fat surrounding, 187
Ethmoidal sinuses, fluid in, 128, *129,* 134
Eustachian tube, orifice of, 144, *146*
Even echo rephasing, 25

f. *See* Frequency
Face, protocol for, 144t
Facial nerve, origin of, 136, *137*
Fallopian tubes, 230
Fat
  in anterior clinoid processes, 134, *134*
  epidural, 239, 241
  surrounding esophagus, 187
  orbital, 128, *130*
  in parapharyngeal spaces, 144, *147*
  in petrous pyramid tips, 76, *78,* 136, *136*
  of scalp, 76, *76*
  T1 relaxation and, 23
Fatty infiltration, effect on image, 54–55, *55*
Femoral head, *231,* 231–232
Ferric ions, effect on images, 56
Ferromagnetic objects, artifacts caused by, 60, *61*
Ferrous ions, effect on images, 56
FID. *See* Free induction decay
Fissures, blood vessels in, *93*
Flowing blood. *See* Blood, flowing
Fluid
  in cysts, 53
  in ethmoidal sinuses, 128, *129,* 134
  urine, effect on image, 209, 211
  in vitreous humor and lens, 128–129
Focus of camera, 60, *63*
Fonar Corporation scanners, 6, *7,* 30
  specifications of, 254–255
Foramen magnum, 234, *236*
Fossa, posterior, *99*
Fossa of Rosenmuller, 144, *146*
Fourier transform, 22
  defined, 259
Free induction decay (FID), 31, 43
  defined, 259
  repeated. *See* Partial saturation
Frequency (f)
  defined, 259
  gradient coils and, 20
  precessional, defined, 260
  resonance, magnetic field strength and, 20, 23
Frequency shift artifacts, *67,* 67–68
Frontal lobes, *102*

G. *See* Gauss
Gallbladder, 207, *208*
γ. *See* Gyromagnetic ratio
Gating, 174
  cardiac, 175–176, *177,* 191
  respiratory, 176, *177,* 180–181, 200
  respiratory and cardiac combined, 176, *177,* 178
  techniques for, 175–176
Gauss (G), 6
  defined, 259–260
General Electric Company scanners, 20, 31
  specifications of, 255
Globe, 128–129
  motion of, 129, *130*
Gradient coils, 8
  changes in frequency and phase produced by, 20
Gradient magnetic field
  defined, 260
  improper, 64, *65*
Gray matter, differentiation from white matter, *91, 94, 125*
Gyromagnetic ratio(s) (γ), 20
  defined, 260
  for paramagnetic nuclei, 20, 20t

Head coil, 10. *See also* Surface coils
Heart, *181–182, 185–187, 189–190. See also* Cardiac gating
  blood flowing within chambers of, 195
  motion artifacts caused by, 58, 60, *60*
  normal anatomy of, *182–183,* 192, 194–195, *195–198*
  pacemakers and, 4
Hemiazygous vein, 187
Hemoglobin, effect on image, 56
Hemorrhage, effect on image, 54, *54*
Hepatic artery, "replaced," *212,* 213
Hepatic veins, 204
  middle, 191
Herringbone patterns, 60, *62*
Hertz (Hz). *See also* Frequency
  defined, 260
Hilar masses, 187
Hilar vessels, 187
Hips, *226, 230–231,* 231–232
  protocol for, 232t
Hydrogen protons
  concentration of, signal strength and, 24, 24t
  magnetic physical properties of, *17,* 17–18, *18*

Hyperostosis frontalis interna, 76, *77*
Hz. *See* Hertz

Iliofemoral ligaments, *226, 230–231,* 231
Image acquisition. *See* Data acquisition
Impedance plethysmography, 176
Infarction, effect on image, 53–54
Inflammatory processes, pancreatic, 209
Infundibulum, *84,* 85
Inhomogeneities, in static magnetic field, spin-echo sequence and, 35
Intercondylar notch, 247, *247*
Intercostal vein, 187
  superior, left, 187
Interleaved slice acquisition, motion artifacts and, 58
Intervertebral disks, T1 and T2 values of, 238–239, 239t
Inversion recovery (IR), 31, 43, *44,* 45, *464–467*
  for brain, 73, *73*
  defined, 260
  for kidney, 209, *210*
  modified, 45
  for pancreas, 209
Inversion spin-echo, 45
Inversion time (TI), 43
  defined, 260
IR. *See* Inversion recovery
Iris, 129
Ischemia, effect on image, 53–54, *54*
Islet cell tumors, 209

Jugular bulb, flowing blood in, 136, *137*
Jugular lymph node chain, internal, 162, *170–172*
Jugular veins, 144, *147*
  flowing blood in, 76, *78*
  internal, 162, *170–172*

Kidneys, 209, *210,* 211
  frequency shift artifacts around, 67, *67*
Knee, 246–247, *246–249*

Larmor equation, 20
Larmor frequency (ω_0), 17, 19
  defined, 260
  calculation of, 20
  re-emission of energy at, 21
Larynx, 158
  musculature of, 162, *163–169*
Lens, 128
Level setting, improper, 60, *63*
Ligament(s). *See specific ligaments*
Ligamentum teres, 207, *208*
Liver, 204, *204,* 207, *208*
  planes for, 204, *204,* 207, 207t
Longitudinal relaxation, 22, *22*
Lungs, appearance of, 24
Lymph node(s)
  abdominal and pelvic, 214
    protocol for, 214t
  jugular, internal, 162, *170–172*
Lymphoma, 209

M & D Technology Ltd. scanners, 253
Magnet(s), 5–6, 6t, *7,* 7–8, *8*
  permanent, 5–6
  proton, random orientation of, 18, *19*
  resistive, 6
    defined, 261
  room containing, *11,* 12, *12*
  superconductive, 6, 8, *8*
    defined, 261
Magnetic field
  gradient
    defined, 260
    improper, 64, *65*
  second, applied at right angles to static field, 19, *19*
  static, inhomogeneities in, 35
  strength of, 6
    resonance frequency and, 20, 20t
Magnetic moment, defined, 260
Magnetic resonance (MR)
  compared with CT, 4t, 4–5
    for abdomen, 200
    for brain, 72
    for cervical spine, 234
    for lumbar spine, 238
    for nasopharynx, 144
    plane and, 30
  contraindications to, 4–5, 5t
  defined, 260
  limitations for imaging of chest, 174
  meaning of, 16–18
  process of, 20
Magnetization
  defined, 260
  macroscopic, 18, *19*
Magnetization vector
  return to original orientation, 21–22, *22*
  rotation of, 21, *21*
Magnet windings, 8, *9*
Mammary veins, internal, 187
Mammography, 243
Mastoid air cells, 144
Matrix (pixel) size
  effect on image, 31, *32*
  specification of, 31
Mediastinum, normal anatomy of, 178, *179–190,* 187, 191
Medulla, lower, *100*
Melanin, effect on images, 56
Meniscal cartilages, 246–247, *247*
Menstrual cycle, 229
Mesenteric arteries
  inferior, 213, *213*
  superior, *206,* 213
Midbrain, *96, 109*
Midpons, *108*
Motion artifacts, 58, *59–60,* 60. *See also* Gating
  cardiac, 58, 60, *60*
  globe and, 129, *130*
  peristaltic, 200
  respiratory, 58
MR. *See* Magnetic resonance
MRI. *See* Magnetic resonance
MR-myelogram, 241

Multiecho nonuniformities, 64, *64*
Muscle(s). *See also specific muscles*
  of hip, 231
  laryngeal, 162, *163–169*
  of skull, 76
Myocardium, *183,* 194–195
Myometrium, 229, *229*

Nasal turbinates, *142,* 143
Nasopharynx, 144, *145–158*
Neck, 158, *159–172,* 162. *See also* Spine, cervical
  axial plane for, 158, *159–162*
  coronal plane for, 162, *163–169*
  protocol for, 162t
  sagittal plane for, 162, *170–172*
Neurovascular bundle, of interior auditory canal, 136, *137*
90° pulse, 21
NMR. *See* Magnetic resonance
NMR Imaging, Inc. scanners, specifications of, 253
Nose, 142–143, *142–143*
Nuclear magnetic resonance (NMR). *See* Magnetic resonance
Nucleon, defined, 260
Nucleus pulposus, T1 and T2 values of, 238, 239t

Oblique images. *See* Plane(s)
Occipital lobes, *114–116*
Oculomotor nerves, 85, *85*
ω_0. *See* Larmor frequency 180° pulse, 21
Operator's console, 11, *11*
Ophthalmic artery, 134, *134*
Ophthalmic vein, superior, 134, *134*
Optic chiasm, *84,* 85, *97,* 134, *135*
  protocol for, 134t
Optic nerve(s), 134, *134–135*
  protocol for, 134t
Optic tract, *84,* 85
Orbit(s), *97, 102*
  anatomy of, 128–129, *129–133*
  techniques for, 128
Orbital fat, 128, *130*
Orbital walls, 128, *129*
Ordered phase encoding, 176
Oropharynx, protocol for, 144t
Orthogonal images. *See* Plane(s)
Ovaries, 230, *230*

Pacemakers, as contraindication to MR, 4
Palmex Instrumentation Oy scanners, specifications of, 253
Pancreas, *208,* 209
Paradoxical enhancement, 25
Paralaryngeal spaces, 158
Paramagnetic, defined, 260
Paramagnetic substances
  effect on image, 55–56, *56,* 56t
  gyromagnetic ratios for, 20, 20t
  with unbalanced nuclear spins, 55–56
Parameters
  weighting in spin-echo, 37–38, 38t
  which must be specified, 30t, 30–34
Paranasal sinuses, 142–143, *142–143*

Parapharyngeal spaces, fat in, 144, *147*
Parasellar regions, 85, *86*
Parenchyma, corporal, 225, *225*
Parotid gland, 140, *141,* 144, *147*
Partial saturation (PS), 31, 43, *43–44*
  for abdominal vasculature, 212
  defined, 260
  for pituitary gland, 83
  for orbit, 128
  for temporal bone, 136
Patient positioning
  asymmetric, 64, *64*
  for oblique images of heart, 191, 192t
Pelvis, 216
  female, 225, *226–228,* 229–230
    protocol for, 216t
  male, 216, *218–225,* 225
    protocol for, 216t
Penis, *220,* 225, *225*
Pericardium, *182,* 192, 194
Peristaltic motion, artifacts produced by, 200
Permanent magnet, 5–6
Petrous pyramid tips, fat in, 76, *78,* 136, *136*
Phantom, defined, 260
Pharyngeal recess, 144, *146*
Phase, defined, 260
Philips Medical Systems, Inc. scanners, *7*
  specifications of, 255–256
Philips surface coil, for knee, 246
Picker International scanners, specifications of, 256
Pincushion distortion, 64, *65*
Pineal gland, *110*
Pituitary gland, 83, *83–85,* 85
Pixel
  defined, 260
  See also Matrix
Plane(s)
  for abdomen, 200, 212–213
  for adrenal glands, 211
  for brain, 72
  for cervical spine, 234
  for chest, 174–175, 175t
  for heart, 191–192
    positioning for, 191, 192t
  for hips, 232
  for kidneys, 209
  for knee, 246, 247, 247t
  for liver, 204, *204,* 207, 207t
  for lumbar spine, 241, 243
  for pancreas, 209
  for pelvis, 216
  for pituitary gland, 83–85, *83–85*
  for seminal vesicles, 225
  for skull, 76, *78–79,* 79
  specification of, 30–31
  for thoracic spine, 237
Portal veins, 204
Precession, defined, 260
Precessional frequency, defined, 260
Pre-epiglottic space, 158
Pregnancy, as contraindication to MR, 4
Preprostatic (Retzius) space, 225
Progressive saturation. *See* Partial saturation
Prostate, 216, *220, 224,* 225
  distinction between rectum and, 225
Protocol(s)
  for abdomen, 214t
  for brain, 73–74, 75t
  for breast, 243t
  for chest, 178, 178t
  for face, sinuses, oropharynx, and nasopharynx, 144t
  for hips, 232t
  for neck, 162t
  for optic chiasm, 134t
  for optic nerves, 134t
  for pelvis, 216t
  for temporal bone, 138t
  for temporomandibular joint, 140t
Proton magnet, random orientation of, 18, *19*
PS. *See* Partial saturation
Pseudocysts, pancreatic, 209
Pulmonary artery, 187
Pulmonary veins, superior, left and right, 187
Pulse(s)
  90°, 21
  180°, 21
  readout, 41, 43
  refocussing, *44,* 45
  rephasing, 35, *36,* 37
  RF, 21
    defined, 261
  synchronizing, 35
Pulse sequence
  defined, 260
  specification of, 31, 33, 33t
Pyriform sinuses, anterior margins of, 158

Quenching, defined, 260

Radio-frequency (RF), defined, 260
Radio-frequency (RF) coil. *See* RF coil
Radio-frequency (RF) interference, 60, *61*
Radio-frequency (RF) pulses, 21
  defined, 261
Readout pulse, 41, 43
Receiver coil, defined, 260
Reconstruction, defined, 260
Rectum, distinction between prostate and, 225
Refocusing pulse, *44,* 45
Relative brightness scale, 39, 41t
Relaxation
  definition of, 22
  from resonance, 21–23
    spin-echo sequence and, 34–35, *36*
  T1, 22, *22*
  T2, 23
Relaxation times, defined, 260–261
Repeated FID. *See* Partial saturation
Repetition time (TR), 37
  defined, 261
Rephasing pulse, 35, *36,* 37
Resistive magnet, 6
  defined, 261
Resonance
  defined, 261
  relaxation from, 21–23
    spin-echo sequence and, 34–35, *36*
  stimulation to, 18–20
Resonance frequency, magnetic field strength and, 20, 20t
Respiratory gating, 176, *177,* 180–181, 200
  cardiac gating with, 176, *177,* 178
Respiratory motion artifacts, 58
Retina, 129
Retzius space, 225
RF (radio-frequency) coil, *9,* 9–10
  improper fields and, 64, *65*
  nonlinearities in, 64, *65*
  tuning of, 13
    improper, 60, *62–63*
Risks, of MR, 4
Rosenmuller, fossa of, 144, *146*

S/N. *See* Signal-to-noise ratio
Sagittal images. *See* Plane(s)
Saturation, defined, 261
Saturation recovery (SR). *See also* Partial saturation
  defined, 261
Scalp, vessels of, 76, *76*
Scalp fat, 76, *76*
Scan, performance of, 13–14
Scanners, 6, *7,* 20, 30, 31
  companies producing, 6
  components of, 7–12, *8–12*
  data acquisition time for, 45, 47t, 47–48
  specifications for, 253–257
Schmorl's nodes, 237, *238*
Sclera, 129
Scrotum, *220,* 225, *225*
SE. *See* Spin-echo
Sella, *106*
  empty, 85, *85*
Semicircular canals, 138, *138*
Seminal vesicles, *218,* 225
Shim coils, 8
Shimming, defined, 261
Siemens Medical Systems, Inc. scanners, 6, 20
  specifications of,
Signal averages, specification of, 31, *32*
Signal generation, 18
Signal strength
  focal changes in, 64, *65*
  hydrogen concentration and, 24, 24t
  properties determining, 23–27
  of spin-echo sequence, 38, *39*
  T1 effects and, 25, *26,* 27, 27t
  T2 effects and, *26,* 27
  velocity effects and, 24–25, *25*
Signal-to-noise ratio (S/N or SNR), defined, 261
Sinus(es)
  cavernous, 85, *86*
  ethmoidal, fluid in, 128, *129,* 134
  paranasal, 142–143, *142–143*
  protocol for, 144t

pyriform, anterior margins of, 158
venous, 82, *82*
Skull, bones and soft tissues of, 76, *76–79,* 79
Slice interleaving, 47
motion artifacts and, 58
Slice thickness, specification of, 31
SNR. *See* Signal-to-noise ratio
Soft tissues, of skull, 76, *76–79,* 79
Spermatic cord, *220,* 225
Sphenoid bone, partial voluming of marrow in body of, 79, *79*
Spheno-occipital synchondrosis, 79, *79*
Spin, defined, 261
Spinal cord, cervical, *101*
Spin-conditioning, 176, *177*
Spine
cervical, 234, *235–236. See also* Neck
lumbar, 238–239, *239–242,* 241, 243, *244–245*
thoracic, 237, *237–238*
Spin-echo (SE), 31, 34–35, *35–36,* 37
for abdominal vasculature, 212
for brain, 73, *74*
for cervical spine, 234
defined, 261
for hips, 232
inversion, 45
for kidneys, 209
for knee, 246
for liver, 204
for lumbar spine, 239, *239*
for neck, 158, 162, *163–169*
for orbit, 128
for pancreas, 209
parameter weighting in, 37–38, 38t
pituitary gland and, 83
for seminal vesicles, 225
short, 37
signal intensity of, 38, *39*
for spleen, 207
tumors and, 53
Spin-lattice relaxation time. *See also* T1 relaxation
defined, 261
Spin-spin relaxation time. *See also* T2 relaxation
defined, 261
Spleen, *205–206,* 207, 209
Splenic vessels, 209
SR. *See* Partial saturation
SSFP. *See* Steady-state free precession
Static field, *16,* 17
Steady-state free precession (SSFP), 31, 176
Sternomanubrial articulation, 187
Sternoxyphoid articulation, 187
Sternum, 187
Stimulating field, turning off, 21, *21*
Stimulation, to resonance, 18–20
Subcarinal space, 191
Subclavian vessels, 187
Sulcus(i), CSF in, *92*
Superconductive magnet, 6, 8, *8*
defined, 261

Surface coil(s), *10,* 10–11
for breasts, *244–245*
defined, 261
for heart, 195, *198*
for knee, 246
for larynx, 158
motion artifacts and, 58, *59*
for orbit, 128, *128,* 129
for temporal bone, 136, *136*
for temporomandibular joint, 140
Syloid process, 144, *147*
Synchronizing pulse, 35
System artifacts, 60, *61–65,* 64
System components, 7–12

T. *See* Tesla
T1
defined, 261
signal strength and, 25, *26,* 27, 27t
T1 relaxation, 22, *22*
defined, 261
T1 value(s)
of brain, 72, 73t
of breast, 243t
of globe, 128
of intervertebral disks, 238–239, 239t
of neck tissues, 158t
of pancreas, 209
T1 weighted sequences
for adrenal glands, 211
for brain, 73
for chest, 178
edema and, 52
for globe, 128–129
for kidneys, 209
for knee, 246
for larynx, 158
for liver, 204
for nasopharynx, 144
pure, 48, *48,* 49
origin of facial and vestibulocochlear nerves and, 136, *137*
for seminal vesicles, 225
tumors and, 53
T2
defined, 261
signal strength and, *26,* 27
T2 interactions, spin-echo sequence and, 35
T2 relaxation, 23
defined, 261
T2 relaxation time, measurement of, 23, *23*
T2 value(s)
of brain, 72, 73t
of breast, 243t
of globe, 128
of intervertebral disks, 238–239, 239t
of neck tissues, 158t
of pancreas, 209
T2 weighted sequences
for brain, 73
for cervical spine, 234
for chest, 178
for cochlea and vestibular apparatus, 138

edema and, 52
for globe, 129
for kidneys, 209
for knee, 246
for liver, 204
for lumbar spine, 241
for nasopharynx, 144
for ovaries, 230, *230*
pure, 48–49, *49*
for seminal vesicles, 225
tumors and, 53
for uterus, 229
TE. *See* Echo time
Technicare Corporation scanners, 6, 30
specifications of, 257
Temporal bone, 136, *136–141,* 138
protocol for, 138t
Temporomandibular joint (TMJ), 140, *141*
protocol for, 140t
Terminology, 14
glossary of, 259–261
Tesla (T), 6
defined, 261
Testis, 225
Thermal relaxation. *See* T1 relaxation
Thomson-CGR Medical Corporation scanners, specifications of, 257
Time, required for imaging, 5, 45, 47t, 47–48. *See also* Echo time; Inversion time; Relaxation time; Repetition time
Tissue characterization, potential of MR for, 5
TMJ. *See* Temporomandibular joint
Torque, defined, 261
Torus tubarius, 144, *146*
TR. *See* Repetition time
Trachea, 191
Transverse relaxation time. *See also* T2 relaxation
defined, 261
Tumor(s)
differentiation from edema, 53
effect on image, 53, *53*
islet cell, 209
Tuning of RF coil, 13
improper, 60, *62–63*
Two-dimensional echocardiography (2DE), 191

Uncooperative patients, contraindication to MR for, 5
Urine, effect on image, 209, 211
Uterus, 229, *229*
broad ligament of, *226,* 230

Vagina, *228,* 230
Vaginal bulb, *226,* 230
Vasculature. *See also specific vessels;* Blood
abdominal, *206,* 212–213, *212–213*
brachiocephalic, 187
cerebral, 80, *81,* 82
in fissures and ventricles, *93*
hilar, 187
of interior auditory canal, 136, *137*

Vasculature (*continued)*
  of scalp, 76, *76*
  splenic, 209
  subclavian, 187
Vector, defined, 261
Vein(s). *See specific veins*
Velocity effects, signal strength and, 24–25, *25*
Vena cava
  inferior, 191
  superior, 187
Venous sinuses, 82, *82*
Ventricles
  blood vessels in, *93*
  fourth, *111*
  lateral, CSF in, *92*
Ventricular wall, 195, *195*
Vermis, cerebellar, *126*
Vertebral bodies, 234
Vestibular apparatus, 138, *138*
Vestibulocochlear nerve, origin of, 136, *137*
Vitreous humor, 128
Voxel, defined, 261

White matter, differentiation from gray matter, *91, 94, 125*
Window setting, improper, 60, *63*
Wraparound artifact, 66, *66*

X-axis control maladjustment, 66, *66*
X-irradiation, lack of, with MR, 4

90000
9 780397 507665